CLINICAL TUBERCULOSIS
Diagnosis and Treatment

CLINICAL TUBERCULOSIS
Diagnosis and Treatment

Rajendra Prasad
MD DTCD FAMS FCCP (USA)
FNCCP FCAI FIAB FIMSA DSC (Honoris Causa)

Director
Vallabhbhai Patel Chest Institute
University of Delhi
Delhi, India

Formerly
Professor and Head
Department of Pulmonary Medicine
King George's Medical University, Lucknow

Director
UP Rural Institute of Medical Science and Research
Saifai, Etawah, Uttar Pradesh, India

Co-author

Nikhil Gupta MD
Assistant Professor
Department of Medicine
Era's Lucknow Medical College
Lucknow, Uttar Pradesh, India

Foreword

SP Agarwal

JAYPEE *The Health Sciences Publisher*

New Delhi | London | Philadelphia | Panama

Jaypee Brothers Medical Publishers (P) Ltd

Headquarters

Jaypee Brothers Medical Publishers (P) Ltd
4838/24, Ansari Road, Daryaganj
New Delhi 110 002, India
Phone: +91-11-43574357
Fax: +91-11-43574314
Email: jaypee@jaypeebrothers.com

Overseas Offices

J.P. Medical Ltd
83 Victoria Street, London
SW1H 0HW (UK)
Phone: +44 20 3170 8910
Fax: +44 (0)20 3008 6180
Email: info@jpmedpub.com

Jaypee-Highlights Medical Publishers Inc
City of Knowledge, Bld. 237, Clayton
Panama City, Panama
Phone: +1 507-301-0496
Fax: +1 507-301-0499
Email: cservice@jphmedical.com

Jaypee Medical Inc
The Bourse
111 South Independence Mall East
Suite 835, Philadelphia, PA 19106, USA
Phone: +1 267-519-9789
Email: jpmed.us@gmail.com

Jaypee Brothers Medical Publishers (P) Ltd
17/1-B Babar Road, Block-B, Shaymali
Mohammadpur, Dhaka-1207
Bangladesh
Mobile: +08801912003485
Email: jaypeedhaka@gmail.com

Jaypee Brothers Medical Publishers (P) Ltd
Bhotahity, Kathmandu, Nepal
Phone: +977-9741283608
Email: kathmandu@jaypeebrothers.com

Website: www.jaypeebrothers.com
Website: www.jaypeedigital.com

Inquiries for bulk sales may be solicited at: jaypee@jaypeebrothers.com

Clinical Tuberculosis: Diagnosis and Treatment

First Edition: **2015**

ISBN 978-93-5152-221-8

Printed at Repro India Limited

Dedicated to

My teachers for their guidance, wisdom and inspiration
My Parents, wife and children for their love and patience

Foreword

Dr. S.P Agarwal
M.S. (Surg.) M.Ch. (Neuro.), FIMSA, FICS, D.Sc (h.c)
(Former Director General Health Service, Govt. of India)
SECRETARY GENERAL
Padma Bhusan Awardee

Indian Red Cross Society

National Headquarters
1, Red Cross Road, New Delhi-110 001 (INDIA)
Tel. : 011-23716424, 23717063
Fax. : 011-23717454
E-mail : spagarwalsg@indianredcross.org
spasgircs@gmail.com

Tuberculosis is a multisystem disease with varied clinical presentations. It has reached epidemic proportions and has tormented mankind for centuries with impact on human beings unparalleled in the history of communicable diseases. One-third of the world's population is infected with *Mycobacterium tuberculosis* and there is 10% lifetime risk of developing tuberculosis and the risk further increases to 10% annual risk in immunocompromised patients. Globally, it was responsible for causing 1.4 million deaths in the year 2011 out of which 0.32 million deaths occurred in India alone. It has re-emerged from oblivion due to pandemic of human immunodeficiency virus although, it never disappeared from developing countries. Additionally, the increasing burden of multidrug resistant (MDR-TB) and extensively drug resistant tuberculosis is posing challenge to tuberculosis control.

Against this backdrop, the publication of *Clinical Tuberculosis: Diagnosis and Treatment* by Professor Rajendra Prasad is a timely and useful addition to the existing literature on tuberculosis. The book summarized the current status of knowledge on tuberculosis and also discusses the latest diagnostic and treatment modalities for pulmonary as well as extra-pulmonary forms of tuberculosis. The chapters in the book have been arranged in a systemic sequence for easy understanding and are based on practical approach with illustrative cases, blended with the most up-to-date knowledge in the field. The chapters have been written on the basis of vast and rich clinical experience gained by the author from day-to-day patient management over the last many years.

Professor Rajendra Prasad is a nationally acclaimed chest physician and tuberculosis expert, possessing over three decades' illustrious teaching, research and administrative experience with proven excellence in quality patient care. Apart from being a clinician par excellence, he is also a very popular medical teacher in pulmonary medicine. He is currently the Director of Vallabhbhai Patel Chest Institute, Delhi. He has earlier served as Professor and Head, Department of Pulmonary Medicine, King George's Medical University, Lucknow, and Director, UP Rural Institute of Medical Science and Research, Saifai, Etawah, Uttar Pradesh. He has devoted all his energy in promoting medical education, patient care and research. His contribution in the field of tuberculosis and multidrug resistant tuberculosis (MDR-TB) are widely acclaimed. He took keen interest in revised national tuberculosis control program (RNTCP) from its inception. His dynamic leadership in academic and administrative areas has earned him a large number of awards from various international and national scientific societies.

This comprehensive well-referenced book contains a plethora of knowledge and would be a valuable source for undergraduate and postgraduate students, clinicians, health authorities, caring for patients with tuberculosis. I am quite hopeful that his book will help in better understanding towards alleviating the suffering of millions by tuberculosis.

SP Agarwal
MS (Surg) MCh (Neuro) FIMSA FICS DSc (hc)
Padma Bhusan Awardee
Secretary General, Indian Red Cross Society
Former Director General Health Service
Government of India

Preface

As a senior author of this book, I look upon tuberculosis as a 100% curable disease and throughout the 38 years of my clinical practice in pulmonary medicine, I have gained an ever-increasing confidence that with proper aid at proper time, disease ends in most instances in healing. However, tuberculosis still continues to be the world's most important infectious cause of morbidity and mortality. Globally, nearly 9 million people develop tuberculosis disease every year and 1.4 million die every year with tuberculosis. In India, nearly 2 million people develop tuberculosis and 0.3 million people are dying every year. It is a cause for concern as India stands first in terms of absolute number of cases closely followed by China. It is real paradox because pathogenesis, transmission, prevention, diagnosis and treatment are well known for tuberculosis. Drug resistant tuberculosis has been reported since the early days of introduction of anti-TB chemotherapy but multidrug resistant tuberculosis and more recently, extensively drug resistant tuberculosis (XDR-TB) has been an area of growing concern and is posing threat to global efforts of tuberculosis control.

This book was written with the aim of defining a practical approach to every aspect of tuberculosis. In total there are 50 chapters in the book. Chapters practically cover all the aspects of tuberculosis ranging from epidemiology, varying presentation of tuberculosis, diagnosis and practical approach to the treatment of pulmonary as well as common extrapulmonary tuberculosis including HIV and TB. It also covers practical approach to drug resistant including multidrug resistant tuberculosis and extensively drug resistant tuberculosis. Chapters also include prevention of tuberculosis and TB control in India. Pharmacokinetics of antituberculosis used in new and retreatment cases of tuberculosis including their doses, regimens, adverse effects are highlighted. Special chapters on case-based approach to treatment of tuberculosis in special situation and MDR-TB have also been included. Chapters on TB in children, TB in elderly, nontuberculous mycobacteria and infection control in TB are also included. Chapters have been written in the background of current literature and practical experience gained from day-to-day dealing with different patients suffering from tuberculosis. Advances up to 2013 have been included making all the chapters well referenced with the latest references.

This book will be useful to both undergraduate and postgraduate medical students, practitioners and program managers of TB control. In toto, this manual will serve as a very useful practical guide regarding all aspects of tuberculosis.

Rajendra Prasad

Acknowledgments

As a senior author of this book, I wish to acknowledge my indebtedness to a number of people who significantly contributed to the publication of this book. The individual to whom I would like to acknowledge first is Prof BK Khanna who as a Head of Department of Tuberculosis at the King George's Medical College, Lucknow, Uttar Pradesh, India while I was postgraduate student in that department, markedly stimulated my interest in tuberculosis. Prof BK Khanna's own tremendous knowledge and wisdom in the field of tuberculosis set an example of thoughtfulness and meticulousness which I have always tried to emulate. I am also indebted to Prof PK Mukherjee, Dr J Nath, Late Dr MS Agnihotri and Late Dr Jafar Jameel, for their great inspiration as a teacher during my postgraduate days. I am greatly indebted to the many postgraduate students who have been trained with me in the department at King George's Medical College, Lucknow and Vallabhbhai Patel Chest Institute, Delhi, especially Dr Sanjay Verma, Dr Kiran Vishnu Narayan, Dr Suneesh C Anand, Dr Giridhar BH, Dr Abhijeet, Dr Jabeed P, Dr Saheer S, Dr Abhishek Agrawal, Dr Shailendra Singh, Dr Mandeep Singh and Dr Pawan Gupta. The efforts of these students in part responsible for generating much of the data that can be incorporated in making the chapters in book more evidence based.

I also wish to express my appreciation to Dr Nikhil Gupta, co-author of this book, for helping me in preparing and correcting the manuscript. I also wish to express my thanks to Mr PP Sharma and Mr Ashish Yadav, for their invaluable help in the preparation and typing of manuscript. I am also thankful to all my patients, who gave me experience in the field of tuberculosis.

My thanks also go to many people of M/s Jaypee Brothers Medical Publishers (P) Ltd, New Delhi, India, especially Shri Jitendar P Vij (Group Chairman), Mr Ankit Vij (Group President) and Mr Tarun Duneja (Director-Publishing), for their coordination in bringing out this book.

Contents

PLATE 1

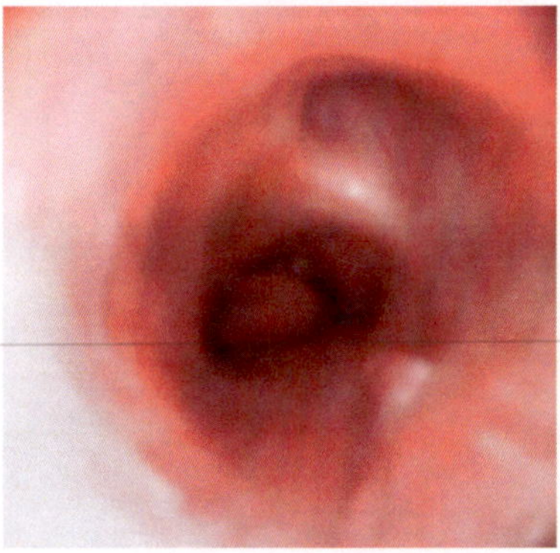

Fig. 6.1: Two nodular growths

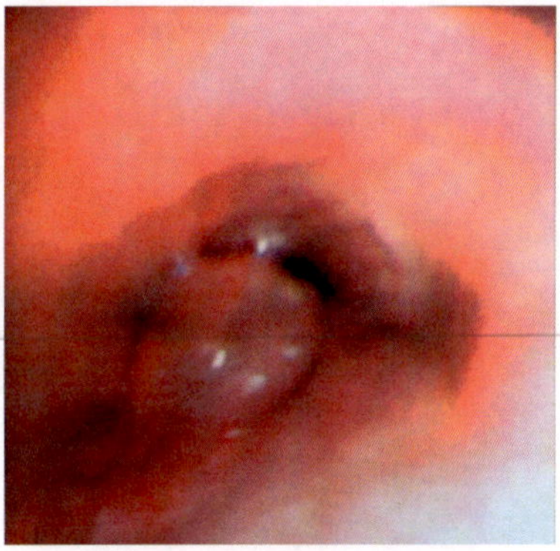

Fig. 6.2: Close view of nodule

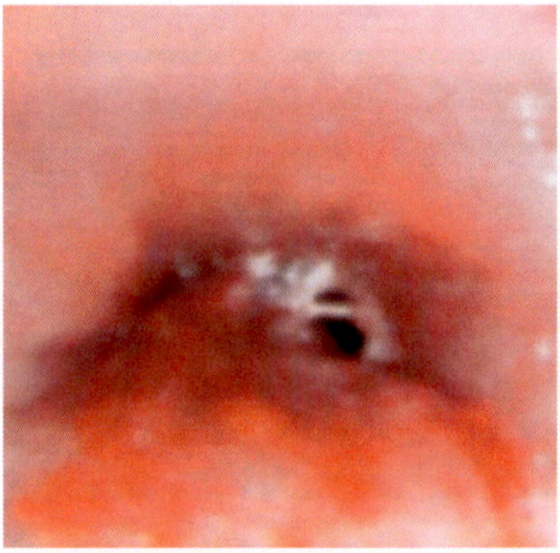

Fig. 6.3: Caseous material after transbronchial needle aspiration

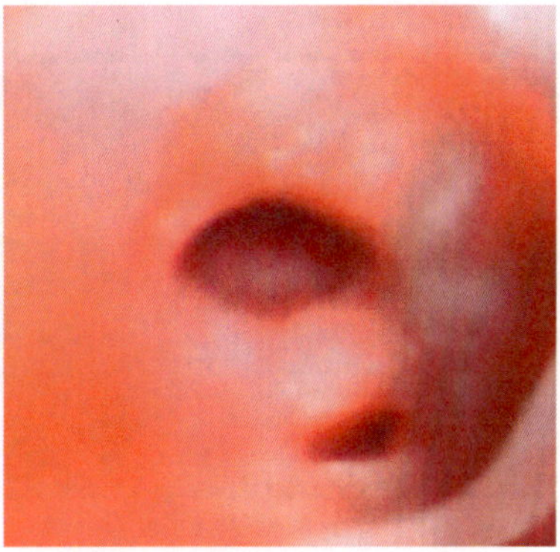

Fig. 6.4: Edematous and hyperemic tertiary carina

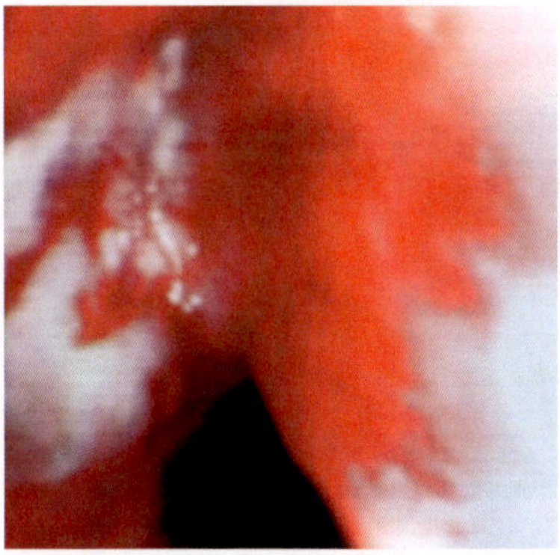

Fig. 6.5: Right upper lobe bronchus obstructed by caseous material and blood

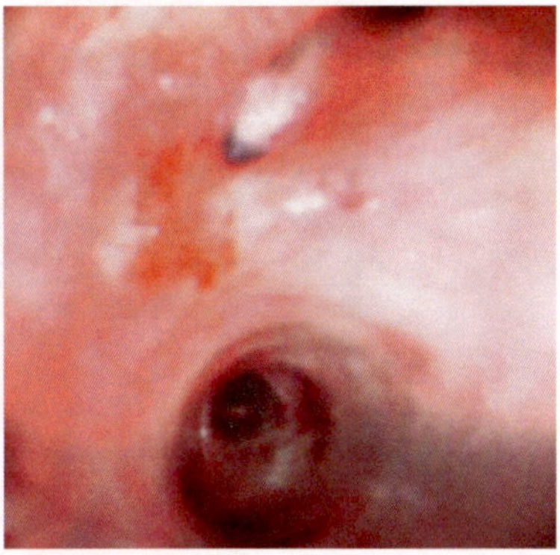

Fig. 6.6: Tuberculous sinus just behind secondary carina

PLATE 2

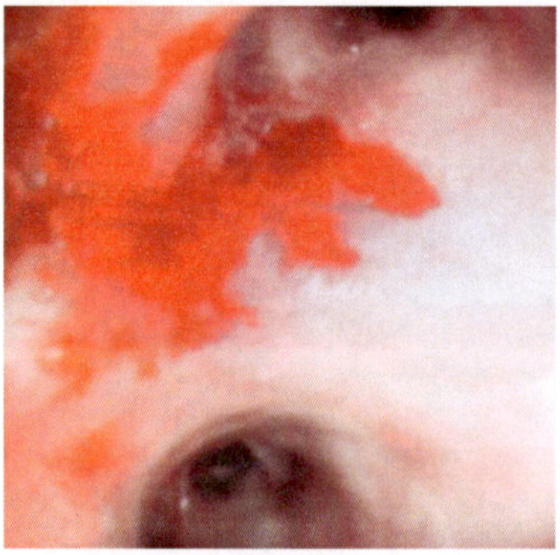

Fig. 6.7: Bleeding after endobronchial biopsy from tuberculous sinus

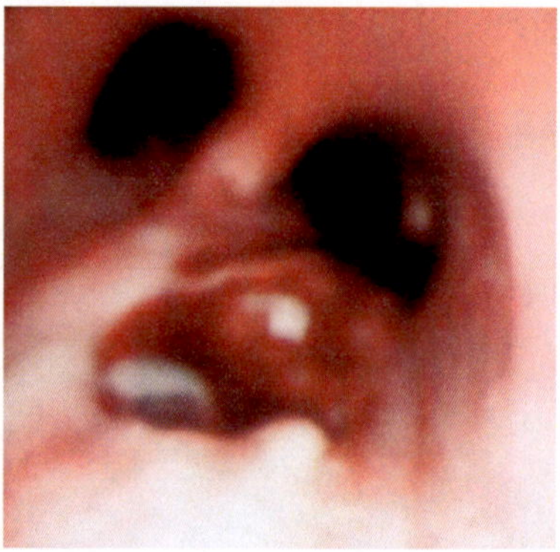

Fig. 6.8: Tracheal fistula surrounded with granulation tissue

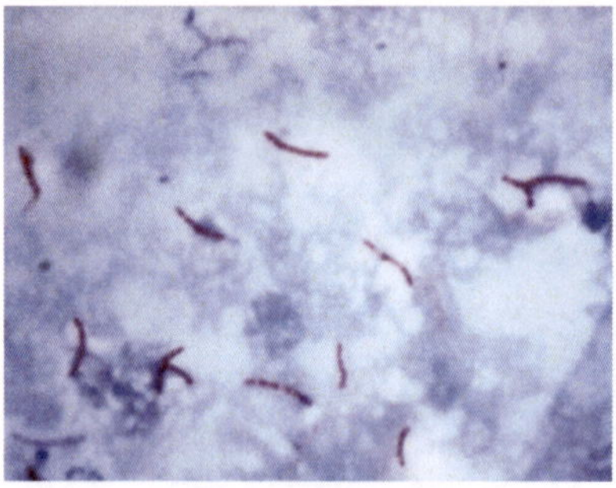

Fig. 9.34: Smear positive for acid-fast bacilli by Ziehl-Neelsen method

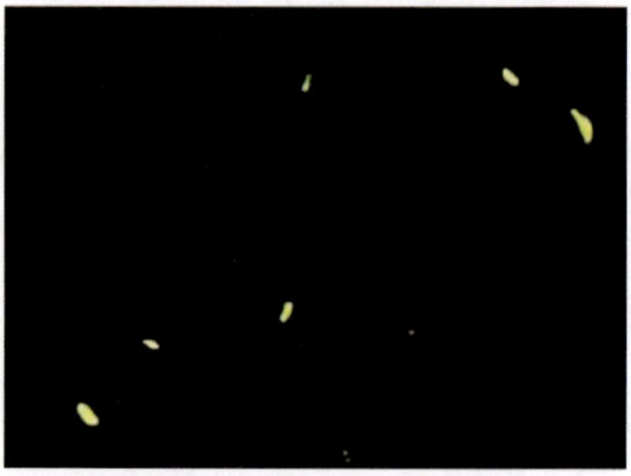

Fig. 9.35: Smear positive for MTB by fluorescence staining method

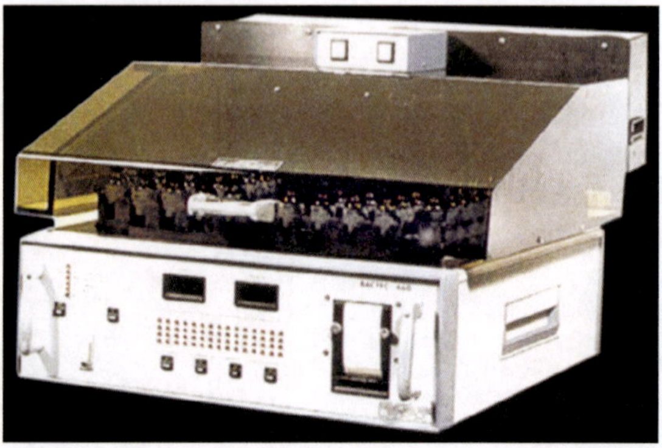

Fig. 9.36: Bactec 460

PLATE 3

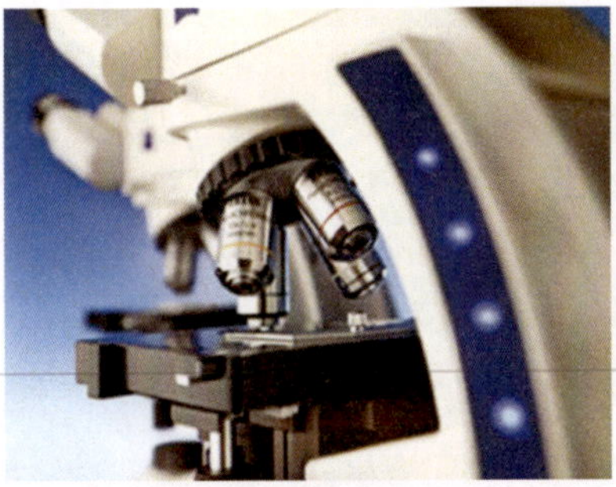

Fig. 9.37: LED microscope

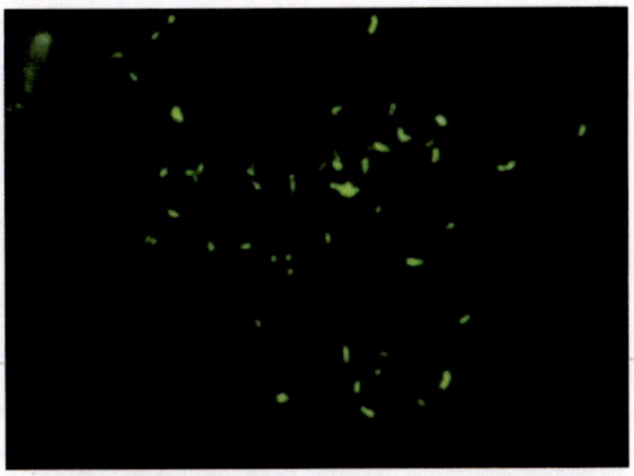

Fig. 9.38: Smear positive for MTB by flourescence staining (done with LED microscope)

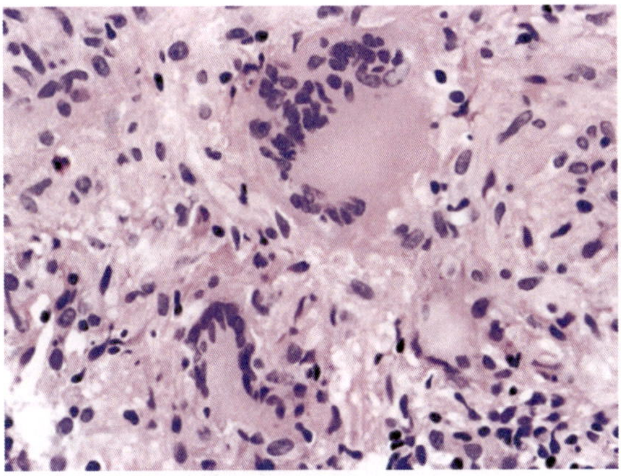

Fig. 9.39: TB granuloma

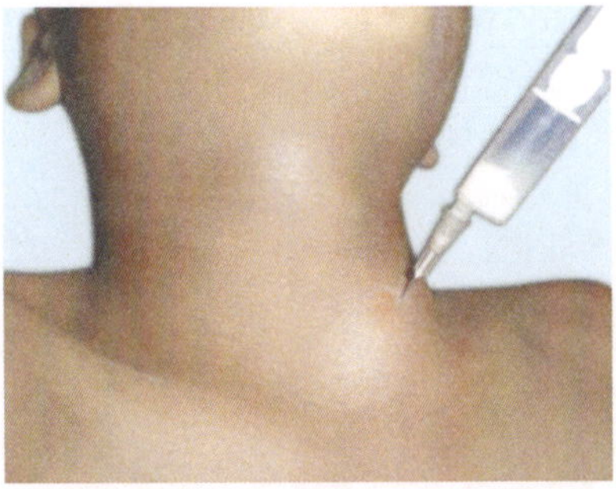

Fig. 9.40: FNAC of lymph node in the neck

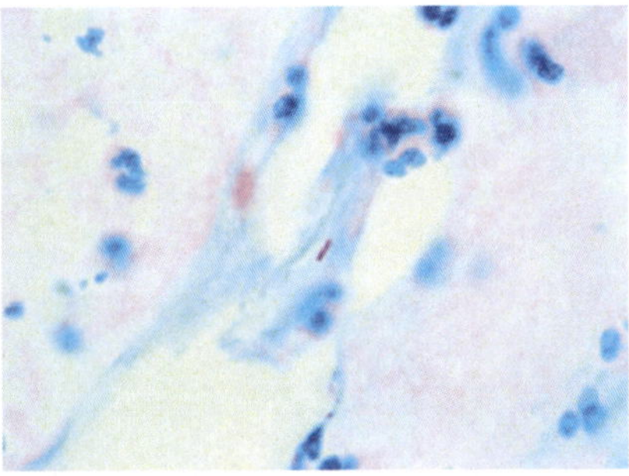

Fig. 9.41: FNAC lymphnode showing AFB

PLATE 4

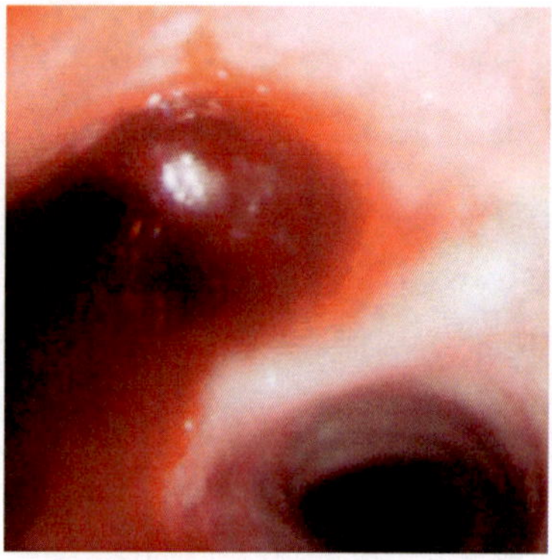

Fig. 10.29: FOB showing growth proven to be squamous cell carcinoma in the left main bronchus

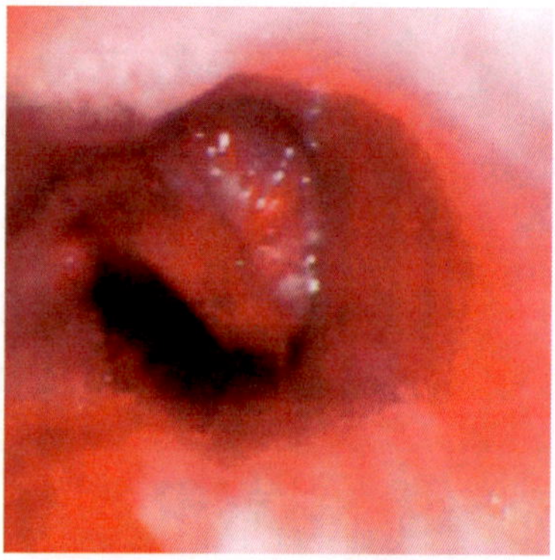

Fig. 10.37: FOB showing irregular growth in left main bronchus just before its bifurcation

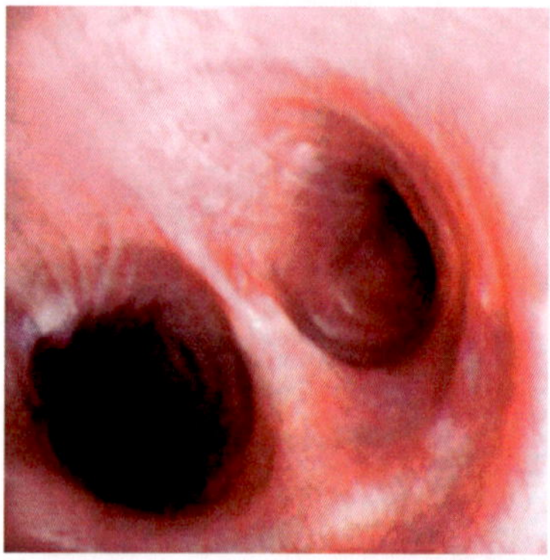

Fig. 10.57: Fiberoptic bronchoscopy showing hyperemic mucosa and endobronchial biopsy from main carina revealed non-caseating granuloma

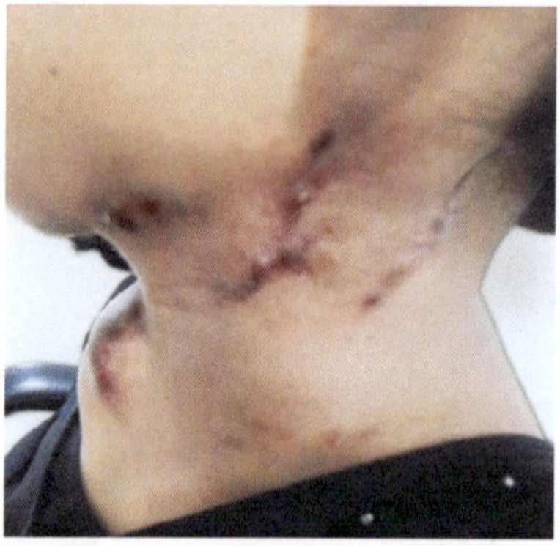

Fig. 42.1: Tuberculous lymphadenitis in the neck with multiple healed sinuses

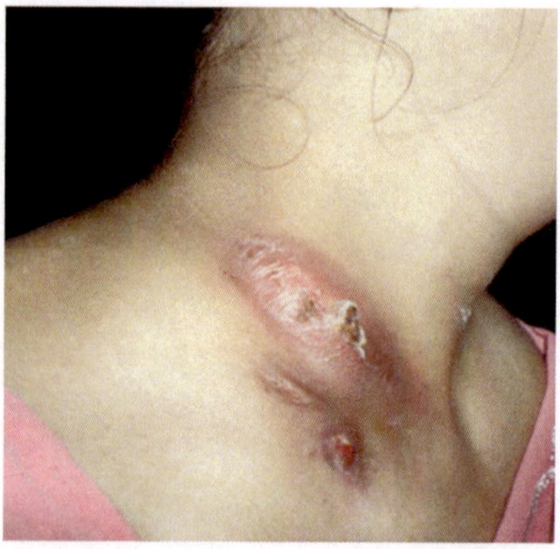

Fig. 42.2: Tuberculous lymphadenitis in the neck showing caseation with abcess formation

PLATE 5

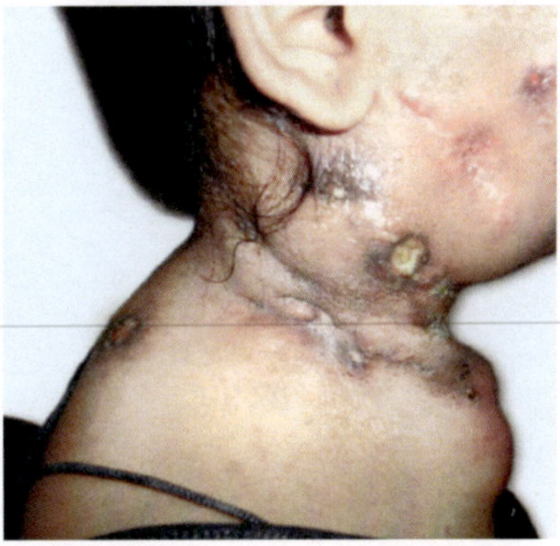

Fig. 42.3: Tubercular cervical lymphadenitis with ulceration in the neck

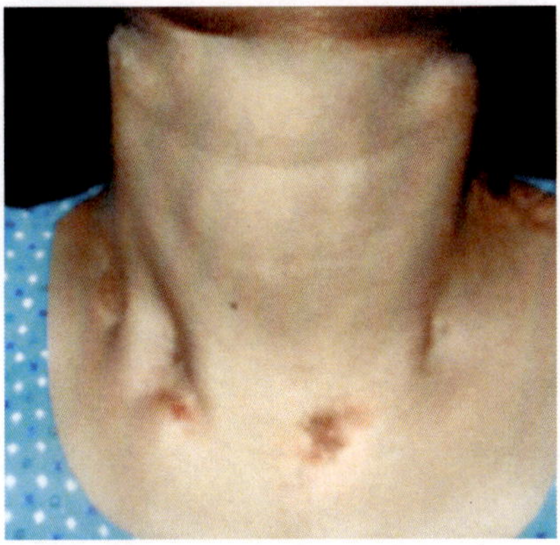

Fig. 42.4: Tuberculous lymphadenitis in the neck showing scarring after treatment

Chapter 1

Landmarks in Tuberculosis Treatment

Aim of the present chapter is to describe important landmarks, which have made impact on management of tuberculosis.

1. Robert Koch's discovered tubercle bacilli as causative agent for tuberculosis in 1882.
2. Roentgen discovered the X-rays in 1895.
3. In 1921, Weill Halle, first used BCG vaccine.
4. Bacteriostatic effect of sulfonamides in guinea pigs infected with tubercle bacilli was discovered in 1940. For the first time, it was demonstrated that a chemotherapeutic agent, a derivative of dapsone, known as promin (glucosulfone sodium), was capable of stopping the progress of otherwise fatal tuberculosis in guinea pigs.[1]
5. Streptomycin, an antibiotic newly isolated by Waksman in 1944 from the soil organism *Streptomyces griseus* which showed a striking therapeutic effect on experimental tuberculosis in guinea pigs.[2,3]
6. Para-aminosalicylic acid (PAS) was discovered in 1949, prevented the emergence of drug resistance if given in combination with streptomycin. Since then, the administration of two or more drugs in combination has been recognized to be essential for adequate tuberculosis treatment.
7. Anti-tuberculosis activity of isoniazid was discovered in 1952. Since its introduction, isoniazid has been an important, component of all primary drug regimen because it is highly effective, of relatively low toxicity and inexpensive.
8. In 1956, Tuberculosis Chemotherapy Center (TCC), now known as Tuberculosis Research Center (TRC) was established in Chennai (then Madras) under the auspices of the Indian Council of Medical Research (ICMR), with assistance of the British Medical Research Council, World

Health Organization and Government of India. Tuberculosis Research Center (TRC) trial demonstrated that ambulatory, domiciliary treatment was highly effective without increasing the risk of infection for family contacts. In this controlled trial, the effect of treatment was compared in two groups of patients—one group treated under good conditions in a sanatorium, the other under poor conditions at home.[4,5] The results in the sanatorium patients, despite good accommodation, nursing care, rich diet, and prolonged bed rest, were not superior to those in patients treated in overcrowded homes, who had a poor diet, much less rest, and often very long working hours. Results for quiescence of the disease at 1 year and relapses in the subsequent 4 years[6] showed no difference between home and sanatorium patients. The risk to close family contacts was studied for 5 years. There was no difference[7,8] in the attack rate of TB between the contact of patients treated at home and those of sanatorium patients, and exposure to the index case under effective treatment appeared to present no major risk to contacts. The study indicated that the major risk to contacts lay in exposure to the infectious index case before diagnosis and the start of treatment. At that point, all the harm the index case could do to family contacts had already been done, so that subsequent isolation in a sanatorium was of little benefit. Thus, domiciliary treatment did not entail any special danger that might have been prevented by sanatorium treatment. In addition, the study showed that treatment in a sanatorium is no safeguard against irregularity of drug taking unless the patient is seen to swallow every dose. These findings prompted a radical departure from the traditional sanatorium treatment to domiciliary treatment as general policy and opened new prospects for nationwide treatment program in developing countries.

9. It was observed that a considerable proportion of patients do not take medications as prescribed, even with extensive health education.[9,10] This finding together with the risk of emergence and spread of drug-resistant tuberculosis eventually led to the recognition of direct observation of tuberculosis treatment as the standard of care.[11,12] Directly observed treatment means that every dose is administered under direct observation, and convenience to the patient is essential for success. The main advantage of directly observed treatment is that treatment is carried out entirely under program supervision. No concealed irregularity can occur. The treatment observer ensures that medicines are taken at the correct intervals and in the correct dosages. Equally important is the dramatic reduction in the development of drug resistance, because direct observation eliminates the patient's ability to intentionally or unintentionally discontinue one or more drugs, with the subsequent emergence of drug-resistant organisms. There is close and continuing contact between the patient and the health worker, adverse effects

and treatment complications can be quickly identified and addressed, especially during the critical initial phase of treatment and confirmed adherence to treatment further reduces the spread of infection in the community. Multiple analyses have demonstrated that the higher personnel and program expenditure associated with directly observed treatment are more than offset by the saving in the cost of re-treatment, the costs of treating drug resistance and the costs associated with the treatment of the new cases of tuberculosis (many with drug resistance) which arise if treatment is not directly observed.[13-15]

10. In 1959, Government of India established the National Tuberculosis Institute (NTI) in Bengaluru with the active cooperation of the WHO, to develop a TB Control Program.
11. In 1962, National Tuberculosis Control Program was formulated in India.
12. The demonstration, in 1964, that intermittent regimens can be as effective as daily regimens, thereby offering the advantage of convenient, directly observed treatment. Intermittent regimens are those in which the individual drugs are given at interval of more than 1 day. It was believed that anti-tuberculosis drugs needed to be given every day to maintain drug concentration continuously at inhibitory levels. However, in vitro studies and animal experiments have demonstrated that certain drugs are also effective when the drug concentration drops temporarily below that level, and indeed even after the drug has disappeared completely from the lesion[16] or the medium.[17] In vitro experiments have demonstrated that, after a culture of *Mycobacterium tuberculosis* is exposed to certain drugs for some time, it takes several days (the "lag period") before new growth occurs. The lag period for growth of *M. tuberculosis* after exposure varies for different drugs. There was no lag period after exposure to thiacetazone and this drug is unsuitable for intermittent treatment. Animal studies[18] have shown conclusively that the longer the chosen interval between doses, the higher the doses need to be for most of the drugs, with the exception of rifampicin. The first such randomized controlled clinical trial on standard intermittent regimens undertaken at the Tuberculosis Research Center, Chennai, India[19] which revealed that twice-weekly regimens containing isoniazid in high dosage (14–15 mg/kg) and streptomycin (0.75–1 g) are highly effective, whether given from the outset or after an initial intensive phase of treatment. Their efficacy in slow and rapid inactivators of isoniazid is similar. These regimens can be highly effective in patients with extensive disease and in populations with a high frequency of rapid inactivators. A once-weekly regimen of isoniazid (15 mg/kg) and streptomycin (1 g), after 4 weeks initial daily therapy with isoniazid and streptomycin, approached the efficacy of the twice-weekly regimen; however, unlike the latter, it was substantially inferior in rapid inactivators of isoniazid and therefore cannot be recommended.

13. The discovery of rifampicin in 1966 as perhaps the most effective medication for tuberculosis,[20] is broad spectrum antibiotic and predominantly use for the treatment of tuberculosis. Use of rifampicin led the emergence of effective short course regimen. The short course chemotherapy trials started in 1971. Monumental work done by the British Medical Research Council and partners around the world led to the development of standard short-course chemotherapeutic regimens.[21,22] The studies established a number of key points that provided the framework for the development of modern treatment. These points include the following: (a) Regimens of 6 and 8 months duration are extremely effective in achieving a high cure rate with a low relapse rate, (b) Rifampicin-containing regimens allow effective short-course treatment even of patients with smear-positive cavitary disease, (c) For 6- and 8-month regimens, both rifampicin and pyrazinamide are necessary, but pyrazinamide is required only for the initial phase of treatment,[23] (d) Relapses with short-course treatment generally occur within the first year and relapses that occur following multidrug therapy are usually caused by organisms that retain their original susceptibility. The development of rifampicin and pyrazinamide prompted studies of intermittent short-course regimens. At first, investigators studied regimens with a daily intensive phase followed by an intermittent continuation phase. The risk of relapse is the key indicator of the effectiveness of a regimen. Many regimens achieve nearly 100% cure; relapse should be less than 5%. The oral regimen of 2 month of isoniazid, rifampicin, pyrazinamide, ethambutol, followed by 4 month of isoniazid, rifampicin, was studied in daily, partial, fully intermittent regimens. Fully intermittent treatment has been found to be highly effective, which make treatment observation more convenient and feasible for health workers and patients; achieve high level of treatment success with low relapse rates.[24] Such regimens have now been widely used, with good results. A twice-weekly, 6 months rifampicin-containing regimen following 2 weeks of daily treatment has also been shown to be highly effective.[25] However, a single missed dose will result in once weekly treatment, which is less effective and potentially more toxic because of immunological mediated adverse effects. Adverse reactions to rifampicin are more frequent in once-daily weekly treatment.
14. The studies in the 1980s that evaluated regimens with a treatment duration of less than 6 months demonstrated high relapse rates (11–40%) in patients with sputum smear-positive pulmonary tuberculosis.[26]
15. National Tuberculosis Control Program was evaluated in 1992 and found wide gap between expected and actual achievement of program.[27] WHO declared tuberculosis as global emergency, in 1993 and decided for categorywise treatment of tuberculosis. The Revised National

Tuberculosis Control Program (RNTCP) adopting the internationally recommended DOTS strategy was started in 1993.

16. Standardized and simplified regimens using fully intermittent, directly observed 6-month treatment have been shown to be effective on a mass basis in India[28] and in China.[29]
17. DOTS-Plus and Green Light Committee was launched in the year 2000 by WHO for control of MDR-TB. DOTS-Plus was launched as a pilot project in the year 2007 in India.[30]
18. Guidelines for programmatic management of drug resistant TB were launched by WHO in 2006 and was revised as an emergency update in the year 2008 and 2011.[31,32]
19. International standards of TB care was launched in 2006[33] and undergone revision in 2009 and 2014.[34]
20. Stop TB Partnership and World Health Organization, the global plan to stop TB 2006–2015 was implemented in the year 2006.[35]
21. The term "XDR-TB" was defined in the year 2006,[36] WHO Global XDR-TB Task Force was established in oct 2006.[37]
22. WHO launched revised treatment of TB guideline in 2009.[38]
23. Standards of TB care in India was launched in 2014.

REFERENCES

1. Barry VC. Development of the chemotherapeutic agent for tuberculosis. In: Bery VC, (Ed). Chemotherapy of tuberculosis. London, Butterworths. 1964.
2. Schatz A, Bugie E, Waksman SA. Streptomycin, a substance exhibiting antibiotic activity against Gram-positive and Gram-negative bacteria. Proceeding of the Society of Experimental and Biological Medicine. 1944;55:66-9.
3. Hinshaw HC, Feldman WH. Streptomycin in the treatment of clinical tuberculosis: a preliminary report. Proceeding of the staff meeting of Mayo Clinic. 1945;20:313-8.
4. Ramakrishnan CV, Rajendran K, Mohan K, Fox W, Radhakrishna S. The role of diet in the treatment of pulmonary tuberculosis. An evaluation in a controlled chemotherapy study in home and sanatorium patients in South India. Bulletin of the World Health Organization, 1961;25:339-59.
5. Tuberculosis Chemotherapy Centre, Madras. A concurrent comparison of home and sanatorium treatment of pulmonary tuberculosis in South India. Bulletin of the World Health Organization, 1959;21:51-145.
6. Dawson JJY, Devadatta S, Wallace Fox, Radhakrishna S, Ramakrishnan CV, Somasundaram PR, et al. A 5-year study of patients with pulmonary tuberculosis in a concurrent comparison of home and sanatorium treatment for one year with isoniazid plus PAS. Bulletin of the World Health Organization. 1966;34:533-51.
7. Andrews RH, Devadatta S, Wallace Fox. Prevalence of tuberculosis among close family contacts of tuberculosis patients in South India, and influence of segregation of the patient on the early attack rate. Bulletin of the World Health Organization. 1960;23:463-510.
8. Kamat SR, Dawson JJ, Devadatta S, Fox W, Janardhanam B, Radhakrishna S. A controlled study of the influence of segregation of tuberculous patients for one year on the attack rate of tuberculosis in a 5-year period in close family contacts in South India. Bulletin of the World Health Organization. 1966;34:517-32.

9. Fox W. The problem of self-administration of drugs with particular reference to pulmonary tuberculosis. Tubercle. 1958;39:269-274.
10. Fox W. Self-administration of medicaments. A review of published work and a study of the problem. Bulletin of the International Union Against Tuberculosis. 1961;31:307-331.
11. Sharbaro JA. The patient-physician relationship: compliance revisited. Annals of Allergy, 1990;64:326-32.
12. Iseman MD, Cohn DL, Sbarbaro JA. Directly observed treatment of tuberculosis—we can't afford not to try it. New England Journal of Medicine. 1993;338:576-8.
13. Weis SE, Slocum PC, Blais FX, King B, Nunn M, Matney GB, et al. The effect of directly observed therapy on the rates of drug resistance and relapse in tuberculosis. New England Journal of Medicine. 1994;330:1179-84.
14. Frieden TR, Fujiwara PI, Washko RM, Hamburg MA. Tuberculosis in New York City—turning the tide. New England Journal of Medicine. 1995;333:229-33.
15. Moore RD, Chaulk CP, Griffiths R, Cavalcante S, Chaisson RE. Cost-effectiveness of directly observed versus self-administered therapy for tuberculosis. American Journal of Respiratory and Critical Care Medicine. 1996;154:1013-9.
16. Canetti G, Grumbach F, Grosset J. Long-term, two-stage chemotherapy of advanced experimental murine tuberculosis with intermittent regimes during the second stage. Tubercle. 1963;44:236-40.
17. Dickinson JM, Mitchison DA. In vitro studies on the choice of drugs for intermittent chemotherapy of tuberculosis. Tubercle. 1966;47:370-80.
18. Grumbach F, Canetti G, Grosset J, Lirzin ML. Late results of long-term intermittent chemotherapy of advanced, murine tuberculosis: limits of the murine model. Tubercle. 1967;48:11-26.
19. A concurrent comparison of intermittent (twice-weekly) isoniazid plus streptomycin and daily isoniazid plus PAS in the domiciliary treatment of pulmonary tuberculosis. Bulletin of the World Health Organization. 1964;31:247-71.
20. Sense P. History of the development of rifampicin. Respiratory and Infectious Disease. 1983; 5:402-6.
21. East African/British Medical Research Council. Controlled clinical treatment of short-course (6 months) regime of chemotherapy for treatment of pulmonary tuberculosis. Third report. Lancet. 1974;2:237-48.
22. Fox W, Ellard GA, Mitchison DA. Studies on the treatment of tuberculosis undertaken by the British Medical Research Council tuberculosis units, 1946–1986, with relevant subsequent publications. International Journal of Tuberculosis and Lung Disease. 1999;3:S231-79.
23. Hong Kong Chest Service/British Medical Research Councils. Controlled trials of 2, 4 and 6 months of pyrazinamide in 6 month, three-times-weekly regimens for smear-positive pulmonary tuberculosis, including an assessment of a combined preparation of isoniazid, rifampicin, and pyrazinamide: results at 30 months. American Review of Respiratory Disease. 1991;143:700-6.
24. Chaisson RE, Clermont HC, Holt EA, Cantave M, Johnson MP, Atkinson J, et al. Six- month supervised intermittent tuberculosis therapy in Haitian patients with or without HIV infection. American Journal of Respiratory and Critical Care Medicine. 1996;154:1034-8.
25. Cohn DL, Catlin BJ, Peterson KL, Judson FN, Sbarbaro JA. A 62-dose, 6 month therapy for pulmonary and extrapulmonary tuberculosis. A thrice-weekly, directly observed, and cost-effective regimen. Annals of Internal Medicine. 1990;112:407-15.
26. East African and British Medical Research Councils. Controlled trials of 5 short course (4-month) chemotherapy regimens in pulmonary tuberculosis. First report of 4th study. Lancet, 1978;2:334-8.
27. Tuberculosis programme review—India, 1992: World Health Organisation, Geneva.1992; National Tuberculosis Institute, Summaries of NTI studies. 1997;101.

28. Khatri GR, Frieden TR. The status and prospects of tuberculosis control in India. International Journal of Tuberculosis and Lung Disease. 2000;4:193-200.
29. China Tuberculosis Control Collaboration. Results of directly observed short-course chemotherapy in 112, 842 Chinese patients with smear-positive tuberculosis. Lancet. 1996; 347:358-62.
30. WHO. DOTS-Plus and the Green Light Committee: Improving access to second-line anti-TB drugs. Geneva: World Health Organization WHO/CDS/TB/2000. 283.
31. World Health Organization. Guidelines for the Programmatic Management of Drug-Resistant Tuberculosis emergency update 2008. WHO/HTM/TB/2008. 402.
32. World Health Organization. Guidelines for the Programmatic Management of Drug-Resistant Tuberculosis update, 2011.
33. Tuberculosis Coalition for Technical Assistance. International Standards for Tuberculosis Care (ISTC). The Hague: Tuberculosis Coalition for Technical Assistance, 2006.
34. World Care Council, The Patients' Charter for Tuberculosis Care, Second Edition, 2009 (revised).
35. World Health Organization. Stop TB Partnership. The Stop TB Strategy. Building on and enhancing DOTS to meet the TB-related millennium development goals. WHO/HTM/TB/2006.368. Geneva: World Health Organization. 2006.
36. Centers for Disease Control and Prevention (CDC). Emergence of *Mycobacterium tuberculosis* with extensive resistance to second-line drugs—Worldwide, 2000–04. MMWR. 2066;55:301-5.
37. Centers for Disease Control and Prevention (CDC). Notice to readers: Revised definition of extensively drug-resistant tuberculosis. MMWR. 2006;55:1176.
38. World Health Organization. Treatment of TB Guidelines, 4th Edition. WHO/HTM/TB/2009.420.

Chapter 2

Case Definitions in Tuberculosis

Aim of the present chapter is to define various definitions used in tuberculosis (TB).

CASE DEFINITIONS

Tuberculosis Suspect

Any person who presents with symptoms or signs suggestive of TB. The most common symptom of pulmonary TB is productive cough for more than 2 weeks, which may be accompanied by other respiratory symptom (shortness of breath, chest pains, hemoptysis) and/or constitutional symptoms (loss of appetite, weight loss, fever, night sweats, and fatigue).[1]

Case of Tuberculosis

A definite case of TB (defined below) or one in which a clinician or other medical practitioner has diagnosed TB and has decided to treat the patients with full course of TB treatment. Any person given treatment for tuberculosis should be recorded as a case. Incomplete trial tuberculosis treatment should not be given as a method for diagnosis.

Definite Case of Tuberculosis

A patient with *Mycobacterium tuberculosis* complex identified from a clinical specimen, either by culture or by a newer method such as molecular line probe assay. In countries that lack the laboratory capacity to routinely identify *M. tuberculosis*, a pulmonary case with one or more initial sputum smear examinations positive for acid-fast bacilli (AFB) is also considered to be a "definite" case, provided that there is a functional external quality assurance (EQA) system with blind rechecking.

The four determinants of case definition are:

- Site of TB disease
- Bacteriology (result of sputum smear)
- Severity of TB disease
- History of previous treatment of TB
- HIV status of the patients.

DISEASE CLASSIFICATION

TB cases are classified as pulmonary and extrapulmonary.

Pulmonary Tuberculosis

Tuberculosis involving only the lung parenchyma.

Extrapulmonary Tuberculosis

Tuberculosis of organs other than the lungs, e.g. pleura, lymph nodes, abdomen, genitourinary tract, skin, joints and bones, meninges. Tuberculous intrathoracic lymphadenopathy (mediastinal and/or hilar) or tuberculous pleural effusion, without radiographic abnormalities in the lungs, therefore, constitutes a case of extrapulmonary TB (EPTB). The definition of an extrapulmonary case with several sites affected depends on the site representing the most severe form of disease. Patients with both pulmonary and extrapulmonary TB should be classified as a case of pulmonary TB.

Pulmonary TB is further classified as smear-positive and smear-negative.

Smear-positive Patient

A case of pulmonary TB is considered to be smear-positive if one or more sputum smear specimens at the start of treatment is positive for AFB [provided that there is a functional external quality assurance (EQA) system with blind rechecking].

A patient with a new sputum smear-positive pulmonary TB is at least one sputum sample in countries with a well functioning EQA system.

In countries without functional EQA, the definition of a smear-positive pulmonary TB case was defined as one with:

- Two or more initial sputum smear examinations (direct smear microscopy) positive for acid-fast bacilli (AFB);

OR

- A patient with one sputum examination positive for AFB and radiographic abnormalities consistent with active pulmonary TB as determined by the treating clinician and other medical practioner.

OR

- A patient with one sputum specimen positive for AFB and culture-positive for *M. tuberculosis*.

Smear-negative Patient

A patient having symptoms suggestive of TB with at least 2 sputum examinations negative for AFB, and radiographic abnormalities consistent with active pulmonary TB as determined by the treating clinician and other medical practioner, followed by a decision to treat the patient with a full course of anti-TB therapy;

OR

A patient whose diagnosis is based on culture-positive for *M. tuberculosis* but sputum smear examinations negative for AFB.

The following forms of smear-negative pulmonary TB are classified as seriously ill:

Seriously ill smear-negative TB[2]

- Miliary TB
- Extensive parenchymal infiltration
- Co-infection with HIV
- Pulmonary disease with cavitations
- All forms of pediatric sputum smear-negative pulmonary TB except primary complex.

Diagnosis of extrapulmonary tuberculosis (EPTB) should be based on:

1. One culture-positive specimen from the site of disease, or
2. Histological evidence of TB, or
3. Strong clinical evidence, consistent with active extrapulmonary TB, followed by the diagnosing medical practitioner's decision to treat the patient with a full course of anti-TB treatment. Depending upon the site of the infection, various diagnostic tools may be used. For example, fine needle aspiration cytology (FNAC)/biopsy is used for diagnosing TB lymphadenitis.

Certain forms of EPTB are considered as seriously ill

Seriously ill EPTB[2]

- Meningitis
- Pericarditis
- Peritonitis
- Bilateral or extensive pleural effusion
- Spinal TB with neurological involvement
- Intestinal
- Genitourinary
- Co-infection with HIV
- All forms of pediatric extrapulmonary TB other than lymph node TB and unilateral pleural effusion are considered to be seriously ill.

Not seriously ill EPTB

- Lymph node
- Pleural effusion (unilateral)

- Peripheral joints
- Skin
- Adrenal gland.

Any patient, with pulmonary or extrapulmonary TB, who is known to be HIV positive based on voluntary sharing of results and/or history of antiretroviral therapy, is considered as seriously ill. For the purpose of categorization, HIV testing should not be done.

TYPES OF TUBERCULOSIS PATIENTS

New

A TB patient who has never had treatment for TB or one who has taken anti-TB drugs for less than one month.

Relapse

Relapse is defined in a person previously treated for TB who has been declared cured or treatment completed, and is diagnosed with bacteriologically positive (smear or culture) tuberculosis.[1,3]

Treatment after Default

A TB patient who received anti-TB treatment for one month or more from any source and returns to treatment after having defaulted, i.e. not taken anti-TB drugs consecutively for two months or more, and who is found to be sputum smear-positive.

Failure

Any TB patient who is smear-positive at 5 months or more after starting treatment. Failure also includes a patient who was treated with Category III regimen but who becomes smear-positive during treatment.

Chronic

A TB patient who remains smear-positive after completing a re-treatment regimen.

Others

TB patients who do not fit into the above-mentioned types. Reasons for putting a patient in this type must be specified.

DIRECTLY OBSERVED TREATMENT

Directly observed treatment (DOT) means that an observer watches the patient swallowing their tablets, in a way that is sensitive and supportive to the patient's needs. This ensures that a TB patient takes the right antitubercular drugs, in the right doses, at the right intervals.[4]

DIRECTLY OBSERVED TREATMENT PLUS

Directly observed treatment plus (DOT-Plus) is an integral component of RNTCP to manage MDR-TB which is to be implemented through program infrastructure of the DOTS program. The strategy is designed to manage MDR-TB using second-line anti-TB drugs within the DOTS strategy in low- and middle-income countries like India.

TREATMENT OUTCOMES OF DOTS

In RNTCP, every patient registered has one and only one of the following six outcomes. This needs to be reported in individual treatment cards. The possible treatment outcomes are as follows:

Cured

Initially sputum smear-positive patient who has completed treatment and had negative sputum smears, on at least two occasions, one of which was at the end of treatment.

Treatment Completed

A sputum smear-positive patient who has completed treatment, with negative smears at the end of IP but none at the end of treatment; or a sputum smear-negative patient who has received a full course of treatment and has not become smear-positive during or at the end of treatment; or an EPTB patient who has received a full course of treatment and has not become smear-positive during or at the end of treatment.

Died

Patient who died during the course of treatment, regardless of the cause of death.

Failure

Failure is defined on the basis of two aspects bacteriologically, i.e. on sputum smear and culture status. In low- and middle-income countries like India where cultures are less frequently used, sputum smears are used to define failures. Failure for initially smear-positive patients (CAT I and CAT II) is defined as sputum smear-positive at the end of the fifth month of treatment or later.[1] Failure for initially smear-negative patients (Category III) regimen is defined as who became smear-positive during treatment.[1]

Based on culture failure is defined as the reappearance, whilst the patient is receiving treatment and after the negative conversion of cultures, of bacteriological activity.[1,3] It is also considered treatment failure when cultures do not become negative during the course of treatment.

Defaulted

A patient who has not taken anti-TB drugs for 2 months or more consecutively after starting treatment.

Transferred Out

A patient who has been transferred to another TB unit or district and for whom the treatment result (outcome) is not known.

DRUG RESISTANT TUBERCULOSIS

Drug resistant tuberculosis is defined as a case of tuberculosis excreting bacilli resistant to one or more antitubercular drugs. DR-TB is confirmed through laboratory tests that show that the infecting isolates of *M. tuberculosis* grow in vitro in the presence of one or more anti-tuberculosis drugs. Four different categories of drug resistance have been established:[4]

Mono-resistance

Resistance to one antituberculosis drug.

Poly-resistance

Resistance to more than one antituberculosis drug, other than both isoniazid and rifampicin.

Multidrug-resistant Tuberculosis (MDR-TB)

Resistant to isoniazid (H) and rifampicin (R) with or without resistance to other drugs.

MDR-TB Suspect

A TB patient who fails an RNTCP Category I or III treatment regimen and any RNTCP Category II patient who is sputum smear-positive at the end of the fourth month of treatment or later.[4] Recently criteria for defining a MDR TB Suspect has been divided into three groups under programmatic management of drug-resistant tuberculosis.[5] The program uses a strategy that screens patients with initially a very high risk of MDR-TB using DST. As laboratory and treatment capacity builds, the program will scale up to achieve universal access to quality assured DST. The MDR Suspects have been divided into three criteria based on the risk of MDR TB. Criteria A includes all failures of new TB cases, smear positive previously treated cases who remain smear positive at 4th month onwards, all pulmonary TB cases who are contacts of known MDR TB case. Criteria B includes in addition to Criteria A all smear positive previously treated pulmonary TB cases at diagnosis, any smear positive follow up result in new or previously treated cases. Criteria C includes in addition to Criteria B all smear negative previously treated pulmonary TB cases at diagnosis, HIV TB co-infected cases at diagnosis. Initially DST will be performed in those patients fulfilling Criteria A and as capacity builds up it will progress to Criteria B and then C.[5]

Confirmed MDR-TB Case

A TB patient whose sputum is culture positive for *Mycobacterium tuberculosis* and is resistant in vitro to isoniazid and rifampicin with or without other anti-tubercular drugs based on DST results from an RNTCP-certified Culture and DST Laboratory. An "MDR-TB suspect" confirmed by an RNTCP-certified Culture and DST laboratory to have MDRTB, or any rifampicin resistance, will be treated with the RNTCP Regimen for MDR TB.[5]

Extensively Drug-resistant Tuberculosis (XDR-TB)

The term extensively drug resistant TB (XDR-TB) is a new term which was provisionally defined as those persons with TB whose isolates were resistant to isoniazid and rifampicin and at least three of the six main classes of second line drugs[6] (SLDs) (Aminoglycosides, Polypeptides, Fluoroquinolones, Thioamides, Cycloserine, and Para-aminosalicylic Acid). But in October 2006, the World Health Organization revised the case definition of XDR-TB as TB with resistance to at least isoniazid and rifampicin as well as further resistance to a fluoroquinolone and a second-line injectable agent (Kanamycin, Amikacin or Capreomycin).[7,8]

XDR-TB Suspect

If the 6th month follow-up culture of MDR patients under DOTS-Plus treatment is found to be positive, then at this time culture isolate should to be sent for second-line DST.[4]

Extremely Drug-resistant Tuberculosis (XXDR-TB) or Total Drug-resistant Tuberculosis (TDR-TB)

The term XXDR-TB or TDR-TD has been proposed for cases resistant to all available first and second-line drugs.[8-11] The term "totally drug-resistant" tuberculosis is not yet recognised by the WHO. For now these cases are defined as extensively drug-resistant tuberculosis (XDR-TB), according to WHO definitions.[12]

TREATMENT OUTCOMES IN DOTS-PLUS[5]

Standardized treatment outcome definitions are to be used following treatment of an MDR-TB case and are as follows:

Cure

An MDR-TB patient who has completed treatment and has been consistently culture negative (with at least 5 consecutive negative results in the last 12 to

15 months). If one follow-up positive culture is reported during the last three quarters, patient will still be considered cured provided this positive culture is followed by at least 3 consecutive negative cultures, taken at least 30 days apart, provided that there is clinical evidence of improvement.

Treatment Completed

A MDR-TB patient who has completed treatment according to guidelines but does not meet the definition for cure or treatment failure due to lack of bacteriological results.

Death

A MDR-TB patient who dies for any reason during the course of MDR-TB treatment.

Treatment Failure

Treatment will be considered to have failed if two or more of the five cultures recorded in the final 12–15 months are positive, or if any of the final three cultures are positive.

Treatment Default

A MDR-TB patient whose MDR-TB treatment was interrupted for two or more consecutive months for any reasons.

Transfer Out

A MDR-TB patient who has been transferred to another reporting unit and for whom the treatment outcome is not known.

Treatment Stopped Due to Adverse Drug Reactions

A patient on MDR-TB treatment who develops severe adverse reactions and could not continue the MDR-TB treatment in spite of the management of the adverse reactions as per the defined protocols and decision has been taken by the DOTS-Plus site committee to stop treatment.

Treatment Stopped Due to Other Reasons

A patient on MDR-TB treatment who could not continue the MDR-TB treatment for any other medical reason (than adverse drug reactions), and a decision has been taken by the DOTS-Plus site committee to stop treatment.

Still on Treatment

A MDR-TB patient who, for any reason, is still receiving their RNTCP CAT IV treatment at the time of the submission of the RNTCP DOTS-Plus Treatment Outcome Report.

HIV SETTING CASE DEFINITIONS[10,13]

The following are suggested case definitions for use in HIV-prevalent settings:

Smear-positive Pulmonary Tuberculosis

- One sputum smear examination positive for acid-fast bacilli (AFB)
- Laboratory confirmation of HIV infection
- Strong clinical evidence of HIV infection.

Smear-negative Pulmonary Tuberculosis

- At least two sputum specimens negative for AFB
- Radiographical abnormalities consistent with active tuberculosis
- Laboratory confirmation of HIV infection
- Strong clinical evidence of HIV infection
- Decision by a clinician to treat with a full course of antituberculosis chemotherapy

OR

- A patient with AFB smear-negative sputum which is culture-positive for *M. tuberculosis*.

Extrapulmonary Tuberculosis

- One specimen from an extrapulmonary site culture-positive for *Mycobacterium tuberculosis* or smear-positive for AFB

OR

- Histological or strong clinical evidence consistent laboratory confirmation of HIV infection
- Strong clinical evidence of HIV infection and
- Decision by a clinician to treat with a full course of antituberculosis chemotherapy with active extrapulmonary tuberculosis.

REFERENCES

1. Training Module for Medical Practitioners 2010. Central TB Division, Directorate General of Health Services, Ministry of Health and Family Welfare, Nirman Bhawan, New Delhi.
2. WHO policy on TB infection control in health care facilities, congregate settings and households. Geneva, World Health Organization. 2009 (WHO/HTM/TB/2009.419).
3. Caminero JA. Guía de la Tuberculosis para Médicos Especialistas. [Tuberculosis Guide for Specialist Physicians]. Paris, International Union Against Tuberculosis and Lung Disease, 2003.
4. Guidlines for the programmatic management of drug resistant tuberculosis; emergency update 2008. Geneva. WHO 2008 (WHO/HTM/TB/2008.402), 2011 (WHO/HTM/TB/2011.6).
5. Guidelines on Programmatic Management of Drug Resistant TB (PMDT) in India 2012. Central TB Division, Directorate General of Health Services, Ministry of Health and Family Welfare, Nirman Bhavan, New Delhi.
6. Centers for Disease Control and Prevention (CDC) Emergence of *Mycobacterium tuberculosis* with extensive resistance to second-line drugs—Worldwide, 2000–2004. MMWR. 2006;55:301-5.

7. Centers for Disease Control and Prevention (CDC) Notice to readers: Revised definition of extensively drug-resistant tuberculosis. MMWR. 2006;55:1176.
8. Migliori GB, Loddenkemper R, Blasi F, Raviglione MC. 125 years after Robert Koch's discovery of the tubercle bacillus: the new XDR-TB threat: is "science" enough to tackle the epidemic? Eur Respir J. 2007;29:423-7.
9. Joshi JM. Preventing Extremely Drug Resistant Tuberculosis: Directly Observed Treatment is the Only Answer. Editorial. Indian J Chest Dis Allied Sci. 2008;50:183-5.
10. Velayati AA, Masjedi MR, Farnia P, et al. Emergence of new forms of totally drugresistant tuberculosis bacilli: super extensively drug-resistant tuberculosis or totally drug-resistant strains in Iran. Chest 2009;136:420–5.
11. Udwadia ZF, Amale RA, Ajbani KK, Rodriguez C. Totally drug-resistant tuberculosis in India. Clin Infect Dis. 2012;54:579-81.
12. WHO Stop TB Department Drug-resistant tuberculosis Frequently Asked Questions. Updated 24 January 2012. Available at: http://www.who.int/tb/challenges/mdr/TDRFAQs160112.
13. Improving the diagnosis and treatment of smear-negative pulmonary and extrapulmonary tuberculosis among adults and adolescents. Recommendations for HIV-prevalent and resource-constrained settings. WHO/HTM/TB/2007.379.

Chapter 3

Epidemiology of Tuberculosis

Epidemiology is the study of frequency, distribution and determinants of health related states or events in specified human populations, and the application of this study to the control of health problems. For the planning and subsequent review of the strategy for control of any communicable disease, information on its epidemiological situation and the trend is a virtual prerequisite. In a chronic infectious disease like tuberculosis, the precise estimate on mortality as well as the prevalence or incidence over long-term needs to be obtained in order to study its time trend. The aim of this chapter is to describe various epidemiological indices in tuberculosis (TB).

EPIDEMIOLOGICAL INDICES

Following are various epidemiologic indices or parameters being needed to measure the TB problem in a community, planning and evaluation of control measures as well as yardsticks for international comparison.

Prevalence of Infection

It is the percentage individuals who show a positive reaction to the standard tuberculin test. The estimation of prevalence of tuberculous infection in the community is based on the interpretation of the results of tuberculin testing of persons without Bacillus Calmette-Guerin (BCG) scar. Prevalence represents a cumulative experience of a population to recent and remote infection with *M. tuberculosis*. Besides the type of tuberculin and their dosages used from survey to survey not being the same, the problem of defining the infected is compounded by the changing levels of demarcation between the infected and uninfected from one survey to the other.[1,2] The problem of changing demarcation levels from survey to survey had no doubt engaged the attention of researchers. It is suggested after a field study that the demarcation line between the infected and noninfected persons would require to be shifted from survey to survey to take care of the observer variations or the rising proportions of BCG scars in the population being wrongly classified as unvaccinated from one survey to the next, thereby affecting the classification between the infected and uninfected. Persons are considered as infected, if the indurations to tuberculin test are observed to lie to the right of the demarcation line as decided on the basis of the distribution of the indurations, for the given study.

Incidence of Infection

Incidence of infection, which gives the most recent tuberculosis transmission situation in the community, is defined as the number of fresh infections occurring in the community between two points in time, among those uninfected initially. It calls for direct measurement of the conversions of uninfected persons to infected status, in the intervening period between two succeeding surveys, say a year or so apart; therefore, it has also been termed tuberculin conversion index. Prevalence figures do not indicate, when in the past, the first infections had occurred.[3]

Annual Risk of Infection (ARI)

It determines the percentage of individuals under study who will be newly infected by *M. tuberculosis* among the noninfected of the preceding survey during the course of one year in a given community.[3] This parameter is considered one of the best indicators for evaluating the TB problem and its trend.[4] It avoids repeat tuberculin testing of the same children essential for correct estimation. Most appropriate age group for ARI surveys are children between 0 and 9 years of age since high prevalence of nonspecific sensitivity in higher ages interferes with interpretation of test results. In developing countries where risk of infection is still high, a relatively small sample of children of the order of 6000–7000 would suffice for baseline estimates of ARI. ARI rates not only provide a measure of the impact of control measures but also enable predictions to be made about the likely magnitude of tuberculosis problem in the following years.

Prevalence of Disease

It is the percentage of individuals whose sputum is positive for tubercle bacilli on microscopic examination. This parameter has been considered to be best in the estimation of the number of infectious cases or case load in a community. The prevalence of smear-positive cases gives information on the magnitude of pool of infectious sources in the community, which is of limited value as an epidemiological index since it depends on quality of chemotherapy of smear-positive cases and the extent of case-finding and therefore is more important indicator of management of tuberculosis control program. Prevalence and incidence of disease are considered in terms of culture with or without smear positivity (C^+), smear-positive cases (SS^+) or, X-ray positive culture/smear negative cases (X^+). Total prevalence is the sum of C^+ and X^+.

Incidence of Disease

It is the percentage of new TB cases (confirmation by bacteriological examination) per 1000 population occurring during one year. It is considered to be a good epidemiological index which reflects the magnitude of the tuberculosis problem in a given community and if observed over the years shows the trend in disease situation. Unfortunately, in developing countries cases detection rates are only a fraction of the true incidence rates and incomplete notification cannot be expected to provide a measure of the burden of tuberculosis. Currently, the only means of estimating incidence of smear-positive cases is the relationship between ARI and the incidence of smear-positive cases that has been obtained by using a variety of data from the Netherlands in pre-chemotherapy era and the number of WHO sponsored surveys in developing countries. According to this parametric relationship, there are 50 incident cases of smear-positive tuberculosis for every one percent of ARI.[3-5]

Prevalence of Drug Resistant Cases

It is the prevalence of patient excreting tubercle bacilli resistant to anti-tubercular drugs. This index is directly related to chemotherapy.

Mortality Rate

It is defined as the number of deaths from TB every year per 1000 or 100,000 population. This parameter has lost its importance since the introduction of an effective ATT and preventive measures. In the Revised National Tuberculosis Program (RNTCP) of the Government of India, deaths reported among registered TB cases are considered to be due to TB unless specified otherwise.

Case Fatality Rate (CFR)

It indicates the proportion of persons in a cohort or group of persons that die due to tuberculosis in a given period of time.

Epidemiological Survery Methods

It is very essential to have a clear vision of burden of TB in a defined population. There are two types of epidemiological survey methods to describe the morbidity which are as follows:

Cross-sectional Survey

This study is based on a single examination of a cross-section of population at one point in time—the results of which can be projected on the whole population provided the sampling has been done correctly. It is the simplest form of an observational study helping in estimation of prevalence of disease therefore, also termed as "prevalence study". It has limitations of providing very little information about the natural history of disease or about the rate of occurrence of new cases (incidence). Till now, only one cross-sectional sample survey has been conducted in our country, i.e. the National Sample Survey (NSS) between 1955–58 under the auspices of Indian Council of Medical Research (ICMR).

Longitudinal Survey

This study involves repeated observations in a defined population over a prolonged period of time by means of follow-up examinations. They are helpful in studying the natural history of the disease and its future outcome, identifying risk factors of disease and also finding out incidence rate in the community. However, these type of studies are difficult to organize and more time-consuming. Several studies have been conducted in various parts of India, major ones being Bangalore Study (1961–86), Chingleput Trial (1968–96) and New Delhi Study (1962–91).

Survey Method in Tuberculosis

Reliable data for estimating the TB burden in any community can be obtained through special techniques such as surveys because mortality as well as morbidity notifications and infection rates have been proved to be unsatisfactory. There are several types of surveys that are described below:

i. *Tuberculin survey*: Survey of a community by tuberculin testing can indicate the time trend of infection provided fresh samples are tested every time to eliminate the possible boosting effect of tuberculin. Epidemiological utility of this testing is marginal as many disadvantages can be observed such as consideration of some of the sputum positive definite cases of TB as nonreactive, interference in the interpretation by nonspecific allergy, artificial conversion caused by mass BCG vaccination in our country and also due to varying dosage and standards of tuberculin conversion.
ii. *Bacteriological surveys*: Sputum examination of persons has great utility in case-finding because of cheapness, feasibility and involvement of less expertization. In under-developed countries where radiological surveys are not possible, this method can provide a quick estimate of the minimum prevalence of TB in a community for initiating a control program. It has high specificity but low sensitivity because of under-estimation as relatively large number of cases would be missed due to difficulty in demonstration of tubercle bacilli in sputum during early stages of disease.
iii. *X-ray surveys*: Radiological examination can detect even the smallest lesions, irrespective of the presence or absence of symptoms. Therefore,

these types of surveys have high sensitivity but low specificity reasons being lack of reasonably accurate objective standards for interpretation, wide inter-individual and intra-individual variations making criterias for assessment liable to change and neither etiology nor activity can always be easily inferred.

GLOBAL BURDEN OF TUBERCULOSIS

Tuberculosis remains a worldwide public heath problem despite the fact that the causative organism was discovered more than 100 years ago and highly effective drugs and vaccine are available making TB a preventable and curable disease. Developed countries like USA have achieved spectacular results in the control of TB as one survey conducted from 1900 to 1980 established the fact that tuberculosis death rate declined from 199 to 0.5 per 100,000. Surveillance and survey data is used to update estimates of incidence. The WHO's 2008 report presents an overview regarding the year 2006 data and estimates, based on the reports from 202 countries representing 99.9% of the world's population.[6] In 2006, globally there were an estimated 9.2 million (139/100,000) new TB cases out of which 4.1 million (62/100,000) were new sputum smear-positive cases and 0.7 millions (7.7%) were HIV co-infected cases. 1.7 million (25/100,000) people died of TB, including 231,000 patients co-infected with HIV. The prevalence rate was estimated to be 14.4 millions (219/100,000). TB prevalence rates appear to be falling globally for several years. It is estimated that about one-third of the current global population is infected asymptomatically with TB, of whom 5–10% will develop clinical disease during their lifetime. The annual risk of TB infection in high burden countries is estimated to be 0.5–2%.[7] Currently, WHO's 2009 report states that there were an estimated 9.4 million incident cases (139/100,000) of TB globally in 2008 out of which 2.7 millions were new sputum smear-positive cases and 1.4 millions (15%) were HIV co-infected cases.[8] Of these HIV-positive cases, 78% were in the African region and 13% were in the South-East Asia region. There were an estimated 11.1 million prevalent cases of TB (164/100,000). It was estimated that 1.3 million deaths (28/100,000) occurred due to TB including 0.5 million deaths among cases who were also HIV-positive. Most of the estimated number of cases in 2008 occurred in Asia (55%) and Africa (30%), with small proportions of cases in the Eastern Mediterranean region (7%), the European region (5%) and the region of the Americas (3%). The five countries that rank first to fifth in terms of total numbers of incident cases in 2008 are India (1.6–2.4 million), China (1.0–1.6 million), South Africa (0.38–0.57 million), Nigeria (0.37–0.55 million) and Indonesia (0.34–0.52 million). India and China alone account for an estimated 35% of TB cases worldwide.

Globally, the rate of treatment success for new smear-positive cases treated in the 2007 cohort was 86%. This is the first time that the treatment success rate has exceeded the global target of 85%, which was set by the World Health Assembly (WHA) in 1991. Three regions the Eastern Mediterranean (88%), Western Pacific (92%), and South-East Asia (88%) regions—exceeded the target, as did 53 countries. The treatment success rate was 79% in the African Region, 82% in the Region of the Americas and 67% in the European Region (where death and failure rates are comparatively high). Between 2006 and 2007, treatment success rates were maintained or improved in all regions with the exception of the European Region. The case detection rate (calculated as the number of notified cases of TB in one year divided by the number of estimated incident cases of TB in the same year, and expressed as a percentage) has been a much-used indicator of progress in TB control for more than a decade. The considerable attention given to the case detection rate was in line with the two principal global targets (case detection and treatment success rates) set for TB control during the period 1991-2005. The target of DOTS program was successful treatment or cure rate of 85% of new smear-positive cases, and detection of 70% of such cases by the year 2000. As these targets were not achieved, the target year was reset to 2005.[9] The WHO has now launched global plan for *Stop TB Strategy* (2006–15) with the objective of reducing the burden of TB in line with global targets set for 2015.[10] DOTS still remains central to the public health approach to TB control in this strategy. The six major components of the strategy are: pursue high-quality DOTS expansion and enhancement, address TB/HIV, MDR-TB, and the needs of poor and vulnerable populations, contribute to health system strengthening based on primary health care, engage all care providers, empower people with TB, and communities through partnership and enable and promote research. Various TB-related Millennium Development Goals has been set: to combat HIV/AIDS, malaria and other diseases (Goal 6), to halt and reverse the incidence of malaria and other major diseases including tuberculosis by 2015 (Target 8), to halve the prevalence and death rates associated with tuberculosis between 1990 and 2015 (Indicator 23) and to detect 70% of new smear-positive TB cases arising annually and to successfully treat 85% of these cases by 2005 (Indicator 24). The *Stop TB Partnership* has set targets to reduce global burden of TB (per capita prevalence and death rates) by 50% relative to 1990 levels by 2015 and also reduction of the global incidence of active TB less than 1 case per million per year by 2050. The best estimate of the case detection rate of new smear-positive cases in 2008 was 62% (range 56–68%), which is 9% less than the milestone of 70% that was set in the Global Plan. The highest rates of case detection in 2008 are estimated to be in the European Region and the Region of the Americas, followed by the Western Pacific Region, with the lowest rate estimated for the African Region. Among the HBCs, the highest rates of case detection in 2008 are estimated to be in Indonesia, Brazil, China, the Russian Federation and the United Republic of Tanzania, with the lowest rate (24%, range 20–30%) in Zimbabwe. Overall, rates of case detection have stagnated since 2006, and renewed efforts to increase case-finding are needed to keep pace with Global Plan milestones. However, global status still remains at high risk reason being increased incidence of HIV co-infection and emergence of acquired drug resistance especially in developing countries.

TUBERCULOSIS BURDEN IN INDIA

Tuberculosis has been known to be in existence more than 2,000 years ago. But no indication of its distribution and extent was available because of lack of data on mortality due to improper death certification and lack of morbidity rates because of inadequate recording and reporting system especially in developing countries. A series of some isolated surveys were conducted in order to estimate TB problem in India in early 1950s. First attempt was carried out by Frimodt-Moller[11] but these surveys were not representative of entire country as they were restricted to a small population group in south India. The only authentic survey, on a country wide basis is the cross-sectional National Sample Survey (1955–58) counducted by the Indian Council of Medical Research (ICMR).[12] Six zones were selected representing 40% of the Indian population. Each zones were comprising of three cross-sections the largest city, medium sized towns and accessible villages covering 80–90% of the population with few exceptions. Methodology included population census and collection of information on economic status, mass miniature radiography of persons aged five years or more as per eligibility, collection of two sputum samples for direct smear for acid-fast bacilli (AFB) and two laryngeal swab specimens for culture of *M. tuberculosis*. Information was analyzed on the basis of active X-ray and bacteriological disease status. No estimation of prevalence of infection was available as tuberculin testing was not done. The data that was generated in order to define the magnitude of TB problem is briefly described below:

1. Prevalence rate of active as well as probably active TB varied from 13 to 25 per 1000 persons aged 5 years and more
2. Rate of bacteriologically positive cases per 1000 population varied from 2 to 8
3. Prevalence in the rural areas was not appreciably less than in the urban areas.
4. Prevalence rates were lower for females than males, especially in age-groups 35 years and above
5. Prevalence rate showed continuous increase with age especially in males
6. Prevalence was higher in overcrowded slums where low income groups of population lived under insanitary conditions
7. A large majority of the active and probably active cases had moderately advanced disease

Various longitudinal surveys were being conducted in order to study the epidemiological trend of TB in India such as at Delhi, Bengaluru, and Chingleput. Several other small-scale surveys have been conducted by various workers—Raj Narain,[13] Pamra[14] and Gothi.[15] All these surveys taken together have thrown considerable light on the TB problem in India though unrepresentative of the entire country.

The National Tuberculosis Institute conducted a longitudinal survey in a rural population in 119 randomly selected villages of Bangalore district for four times from 1961-68 using mass miniature radiography, tuberculin testing as well as bacteriological examination.[1] Fifth survey was carried in 1977 with implementation of National Tuberculosis Program (NTP) and further follow-up was undertaken between 1984 and 1986. It was observed that TB situation is supposed to be presenting a steady state. Without active intervention, one-third of bacillary cases get eliminated through death and natural cure annually but the same proportion gets added to it. Salient findings are as follows:

1. Prevalence and incidence rates of culture-positive cases and radiologically active abacillary cases revealed no change in the period of 12 years (1961–68 to 1977–78)
2. Mean age of cases was higher at later surveys
3. ARI declined from 1.1 to 0.65% from 1961–84, average being 2.35 per year
4. Incidence of smear-positive cases declined from 65/100,000 to 23/100000 from 1961–84
5. Very large population sizes would be required to be surveyed repeatedly to appreciate a change
6. High levels of intervention could result in marked change in the prevalence rates

Subsequently, Tuberculosis Research Center (TRC) Chennai carried out a longitudinal survey in a rural population of Chingleput (360,000) in Tamil Nadu from 1968 to 1984 and in a subset of population, again in 1991-92 and 1994-96.[16] Methodology included mass miniature radiography, bacteriological examination and BCG vaccination to study its efficacy in preventing incidence of TB in the noninfected, by different strains of BCG and their dosages. This survey is the longest of all well-known surveys conducted in India.

1. ARI had remained unchanged for the entire period as its value was between 1.8% and 1.9% in earlier period and between 2.9% and 3.2% in later period
2. No change in culture-positive case prevalence during the period (1968–75), but a decline of 2.3% per year for the later period (1984–86). However, overall rate was recorded 1.4% per annum
3. There was declining trend in culture-positive cases in all ages, especially in 10–14 years
4. No change in smear-positive case prevalence for all ages but a declining trend was observed in younger population aged up to 35 years
5. There was strong evidence of decline in both culture-positive as well as smear-positive case prevalence in females (3.8% and 2.8% annually)
6. The culture-positive cases had shown decline at a later period (1975–78 and 1979–81) for males without any significant change in trend of smear-positive cases
7. The male/female ratio in culture-positive cases had increased from 3.5 in 1968–70 to 5.2 in 1984–86 (average 4.7) whereas average for smear-positive cases for the entire period was found to be 1.7
8. There was a steady decline in the incidence of culture-positive cases from 352/100,000 to 189/100,000 as going from earlier to later period irrespective of age and sex

Contd...

Contd...

9. Incidence of smear-positive cases has shown a tendency for decline
10. Ratio of prevalence and incidence of smear-positive cases was found to be 3.6 at the surveys
11. Significant decline in prevalence rate of radiologically active abacillary cases from 1289/100,000 to 827/100,000 from 1968–86 (average decline being 3.2% per annum)

The New Delhi Tuberculosis Center (NDTBC) has conducted a longitudinal survey (New Delhi study) in an area inhabited by urban population of 30,000 in Delhi for a period of 30 years (1962–91).[17] Seven more surveys were carried out following the baseline survey in 1962. Methodology included population census on house to house visit, radiological as well as bacteriological assessment, clinical observation for a defined period and treatment of all diagnosed patients. In fact, this is the only other source apart from the NSS, from which TB situation for an urban metropolitan area in India could be observed.

1. There was considerable decline in prevalence of radiologically active abacillary cases (all ages and both sexes) at later survey in 1991 (5.4/1000) as compared to earliest survey in 1962 (13.2/1000)
2. The prevalence of radiologically active/probably active abacillary cases increased with age, the lowest being in those aged 5–14 years (1.61 per 1000) and the highest in those aged 55+ years (26.14 per 1000), both the rates were more in males than females, in all the age groups except 5–15 years
3. Reduction in incidence rate of radiologically active abacillary cases was not observed in last two surveys
4. Majority of the bacillary and X-ray active cases studied at last survey had come from the radiologically normal group of the previous survey
5. Of the 62 bacillary cases of last survey, 34 (54.8%) had come from the radiologically normals, 15 (24.2%) from the active abacillary group, 8 (12.9%) from the group with inactive TB shadows of seventh survey and 5 (8.06%) had continued as bacillary cases beween seventh and last survey
6. The overall culture-positive case rate at the last survey was 3.30 per 1000, risen for both the sexes with age (0.35 per 1000 in age group 5–14 years to 8.26 per 1000 in 55+ age group)
7. The fate of 70 bacteriologically positive cases in seventh survey was followed up in last survey–21 (30%) expired and majority of the remaining 49 cases had inactive lesions in chest X-ray (85.7%) while a small proportion had remained either as bacillary cases (8.2%) or as radiologically active abacillary cases (6.1%)
8. The overall prevalence rates remained unchanged in the area over 30 years after adjusting for the population changes observed despite of good program service (80% in 1962 and 90% in 1995–96)

A longitudinal survey was also conducted in a rural population of 15,575 in Car Nicobar which is an island situated in the Bay of Bengal through an intensified TB control project launched in 1986.[18] The study included detection of SS^+ and C^+ cases on house to house survey along with provision of adequate treatment, six to nine months chemoprophylaxis after tuberculin testing in children aged 5 years and above and BCG vaccination in children less than 4 years of age. This survey describes the trend of TB in a tribal area (1986–2002).

1. Prevalence of infection was 10% among children under 14 years of age
2. Prevalence rate of smear-positive cases were found to be 4.1/1000 as well as of radiologically active abacillary cases 7.9/1000
3. Conversion rate of 94% among smear-positive cases after short-course chemotherapy
4. No freshly infected children were detected during follow-up survey conducted after 16 months
5. Number of new smear-positive cases in the period of 16 months was only one-third of previous prevalence
6. Total newly diagnosed smear-positive cases were estimated to be 2,254,943 and expected incidence of smear-positive rate was 25-35/100,000 at repeated survey in 2001–2002
7. According to the re-survey (2001–2002), prevalence of infection increased to 25.1%,ARI increased to 3.50% (1.53% in 1986) and prevalence of smear-positive cases was significantly higher (7.1%)
8. The accumulation of cases over the years occurring due to the failure of National Tuberculosis Program (NTP) had made the epidemiological trend worse than that in 1986

Chakraborty, et al. has described the outcome of several surveys, conducted from time to time in different areas of the country, since 1955–1958 to estimate the burden of TB in India which undergone further necessary corrections and refinement.[19,20] The average rates of disease and infection (both prevalence and incidence), as well as death were computed. The estimation of TB burden (both prevalence and incidence) was based on a population of 1000 million of which 850 million were above 5 years of age (85%) as per 1991 census. The results were as follows: Prevalence rate of infection—38% (380 million), prevalence of radiologically active abacillary pulmonary tuberculosis 16/1000 (13.6 million), prevalence of culture-positive cases (C^+)- 4/1000 (3.4 million), prevalence of total pulmonary TB cases—20/1000 (17 million), new annual culture-positive cases—1.3/1000 (1.1 million), annual mortality rate—50-80/100,000 (0.43-0.68 million) and annual case fatality rate 14% of untreated C^+ cases. The survey results were revised to study and correct the observed inaccuracies and inconsistencies in the previous estimates are relied upon. A more detailed and extensive exercise was conducted by Dye et al[21] directed towards providing an average estimate for the country which was a part of global task, in order to make a consensus statement of the problem. The modified findings were described as follows: Prevalence rate of infection—44% (440 million), prevalence of all forms of TB disease—5.05/1000 (5.05 million), prevalence of smear-positive cases (SS^+)—2.27/1000 (1.93 million), new annual smear-positive cases—0.84/1000 (0.71 million), annual mortality rate—28-71/100,000 (0.24-0.60 million) and annual case fatality rate—24% of all TB cases (0.48-1.21 million). This method for computation of average rate is adopted, since a representative sample for the country as a whole, has so far eluded the researchers, as also the sample, sensitive enough to discriminate prevalence or incidence rates between one area and the other. As already explained, notification of sputum-positive or other diagnosed cases of tuberculosis is not yet the source of data on incidence and prevalence in India.

WHO Estimate of TB Burden

India is the second-most populous country in the world having more new TB cases annually than any other country and accounting for one-fifth of the global incidence. About 40% of Indian population is infected with TB bacillus. Patients with infectious disease can infect 10–15 persons in a year. India has been ranked 17th among 22 High Burden Countries (HBC) in terms of TB incidence rate. According to WHO 2009 report, the global annual incidence estimate is 9.4 million cases out of which it is estimated that 1.98 million cases are from India. Every year, 1.8 million persons develop TB, of which about 0.8 million are new smear-positive highly infectious cases. The incidence of TB in India is estimated based on findings of the nationwide annual risk of tuberculosis infection (ARTI) study conducted in 2000–2003.[22] Annual risk of becoming infected with TB is 1.5% (75/100,000) and once infected there is 10% life-time risk of developing TB disease. The prevalence of TB has been estimated at 3.8 million bacillary cases for the year 2000, by an expert group of Government of India. However, the recent estimate by WHO in 2008 gives a prevalence of 2.186 million. With respect to the progress towards indicator 23 of TB-related Millennium Development Goals, as per the WHO estimates in the year 1990, the prevalence of TB in India was 586 per 100,000 populations and the mortality due to TB was 42 per 100,000 populations. In comparison, in the year 2008, the prevalence of TB in India was estimated by WHO to be 185 per 100,000 populations, and the mortality due to TB is 24 per 100,000 populations. The estimates show that India has progressed in reducing the prevalence rate by 68% and mortality rate by 43%. Besides the disease burden, TB also causes an enormous socioeconomic burden to India. TB primarily affects people in their most productive years of life with important socioeconomic consequences for the household and the disease is even more common among the poorest and marginalized sections of the community. Almost 70% of TB patients are aged between the ages of 15 and 54 years of age. The tuberculosis situation in the country is further threatened by the emergence and spread of HIV and drug-resistant tuberculosis. India, the third highest HIV burdened country, had an estimated 2.31 million (0.36% of adult population in the country) people living with HIV/AIDS (PLHAs) in 2007 (estimates revised from the earlier 5.2 million PLHAs in the country, based on the findings of the comprehensive National Family Health Survey - NFHS 3), emphasizing the enormous challenge ahead.[23]

Annual Risk of TB Infection in India: Current Status

Most TB epidemiological studies, subsequent to the ICMR disease survey of 1955–58, including tuberculin surveys have been conducted in limited geographical areas mostly in southern parts of the country as stated above. Hence, the information on the prevailing epidemiological situation of TB was lacking for most parts of India. It was, therefore, planned to assess the prevailing epidemiological situation of tuberculosis by conducting a nation-wide tuberculin (1TU PPD RT23 with Tween 80) survey during 2000–2003, at a time when the tuberculosis control activities in the country were being intensified under the RNCTP.[22] The objective of the survey was to estimate the prevalence of infection among children one to nine years of age residing in 1668 selected villages (rural clusters) and 645 urban blocks (urban clusters) in 26 districts of 19 states and to compute average ARI for TB in each of the four defined zones (North, South, East and West) into which the country was stratified for the purpose of the survey. The survey was conducted independently in each zone while following a uniform methodology, with NTI as the nodal center and TRC, Chennai as the collaborating center with local support from state health authorities. The estimation of prevalence of infection was done by two different methodologies for each zone as a whole as well as separately for rural and urban areas. Method I was based on identifying a cut-off point (anti-mode) from the frequency distribution of reaction sizes. The prevalence was estimated as the proportion of children with reactions equal to or greater than this cut-off point. The anti-modes varied from 14–16 mm in rural areas and 12–16 mm in urban areas, in the four zones whereas method II was based on identifying the mode of reactions attributable to infection with tubercle bacilli and obtaining the estimates by mirror-image technique. The modes were observed at 20 mm in north, west and east zones and 19 mm in south zone. It is noteworthy that the anti-modes and modes of reactions attributable to infection with tubercle bacilli did not differ significantly in the four zones. The estimates of prevalence obtained by either method were found to be similar in all zones except in the west where it was marginally lower by method II. The average prevalence of infection was observed to be 8.2% by method I and 7.9% by method II. ARI was computed from the estimated prevalence of infection by using the appropriate equation (1.5%). The estimated ARI showed regional variations and was higher in the northern and western zones compared with the eastern and southern zones. The proportion of infected children was found to be significantly higher in urban (2.2%) than in rural areas (1.3%) in all zones (Tables 3.1 and 3.2). The ARI estimates obtained in the present study also imply that the incidence of fresh cases will continue to be high in the years to come and a drastic reduction in the disease situation cannot be expected within a short time. Therefore, the efficiency of TB control measures will have to be sustained over a prolonged period, in order to reduce the risk of infection and control tuberculosis in this country. The results of the study provide, for the first time, vital information on the prevailing epidemiological situation of TB across the country and would serve as the baseline data for the study of epidemiological trends of TB at the zonal levels in the future.

Table 3.1: Average prevalence of infection among children 1–9 years of age and computed ARI in India

	Method I		Method II	
	Prevalence % (95% CI)	ARI % (95% CI)	Prevalence % (95% CI)	ARI % (95% CI)
Rural	7.0 (6.2–7.8)	1.3 (1.2–1.5)	6.8 (5.6–7.9)	1.3 (1.0–1.5)
Urban	11.6 (9.9–13.2)	2.2 (1.9–2.5)	11.4 (9.4–13.4)	2.2 (1.8–2.6)
Total	8.2 (7.4–8.9)	1.5 (1.4–1.7)	7.9 (7.4–8.5)	1.5 (1.4–1.6)

Table 3.2: Estimated prevalence of infection in 4 zones of India

	Method I			Method II		
	Rural % (95% CI)	Urban % (95% CI)	Total % (95% CI)	Rural % (95% CI)	Urban % (95% CI)	Total % (95% CI)
North	9.1 (7.1–11.0)	14.1 (12.6–15.7)	10.3 (8.4–12.2)	8.2 (5.1–11.4)	17.4 (14.9–19.9)	10.5 (7.4–13.5)
West	7.8 (5.9–9.7)	12.6 (8.3–17.0)	9.3 (6.8–11.8)	7.4 (4.9–9.9)	11.0 (6.0–16.0)	8.5 (5.4–11.6)
South	4.5 (3.0–5.9)	9.8 (8.1–11.5)	6.1 (4.9–7.2)	4.7 (2.5–6.8)	8.8 (5.1–12.4)	5.9 (4.0–7.7)
East	6.5 (5.3–7.7)	9.0 (5.8–12.2)	6.9 (5.6–8.3)	6.5 (5.2–7.9)	8.3 (7.2–9.3)	6.9 (5.5–8.2)

Tuberculosis Mortality

Tuberculosis mortality is an important indicator in the trend in the history of the epidemic. The risk of dying due to TB depends upon the site, type and severity of the disease as well as timeliness and the initiation of appropriate treatment. In the Madanapalle area, the mortality was reported to have declined from 253 (in 1949) to 64 (1952-53) and then to about 21 per 100,000 (in 1954-55) the latter hypothetically attributed to be due to a well-organized program.[11] Nearly 10% of all causes crude mortality in the community was shown to be due to tuberculosis in the National Tuberculosis Institute Longitudinal Survey area (Proportional mortality due to tuberculosis). Mortality rate due to tuberculosis in the community especially in the National Tuberculosis Institute Longitudinal Survey area was reported to be 95/100,000, not changing with time in 5 years (1967-68).[24] In the New Delhi area, between 1972 and 1976, the rates were about 40 per 100,000, consequent on a well-organized program.[14] Murray CJL, in his draft tripreport (Geneva WHO CDS 1992) estimated that women in their reproductive age (15-44 years) had about 70,000 deaths from tuberculosis, every year, higher than that attributed to perinatal causes related to pregnancy and childbirth (unpublished). Further, unpublished report derived from the sample registration system (SRS), and available with the TB section, Government of India, estimates around 400,000 annual deaths from tuberculosis in India. The currently estimated mortality due to tuberculosis could be in the range of 50–80 per 100,000. The above projection agrees with that by Dholakia.[25] According to WHO 2004 report, TB accounts for 17.6% of deaths from communicable disease and for 3.5% of all causes of mortality. More than 80% of the burden of tuberculosis is due to premature death, as measured in terms of disability-adjusted life years (DALYs) lost. In India, two persons die of TB every three minutes, more than 1000 people die everyday and almost 0.4 million die every year. It was estimated that the TB mortality was over 500,000 annually at the beginning of the revised National TB Control Program (RNTCP). WHO estimated TB mortality in India as 276,000 (24/100,000 population) in 2008. With RNTCP implementation, there is 43% decline in death due to TB in India by 2008 is compared to 1990 data from specific surveys, however, suggest that case fatality rates prior to RNTCP were generally greater than 25%. In the era of RNTCP, case fatality has remained less than 5% for new cases registered under the program. Death rates are declining since the last two decades in many areas where DOTS has been fully implemented. Most of the developing countries do not have efficient system for monitoring and surveillance. Consequently, real picture of mortality due to this disease is not furnished.

REFERENCES

1. National Tuberculosis Institute, Bengaluru. Tuberculosis in a rural population of South India: A five year epidemiological study. Bull World Health Organ. 1974;51:473-88.
2. Chakraborty AK, Choudhari K, Sreenivas TR, Krishnamurthy MS, Shashidhara AN, Channabasavaiah R. Tuberculosis infection in a rural population of south India: 23-year trend. Tuber Lung Dis. 1992;73:213-8.
3. Styblo K, Meijer J, Sutherland I. The transmission of tubercle bacilli. Its trend in a human population. Bull Int Union Tuberc. 1969;41:137-78.
4. Styblo K. Recent advances in epidemiological research in tuberculosis. Adv Tuberc Res. 1980;20:1-63.
5. World Health Organization. WHO weekly epidemiological record. 1981;56(50):393-400.
6. World Health Organization. WHO report 2008. Global tuberculosis control: surveillance, planning, financing. WHO/HTM/TB/2008.393. Geneva: World Health Organization. 2008.
7. World Health Organization. WHO weekly epidemiological record. 23rd Jan 2004, No.4.
8. World Health Organization. WHO report 2009. Global tuberculosis control: epidemiology, strategy, financing. WHO/HTM/ TB/2009.411. Geneva: World Health Organization. 2009.
9. World Health Organization. The global plan to stop tuberculosis. WHO/CDS/STB/2001.16. Geneva: World Health Organization; 2001. Accessed on October 7, 2008.
10. World Health Organization. Stop TB Partnership. The Stop TB Strategy. Building on and enhancing DOTS to meet the TB-related Millennium Development Goals. WHO/HTM/ TB/2006.368. Geneva: World Health Organization. 2006.
11. Frimodt-Moller J. A community wide tuberculosis study in a south Indian rural population, 1950-55. Bull World Health Organization. 1960;22:61-70.
12. Indian Council of Medical Research. Tuberculosis in India (Special Report series No. 34) – A sample survey, 1955-58. New Delhi: ICMR;1959:1-121.

13. Raj Narain, Geser A, Jambunathan MV, Subramaniam M. Tuberculosis prevalence survey in Tumkur district. Ind J Tuber. 1963;10:85-116.
14. Goyal SS, Mathur GP, Pamra SP. Tuberculosis trends in an urban community. Indian J Tuberc. 1978;25:77-82.
15. Gothi GD, Chakraborty AK, Nair SS, Ganapathy KT, Banerjee GC. Prevalence of tuberculosis in a south Indian district twelve years after initial survey. Ind J Tuber. 1979;26:121-35.
16. Tuberculosis Research Centre, Chennai. Trends in the prevalence and incidence of tuberculosis in South India. Int J Tuberc Lung Dis. 2001;5:142-57.
17. New Delhi Tuberculosis Centre. Study of epidemiology of tuberculosis in an urban population of Delhi. Report on 30 year follow-up. Indian J Tuberc. 1999;46:113-24.
18. Directorate of Health Services A & N Administration. Intensified TB control programme in the isolated tribal population of Car Nicobar. WHO-HSR GOI Project No. IND/HSR 001/D.1989. p1-64 (unpublished).
19. Chakraborty AK. Epidemiology of tuberculosis: current status in India. India J Med Res. 2004;120:248-75.
20. Chakraborty AK. Prevalence and incidence of tuberculosis infection and disease in India: a comprehensive review. WHO/TB/97.231. Geneva World Health Organization. 1997:1-26.
21. Dye C, Scheele S, Dolin PJ, Pathania V, Raviglione MC. Consensus statement. Global burden of Tuberculosis: estimated incidence, prevalence and mortality by country. WHO Global Surveillance and Monitoring Project. JAMA. 1999;282:677-86.
22. Chadha VK, Kumar P, Jagannatha PS, Vaidyanathan PS, Unnikrishnan KP. Average annual risk of tuberculous infection in India. Int J Tuberc Lung Dis. 2005;9:116-8.
23. National AIDS Control Organization. http://www.nacoindia.org
24. Chakraborty AK, Gothi GC, Dwarkanath S, Singh H. Tuberculosis mortality rate in a south Indian rural population. Ind J Tuber. 1978;25:181-6.
25. Dholakia R. The potential economic benefits of the DOTS strategy against TB in India. WHO/TB/96.218. Geneva: World Health Organization; 1996.

Chapter 4

Clinical Presentation of Tuberculosis

INTRODUCTION

Based on sequence of events following the first exposure to the tubercle bacilli, tuberculosis can be classified as primary tuberculosis and post-primary tuberculosis. This chapter aims to describe the clinical presentation of congenital, primary and post-primary tuberculosis.

CONGENITAL TUBERCULOSIS

Congenital tuberculosis is defined as tuberculosis occurring in newborn/infants as a result of infection with *M. tuberculosis* during intrauterine life. It is a very rare condition with fewer than 300 cases reported in the literature.[1] Congenital tuberculosis is usually diagnosed by the criteria put forward by Cantwell, et al[2] in 1994. Congenital tuberculosis is diagnosed if the infant has proven tuberculosis lesions and at least one of the following 4 criteria: (i) Appearance of lesion in the first week of life, (ii) A primary hepatic complex or caseating hepatic granulomas, (iii) Tuberculous infection of the placenta or the maternal genital tract and (iv) Exclusion of the possibility of postnatal transmission by the thorough investigation of the contacts including the infant's hospital attendants or birth attendant. Possible modes of infection of the fetus can be hematogenous infection via the umbilical vein, fetal aspiration of the infected amniotic fluid and fetal inhalation of the infected amniotic fluid. The primary lesions are usually seen in the liver and lungs. Liver is the major site of involvement reflecting the hematogenous spread via the fetal circulation.[3] The lungs are almost always involved, possibly due to the passage of the tubercle bacilli from the umbilical vein through the ductus venosus or by aspiration of the tuberculous amniotic fluid or tuberculous matter present in the birth canal. The disease is usually widespread with multiple organ involvement and the baby is often premature. Symptoms are usually delayed till second or third week of life or later.[4] The most common signs are respiratory distress, fever, hepatosplenomegaly, poor feeding, lethargy and irritability, lymphadenopathy and failure to thrive. Meningitis and jaundice are uncommon, obstructive jaundice can occur due to glands in the porta hepatis. In a small percentage of cases, otitis media with or without mastoiditis is the first sign of congenital tuberculosis. Papular or pustular skin lesions may be present. Montoux test is usually negative, positive smear and/or culture results can be obtained from gastric washings, liver, lymph node, lung biopsy or tracheal aspirates. On chest X-ray, there is frequently a miliary pattern or nonspecific changes. Without waiting for laboratory confirmation treatment of the infant should begin as soon as congenital tuberculosis is suspected. Since congenital tuberculosis is rare, no therapeutic trials have determined the optimal treatment. A six-month course of isoniazid (H), rifampicin (R), pyrazinamide (Z) and streptomycin (S) for two months and rifampicin and isoniazid for four months daily or thrice weekly has shown good results with a relapse of only one percent and no deaths from the disease. Corticosteroids may be given empirically if the baby is very ill. The prognosis is poor with only 54% of 26 treated cases survived in a recent study.[2] The mortality rate is high probably because the diagnosis is often missed. The only hope of preventing this rare but often fatal condition lies in the screening of the high-risk groups and appropriate treatment of those found to be suffering from tuberculosis.[1,3,5]

PRIMARY TUBERCULOSIS

When infection with *M. tuberculosis* occurs in a person who has had no previous exposure to tubercle bacillus, it is referred to as "primary infection".[6] The usual route of invasion is by the lungs. The bacilli will be deposited in the alveoli and a small patch of caseous bronchopneumonia develops. This encapsulates later and is called as "primary focus" or "Ghon's focus." The regional lymph node is soon involved and together they are called the "primary complex" (parenchymal lesion + lymph node). Deposition of tubercle bacilli in the alveoli of the lungs is followed by vasodilatation and an influx of polymorphonuclear leukocytes and macrophage to the area. After several weeks, the polymorph numbers diminish and macrophages predominate. The macrophages develop pale foamy cytoplasm rich in lipid and crowd together as epithelioid cells to form the tubercle or unit lesion of tuberculosis. Some mononuclear cells fuse to form the multinucleated or Langhan's giant cell. Lymphocytes surround the outer margin of the tubercle and in the center of the lesion, a zone of caseous necrosis may appear that may subsequently calcify. Classical features of a primary complex in the lung are a small usually less than one centimeter often inapparent parenchymal lesion (Ghon's focus) coupled with enlarged, ipsilateral hilar and less commonly paratracheal nodes. The lymph nodes are generally much larger than the parenchymal focus. The location of the parenchymal lesion is usually towards the middle of the lung (upper part of the lower lobe or the lower region of the middle or upper lobe). Certain sites such as the apical and posterior segments of the upper lobe, apical segment of the lower lobe or upper portion of right middle lobe are described as likely sites of primary infection, however, no part of lungs is exempt.[7] A typical primary or Ghon's focus is single, two millimeters or more in size and located within one centimeter of the pleura of the collapsed lung. Lesions within the lung are relatively uncommon. A majority of the primary foci calcify (85%) and a minority show caseous necrosis (15%). Lymph node enlargement is easily identified in a large majority (87%). Bilateral adenopathy is uncommon except with left sided primary foci.[8]

Timetable of Tuberculosis

The natural history of tuberculosis in the human host is influenced by age, sex, mycobacterial virulence, infecting dose, natural and acquired resistance, certain host factors resulting in a tendency of the disease to follow a pattern of progression according to Wallgren's timetable[9] described in Sweden in 1948 in the era before chemotherapy or BCG. Early in the course of disease, tuberculin conversion after primary infection may result in mild illness, minority of those infected experience febrile episodes and erythema nodosum. Miliary tuberculosis and tuberculous meningitis occurred usually within six months of primary infection and were especially common in children under five years. Pleural effusion presumably due to seeding of the pleura from a lung focus also occurred early usually within six to twelve months and was commoner in young adults and unusual in small children. In young adults, the primary disease could progress with increasing infiltration and cavitation evident in one to two years or even later after the primary infection. This type of disease was labeled progressive primary or postprimary disease and occurred most commonly at puberty. Skeletal tuberculous lesions most commonly of the spine could also present one to five years after the primary infection. Lesions of the genitourinary tract and the skin made their appearance much later, commonly five to fifteen years after the primary infection. There are some limitations of this timetable. Every case of primary infection need not necessarily pass through all the stages enumerated above. Following the institution of chemotherapy the time interval between the various stages may not be followed faithfully. In fact, the progress of the lesion may be aborted at any stage.

Further Changes of the Primary Complex

Healing of the primary lesions is the rule and most primary foci become quiescent and calcify. The caseous focus is gradually replaced by reticulin and collagen deposition. Eventually, hyalinization and calcification are common. Some of the calcified foci, especially those in the lymph nodes may recrudesce at a later age and become the source of progressive pulmonary or extrapulmonary tuberculosis. Early generalization or dissemination is an invariable accompaniment of primary infection. The primary infection is accompanied by early lymphohematogenous spread within hours or days from the site of initial implantation.[10] Huebschman[11] (1928) observed a group of nodular lesions in one or both apices of the lung that occasionally follow primary tuberculosis in children. These Huebschman foci heal and cause no further disease. Simon foci which are larger, single or multiple apical caseous nodules with a tendency to calcification are exaggerated form of these smaller foci. The importance of Simon foci lies in the pathogenesis of post-primary tuberculosis. Liquefaction of solid caseous foci is thought to be related to the onset of delayed type hypersensitivity with the release of hydrolytic enzymes by macrophages.[12] Liquefaction may result in a caseous mass that may include the enlarged lymph nodes. Within the liquefied area there are multiplying tubercle bacilli, and therefore there is a risk of transmission of disease. Due to the liquefactive necrosis, there is extensive parenchymal destruction and cavitation. The cavity may communicate with an airway and thus promote bronchial spread to other parts of the lung, larynx, and the alimentary tract. An acute fatal bronchopneumonia may result. In some of these cases, the inflammatory reaction is neutrophilic like in the case of bacterial pneumonia but AFB are demonstrable. Discharge of the liquefied material through the adjacent pleura results in pleural effusion, pneumothorax or empyema. Rupture of a caseous pulmonary focus into a blood vessel may result in a miliary tuberculosis, with the formation of multiple 0.5–2 mm tuberculosis foci in the lung and in the other organs of the body. Encroachment on bronchi of pulmonary or lymph node caseous material may give rise to tuberculous bronchitis. Rupture of caseous glands into trachea or major bronchi causes collapse of lung or even sudden death by suffocation in young children.

Clinical Features

In majority of cases, the primary infection is symptomless and is passed of unnoticed. The only indication will be a Mantoux conversion from a negative one to positive. This will only be possible if the previous status is known. A proportion will experience a short febrile illness at the time of tuberculin conversion, which is similar to many other febrile illness of childhood. Only a small minority with severe infection or low host resistance will manifest features of unwell with anorexia, fretfulness and failure to gain weight. Cough and wheeze may present because of compression of bronchial wall due to enlarged lymph nodes. Expectoration is not usual in children. Auscultation of the chest is usually unrewarding but occasionally crepitations may be heard over an extensive primary focus.

Complications

Epituberculosis

It is a rare but more frequent in infants and children than in adults. The term epituberculosis is coined by Eliasberg and Neuland to describe the development of dense homogeneous shadows in the lungs of children with tuberculosis. These radiological appearances are due to lobar or segmental consolidation/collapse, and are associated with enlarged tuberculous lymph nodes at the hilum, and may rarely occur in elderly subjects who have lost their tuberculin sensitivity. The middle lobe is most often affected. Segmental lesions are seen in 43% of infected infants. The radiological appearances may be due to a collapse, inflammatory exudation, caseous pneumonia or any combination of these three. Collapse is produced by pressure of the lymph node on the bronchus, by the spread of tuberculous granulation tissue into the bronchus with resultant stenosis or by discharge of caseous material from the lymph node through the bronchial wall.[13-15] Later, the bronchial lesion may heal with residual scarring or fibrous stenosis. The most common pathological cause for the appearance is inflammatory exudate, either monocytic or polymorphonuclear. Epithelioid tubercles may also be present. The exudate is probably due to the discharge of caseous material into the bronchial lumen, with aspiration into a segment or lobe and a resultant exudative hypersensitivity reaction to the contained tuberculoprotein. It is not possible purely on radiological grounds to distinguish this appearance from caseous pneumonia, although the latter may be inferred from the absence of clinical illness and the later development of calcification. Clinically, there is a greater likelihood of wheeze or paroxysmal cough, dullness to percussion and diminished air entry. Bronchial breathing or crepitations may be found. In infants and young children sudden asphyxia resulting in death may occur. Treatment does not differ from that for primary tuberculosis, except that corticosteroids are utilized on the basis that a hypersensitivity reaction is often involved.[16,17] The daily dose should be equivalent to prednisolone 1–2 mg/kg and this should be continued for 4–6 weeks with a gradual reduction thereafter. Steroid therapy may need to be resumed if there is any subsequent radiological or febrile relapse. Steroid therapy may reduce the rate of residual bronchiectasis following this complication of primary pulmonary tuberculosis.[16]

Bronchiectasis

Distension by mucus, caseous tissue or secondary infection beyond a bronchial stenosis may result in bronchiectasis, especially following lobar or segmental lesions.[18] The incidence is reduced by prompt chemotherapy and use of corticosteroid drugs.[16]

Obstructive Emphysema

Occasionally, a bronchus is compressed in such a way that a valve action results, with air being admitted to a portion of lung on inspiration but unable to escape on expiration. This results in distension of a segment or lobe, often with depression of the horizontal fissure or diaphragm and deviation of the mediastinum on expiration. The phenomenon is best shown on a chest film taken on expiration. The condition is rare but is more common in children under the age of 2 years. It usually resolves with chemotherapy and may be an indication for the use of corticosteroid drugs.[19,20]

Broncholith

Calcification in a primary focus, or more commonly in a lymph node, may later be extruded into a bronchus as a 'broncholith' which may present itself with hemoptysis.

Erythema Nodosum (EN)

This complication of primary tuberculosis has a characteristic racial distribution. It occurs in 1–2% of British, and 5–15% of Scandinavian patients. It is very unusual in Asians or Black population. It is also rare below the age of 7, with an increase in frequency up to puberty. It is more common in girls than boys in all ages and 80–90% of cases are females after puberty. The skin lesion is a manifestation of the Arthus phenomenon. Most commonly tuberculin conversion precedes the eruptions by few days to few weeks. However, EN may also occur later in primary or even postprimary disease. The characteristic EN lesions are tender, dusky red, and nodular in nature and are present on the anterior surface of the legs. They may occasionally be present on the anterior surfaces of thighs, the extensor surfaces of forearms, and rarely on the face and breasts. The nodule vary in size from 5–20 mm, with ill-defined margins they may become confluent. The lesions usually resolve over a week or two, with fading of the red color to purple, then brown with persistence of brownish pigments for several weeks. The lesions may recur. Systemic features like fever and arthralagias may accompany or precede the skin lesions. Erythrocyte sedimentation rate (ESR) is usually very high. Tuberculin test is always positive, and a negative test rules out the cause of EN as tubercular in orgin.

Phlyctenular Conjunctivitis

This, like erythema nodosum, is also a manifestation of hypersensitivity to the tubercle bacilli. Unlike erythema nodosum, which occurs in the first week of infection, it occurs within the first year. It is common in children, particularly from poor socio-economic background. Usually, one eye is involved but both eyes may be involved either simultaneously or successively. It is manifested as irritation, lacrimation or photophobia. The characteristic finding is small 1–3 mm shiny yellowish or gray bleb at the limbus with a sheaf of dilated vessels running out towards it from the edge of the conjunctival sac. The reaction subsides in a week or so, but recurrences are common. Any underlying tuberculosis should be treated by chemotherapy. Locally, the pupil is dilated with atropine, and 1% hydrocortisone drops rapidly relieve the symptoms.

Pleural Effusion

Pleural effusion may sometimes accompany primary pulmonary tuberculosis in children under the age of puberty.[21, 22] Such effusions are usually small and transient, resolving with chemotherapy. Larger effusions are more common after puberty.

Primary Tuberculosis in Adults

The radiological and other features of adult primary tuberculosis are essentially similar to childhood primary disease.[23] Primary tuberculosis poses diagnostic problems in adults.[24] Prominent hilar and mediastinal glands and caseation are less frequent in adults except in patients with AIDS. Bronchial obstruction and dissemination are less common. As in children, endobronchial tuberculosis can complicate postprimary tuberculosis in adults. With increasing primary adult tuberculosis, endobronchial tuberculosis may occur as sequelae of adjacent parenchymal disease from which submucosal lymphatic spread lead to mucosal ulceration, hyperplastic polyp formation or fibrostenosis with atelectasis of the subtended lobe.[25]

POSTPRIMARY TUBERCULOSIS

Postprimary tuberculosis is by far the most important type of tuberculosis, partly because it is much frequent and partly because smear-positive sputum is the main source of infection responsible for the persistence of the disease in the community. The disease is transmitted by contaminated aerosols smaller than 5 microns in size and can bypass the bronchial defense mechanism and reach the alveoli. In most of the cases (> 90%), the alveolar macrophages and specific cell-mediated immunity prevent further multiplication of Mycobacteria and hence the development of disease. The infected individuals usually remain asymptomatic and can be diagnosed only with a positive tuberculin reaction. In about 5% of individuals, the infection overcomes the above defense mechanisms and develops into primary tubercular disease (see above) within several weeks or months. In another 5–10% of individuals, late reactivation of an earlier asymptomatic infection leads to a predominantly chronic wasting disease after many months or years and the condition is called *the postprimary or reactivation tuberculosis.*

	Primary tuberculosis	Postprimary tuberculosis
Site	Anywhere in lung	Infraclavicular areas
Glands	Regional lymph nodes enlarged	May not be enlarged
Cavitation	Uncommon	Common
Modes of spread	Lymphatics and blood vessels	Bronchi (Bronchogenic spread)
Healing	By calcification	By fibrosis
Age	Infants and children	Adults and adolescents

Pathogenesis

Postprimary pulmonary tuberculosis may arise in one of the three ways.

- Direct progression of a primary lesion.
- Reactivation of a quiescent primary or postprimary lesion
- Exogeneous reinfection.

i. **Direct progression of a primary lesion:** This is most likely to occur if the primary infection has occurred around the time of puberty.[26, 27]

ii. **Reactivation of a quiescent primary or postprimary lesion:** This can occur at any time in patient's life. The original lesion need not necessarily be visible radiographically and the only evidence that it has occurred is a positive skin test. It is probable that the great majority of middle-aged and elderly men who develop postprimary tuberculosis do as a result of reactivation of lesions contracted many years previously. Waning of individual defenses at any time of life may result in the development of postprimary pulmonary tuberculosis. The risk factors and predisposing conditions for tuberculosis are given below in a tabulated form.[28,29]

Risk Factors

- Exposure/close contacts of active tuberculosis (family members)
- Low socioeconomic status (overcrowding)
- Recent tuberculin conversion
- Untreated/inadequately treated tuberculosis
- Homelessness, living in institutions
- Prisons
- Infancy and old age.

Predisposing Factors

- HIV infection
- Silicosis
- Diabetes mellitus
- Renal insufficiency (chronic dialysis and renal transplant)
- Steroid/immunosuppressive drugs

- Malignancy/lymphoma
- Postgastrectomy
- Alcoholism/drug abuse
- Massive weight loss.

iii. **Exogenous reinfection:** Most tuberculin positive individuals have sufficient immunity to control an episode of reinfection with tubercle bacilli and prevent the development of disease. Disease from reinfection may be more common in populations with a high prevalence of tuberculosis. Most cases of primary tuberculosis arise either from a progressive primary lesion (in young people) or from reactivation of a dormant primary or postprimary lesion (in the middle aged or elderly).[30]

Pathology

In contrast to primary tuberculosis (TB), the localization of postprimary TB is apical or subapical. This area has been referred to as the 'Vulnerable region' by Medlar.[7] This site probably relates to the relatively higher oxygen tension in the region resulting from the effect of gravity on the ventilation-perfusion ratio in the upright lung. Presently, evidence suggests that this is possibly because of better survival of bacillus at this region as the higher oxygen tension has an unfavorable effect on the macrophage and thereby permits intracellular growth.[31] This may also influence progressive primary disease that is more frequent in the apical and posterior segments of the upper lobe. Higher vascularity and consequently increased oxygen tension may determine the preferential multiplication of bacilli at other sites also, such as ends of long bones, vertebrae and the renal cortex. Similarly, mitral stenosis, which results in higher pulmonary arterial pressure and increased apical blood flow, confers a protective effect. Lowered blood flow may also be associated with decreased lymph flow and thus lesser antigen clearance. The pathological lesions seen in postprimary tuberculosis are based on the findings of Medlar[7] and Nayak, et al.[32]

Pulmonary Lesions

Lobular Pneumonia

The earliest lesion is probably an apical or subapical lobular pneumonia.[33] These lesions are not well documented because it is believed that the pneumonia gives way to a granuloma rapidly. An outline of the alveolar reticulin framework in the center of some of these granulomas may suggest such a transition. Assmann drew attention to the fact that the earliest lesions clearly visible in clinical TB consist of infiltrates not at the apex, but at the subapical and infraclavicular region. These infiterates are known as *Assmann infiltrates or foci.*[11] The histopathological counterpart of these lesions is not known.

Nodular Lesions

Nodular lesions (coin lesions, tuberculomas) are localized, well-defined areas of TB wherein the adjacent pulmonary parenchyma is usually normal or may show some scarring. A small nodule is less than a centimeter in diameter whereas larger nodule is more than a centimeter in diameter. Grossly, nodules are white to yellow in color and may vary in consistency from soft lesions that are largely necrotic to firm or hard lesions that are fibrosed or calcified. Small nodules have a central area of caseation, are surrounded by epithelioid cells and giant cells and are encapsulated by a fibrous wall. Large nodules are similar but show more caseation and less encapsulation. Healed nodules are of the size of small nodules and are fibrosed or hyalinized or calcified. In the nodules, anthracotic pigment may be identified. Active nodules especially of the small size are predominantly located in the apical and subapical regions and may be single or multiple.

Fibrocaseous Tuberculosis

Fibrocaseous TB includes lesions that reveal well-known features of TB such as caseation, consolidation, liquefaction and fibrosis. Grossly, various patterns are seen. The apical and posterior segments of the upper lobes are predominantly involved.[34-36] Lymph node involvement is slight in comparison to primary TB. Retraction of lung parenchyma is often associated with pleural thickening. The most striking feature is the presence of one or more cavities. Cavities may assume varying sizes and may be so large so as to result in a severe loss of lung parenchyma. The wall of the cavity may be lined by TB granulation tissue or show varying fibrosis. Communication may or may not have been established with a bronchus. Traversing the wall or lumen along fibrous bands, are bronchi and branches of pulmonary artery. The caseous material may soften the wall of the arteries giving rise to Rasmussen's aneurysms. This may give rise to hemoptysis that may be fatal. Microscopically variable caseous necrosis, extensive fibrosis, numerous palisades of epithelioid cells and fibroblasts together with Langhan's giant cell are seen. Cavities are lined by necrotic TB granulation tissue and show fibrosis. Occasional cavities may be lined in part by columnar or squamous epithelium. Acid-fast bacilli can be demonstrared more frequently in fibrocaseous lesions than in nodular TB. Acid-fast bacilli were found more frequently in cavitary lesions in comparison to noncavitatory lesions. Smaller cavities may heal. Healing in general results in fibrosis and cicatrization extending between the upper pole of the hilum and apex, thus elevating the hilum on that side. This causes volume loss on the ipsilateral side. Simultaneously, the upper mediastinum would be pulled towards the side of the lesion distorting the trachea and giving a characteristic radiological appearance.

Tuberculous Bronchopneumonia

Tuberculous bronchopneumonia occurs as a consequence of a larger dose of virulent organisms disseminating through the bronchus. Most of the time the host immunity is compromised in these conditions.

Bronchial Lesions

Despite being closely associated with the lung parenchyma, bronchi do not appear to be frequently affected in pulmonary TB.[7] In a majority of cases, the inflammation is nonspecific and typical granulomas may not been seen. In some cases endobronchial TB, as discussed under primary pulmonary TB, may follow post-primary lesions[37] and this is characterized by bronchial inflammation, ulceration, granuloma, small pseudopolyps and eventual healing by fibrosis. Bronchostenosis may give rise to poststenotic dilatation of the bronchus. Bronchiectasis directly attributable to pulmonary TB is rare.[7] In those instances when this is found, it usually occurs in the upper lobe and is relatively asymptomatic.

Whole Lung Tuberculosis

Rarely, TB affects the whole lung. This condition has a high mortality and results from diffuse bronchogenic spread or hematogeneous dissemination.[38]

Clinical Features

In the developed countries, the majority of patients with postprimary pulmonary tuberculosis are middle aged or elderly, but in developing countries the age distribution is strikingly different with a predominance of young and middle-aged patients.[39] Classically, the onset of symptoms occur over weeks to months. General symptoms like tiredness, malaise, weight loss, anorexia and weakness are very common and reported by majority of patients. Fever with night sweats is a classical symptom of tuberculosis and are more common in patients with more advanced form of the disease. Prolonged undiagnosed fever (PUO-pyrexia of unknown origin) is one of the common presentations of tuberculosis. Fever is present in up to 60% of patients, which disappears rapidly within 1–2 weeks with therapy.[40,41] Symptoms related to respiratory system include most importantly cough. Sputum may be mucoid, purulent or blood stained. Hemoptysis is a classical symptom of pulmonary tuberculosis and may vary from mere blood staining of sputum to massive amount of hemoptysis. Chest pain is common and may vary from dull ache or tightness to pleuritic pain, but distinctly different form due to lung cancer. Elderly patients (> 65 years) with TB are more likely to present with nonspecific complaints and atypical radiographic appearances.[42] They usually have a lower body weight, less hemoptysis and more nonspecific symtoms. There may be no physical signs in pulmonary tuberculosis even with relatively advanced disease. Fever, anemia and cachexia will be present. Finger clubbing is seen in advanced cases of tuberculosis. The earliest chest sign is post-tussive crepitation in the upper lobes or apices. With advanced disease fibrosis with cavity is the most common finding in postprimary tuberculosis. The findings are most often bilateral. There may be signs of consolidation also when the presentation is like pneumonia. Loss of lung volume in chronic cases is very common with shifting of mediastinum to the same side. Clinical findings of collapse are not the findings of tuberculosis except in very young individuals where the node may compress a lobe. Occasionally bronchostenosis may produce collapse. Localized wheezes are heard sometimes as a result of associated chronic bronchitis or rarely due to tubercular bronchostenosis. Associated findings of pleural disease in the form of pleural effusion or pleural thickening may aiso be present. Fibrothorax may be present in more advanced and chronic cases. Empyema or bronchopleural fistula is other clinical findings. Post tubercular bronchiectasis is another sequel of tuberculosis. Examination of the respiratory system is very important and findings of a cavity with fibrosis in association of history will strongly point towards tuberculosis as the underlying cause particularly in countries with high prevalence of the disease.

REFERENCES

1. Snider DE, Block AB. Congenintal tuberculosis. Tubercle. 1984;65:81-2.
2. Cantwell MF, Shehab ZM, Costello AM, Sands L, Green WF, Ewing Ep Jr., et al. Brief report. Congenital tuberculosis. N Eng J Med. 1994;330:1051-4.
3. Hageman J, Shulman S, Schreiber M, et. al. Congenital tuberculosis: critical appraisal of clinical findings and diagnostic procedures. Pediatrics. 1980;66:980-4.
4. Neemir RL, O' Hare D. Congenital tuberculosis. Review and diagnostic guidelines. Am J Dis Child. 1985;139:284-7.
5. Snider De, Layde PM, Thomson MW, Lyle MA. Treatment of tuberculosis during pregnancy. Am Rev Respir Dis. 1980;122:65-79.
6. Nayak NC. Nature and evolution of pulmonary tuberculosis. J AIIMS. 1976;1:190-4.
7. Medlar EM. The behavior of pulmonary tuberculosis lesion: a pathological study. Am Rev Tuberc. 1955;71:1-244.
8. Lincolin EM, Swell BH. Tuberculosis in Children. New York: Mc graw-Hill; 1963. p.19-83.
9. Wallgren A. The timetable of tuberculosis. Tubercle. 1948;29:245-51.
10. Bates JH. Transmission and pathogenesis of tuberculosis. Clin Chest Med. 1980;1:167-74.
11. Rich AR. The pathogenesis of tuberculosis. 2nd edn. Illinois: Charles C. Thomas. 1951.
12. Dannenberg AM Jr, Sugimoto M. Liquefaction of caseous foci in tuberculosis. Am Rev Respir Dis. 1976;113:257-9.
13. Lincolin EM, Harris LC, Bovornkitti S, Caretto R. The course and prognosis of endobronchial tuberculosis in children. Am Rev Tuberc. 1956;74:246-55.
14. Lorriman G, Bentley FJ. The incidence of segmental lesions in primary tuberculosis in childhood. Am Rev Tuberc. 1959;79:756-63.

15. Morrison JB. National history of segmental lesions in primary pulmonary tuberculosis. Arch Dis Child. 1973;48:90-8.
16. Gerbeaux J, Bacülard A, Couvreur J. Primary tuberculosis in childhood. Indications and contraindications for corticosteroid therapy: observations on 577 treated cases. Am J Dis Child. 1965;110:507.
17. Nemir RL, Cardona J, Vaziri F, Toledo R. Prednisone as an adjunct in the chemotherapy of lymph node tuberculosis in childhood. A double blind study II. Further team observation. Am Rev Respir Dis. 1967;95:402-10.
18. Roberts JC, Blair LG. Bronchiectasis in primary tuberculosis associated with segmental collapse. Lancet. 1950;1:386.
19. Miller FJW, Seal RME, Taylor MD, et al. Tuberculosis in children. London: Churchill, 1963;163:87.
20. Giammona ST, Poole CA, Zelowitz P, Skrovan C. Massive lymphadenopathy in primary tuberculosis in children. Am Rev Respir Dis. 1969;100:480-9.
21. Aderele WI. Radiological patterns of tuberculosis in Nigerian children. Tubercle. 1980;61:157-63.
22. Pineda PR, Leung A, Muller NL, Allen EA, Black WA, Fitzgerald JM. Intrathoracic paediatric tuberculosis: a report of 202 cases. Tubercle Lung Dis. 1993;74:261-6.
23. Choyke PL, Sostman HD, Curtis AM, Ravin CE, Chen JT, Godwin JD, et al. Adult onset pulmonary tuberculosis. Radiology. 1983;148:357-62.
24. Tead WW, Kerby GR, Schleuter DP, Jordahl CW. The clinical spectrum of primary tuberculosis in adults. Confusion with reinfection in the pathogenesis of chronic tuberculosis. Ann Intern Med. 1968;68:731-45.
25. Smith LS, Schillaci RF, Sarlin RF. Endobronchial tuberculosis serial fiberoptic bronchoscopy and natural history. Chest. 1987;91;644-7.
26. Holm S. Om der Friske Tuberculose Infection den Klinik, Prognose og Behandlung. Cogenhagen: Rosenkilde, 1947.
27. Lincoln EM, Gilbert L, Morales SM. Chronic pulmonary tuberculosis in individuals with known previous primary tuberculosis. Dis Chest. 1960;38:473-82.
28. McDormott LJ, Glassroth. Natural history and epidemiology. Tuberculosis, Part I. Dis Month 1997;43:131-55.
29. Gryzbowski S, Barnett GD, Stybo K. Contacts of active pulmonary tuberculosis. Bull Int Union Tuberc. 1975;50:90-106.
30. Stead WW. Pathogenesis of a first episode of chronic pulmonary tuberculosis in man: recrudescence of residuals of the primary infection or exogeneous reinfection. Am Rev Respir Dis. 1967;95:729-45.
31. Meylan PRA, Richman DD, Kornbluth RS. Reduced intracellular growth of mycobacteria in human macrophages cultivated at physiologic pressure. Am Rev Respir Dis. 1992;145:947-53.
32. Goodwin RA, Des Prez RM. Apical localisation of pulmonary tuberculosis, chronic pulmonary histoplasmosis and progressive massive fibrosis of the lung. Chest. 1983;83:801-5.
33. Nayak NC, Sabharwal BD, Bhathena D, Mital GS, Ramalingaswami V. The pulmonary tuberculous lesion in north India: a study in medicolegal autopsies I. Incidence, nature and evolution. Am Rev Respir Dis. 1970;101:1-17.
34. Woodring JH, Vandiviere HM, Lee C. Intrathoracic lymphadenopathy in postprimary tuberculosis. South Med J. 1998;81:992-7.
35. Lung AN, Muller NL, Pineda PR, Fitgerbld JM. Primary tuberculosis in childhood: radiographic manifestations. Radiology. 1992;182:87-91.
36. Sweany HC, Cook CE, Kegeggereis R. A study of the position of primary cavities in tuberculosis. Am Rev Tuberc. 1931;24:558-82.

37. Van den Brande PM, Van de Mierop F, Verbeken EK, Demedts M. Clinical spectrum of endobronchial tuberculosis in elderly patients. Arch Intern Med. 1990;150:2105-8.
38. Tsao TC, Juang YC, Tsai YH, Lan RS, Lee CH. Whole lung tuberculosis, a disease with high mortality which is frequently misdiagnosed. Chest. 1992;101:1309-11.
39. Graf P. Tuberculosis control in high prevalence countries. In: Davies PDO (Ed). Clinical tuberculosis. London; Chapman 7 Hall, 1994.
40. Poulson A. Some clinical features of tuberculosis. Acta Tuberc Scand. 1957;33:37-92.
41. Chan CHS, Woo J, Or KKH, Chan RCY, Cheung W. The effects of age on the presentation of patients with tuberculosis. Tubercle Lung Dis. 1995;76:290-4.
42. Barnes PF, Verdegem TD, Vachon LA, Leedom JM, Overturf GD. Chest roentgenogram in pulmonary tuberculosis. New data on an old test. Chest. 1988;94:316-21.

Chapter 5

Miliary Tuberculosis

INTRODUCTION

Miliary tuberculosis (TB) is the widespread dissemination of *Mycobacterium tuberculosis* via hematogenous spread. In high-prevalence areas, the majority of cases follow shortly after initial infection, but in low-prevalence areas, the majority of cases are in the elderly, representing reactivation. The lung is always involved, other organs variably so. Classic miliary TB is defined as millet like (mean, 2 mm; range, 1–5 mm) seeding of TB bacilli in the lung, as evidenced on chest radiography. This pattern is seen in 1–3% of all TB cases. Although, the overt case is relatively easily diagnosed, cryptic forms are not at all uncommon. In communities where tuberculosis is now greatly decreased, these cryptic forms in older people contribute an important proportion of cases of miliary tuberculosis and are sometimes diagnosed only at postmortem. Therefore, a high index of clinical suspicion is important to obtain an early diagnosis and to ensure improved clinical outcomes. The aim of this chapter is to describe the pathogenesis, pathology, diagnosis and treatment of miliary tuberculosis.

PATHOGENESIS

When tuberculosis was widespread in the community the majority of cases of miliary tuberculosis closely followed the primary tuberculous infection in young children, more than one-third in one series being aged less than 3 years.[1]

If the initial infection is overwhelming or the patient's defenses are poor due to malnutrition, intercurrent disease or corticosteroid or immunosuppressive drug therapy, then the hematogenous phase of the primary infection may give rise to acute miliary tuberculosis. Seeding of bacilli into vessel walls may cause a caseous vasculitis of the intima, with subsequent discharge of bacilli into the bloodstream. Such lesions are said to be more common in the large veins and the thoracic duct but less so in the arterial system, aorta or endocardium.[2] Miliary dissemination may also follow recrudescence of an old primary lesion, which may discharge itself into a vessel wall. Vascular invasion presumably also occurs from other active postprimary lesions, thus explaining the now relatively more frequent occurrence of miliary tuberculosis in the middle-aged and elderly.

PATHOLOGY

Microscopically, the miliary lesions consist of Langhan's giant cells, epithelioid cells and lymphocytes, and contain acid-fast bacilli, sometimes with central caseation. The distribution of the lesions in the body is variable but the lungs are virtually always affected, sometimes only microscopically. Involvement of other organs varies from case to case. Lesions may occur in any of the serous sacs with resultant effusions. In elderly or immunosuppressed patients, nonreactive pathological appearances are described with necrotic lesions containing no specific tuberculous features, but teeming with acid-fast bacilli. The spleen and liver may be enlarged and studded with irregular necrotic foci, usually less than 1 cm in diameter or only visible microscopically. Any organ may be affected.

Acute or Classical Miliary Tuberculosis

The disease is most common in infants and young children.[3] In children, the onset may be associated with an acute or subacute febrile illness but often, especially in adults, the onset is insidious with gradual development of vague ill-health, malaise, anorexia, weight loss and fever. Cough, breathlessness, hemoptysis and night sweats are less common. In addition to the general symptoms, headache from coexistent tuberculous meningitis occurs frequently and should alert the clinician to perform a lumbar puncture. Physical signs are few; the chest almost invariably sounds clear on auscultation. Enlargement of the liver, spleen or lymph nodes may be found in a small number of cases.[4] Involvement of the serosal surfaces can lead to the development of small pericardial or pleural effusions or ascites. Fundal examination should be carried out to detect choroidal tubercles, which are more commonly seen in children. Skin lesions may also occur in the form of papules, macules and purpuric lesions. These probably represent local vasculitic lesions caused by reaction to mycobacterial antigen. The typical X-ray shows an even distribution of uniform-sized lesions 1–2 mm throughout all zones of the lung. Small bilateral pleural effusions may also be seen.

Cryptic Miliary or Disseminated Tuberculosis

As tuberculosis declines in incidence in the native populations of developed countries, a form of miliary tuberculosis without typical X-ray shadowing, so-called 'cryptic' miliary tuberculosis has been seen more frequently. This is usually seen in patients aged over 60 years, but may be seen in young patients in some immigrant groups. The symptoms are usually insidious, with weight loss, lethargy and intermittent fever.[5] Meningitis and choroidal tubercles are rarely found; mild hepatosplenomegaly may be found but physical signs are usually absent. Because of this, a high index of suspicion is required to reach a diagnosis, and commonly the diagnosis is not made until postmortem.[6] The main differential diagnosis is disseminated carcinoma. Table 5.1 contrasts the features of classical 'acute' and 'cryptic' forms of miliary disease.

DIAGNOSIS

The classical form of the disease is usually easy to diagnose because of the typical X-ray appearances, which are only absent in the early stages, but which may be detected earlier on high-resolution CT scanning. The tuberculin test is usually positive, and bacteriological confirmation may be obtained from sputum, urine and cerebrospinal fluid. The detection of the cryptic form rests initially on having clinical suspicion of the diagnosis and then carrying out specific tests or monitoring response to a trial of antituberculosis drugs. Blood dyscrasias are not uncommonly seen in the cryptic form, pancytopenia, leukemoid reactions, and other granulocyte abnormalities, have all been reported. Bone marrow aspiration may yield both granulomata on biopsy

Table 5.1: Comparison between classical and cryptic forms of miliary tuberculosis

Feature	Classical acute	Cryptic
Age	Majority under 40 years	Majority over 60 years
TB history or contact	Upto 33%	Up to 25%
Malaise/weight loss	75%	75%
Fever	75%	90%
Choroidal tubercles	Up to 20%	Absent
Meningitis	Up to 20%	Rare unless terminal
Lymphadenopathy	Up to 20%	Absent
Miliary shadowing on X-ray	Usual except in early stages	Rare
Tuberculin test	Usually positive	Usually negative
Pancytopenia/ Leukemoid reaction	Rare	Common
Bacteriological confirmation	Sputum, cerebrospinal fluid	Urine, sputum, bone marrow
Biopsy evidence	Seldom required	Liver up to 75%; bone marrow, lymph node

and acid-fast bacilli on culture, and should be considered if a blood dyscrasia is present. Liver biopsy has the highest yield of granulomata which have been reported in up to 75% of biopsies. In cases where the patient is unwilling, or where facilities for them do not exist, a clinical trial of antituberculosis drugs should be given. The fever usually responds within 7–10 days, followed by clinical improvement in 4–6 weeks.

TREATMENT

Early therapy for suspected miliary tuberculosis (TB) is prudent and any delay will contribute to a high mortality rate. There is no consensus regarding the optimum duration of treatment in patients with miliary TB. According to WHO guidelines miliary TB is included under treatment category I and patients receive six months of treatment.[7,8] In the absence of associated meningeal involvement, the American Academy of Pediatrics (AAP) advocates nine months of treatment.[9] However the American Thoracic Society (ATS), the Center for Disease Control and Prevention (CDC), the Infectious Disease Society of America (IDSA),[10] and the National Institute for Health and Clinical Excellence (NICE) TB guidelines[11] state that six months of treatment is adequate for miliary TB. In the presence of associated TB meningitis, treatment needs to be given for at least 12 months.[9-11] Under the Revised National Tuberculosis Control Program (RNTCP) of Government of India, patients with miliary TB get treated with category I DOTS for six months.

Sparse published data are available regarding the usefulness of adjunct corticosteroid therapy in patients with miliary TB with conflicting results. A beneficial response was observed in one study[12] although such benefit could not be documented in another study.[13] Presence of associated adrenal insufficiency is an absolute indication for their administration. Adjunctive corticosteroid treatment may be beneficial in miliary TB with TB meningitis, large pericardial effusion, dyspnea, disabling chest pain, immune reconstitution inflammatory syndrome (IRIS), adult respiratory distress syndrome (ARDS) and immune complex nephritis.[14]

COMPLICATIONS

Adult Respiratory Distress Syndrome

Miliary tuberculosis may present with all the features of the adult respiratory distress syndrome or the syndrome may even develop after treatment has been initiated.[15,16] Therapy should be directed to both conditions.

Immune Complex Nephritis

Immune complex nephritis complicating miliary tuberculosis has been described.[17]

Tuberculous Meningitis

Tuberculous meningitis may complicate miliary tuberculosis and is a manifestation of acute hematogenous spread. It occurs overtly in up to 20% of cases. Lumbar puncture should be performed if there are any symptoms of meningism or headache. A positive microscopy for acid-fast bacilli from the CSF may be the most rapid way of confirming the clinical diagnosis of miliary tuberculosis.

REFERENCES

1. Debre R. Miliary tuberculosis in children. Lancet. 1952;2:545.
2. Pagel W, Simmonds FAH, Macdonald N, Nassau E. Pulmonary Tuberculosis. London: Oxford University Press. 1964.
3. Hussey G, Chisholm T, Kibel M. Miliary tuberculosis in children: a review of 94 cases. Pediatr Infect Dis J. 1991;10:832.
4. Sahn SA, Neff TA. Miliary tuberculosis. Am J Med. 1968;56:495-505.
5. Proudfoot AT. Cryptic disseminated tuberculosis. Br J Hosp Med. 1971;5:773-80.
6. Grieco MH, Chmel H. Acute disseminated tuberculosis as a diagnostic problem. Am Rev Resp Dis. 1974;109:554-60.
7. World Health Organization. Treatment of tuberculosis: Guidelines for national programmes. WHO/CDS/TB/2003.313. Third edition. Geneva. World Health Organization. 2003.
8. World Health Organization. Revised guidelines for national programmes. WHO/CDS/TB/2003.313. Third edition 2003. Revision approved by STAG, June 2004. Available at URL:http//www.who.int/docstore/gtb/publications/ttgnp/PDF/tb_2003_313chap4_rev.pdf. Accessed on December. 29, 2010.
9. American Academy of Pediatrics Committee on Infectious Diseases. Chemotherapy for tuberculosis in infants and children. Pediatrics. 1992;89:161-5.
10. American Thoracic Society/Centre for Disease Control and Prevention/Infectious Diseases Society of America. Treatment of Tuberculosis. Am J Respir Crit Care Med. 2003;167:603-62.
11. National Institute for Health and Clinical Excellence, National Collaborating Centre for Chronic Conditions. Management of non-respiratory tuberculosis. Tuberculosis: Clinical diagnosis and management of tuberculosis, and measures for its prevention and control. London: Royal College of Physicians. 2006.p.63-76.
12. Sun TN, Yang JY, Zheng LY, Deng WW, Sui ZY. Chemotherapy and its combination with corticosteroids in acute miliary tuberculosis in adolescents and adults: analysis of 55 cases. Chin Med J. 1981;94:309-14.
13. Massaro D, Katz S, Sachs M. Choroidal tubercles. A clue to hematogenous tuberculosis. Ann Intern Med. 1964;60:231-41.
14. Sharma SK, Mohan A, Sharma A, Mitra DK. Miliary tuberculosis: new insights into an old disease. Lancet. Infect Dis. 2005;5:415-30.
15. Zimmermann HM, Wertheimer DE, Rosner E. Miliary tuberculosis and the adult respiratory distress syndrome. NY State J Med. 1981;81:787-9.
16. So SY, Yu D. The adult respiratory distress syndrome associated with miliary tuberculosis. Tubercle. 1981;62:49-53.
17. Shribman JH, Eastwood JB, Uff J. Immune complex nephritis complicating miliary tuberculosis. Br Med J. 1983;287:1593-4.

Chapter 6

Endobronchial Tuberculosis

INTRODUCTION

Endobronchial tuberculosis (EBTB) also known as tubercular tracheobronchitis is the involvement of trachea and bronchi by the tubercular pathological processes.[1] Till the last years of the second decade of 20th century, endobronchial TB was diagnosed mostly at autopsy.[2-4] However, with the introduction of bronchoscopy in the field of pulmonary medicine, its antemortem reporting became frequent. With the advent of effective antitubercular chemotherapy, reporting of endobronchial TB diminished to almost nil.[5-9] Re-emergence of interest in this area has occurred due to current reporting of several cases of endobronchial TB.[10-20] This chapter aims to illustrate the epidemiology, pathophysiology, diagnosis and treatment of endobronchial tuberculosis.

EPIDEMIOLOGY

There is a huge variation in reporting of the prevalence of endobronchial TB, ranging from 3%[21], to a whopping 72%[22] with an average serial reporting rate of nearly 40%.[23,24] In nonendemic areas, the current prevalence may be less than 0.2%. Through the decades, a significant reduction in the reporting rate of endobronchial TB has occurred most probably due to advent of effective ATT and timely management of cases.[5-9] Involvement of smaller distal airways which are frequently out of bronchoscopic reach may be the reason behind an increased postmortem reporting of endobronchial TB.[22] Female predominance[4,12,14,18,22,24] has been reported in several studies most likely due to comparatively smaller airway size in them. 'Lady Windermere syndrome' which is habitual voluntary cough suppression in females, leads to failure to clear airway secretions thereby causing retention of infected sputum leading to tracheobronchial dissemination of the disease may also be a contributing factor to this female predominance.[19,25,26]

PATHOPHYSIOLOGY

Five potential mechanisms have been suggested for the development of endobronchial infection due to *M. Tuberculosis*.[3]

1. *Direct extension from lung parenchyma:* The bronchi immediate to an infected part of lung parenchyma get involved probably due to direct infiltration. Ulceration of the tracheobronchial tree is frequently seen adjacent to a parenchymal focus.[22]
2. *Implantation of bacilli from infected sputum:* The passage of sputum containing bacilli over the mucous membranes of tracheobronchial tree may lead to implantation of organisms. This may serve as a reason behind presence of gross ulcerations in the airways adjacent to the cavitations.[22]
3. *Hematogenous spread:* A rare phenomenon. Hematogenous dissemination may be seen in a few cases of miliary tuberculosis[22].
4. *Lymphatic dissemination:* Myerson[27] has suggested alternative mechanism of retrograde passage of tubercle bacilli through lymphatics from bronchioles and subsegmental bronchi to the main stem bronchus.
5. *Lymph node erosion into the bronchus:* Perforation of a tuberculous lymph node into the bronchi has been considered in some adults.[28] However, this phenomenon of endobronchial spread is more common in children with primary tuberculosis where an infected lymph node gets attached to the bronchial wall due to inflammation leading to spread of infection to the bronchial mucosa. Endobronchial involvement has been reported in most of the cases of intrathoracic TB lymphadenitis.

Gross Appearance

The earliest feature visualized bronchoscopically is erythema of mucous membranes.

EBTB usually starts as a submucosal tubercle that progresses to ulcer formation whose depth progresses from shallow to deep. Granulation tissue that is generally formed looks like polypoidal mass which when extensive mimicks a tumorous growth in the lumen of bronchus. The ulcers heal by fibrosis. The degree of fibrostenosis depends on the depth of the ulcer. Once ulceration occurs, there is some degree of residual fibrosis even with treatment. Stenosis may also be secondary to hyperemia of mucous membrane or by a lymph node compressing extrinsically.[22] Ulcers have been described more commonly in the carina and posterior surface of tracheobronchial tree in post-mortem studies.[22] Cartillage may be partially visible due to progressive growth and gradual coalescence of these ulcers.[22]

Microscopic Appearance

Typical granulomatous inflammatory foci with central necrosis pertaining to tuberculosis are evident in the subepithelium and mucus glands in the early phase of disease. In the later course, these changes are also evident in the adventitia. Rarely only adventitia may show these changes.[22] Cartilaginous involvement is usually limited to very extensive disease. Ulceration results from rupture of submucosally located foci leading to gradual destruction of the bronchial wall. Ingrowth of the peripherally surrounding vascular granulation tissue into the central necrosed area occurs during healing. This granulation tissue is subsequently replaced by fibrous connective tissue leading to scarring and if the process involves substantial circumference of the airway, stenosis takes place.

NATURAL HISTORY

Endobronchial TB can present variably. Endobronchial tuberculosis is more common in young adults with a female predominance.[10,12] Both primary and reactivation TB can manifest as endobronchial TB in adults. Among children EBTB is commonly a complication of primary tuberculosis and is usually caused by encroachment of enlarged lymph nodes on bronchi.

EBTB may have insidious onset, simulating bronchogenic carcinoma, or may be acute, mimicking asthma, foreign body aspiration and pneumonia. Symptoms of EBTB may develop even after years of diagnosis and completion of antitubercular therapy. The barking cough that is not responsive to an antitussive medication, but responds to steroids along with antituberculosis treatment may be a feature of EBTB.[9] Bronchorrhea can occur in active endobronchial tuberculosis.[29] Sputum production is variable. Hemoptysis may occur but is seldom massive. Lymph node rupture may cause chest pain that may be sharp or dull in sternal or parasternal region. Dyspnea is often associated with atelectasis of the lung. Physical examination may reveal diminished breath sounds and localized low-pitched wheeze or rhonchi. Up to 25–35% of EBTB may have features of collapse. Classical monophonic wheeze may be heard in about 15% of the patients.[12] Endobronchial tuberculosis with expectoration of tracheal cartilage has been reported.[30] Dull and sharp chest pain can occur anteriorly due to enlargement and rupture of the lymph nodes. Constitutional symptoms including fever, weight loss, anorexia and night sweat are not usually prominent in EBTB. Serious sequelae especially with tracheal involvement such as respiratory failure, collapse of dependent portion of lungs, failure of endobronchial intubation for general anesthesia, the need of tracheostomy, or death by suffocation have been reported.[31,32] Simultaneous involvement of other organ systems has been reported. "Tract tuberculosis" hypothesis given by Auerbach explains the tendency towards development of TB of hollow viscera (e.g. Koch's abdomen) in the body.[22]

DIAGNOSIS

Although sputum examination is the essential and first step towards the diagnosis of EBTB, bronchoscopy and computed tomography are the methods of choice for accurate diagnosis of bronchial involvement and assessment for surgical intervention. Fiberoptic bronchoscopy is indicated in patients in whom chest radiographs, physical signs or symptoms suggest the possibility of endobronchial tuberculosis. Due to the potential utility of early antituberculosis treatment and use of corticosteroids in reducing the lymph node size and mucosal swelling, the above procedures should be carried out at the earliest. Typical bronchoscopic finding is the presence of white gelatinous granulation tissue. The mucosa is nodular, red, vascular and some times ulcerated. It may simulate a bronchogenic carcinoma.[12,33] Nucleic acid amplification tests, such as PCR and other methods for amplifying DNA and RNA, may facilitate rapid detection of *M. tuberculosis* in respiratory tract specimens. Recommendations for interpretation and use of nucleic acid amplification have been recently updated by the Centers for Disease Control and Prevention.[34]

Sputum Examination

Sputum smear microscopy yield is low for enobronchial TB. However, all suspected patients of EBTB should be subjected to sputum smear and culture examination for *M. tuberculosis*. Yield of sputum smear for AFB is not as high as in parenchymal involvement even in an optimal laboratory setup with meticulous sputum examination. In recent studies, sputum positivity in EBTB has been demonstrated from 16–53.3%.[18,35,36] However, EBTB with ulceration and mucosal involvement has higher sputum positivity and yield is even greater with sputum culture when compared to smear (73.6 vs 53.3%).[12,18]

Chest Roentgenography

A clear chest radiograph does not exclude the diagnosis of endobronchial TB as 10–20% cases may exhibit a normal chest roentgenogram.[12] Bronchial stenosis occurs in 10–40% of patients with active pulmonary tuberculosis exhibiting radiological manifestations of persistent segmental or lobar collapse, lobar hyperinflation, obstructive pneumonia and mucoid impaction.[37] Volume loss on chest radiography may indicate development of bronchial stenosis, and fiberoptic bronchoscopy should be considered in such cases.[2] Erosion of calcified hilar nodes into adjacent bronchi, known as broncholithiasis, may also result in segmental collapse or overinflation.[38] Bronchiectatic changes may be evident usually in the upper lobes. Other radiographic features include cavity formation, pleural effusion, military infiltrates and mediastinal lymphadenopathy.[1,10]

Computed Tomography

High resolution computed tomography (HRCT)[39] has become one of the best tools for evaluation of endobronchial TB. It may exhibit involvement of the large as well as small airways which as compared to the large airways have been seen to get involved more substantially.[39-42] Characteristic HRCT findings of EBTB are patchy asymmetric centrilobular nodules and branching lines that may have unilateral or bilateral distribution.[40,43] Multiple branching linear structures of similar caliber originate from a single stalk (the 'tree-in-bud' appearance). The stalk is thought to represent a lesion that affects the last order bronchus within the secondary pulmonary lobule and the bud is thought to represent a lesion that is in the bronchioles and alveolar ducts.[40] In CT scan, there are foci of ill-defined nodular densities which are peribronchiolar in location and markedly variable in size, including the lesions as small as 2–3 mm. These nodular densities may become confluent.[44] Other CT findings include stenosis or obstruction of major airways, soft tissue peribronchial cuffing, mediastinal lymphadenopathy (low density-typical of caseation or necrosis) compressing the airways. The chest CT may also depict parencymal lesions like segmental collapse, cavitations and low density round lesions due to mucus impaction distal to obstruction. A low density polypoidal mass in the airway lumen may also be visualized on CT.[42,45-47] The drawbacks of CT is its inability in the accurate prediction of the lesion being endobronchial, submucosal or outside the airway and in accurate assessment if the thickness of bronchial wall.[42,45] It is also difficult to differentiate endobronchial TB from bronchogenic carcinoma on a chest CT. However, CT is advantageous in determining the length of bronchial stenosis and visualization of areas beyond stenosis for parenchymal and lymphatic involvement.[19,48] Hence, CT thorax has emerged as a complementary tool to fiberoptic bronchoscopy in evaluation of EBTB cases and monitoring response to chemotherapy.[48] The differential diagnosis of radiologic findings on CT are sarcoidosis, amyloidosis, relapsing polychondritis and tracheopathia osteoplastica which may present with bronchial wall thickening and stenosis.[46] Newer radiologic techniques such as virtual bronchoscopy and three-dimensional helical CT are being looked forward as better aids in diagnosing EBTB.[46,47,49,50]

Spirometry

Restrictive pattern is the one most commonly encountered due to luminal fixation resulting from fibrostenosis of the airways in endobronchial TB. A study revealed restrictive abnormality to be the most common (47%). Obstructive pattern was evident in 5.9%, mixed in 23.5% and normal spirometry in 23.5% of the patients.[19] Patients of endobronchial TB do not exhibit hyperreactivity to inhaled histamine unlike those having bronchial asthma.[51]

Fiberoptic Bronchoscopy

Bronchoscopic sampling has been the key to the diagnosis of EBTB, producing more than 90% yield on smear as well as on culture.[3,10,12,22,23,52-54] In diagnosing EBTB, the experience of the bronchoscopist is also of great importance for eliciting the bronchoscopic findings that contribute to the diagnosis. Even if biopsy fails to supply tangible results, the bronchoscopic changes, supported by clinical and radiological findings, may be sufficient to establish the diagnosis of EBTB. Endobronchial biopsies usually reveal the classic histologic features of tuberculosis. Non-necrotic granulomas with no bacilli or granulomas with caseation and high bacillary load may be evident on bronchoscopy. A brush smear taken with the biopsy may increase the diagnostic yield many folds. Bronchial biopsy may be positive in 30.35 to 84% patients.[17,35] Bronchial brushing has provided a high yield of 84.88% in a study from China.[21] Similarly, bronchial washings have also yielded variable results ranging from 10–37.5%.[17,36] A widely accepted classification defining EBTB by FOB has the following seven subtypes:

i. *Actively caseating form:* This is the most commonly encountered form of EBTB on bronchoscopy and is evident by hyperemic and edematous mucosa with a diffuse covering of cheesy necrosed tissue. Diffuse mucosal congestion with edema (suggestive of inflammation) and mass lesion were most common bronchoscopic findings in three different studies.[1,15,17] Luminal narrowing at diagnosis is seen usually and 65% of the cases progress to stenotic changes despite adequate treatment.
ii. *Ulcerative:* Ulcers which may range from shallow to deep are visualized in this form in the tracheobronchial tree. Prognosis is good with many cases resolving completely with proper therapy within three months.
iii. *Edematous hyperemic:* Severe mucosal swelling with adjacent hyperemia leading to luminal narrowing is evident. It is a poor prognostic marker as 60% of the cases progress to fibrostenosis within 2–3 months after treatment and 30% progress to complete luminal narrowing.
iv. *Granular:* This form presents with grains simulating those of boiled rice scattered in the tracheobronchial tree with evidence of severe inflammatory changes in the underlying bronchial mucosa. Prognosis is good with only 20% of cases progressing to fibrostenotic changes.
v. *Fibrostenotic:* Substantial luminal narrowing secondary to fibrotic changes is evident with the patients not responding to treatment. Progressive fibrosis despite treatment may result in complete luminal obstruction.
vi. *Tumorous:* This type often mimicks bronchogenic carcinoma. Tumor like granulation tissue often covered with caseous matieral protruding into the bronchial lumen is seen. The prognosis is grave and unpredictable. In a study, 70% of the patients with tumorous endobronchial TB progressed to fibrostenotic changes despite appropriate treatment. Development

of other tumorous lesions can occur subsequently elsewhere in the tracheobronchial tree.

vii. *Nonspecific bronchitic:* In this form, only mild mucosal edema with or without hyperemia is evident bronchoscopically. This type corresponds to the initial lesion, with simple erythema and edema of the bronchial mucosa with lymphocytic infiltration. The overall prognosis is good with cases responding to treatment within 2 months.

Rarely, rupture of inflamed lymph nodes occurs.[55] Obstruction of the lumen by a grayish-yellow mass protruding through the mucosa represents an early stage. Gradual hemorrhage and granulation tissue formation may occur subsequently leading to fistula formation and discharge of necrosed material into the bronchial lumen. At this point of time, inflammation of of mucous membrane is reduced and lymph node evacuation takes place followed by gradual closure of fistula and subsequent development of bronchial fibrostenosis. A perforated lymph node may present mass or a hyperpigmented mucosa[11,56-60] with stenosed bronchus due to anthracotic material in the node termed as "anthracofibrosis"[60] (Figs. 6.1 to 6.8).

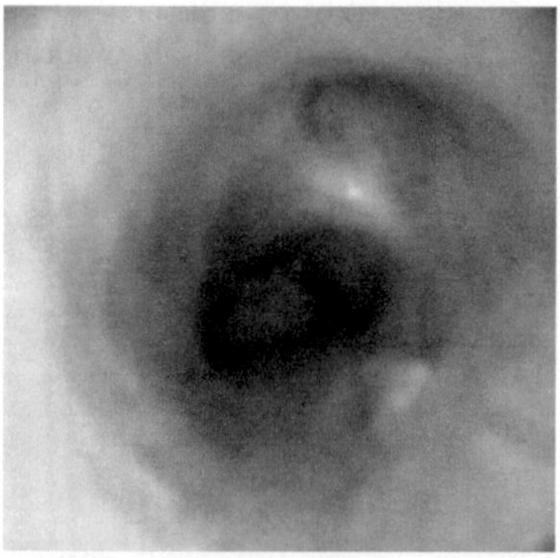

Fig. 6.1: Two nodular growths (For color version, see Plate 1)

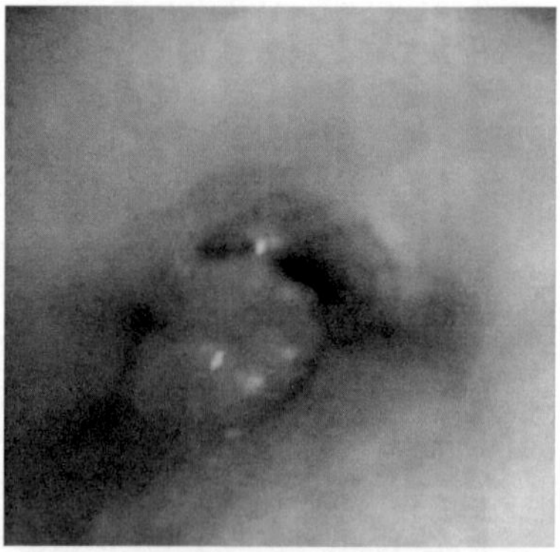

Fig. 6.2: Close view of nodule (For color version, see Plate 1)

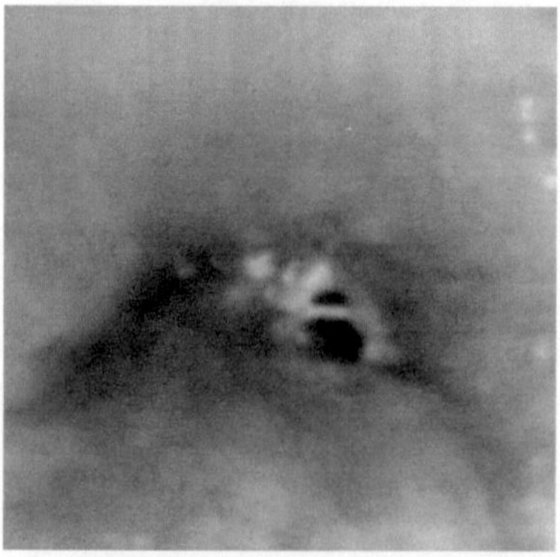

Fig. 6.3: Caseous material after transbronchial needle aspiration (For color version, see Plate 1)

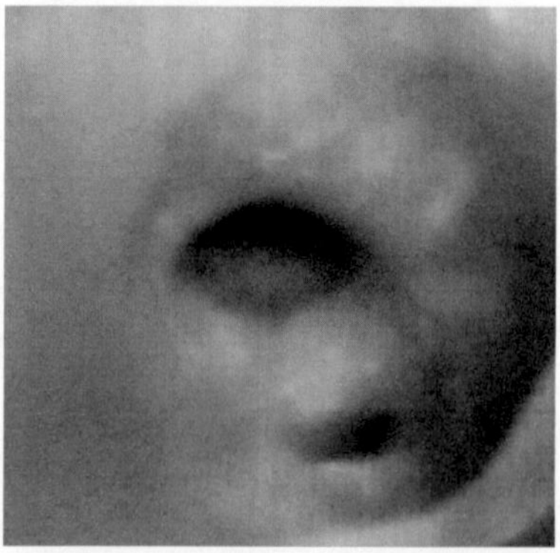

Fig. 6.4: Edematous and hyperemic tertiary carina (For color version, see Plate 1)

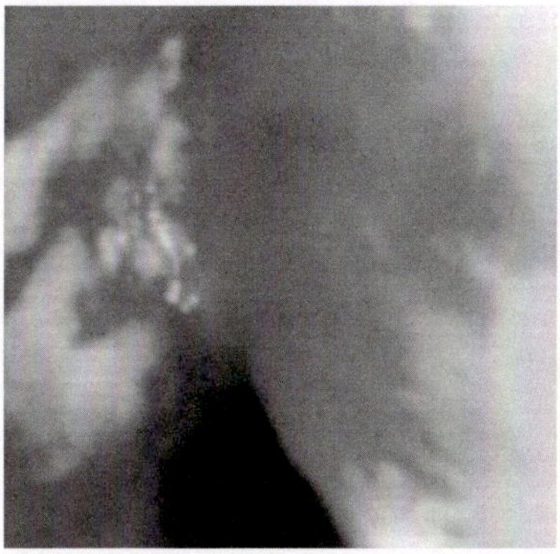

Fig. 6.5: Right upper lobe bronchus obstructed by caseous material and blood (For color version, see Plate 1)

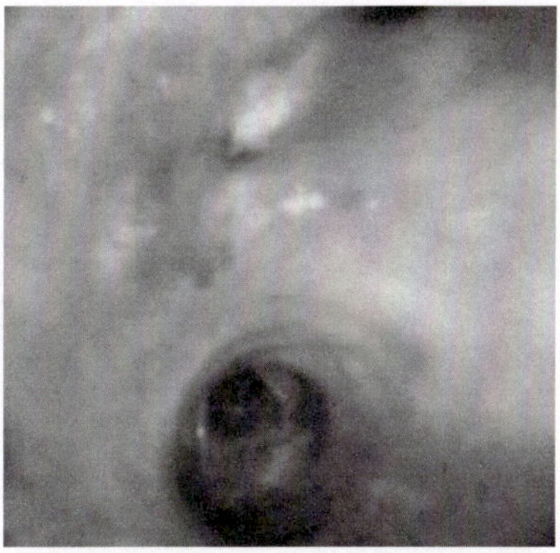

Fig. 6.6: Tuberculous sinus just behind secondary carina (For color version, see Plate 1)

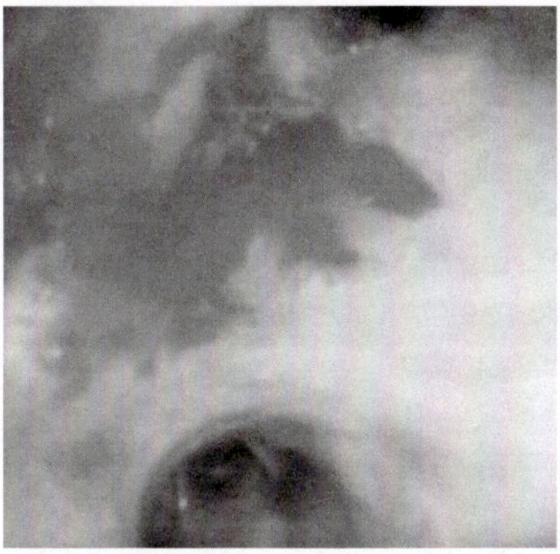

Fig. 6.7: Bleeding after endobronchial biopsy from tuberculous sinus (For color version, see Plate 2)

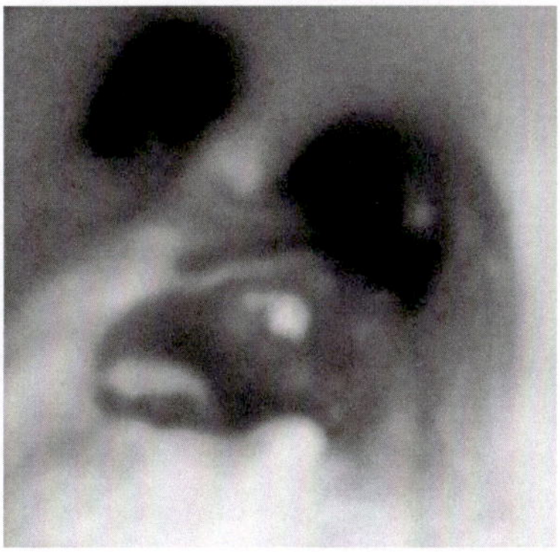

Fig. 6.8: Tracheal fistula surrounded with granulation tissue (For color version, see Plate 2)

Bronchography

Contemporary diagnostic techniques have now rendered this once widely utilized procedure to be obsolete. Bronchography used to be an aid for the diagnosis and preoperative evaluation of bronchial stenosis.[21,61]

DIFFERENTIAL DIAGNOSIS

Lung cancer is most important differential diagnosis. However, other differential diagnoses are simple inflammation, sarcoidosis, bronchial asthma, atelectasis, foreign body aspiration, pneumonia and endobronchial actinomycosis,[62] papillomatosis[63] and infection with nontuberculous mycobacteria (NTM).[64-66] Sarcoidosis also involves the bronchi and may manifest with endobronchial inflammation closely resembling EBTB. Bronchostenosis due to sarcoidosis that may develop in certain cases needs to be differentiated from EBTB carefully.[67] There is a need to have a high index of suspicion to exclude atelectasis due to EBTB in children with either acute or chronic respiratory tract symptomatology. However, in patients with acquired immune deficiency syndrome (AIDS), endobronchial Kaposi's sarcoma (EKS) should be considered.[68] Previous endotracheal intubation and systemic diseases as Crohn's disease and Behset's syndrome may also present with focal stenotic lesions.[63] Diffuse stenosis of tracheobronchial tree may be evident in Wegner's granulomatosis, relapsing polychondritis, tracheobronchopathia osteochondroplastica, amyloidosis, papillomatosis and rhinoscleroma.[63]

TREATMENT

It has been demonstrated that adequate treatment of parenchymal disease leads to spontaneous healing of many endobronchial TB ulcers.[23] With the advent of effective chemotherapy, the natural course of EBTB has been altered.[69,70] In the pre-chemotherapy era, endobronchial lesions used to be treated by painting caustic soda or silver nitrate on small ulcers thus enhancing fibrosis.[3,71,72]

Antitubercular Chemotherapy

Early introduction of conventional chemotherapy containing INH, rifampicin, pyrazinamide and ethambutol should control the progression. Duration and regimens are the same as for standard short course chemotherapy and most of the studies have advocated six to nine months duration for chemotherapy.[1,18,40,73-77] Role of DOT (Directly Observed Treatment) in EBTB is not extensively studied, although one recent study has shown favorable results.[40] Addition of aerosol therapy with streptomycin and isoniazid (200 mg/day)[78,79] to the standard regimen have shown to improve outcomes in some studies.

Corticosteroids

Inhaled corticosteroid therapy is useful in the treatment of EBTB. Time to healing of ulcerous lesions is shorter and bronchial stenosis is less severe in patients on aerosol therapy with corticosteroids. Progression to bronchial stenosis may be prevented if the therapy is initiated as soon as possible.[74] Empirical use of systemic corticosteroids along with antitubercular chemotherapy is done in some cases to prevent stenosis.[10,12,18] Systemic steroids may suppress the barking cough associated with EBTB.[12,80-82] Some studies suggest a positive role of steroids in bronchial obstruction associated with childhood TB lymphadenitis.[83,84]

Bronchoscopy

Various bronchoscopic procedures are being employed alone or as an adjuvant to chemotherapy for relieving bronchial stenosis. Endoluminal dilatation and stenting is currently recommended as the first line intervention for the stenosis in EBTB. Narrowed airways can be dilated by using dilators, balloons or the bronchoscope itself. Balloon dilatation is successful in dilating short stenotic segments.[14,85] Repeated dilatation may be required.[22,86] Verhaeghe, et al[91] have demonstrated rapid healing and complete resolution of endobronchial tuberculosis by local endoscopic injection of corticosteroids in different sittings. Laser bronchoscopy is a newly established procedure employed in interventional bronchoscopy. A small series by Tscheikuna has demonstrated the benefit of laser bronchoscopy is patients with high-risk endobronchial obstructive lesions.[87] In another Russian study, endobronchial laser therapy along with α-tocopherol and endobronchial instillation of sodium thiosulfate in nine patients of post-tuberculous fibrous stenosis of large bronchi provided a steady-state dilatation of the airway lumen.[88] Removal of excess fibrous tissue by forceps and CO_2 laser or Nd:YAG laser is useful.[89] Patency of the stenosed region can be maintained by metallic stent placement.[90]

Surgery

Surgical treatment such as bronchoplasty (sleeve resection with end-to-end anastomosis)[92,93] may be contemplated for EBTB particularly when the response to antituberculosis chemotherapy is poor. In addition to checking progression of the disease, bronchoplasty helps to preserve lung function. Appropriate chemotherapy should be given perioperatively to prevent a recurrence of disease and re-stenosis.[94] Bronchoplastic surgery is the best treatment for bronchial stricture involving both the main bronchi.[52] Bronchoscopic curettage with forceps of the pseudomembranes coupled with systemic steroid therapy has been reported to enhance the drainage among selective patients.[12] The surgical modality that should be used depends upon the location, extent and degree of stenosis.[93] Involvement of lobar or segmental bronchi may be treated by performing a lobectomy. Lesions involving trachea or main stem bronchus, bronchoplasty with or without lobectomy is the treatment modality. The amount of lung parenchyma resected must be as minimal as possible, as the objective of surgery is to restore maximum possible lung function of the hypoventilated lung. Pneumonectomy should be the last resort when the involved lung shows extensive damage or bronchiectatic changes or when the main stem bronchus is completely obliterated.[92]

ENDOBRONCHIAL TUBERCULOSIS IN SPECIAL SITUATIONS

Endobronchial Tuberculosis in Children

Most cases of primary infection with tuberculosis remain asymptomatic. However, with the progression of the disease the lymph nodes located in hilar and paratracheal regions become enlarged due to host inflammatory response and may encroach upon the regional bronchus. Partial obstruction caused by external compression by the enlarged lymph node leads to hyperinflation of the distal lung segment. Occasionally, these lymph nodes lead to complete obstruction of the bronchus resulting in atelectasis of the segment.[95] More often the inflamed caseous nodes attached to the bronchial wall erode through it, leading to EBTB or a fistulous tract.[96] Consequent upon these changes EBTB in children often presents with localized wheezing and sublobar atelectasis and consolidation attributable to the erosion of the inflamed lymph nodes into the bronchial lumen. The extrusion of infected material into the bronchus can spread infection to the lung parenchyma. At times EBTB manifests clinically as foreign body aspiration in children.[97,98] Because of the short- and long-term sequelae of EBTB, including bronchial stenosis and postobstructive bronchiectasis, therapy is indicated to relieve peribronchial obstruction. In a small series of 29 pediatric cases with primary tuberculosis and bronchial obstruction, randomization to prednisolone was associated with a favorable outcome by both radiographic and bronchoscopic appearances.[99]

Endobronchial Tuberculosis in Geriatric Age

Approximately 90% of cases of tuberculosis involving elderly persons are caused by reactivation of primary infection.[100] Endobronchial tuberculosis occurs in adults mostly by superficial ulceration in the bronchus caused by secretions containing high numbers of live TB bacilli from cavitary lesions. EBTB is observed in about 15% of elderly patients with pulmonary TB and bronchial stenosis may occur in about 60% of cases.[107] As malignancy and pneumonia are common among the elderly, EBTB is perhaps underestimated. Cough usually is the main symptom. Chest pain, wheeze, hemoptysis may be seen in addition to constitutional symptoms of tuberculosis. Constitutional symptoms of tuberculosis such as weakness, anorexia and fatigue are marked with no difference in the bronchoscopic findings when compared to other age groups.

Endobronchial Tuberculosis in HIV Patients

Human immunodeficiency virus (HIV) leads to marked depression of cellular immunity with progressive destruction of $CD4^+$ lymphocytes. The absence or incomplete formation of granulomata and dissemination of mycobacteria in HIV-infected patients appears to be directly proportional to the circulating $CD4^+$ lymphocytes. There is no firm conclusion from the available literature that EBTB is more common in subjects with HIV infection. However, it is expected that EBTB should be more frequent in association with HIV infection because, it is a frequent manifestation of primary tuberculosis due to depressed cell-mediated immunity and also, the usual mechanism for development of

EBTB is a direct airway infiltration from adjacent tuberculous mediastinal lymph nodes that are commonly noticed in patients with HIV infection. On the other hand, a possible explanation for underestimation of EBTB in HIV infected patients may be the infrequent use of fiberoptic bronchoscopy in patients with positive acid-fast bacilli on sputum smear examination; and therefore, endobronchial pathology may go undetected.[68,101] Certain specific diseases may present with endobronchial abnormalities, including EBTB. It is important to know the bronchoscopic appearances of the lesions such as Kaposi's sarcoma, aspergillosis, lymphoma and lung cancer because some of these lesions may require biopsy and special stains. In the setting of HIV, it is also important to consider the risks and benefits of the biopsy of endobronchial lesions.[99]

Endobronchial Tuberculosis in Patients with Lower Lung Field Involvement

Involvement of the right middle lobe, lingular division of left upper lobe and bilateral lower lobes is seen commonly in patients having concomitant diabetes mellitus, pregnancy, chronic renal failure and malignancy. Reports show that up to 75% of these patients may have associated endobronchial changes.[102-104]

Endobronchial Involvement by Nontuberculous Mycobacteria

Nontuberculous mycobacteria (NTM) are rarely seen to involve the tracheobronchial tree. Such instances are mostly seen with concomitant HIV infection and most cases respond well to the therapy without leaving any residual bronchostenosis.[64-66,105]

Drug Resistance in Endobronchial Tuberculosis

No definite study of EBTB and multidrug resistant tuberculosis is available. As EBTB is associated with pulmonary tuberculosis, the pattern of drug resistance is likely to be similar. Factors responsible for drug resistance in pulmonary tuberculosis should also be applicable to EBTB. Sputum for culture and sensitivity should be sent if sputum remains positive for acid-fast bacillus after sufficient appropriate treatment.[106]

REFERENCES

1. Hoheisel G, Chan BK, Chan CH, et al. Endobronchial tuberculosis: Diagnostic features and therapeutic outcome. Respir Med. 1994;88:593-7.
2. Cohen AG, Wessler H. Clinical recognition of tuberculosis of major bronchi. Arch Intern Med. 1939;63:1132-57.
3. Smart J. Endobronchial tuberculosis. Br J Tuberc Chest Dis. 1951;45:61-8.
4. Wilson NJ. Bronchoscopic observations in tuberculosis tracheobronchitis; clinical and pathological correlations. Dis Chest. 1945;11:36-59.

5. Danek SJ, Bower JS. Diagnosis of pulmonary tuberculosis by fiberoptic bronchoscopy. Am Rev Respir Dis. 1979;119:677-9.
6. Jett JR, Cortese DA, Dines DE. The value of bronchoscopy in the diagnosis of mycobacterial disease: a five year experience. Chest. 1981;80:575-8.
7. Wallace JM, Deutsch AL, Harrel JH, Moser KM. Bronchoscopy and transbronchial biopsy in patients with suspected active tuberculosis. Am J Med. 1981;70:1189-94.
8. Willcox PA, Benatar SR, Potgeiter PD. Use of flexible fibreoptic bronchoscope in the diagnosis of sputum negative pulmonary tuberculosis. Thorax. 1982;37:598-601.
9. Stenson W, Aranda C, Bevelaqua FA. Transbronchial biopsy culture in pulmonary tuberculosis. Chest. 1983;83:883-4.
10. Ip MS, So SY, Lam WK, Mok CK. Endobronchial tuberculosis revisited. Chest. 1986;89: 727-30.
11. Smith LS, Shillaci RF, Sarlin RF. Endobronchial tuberculosis. Serial fibreoptic bronchoscopy and natural history. Chest. 1987;91:644-7.
12. Lee JH, Park SS, Lee DH, Shin DH, Yang SC, Yoo BM. Endobronchial tuberculosis: clinical and bronchoscopic features in 121 cases. Chest. 1992;31:593-8.
13. Kurasawa T, Kuze F, Kawai M, Amitani R, Murayama T, Tanaka E, et al. Diagnosis and management of endobronchial tuberculosis. Intern Med. 1992;31:593-8.
14. Kim YH, Kim HT, Lee KS, Uh ST, Chung YT, Park CS. Serial fibreoptic bronchoscopic observations of endobronchial tuberculosis before and early after antituberculosis chemotherapy. Chest. 1993;103:673-7.
15. Wang SY, Zhang XS. Endobronchial tuberculosis: report of 121 cases. Chest. 1994;105:1910-1.
16. Singla R, Kumar A, Chauhan D, Juneja D, Tyagi VN, Arora VK. Endobronchial tuberculosis prenting as a tumorous mass. Indian J Chest Dis Allied Sci. 2007;49:45-7.
17. Altin S, Cikrikcioglu S, Morgul M, Kosar F, Ozyurt H. Fifty endobronchial tuberculosis cases based on bronchoscopic diagnosis. Respiration. 1997;64:162-4.
18. Chung HS, Lee JH. Bronchoscopic assessment of the evolution of endobronchial tuberculosis. Chest. 2000;117:385-92.
19. Lee JH, Chung HS. Bronchoscopic, radiologic and pulmonary function evaluation of endobronchial tuberculosis. Respirology. 2000;5:411-7.
20. Flance IJ, Wheeler PA. Postmortem incidence of tuberculous tracheobronchitis. Am Rev Tuberc. 1939;39:633-6.
21. Sweany HC, Behm H. Tuberculosis of the trachea and major bronchi. Dis Chest. 1948;14:1.
22. Auerbach O. Tuberculosis of trachea and major bronchi. Am Rev Tuberc. 1949;60:604-10.
23. Salkin D, Cadden AV, Edson RC. The natural history of tuberculous tracheobronchitis. Am Rev Tuberc. 1943;47:351-69.
24. Stone MJ. Clinical aspects of endobronchial tuberculosis. Dis Chest. 1945;11:60-71.
25. Dhillon SS, Watanakunakorn C. Lady Windermere Syndrome: middle lobe bronchiectasis *Mycobacterium avium* complex infection due to voluntary cough suppression. Clin Infect Dis. 2000;30:572-5.
26. Reich JH, Johnson RE. *Mycobacterium avium* complex pulmonary disease presenting as an isolated lingular or middle lobe pattern. The Lady Windermere Syndrome. Chest. 1992;101:1605-9.
27. Myerson MC. Tuberculosis of the Trachea and Bronchus. Springfield: Charles C. Thomas. 1944:250-75.
28. Chang SC, Lee PY, Perng RP. Clinical role of bronchoscopy in adults with intrathoracic tuberculous lymphadenopathy. Chest. 1988;93:314-7.
29. So SY, Lam WK, Sham MK. Bronchorrhoea: A presenting feature of pulmonary tuberculosis. Chest. 1984;86:642-4.

30. Park MJ, Woo IS, Son JW, et al. Endobronchial tuberculosis with expectoration of tracheal cartilages. Eur Respir J. 2000;15:800-2.
31. Tse CY, Natkunam R. Serious sequelae of delayed diagnosis of endobronchial tuberculosis. Tubercle. 1988;69:213-6.
32. Volckaert A, Roels P, Vawder Niepen P, Schandevyl W. Endobronchial tuberculosis: Report of three cases. Eur J Respir Dis. 1987;70:99-101.
33. Matthews JI, Matarese SL, Carpenter JL. Endobronchial tuberculosis simulating lung cancer. Chest. 1984;86:642-4.
34. Centers for Disease Control and Prevention. Nucleic acid amplification tests for tuberculosis. MMWR. 2000;49:593-4.
35. Yu W, Rong Z. Clinical analysis of 90 cases with endobronchial tuberculosis. Zhonghua Jie He He Hu Xi Za Zhi. 1999;22:396-8.
36. Aggarwal AN, Gupta D, Joshi K, Behera D. Endobronchial involvement in tuberculosis: A report of 24 cases diagnosed by fibreoptic bronchoscopy. J Bronchol. 1999;6:247-50.
37. Fraser RG, Pare JAP, Pare PD. Diagnosis of Diseases of the Chest; Vol. 2. Philadelphia: WB Saunders Co. 1988:883-929.
38. Winner-Muram HT, Rubin SA. Thoracic complications of tuberculosis. J Thoracic Imag. 1990;5:46-63.
39. Gruden JF, Webb WR, Warnock M. Centrilobar opacities in the lung on high resolution CT: diagnostic considerations and pathologic correlation. AJR Am J Roentgenol. 1994;162: 569-74.
40. Long R, Maycher B, Dhar A. Pulmonary tuberculosis treated with directly observed therapy: Serial changes in lung structure and function. Chest. 1998;113:933-43.
41. Im JG, Itoh H, Shim YS, Lee JH, Ahn J, Han MC. Pulmonary tuberculosis: CT findings-early active disease and sequential change with antituberculous therapy. Radiology. 1993;186:653-60.
42. Lee KH, Kim WS, Hwang SH, Kim PN, Lee BH. Endobronchial tuberculosis: CT features. J Comput Assist Tomogr. 1191;15:424-8.
43. Muller NL, Fraser RS, Colman NC, Pare PD. Radiologic Diagnosis of Diseases of the Chest. Philadelphia: WB Saunders Co. 2001;78-80.
44. Itoh H, Tokunaga S, Asamato M. Radiologic-pathologic correlations of small lung nodules with special reference to peribronchial nodules. Am J Roentgenol. 1978;130:223-31.
45. Naidich DP, Lee JJ, Garay SM, McCauley DI, Aranda CP, Boyd AD. Comparision of CT and fiberoptic bronchoscopy in the evaluation of bronchial disease. Am J Roengenol. 1987;148: 1-7.
46. Km Y, Lee KS, Yoon JH, Chung MP, KIM H, Kwon OJ. Tuberculosis of the trachea and main bronchi: CT findings in 17 patients. Am J Roengenol. 1997;168:1051-6.
47. Moon WK, Im JG, Yeom KM, Han MC. Tuberculosis of the central airways: CT findings of active and fibrotic disease. Am J Roengenol. 1997;169:649-53.
48. Choe KO, Jeong HJ, Sohn HY. Tuberculous bronchial stenosis: CT findings in 28 cases. Am J Roengenol. 1990;155:971-6.
49. Finkelstein SE, Summers RM, Nguyen DM, Stewart JH, Tretler JA, Schrump DS. Virtual bronchoscopy for evaluation of malignant tumours of the thorax. J Thorac Cardiovascular Surg. 2002;123:967-72.
50. Lee KS, Yoon JH, Kim TK, Kim JS. Evaluation of tracheobronchial disease with helical CT with multiplanar and three dimensional reconstruction: Correlation with bronchoscopy. Radiographics. 1997;17:555-70.
51. Park CS, Km Ku, Lee SM, Jeong SW, Uh S, Kim HT. Bronchial hyperreactivity in patients with endobronchial tuberculosis. Respir Med. 1995;89:419-22.
52. Lincoln EM, Haris LC, Bovornkiti S, Caraterro R. The course and prognosis of endobrochial tuberculosis in children. Am Rev Tuber. 1955;71:246-56.

53. Fortasd S. Segemental atelectasis in children with primary tuberculosis. Am Rev Respir Dis. 1959;79:597-605.
54. Smith LS, Schillaci RF, Sarlin RF. Endobronchial tuberculosis: Serial fibreoptic bronchoscopy and natural history. Chest. 1987;91:644-7.
55. Kraan JK, Muller S. Perforation of tuberculosis gland into a bronchus. Acta Tuber Scand. 1950;24:88-102.
56. Arnstein A. Nonindustrial pneumoconioses, pneumoconio-tuberculosis and tuberculosis of the mediastinal and bronchial lymph glands in old people. Tubercle. 1941;22:281-95.
57. Van den Brande P, Lambrechts M, Tack J, Demets M. Endobronchial tuberculosis mimicking lung cancer in elderly patients. Respir Med. 1991;85:107-9.
58. Yee A, Hardwick JA, Wasef E, Sharma OP. Pigmented polypoid obstructive endobronchial tuberculosis. Chest. 1985;87:702-3.
59. Abraham GC. Atelectasis of right middle lobe resulting from perforation of tuberculous lymph node into bronchi in adults. Ann Intern Med. 1951;35:820-35.
60. Chung MP, Lee KS, Han J, Kim H, Rhee CH, Han YC, et al. Bronchial stenosis due to anthracofibrosis. Chest. 1998;113:344-50.
61. Rose RM, Cardona J, Daly JF. Bronchographic sequelae of endobronchial tuberculosis. Ann Otol Rhinol Laryngol. 1965;74:1133-43.
62. Lee SH, Shim JJ, Kang EY. Endobronchial actinomycosis simulating endobronchial tuberculosis: A case report. J Korean Med Sci. 1999;14:315-8.
63. Prince JS, Duhamel DR, Levin DL, Harrel JH, Friedman PJ. Nonneoplastic lesions of tracheobronchial wall: Radiologic findings with bronchoscopic correlation. Radiographics. 2202;22:S215-30.
64. Connolly MG Jr, Baughman RP, Dohn MN. *Mycobacterium kansasii* presenting as an endobronchial lesion. Am Rev Respir Dis. 1993;148:1405-7.
65. Quieffin J, Poubeau P, Laaban JP, Brechot JM, Capron F, Rochemaure J. *Mycobacterium kansasii* infection presenting as an endobronchial tumour in a patient with acquired immunodeficiency syndrome. Tuber Lung Dis. 1994;75:313-5.
66. Asano T, Itoh G, Itoh M. Disseminated *Mycobacterium* intracelular infection in an HIV negative, nonimmunocompromised patient with multiple endobronchial polyps. Respiration. 2002;69:175-7.
67. Udwadia ZF, Pilling JR, Jenkins PF, Harrison BDW. Bronchoscopic and bronchographic findings in 12 patients with sarcoidosis and severe progressive airway obstruction. Thorax. 1990;45:272-5.
68. Judson MA, Sahn SA. Endobronchial lesion in HIV infected individuals. Chest. 1994;105: 1314-23.
69. Medical Research Council. Streptomycin treatment of tuberculous lesions of the trachea and bronchi. Lancet. 1951;1:253-7.
70. Brewer LA, Bogen E. Streptomycin in tuberculous tracheobronchitis. Am Rev Tuberc. 1947;56:408-14.
71. Judd AR. Tuberculous tracheobronchitis. J Thoracic Surg. 1947;16:512-23.
72. Lukomsky GI, Tetarchenko VE. Bronchology. St Louis: CV Mosby Co. 1979:287-305.
73. Rikimaru T, Kinosita M, Yano H, et al. Diagnostic features and therapeutic outcome of erosive and ulcerous endobronchial tuberculosis. Int J Tuberc Lung Dis. 1998;2:558-62.
74. Rikimaru T, Koga T, Sueyasu Y. Treatmentof ulcerative endobronchial tuberculosis and bronchial stenosis with aerosolized streptomycin and steroids. Int J Tuberc Lung Dis. 2001;5:769-74.
75. Park IW, Choi BW, Hue SH. Prospective study of corticosteroid as an adjunct in the treatment of endobronchial tuberculosis in adults. Respirology. 1997;2:275-81.
76. Takahashi N, Horie T. Medical treatment for bronchial stenosis due to endobronchial tuberculosis. Kekkaku. 1999;74:885-9.

77. Kurasawa T, Kuze F, Kawai M. Diagnosis and management of endobronchial tuberculosis. Intern Med. 1992;31:593-8.
78. Yokota S, Miki K. Effects of INH (isoniazid) inhalation in patients with endobronchial tuberculosis (EBTB). Kekkaku. 1999;74:873-7.
79. Miki K, Yokota S, Hiraga T. Effectiveness of isoniazid inhalation in patients with endobronchial tuberculosis. Nihon Kokyuki Gakkai Zasshi. 1999;37:31-5.
80. Williams DJ, York EL, Nobert EJ, Sproule BJ. Endobronchial tuberculosis presenting as asthma. Chest. 1988;93:836-8.
81. Chan HS, Pang JA. Effect of corticosteroids on deterioration of endobronchial tuberculosis during chemotherapy. Chest. 1989;96:1195-6.
82. Chan HS, Sun A, Hoheisel GB. Endobronchial tuberculosis is corticosteroid treatment useful? Areport of 8 cases and review of literature. Postgrad Med J. 1990;66:822-6.
83. Toppet M, Malfroot A, Derde MP. Corticosteriods in primary tuberculosis with bronchial obstruction. Arch Dis Child. 1990;65:1222-6.
84. Nemir RL, Cardona J, Lacoius A, David M. Prednisone therapy as an adjunct in the treatment of lymph node bronchial tuberculosis in childhood. Am Rev Tuberc. 1963;88:189-98.
85. Ball JB, Delaney JC, Evans CC, Donnelly RJ, Hind CR. Endoscopic bougie and balloon dilatation of multiple bronchial stenoses: 10 year follow up. Thorax. 1991;46:933-5.
86. Guleria R, Behera D, Dhaliwal RS, Jindal SK. Tracheobronchial stenosis—report of 3 cases. Indian J Chest Dis Allied Sciences. 1991;33:165-70.
87. Tscheikuna J. Laser bronchoscopy: Experience at Siriraj Hospital. J Med Assoc Thai. 2001;84:1661-6.
88. Agaev FF. Endobronchial laser therapy in the surgery of pulmonary tuberculosis. Probl Tuberk. 1998;1:33-6.
89. Tong MC, van Hasselt CA. Tuberculous tracheobronchial strictures: clinicopathologigal features and management with the bronchoscopic carbon dioxide laser. Eur Arch Otorhinolaryngol. 1993;250:110-4.
90. Wan IY, Lee TW, Lam HC, Abdullah V, Yim AP. Tracheobronchial stenting for tuberculous airway stenosis. Chest. 2002;122:370-4.
91. Verhaeghe W, Noppen M, Meysman M. Rapid healing of endobronchial tuberculosis by local endoscopic injection of corticosteroids. Monaldi Arch Chest Dis. 1996;51:391-3.
92. Watanabe Y, Murakami S, Oda M. Treatment of bronchial stricture due to endobronchial tuberculosis. World J Surg. 1997;21:480-7.
93. Kato R, Kakizaki T, Hangai N, Sawafuji M, Yamamoto T, Kobayashi T. Bronchoplastic procedureus for tuberculos bronchial stenosis. J Thoracic Cardiovascular Surg. 1993;106:1118-21.
94. Hsu HS, Hsu WH, Huang BS, Huang MH. Surgical treatment of endobronchial tuberculosis. Scand J Cardiovasc Surg. 1997;31:79-82.52.
95. Lincoln EM, Harris LC, Bovornkitti S. Endobronchial tuberculosis in children. Am Rev Tuberc Pulm Dis. 1958;77:39.
96. Daly JF, Brown DS, Lincoln EM. Endobronchial tuberculosis in children. Dis Chest. 1952;22:380.
97. Wood GS, Gonzalez C, Done S, Albus RA. Endobronchial tuberculosis in children. Int J Pediatr Otorhinolaryngol. 1990;20:241-5.
98. Park AH, Fowler SS, Challapalli M. Suspected foreign body aspiration in a child with endobronchial tuberculosis. Int J Pediatr Otorhinolaryngol. 2000;53:67-71.
99. Toppet M, Malfroot A, Derde MP. Corticosteroids in primary tuberculosis with bronchial obstruction. Arch Dis Child. 1990;65:1222-6.
100. Yoshikawa TT. Tuberculosis in aging adults. Am Geriatr Soc. 1992;40:178-87.

101. Calpe JL, Chiner E, Larramendi CH. Endobronchial tuberculosis in HIV-infected patients. AIDS. 1995;9:1159-64.
102. Chang SC, Lee PY, Perng RP. Lower lung field tuberculosis. Chest. 1987;91:230-2.
103. Rothstein E. Pulmonary tuberculosis involving the lower lobes. Am Rev Tuberc. 1949;59: 39-49.
104. Parmar MS. Lower lung field tuberculosis. Am Rev Respir Dis. 1967;96:310-3.
105. Lambert GW, Baddour LM. Right middle lobe syndrome caused by *Mycobacterium fortuitum* in a patient with human immunodeficiency virus infection. South Med J. 1992;85:767-9.
106. Kashyap S, Mohapatra PR, Saini V. Endobronchial tuberculosis. Indian J Chest Dis Allied Sciences. 2003;45:254-5.
107. Brande PM Vanden, Mierop FV, Verbeken EK, Demedts M. Clinical spectrum of endobronchial tuberculosis in elderly patients. Arch Intern Med. 1990;150:2105-8.

Chapter 7

Lower Lung Field Tuberculosis

INTRODUCTION

It was the prevailing opinion at the turn of the century that pulmonary tuberculosis almost always originated from the apices.[1-4] This idea plus the universal experience that chronic upper lung lesions were always tuberculous in nature have made lower lobe location of this disease virtually nonexistent among the early clinicians.[1-4] Slowly, however, data began to accumulate that proved the presence of this problem and by the first half of this century, published reports had not only attempted to characterize the clinical features of tuberculosis in the lower lobes but also expounded on its possible pathogenesis. Aim of this chapter is to describe the pathogenesis, clinical features, investigations and treatment of lower lung field tuberculosis.

DEFINITION

Lower lung field tuberculosis is defined as "tuberculous disease found below an imaginary line traced across the hila and including the parahilar regions on a standard posterior-anterior (PA) chest roentgenogram".[5] Ossen[6] subdivided his cases into pure and impure groups: the pure group having no visible lesions in the upper lung fields and the impure group having nodular or fibrotic infiltrations in one or both apices. Other terms used for the same entity have been "basal, lower lobe, hilar, parahilar, and perihilar tuberculois".[4,7,8] The term 'hilar and perihilar TB' was used in the view of the proximity of the lesion to hilum.[9,10] Lower lung field tuberculosis is not all that uncommon and it was Kidd in 1886 who noticed the vulnerability of the apex of lower lobe even before the apex of upper lobe was involved.[11] Without a lateral chest X-ray film, it is quite difficult to localize a lesion topographically, i.e. whether the disease is confined to the lower lobe only or has extensions in the middle lobe or lingula also. Due to this fact the term 'lower lung field tuberculosis' has been coined which in a PA radiograph of the chest, includes the lesions involving the middle lobe and lingula in addition to the lower lobe.[12]

PREVALENCE

There has been no agreement on the exact prevalence of lower lung field tuberculosis. A review of literature shows a great variation in the reported frequency of lower lung field tuberculosis. It varies from 0.003[13]–19.8%.[14] The prevalence of lower lung field tuberculosis in India ranges from 0.63%[15] to 10.5%.[16] The discrepancies in the reported prevalence may be due to confusion in the terms and definitions used, such as basal, lower lobe, or lower lung field tuberculosis.[17] Also, the studies from TB sanatoria reported a lower percentage[4,18] than general hospitals.[19,20] HIV/AIDS epidemic has also caused an increase in the prevalence. A higher prevalence of lower lung field TB has been reported in various studies fron India as compared to the Western studies.[12]

PATHOGENESIS

The most likely explanation for the development of lower lung field tuberculosis is transbronchial perforation of a hilar lymph node, with spread to the adjacent lung.[4,21,22] Thus, lower lung field disease occurs as a continuation of the primary tuberculous infection or soon afterwards in the postprimary period.[8,18] This explanation is consistent with the high incidence of endobronchial involvement and with reported clinical and radiologic observation.[18] A diagnosis of endobronchial disease is made when bronchoscopic evidence of stenosis or severe tracheobronchitis is detected or when there is roentgenographic evidence of atelectasis or tension cavities.[23] It has been proposed that lower lung field TB occurs as a consequence of primary TB or earlier in the postprimary phase.[4,18] Other mechanisms postulated in the pathogenesis of lower lung field tuberculosis have been restricted ventilation, costal breathing, and retrograde lymphatic flow from involved hilar nodes.[21,22,24,25]

CLINICAL FEATURES

Age, Sex and Race

The majority of studies have revealed that lower lung field tuberculosis occurs more frequently in patients younger than 40 years of age when compared to upper lobe disease.[8] Segarra et al[5] reported that 89% of patients with lower lung field tuberculosis were less than 40 years old compared to 53% in patients as a whole. In the study conducted by Berger and Grenada, 30%

patients with lower lung field TB were 21–30 years old and 22% were 31–40, with a total of 59% under 40 years of age.[26] Not uncommonly though, lower lung field tuberculosis may be encountered among patients of advanced age.[25,26] Few studies have reported as lower lung field TB now no longer being an entity of the younger age group.[20 ,26,27] The predominance of lower lobe tuberculosis in women has been a common observation. A male to female ratio of 1:1. 2–6 was reported in the literature.[1,3-6,18,25] The reason for this predilection remained obscure.[4,6] Various investigators postulated that this female predilection was due to a difference in the pattern of breathing between males and females and the resultant inadequate ventilation of the involved lung area.[21,25] At least one author discarded this proposed theory because of inadequate supporting evidence.[18] There is no racial preference for lower lung field disease compared to upper lobe involvement.[5] Only Dunham and Norton[28] mentioned a higher incidence in Negroes.

Symptoms and Signs

The symptoms in lower lung field tuberculosis are similar to those in upper lobe disease except for variations associated with the higher incidence of endobronchial involvement, which has ranged from 42–90% in several reports.[1,4,18] Cough with or without expectoration has been reported to be as the most common symptom in some studies.[1-3,21,29] Hemoptysis and chest pain have also been identified as important symptoms associated with lower lung field TB.[1,2,4,5,18,21,25,26,30,31] Other manifestations associated with tubercular infection such as fever with or without chills, weight loss, malaise, loss of appetite and generalized weakness are also seen frequently.[2,5,26,27,32] Previous reports have shown that in most patients, the duration of the illness was short; the onset, usually acute. Berger, et al. and Segarra, et al. reported that 96% and 90%, respectively had been ill for less than six months.[5,26] Similarly, 68% cases in the study conducted by Estrada, et al. presented with manifestations equal to or less than six weeks.[27] On physical examination, signs are usually pronounced and easily detectable in patients who show extensive involvement of the lower lobe(s).[25] However, the signs may be peculiarly minimal or even completely absent and therefore markedly incompatible with the roentgenologic findings.[25] However, physical signs are encountered more often in cases with a lower lung field involvement as compared with the classical form involving the upper zones.[26]

INVESTIGATIONS

Sputum for Acid-fast Bacilli

It is emphasized that the diagnosis should not be made unless a positive sputum is obtained.[6] It has often been reported, however, that the tubercle bacilli, even in cases with cavitary lesions and/or endobronchial disease may be difficult to demonstrate on sputum smear or culture and that multiple examinations are often necessary.[1-3,26,27,33] Isolation of *M. tuberculosis* in sputum smear or culture is, however, the most definite tool. Ahmad, et al. and Pandya, et al. have reported a higher sputum positivity in lower lung field tuberculosis compared to all cases of pulmonary tuberculosis.[16,34]

Chest Roentgenography

The radiographic findings in lower lung field tuberculosis differ significantly from those found in upper lobe disease and often resemble bacterial or viral pneumonia more than tuberculosis.[5,8] Consolidation in lower lung field disease tends to be more confluent and extensive than that found in upper lobe disease, and acinar shadows are less prominent. Homogeneity of the consolidation may range from patchy to frankly confluent.[26] Data from roentgen examinations in previous studies point to a predominant involvement of the right lung.[2-6,18,21,25-27] Most authors[6,22,23] have noted a preference for the superior segment of the lower lobes, with the exception of Pratt-Johnson[8] who stated that the apical and subapical segments were rarely involved except for cavitation. Cavitations have been noted to occur early and frequently in lower lung field disease.[3,4,18,23,25,26] Cavities in lower lung field tuberculosis are usually single but may be multiple and may either be isolated or lie within an area of consolidation.[3,5] Previous reports have stressed that the cavities in lower lung field tuberculosis tend to be large tension cavities, usually greater than 3–4 cm in diameter.[8,35] Larger tension cavities have been described as having a wall that is usually thin, with fluid present more often than in upper lobe disease.[18,25,36] Few of the reports have suggested the cavities being thick walled.[26] The cavities also tend to occur earlier in the course of the disease than in upper lobe tuberculosis.[8,18] Pleural effusion occurs more frequently in lower lung field disease than in upper lobe disease. Segarra, et al.[5] reported pleural effusion in 16% patients. Hilar lymph node enlargement, which is also said to occur frequently in lower lung field disease[8] must not be confused with a prominent hilum due to consolidation in front of or behind the lung root superimposed upon the vascular shadows.[26] Other roentgenologic findings include atelectasis or solitary mass with intrathoracic lymphadenopathy.[12] Lung collapse or pulmonary consolidation associated with lower lung field TB if evident on chest radiogram is an unfavorable prognostic marker (Figs. 7.1 to 7.6).[29,37]

Fiberoptic Bronchoscopy

Flexible fiberoptic bronchoscopy significantly increases the recovery rate of acid-fast bacilli from 47–94% in those patients suspected of having active pulmonary tuberculosis.[38-43] Microscopic examinations of bronchoscopic specimens were found positive for acid-fast bacilli in 48–67%. Of these specimens, bronchial brush gave the highest diagnostic yield.[38] Wallace reported that transbronchial biopsy had the best yield.[41] Hence, around 50–75% of cases would have an immediate microscopic evidence of

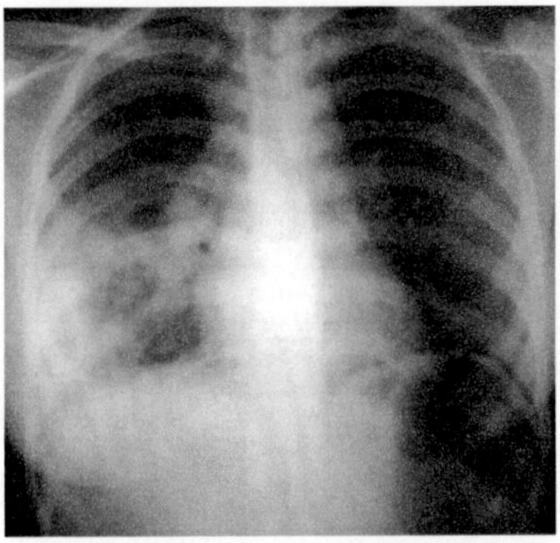

Fig. 7.1: Lower lung field TB with sputum smear positive for AFB

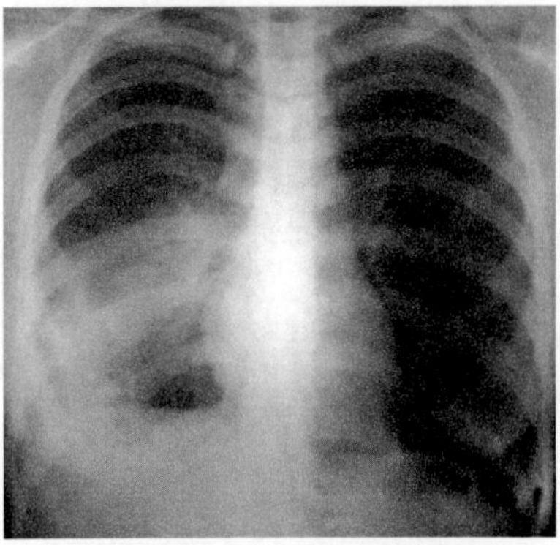

Fig. 7.2: Lower lung field TB under treatment

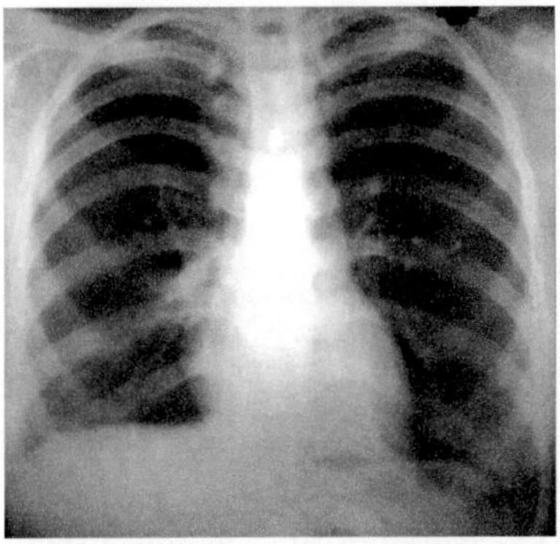

Fig. 7.3: Lower lung field TB after treatment

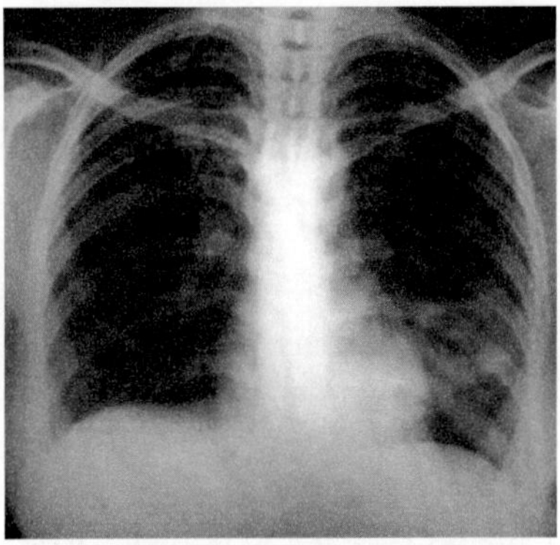

Fig 7.4: Cavity in the left lower zone with sputum smear positive for AFB

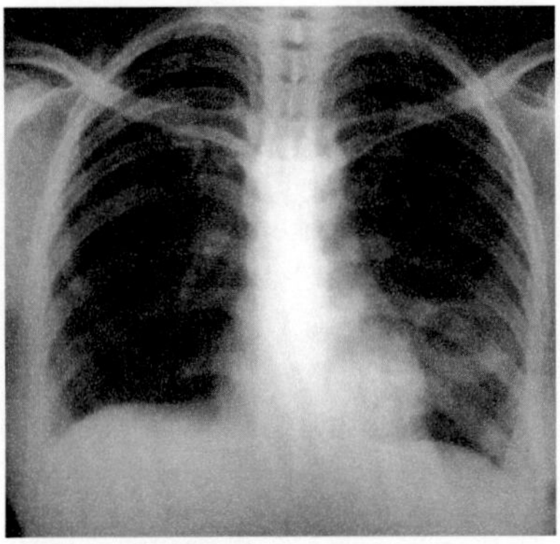

Fig. 7.5: Cavity in the left lower zone under treatment

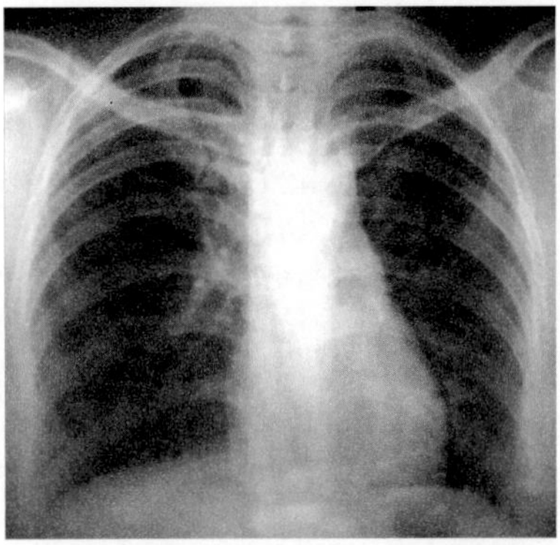

Fig. 7.6: Cavity disappeared in the left lower zone after treatment

mycobacterial infection. Post-bronchoscopy sputum smears for acid-fast bacilli (AFB) also proved to be useful.[38-44] Bronchoscopic specimens submitted for mycobacterial cultures had lower diagnostic yield ranging from 39-63%.[38-44] This was attributed to the inhibitory effect of local anesthetics, such as xylocaine spray which is commonly used during the procedure. Thus, this agent should be used in the lowest possible quantities compatible with adequate analgesia.[39-42] Schmidt and Rosenkranz reported that most strains of *M. tuberculosis* were inhibited by a concentration of 0.5%.[45] Correlated with roentgenographic patterns, bronchoscopy has resulted in more positive specimens most frequently in patients with cavitary disease.[38,41] On the other hand, a correlation with bronchial mucosal abnormality was noted as positive bronchoscopic specimens were obtained in those with inflamed mucosa or endobronchial plaque.[38] Besides its diagnostic merit, bronchoscopy can likewise assess the severity of the endobronchial lesions and provide a guide to early surgical intervention especially in those with severe fibrostenosis. Nevertheless, bronchoscopy should be performed early to make a diagnosis of tuberculosis in patients with lower lung field lesions despite negative smear or culture for acid-fast bacilli.[18-20,46]

ASSOCIATED MEDICAL CONDITIONS

Diabetes mellitus, pregnancy, silicosis and kyphoscoliosis have been reported to occur more frequently in patients with lower lung field disease than in the general population.[5,25,26] In addition to diabetes, Kahn, et al. found pulmonary malignancy and alcohol abuse[19] to be common among their subjects. Although, it is well documented that carcinoma and tuberculosis may coexist, there remains a controversy regarding the significance of the relationship. It may be coincidental, but it is also possible that scars of infection may play a role in carcinogenesis.[33]

MANAGEMENT

Lower lung field tuberculosis often is confused initially with bacterial or viral pneumonia, lung cancer, bronchiectasis or lung abcess.[12,26] Hamilton stressed that when the radiologic picture suggests unresolved pneumonia, abscess, tumor, bronchiectasis or chronic pneumonitis, tuberculosis should be included as a differential diagnosis.[1] TB should also be considered as a diagnostic possibility in cases with lower lung field involvement having concomitant conditions as diabetes mellitus, advanced age, steroid treatment and renal or hepatic disease.[12,29,47] Tuberculosis should be considered a diagnostic possibility in patients with "lower lung field pneumonia" who do not appear acutely ill or have had symptoms for more than several days and particularly several weeks before seeking medical aid. Important clues to the diagnosis of tuberculosis are hemoptysis, normal white blood cell count, cavitation, hilar nodes, pleural effusion, evidence of old tuberculosis, and especially failure to improve radiologically with treatment for pneumonia.[26] Treatment is same like other tuberculosis and the response to treatment with antituberculosis drugs is similar to that seen in upper lobe disease.

An important complication of lower lung field TB that must be looked upon closely is tracheobronchial stenosis which presents with a poor outcome. Such patients must be followed up closely by fiberoptic bronchoscopy if the chest skiagram or clinical features show insignificant improvement with proper antitubercular chemotherapy after a few months of treatment. Surgical intervention in the form of sleeve resection is recommended earlier in the course if repeat bronchoscopic examinations show insignificant improvement in the setting of severe fibrostenosis.[12,26,37]

REFERENCES

1. Hamilton CE, Fredd H. Lower lobe tuberculosis. JAMA. 1935;105:427-30.
2. Tirona JP. Basal lesions of pulmonary tuberculosis among Filipinos. Dis Chest. 1940;6: 172-81.
3. Sokoloff MJ. Lower lobe tuberculosis. Radiology. 1940;34:589-94.
4. Romendick SS, Friedman B, Schwartz HF. Lower lung field tuberculosis. Dis Chest. 1944;10:481-8.
5. Segarra F, Sherman DS, Rodriguez-Aguem J. Lower lung field tuberculosis. Am Rev Resp Dis. 1963;87:37-40.
6. Ossen EZ. Tuberculosis of the lower lobe. N Engl J Med. 1844;230:693-8.
7. Busby LF. Basal tuberculosis. Am Rev Tuberc. 1939;40:692-703.
8. Pratt-Johnson JH. Observations on lower lobe tuberculosis. Br J Dis Chest. 1959;53:385-9.
9. Bernard M, Lelong M, Renard G. La localisation perihilarede la tuberculose pulmonaire chronique de la adulate. Ann de Med. 1927;21:366.
10. Faber K. Perihilar pulmonary tuberculosis in adults. Acta Med Scand. 1931;75:403.
11. Kidd P. Basic tuberculous pthisis. Lancet. 1886;2:616.
12. Sharma SK, Mohan A. Tuberculosis, 2nd edn. Jaypee Brothers Medical Publishers (P) Ltd., New Delhi. pp.227-31.
13. Colton WA. Basal lesions in pulmonary tuberculosis with a report of seven cases. US Vet Bureau Med Bull. 1928;4:503.
14. Ayatollahi J. Clinical study of lower-lung field tuberculosis. Iran J Med Sci. 2006;31:79-81.
15. Mathur KC, Tanwar KL, Razdan JN. Lower lung field tuberculosis. Ind J Chest Dis. 1974;16: 31-41.
16. Ahmad Z, Zaheer MS. Lower lung field tuberculosis—a clinical study. J Ind Acad Clin Med. 2003;4:116-20.
17. Satya Sris. Textbook of Pulmonary and Extrapulmonary tuberculosis. 3rd edn. New Delhi. Interprint Publication. 1998;120.
18. Parmar MS. Lower lung field tuberculosis. Am Rev Respir Dis. 1967;95:310-3.
19. Kahn MA, Kovnat DM, Bachus B. et al. Clinical and roentgenographic spectrum of pulmonary tuberculosis in the adult. Am J Med. 1977;62:31-8.
20. Chang SC, Lee PY, Perng RP. Lower lung field tuberculosis. Chest. 1987;91:230-2.
21. Viswanathan R. Tuberculosis of the lower lobe. Br Med J. 1936;2:1300-2.
22. Andosca JB, Foley JA. Basal tuberculosis. J Thorac Surg. 1943;12:259-66.
23. Rothstein C. Pulmonary tuberculosis involving the lower lobes. Am Rev Tuberc. 1949;59: 39-49.

24. Fries JW, Groves W. Lower lobe tuberculosis. Mich Med. 1955;54:1310-4.
25. Reisner D. Pulmonary tuberculosis of the lower lobe. Arch Intern Med. 1935;56:258-80.
26. Berger HW, Granada MG. Lower lung field tuberculosis. Chest. 1974;65;522-6.
27. Estrada DR, Alora BD. Lower lung tuberculosis. Phil J Microbiol Infect Dis. 1985;14:58-64.
28. Dunham K, Norton W. Basal tuberculosis. JAMA 1927;89:1573-5.
29. Kobayashi Y, Matsushima T. Clinical analysis of recent lower lung field tuberculosis. J Infect Chemother. 2003;9:272-5.
30. Du Fault P. Basal pulmonary lesions. Am Rev Tuberc. 1932;25:17-23.
31. Gordon BL, Charr R, Sokoloff MJ. Basal pulmonary tuberculosis. Am Rev Tuberc. 1944;49:432-6.
32. Tripathy SN, Nanda CN. Lower lung field tuberculosis in adults. J Assoc Physicians India. 1970;18:999-1008.
33. Kaplan MH, Armstrong D, Rosen P. Tuberculosis complicating neoplastic disease. Cancer. 1974;33:850-8.
34. Pandya L, Al-Sharif N, Maraey MA. Lower lung field tuberculosis in Saudi Arabia. An Saud Med. 1990;4:374-7.
35. Vivas JR, Laubach CA Jr. Observations on lower lobe disease in pulmonary tuberculosis. Am Rev Tuberc. 1949;80:15-24.
36. Weidman WH, Campbell HB. Lower lobe tuberculosis. Am Rev Tuberc. 1937;36:525-41.
37. Chang SC, Lee PY, Perng RP. The value of roentgenographic and fiber bronchoscopic findings in predicting outcome of adults with lower lung field tuberculosis. Arch Intern Med. 1991;151:1581-3.
38. Wongthim S, Limthongkul S, Udompanich J, et al. Fiberoptic bronchoscopy in diagnosis of patients with suspected active pulmonary tuberculosis. J Med Assoc Thai. 1989;72:154-9.
39. Willcox PA, Benatar SR, Potgieter PD. Use of the flexible fiberoptic bronchoscope in diagnosis of sputum-negative pulmonary tuberculosis. Thorax. 1982;37:598-601.
40. Jett JR, Cortese DA, Dines DE. The value of bronchoscopy in the diagnosis of mycobacterial disease. Chest. 1981;80:575-8.
41. Wallace J, Deutseh A, Harrell J, Moser K. Bronchoscopy and transbronchial biopsy in evaluation of patients with suspected active tuberculosis. Am J Med. 1981;70:1189-94.
42. Unddenfeldt M, Lundgren R. Flexible fiberoptic bronchoscopy in the diagnosis of pulmonary tuberculosis. Tubercle. 1981;62:197-9.
43. Sarkar SK, Sharma GS, Gupta PR, Sharma RK. Fiberoptic bronchoscopy in the diagnosis of pulmonary tuberculosis. Tubercle. 1980;61:97-9.
44. Mitchell SM, Emerson CJ, Collins JV, Stableforth DE. Transbronchial lung biopsy with the fiberoptic bronchoscope: Analysis of results in 433 Patients. Br J Dis Chest. 1981;75:258-62.
45. Schmidt RM, Rosenkranz IIS. Antimicrobial activity of local anesthetics: lidocaine and procaine. J Infect Dis. 1970;121:597-607.
46. Varkey B, Politis J. Pulmonary tuberculosis: A multifaceted disease. Postgrad Med. 1981; 69:117-7.
47. Bacakoglu F, Basoglu OK, Cok G, Sayiner A, Ates M. Pulmonary tuberculosis in patients with diabetes mellitus. Respiration. 2001;68:595-600.

Chapter 8

Hemoptysis

INTRODUCTION

The expectoration of blood has for centuries been regarded as pathognomonic of tuberculosis. Many nontubercular patients were sent to tuberculosis sanatoria merely because of this symptom. Even today many physicians consider hemoptysis invariably as tubercular in origin, despite the constantly expanding categories of disease known to be associated with it. This chapter aims to review the etiology, pathogenesis, diagnostic workup and treatment of hemoptysis.

Hemoptysis is defined as the coughing up of blood from lower respiratory tract.[1] It is encountered in 10–15% of respiratory disease patients. It has to be distinguished from hematemesis. The distinguishing points are reproduced below in tabulated form (Table 8.1).

Table 8.1: Distinguishing points between hemoptysis and hematemesis

		Hemoptysis	Hematemesis
1.	History of past illness	Lung diseases	Upper gastrointestinal tract
2.	Predisposing factors	Physical strain, severe bout of cough	Vomiting
3.	Preceding symptoms	Tickling in forces and cough	Nausea and vomiting
4.	Nature of blood	Fresh, frothy and red in color	Clotted and altered
5.	pH of blood	Alkaline	Acidic
6.	Mixed with	Froth	Food particles
7.	Post symptoms	Blood tingling of sputum	Blood may be detected in stool
8.	Hemosiderin laden macrophages in sputum	Present	Absent

PSEUDO OR SPURIOUS HEMOPTYSIS

This term is implied when source of bleeding is above the larynx and the causes are as follows:

- Blood form oral cavity, nares, pharynx and tongue
- Aspirated blood from hematemesis
- When oropharynx is colonized with a red pigment producing aerobic gram-negative rod—serratia marcescens.[2] This colonization is more in hospitalized patients who have received broad-spectrum antibiotics and mechanical ventilatory support
- Oxidation of inhaled bronchodilaters occasionally results in a brownish red color that can impart a pink color to expectorated sputum
- Self-inflicting injuries and malingering.

GRADES OF HEMOPTYSIS

There are three grades of hemoptysis:

1. *Mild:* When there is streak of bright red blood in the sputum.
2. *Massive:* It has been arbitrarily defined as the expectoration of greater than 600 mL of blood in 24 hours or greater than 500 mL[3] of blood in single bout. It is present in 4–10% of all the patients of hemoptysis. All too often massive hemoptysis is medical catastrophe. It is serious and potentially fatal problem. Patient may die within few minutes from asphyxiation before any treatment can be carried out. Also beyond the actual quantity of expectorated blood, rate of bleeding appears to be clinically imporatant.[4]
3. *Moderate:* When quantity of expectorated blood is between mild and massive hemoptysis.

RECURRENT HEMOPTYSIS

Bleeding episode that recur at an interval of less than one year.[5]

ETIOLOGY OF HEMOPTYSIS

1. Inflammatory:
    - Pulmonary tuberculosis
    - Pneumonia
    - Bronchitis
    - Bronchiectasis
    - Lung abscess
    - Necrotizing lesions
        - *Klebsiella pneumoniae*
        - *Staphylococcal pneumonia*
        - *E. coli*
        - *Anaerobic infection.*

2. Neoplasm:
    - Bronchogenic carcinoma
    - Bronchial adenoma
    - Secondaries (rare)
    - Kaposi sarcoma.
3. Cardiovascular:
    - Mitral stenosis
    - Pulmonary thromboembolism
    - Pulmonary infarction
    - Eisenmenger syndrome
    - Pulmonary arteriovenous malformation
    - Left ventricular failure
    - Rupture of aneurysm of aorta into trachea
    - Pulmonary hypertension
    - Hepatopulmonary syndrome.
4. Injury to lungs:
    - Pulmonary contusion
    - Foreign body in respiratory passages.
5. Iatrogenic:
    - After bronchoscopy/pleural biopsy/lung biopsy.
6. Parasitic infections:
    - Pulmonary amebiasis
    - Hydatid cyst
    - Tropical pulmonary eosinophilia
    - Paragonimiasis.
7. Mycotic infection:
    - Candidiasis
    - Aspergillosis
    - Blastomycosis.
8. Hemorrhagic diathesis:
    - Anticoagulant therapy
    - Thrombocytopenia
    - Coagulopathies.
9. Granulomatous lesions:
    - Vasculitis
    - Goodpasture's syndrome
    - Systemic lupus erythematosus
    - Idiopathic pulmonary hemosiderosis.
10. Pneumoconiosis
11. Miscellaneous:
    - Broncholith
    - Cyst, bullae
    - Cystic fibrosis

- Catamenial hemoptysis
- Idiopathic pulmonary hemosiderosis
- Malingering.

12. Idiopathic or essential hemoptysis—like essential hypertension there is essential or idiopathic hemoptysis where cause of hemoptysis is unknown despite best possible investigations. Its prevalence varies from 2–18%[6,7] of total hemoptysis. It is most common in men between age of 30 and 50 years. Prolong follow-up of these patients almost always fails to reveal the source of bleeding even though 10% of them continue to have episodes of hemoptysis. Antituberculous drugs should not be given for mere presence of this symptom unless some definite proof of tuberculosis is forthcoming.

The most common causes of hemoptysis in India are:

1. Pulmonary tuberculosis
2. Bronchiectasis
3. Chronic bronchitis
4. Bronchogenic carcinoma
5. Mitral stenosis

HEMOPTYSIS WITH NORMAL CHEST X-RAY

The expectoration of blood is always an alarming symptom. Most serious causes of hemoptysis produce significant radiographic changes that will point the way to subsequent investigations. A normal radiograph reduces the possibilities considerably but malignancy, pulmonary emboli, bronchitis and other minor infective causes remain possible. The history may help but there will remain a group of patients with hemoptysis that could due to malignancy or could be due to bronchitis or another nonthreatening condition.

MECHANISM OF BLEEDING

Lung has a dual blood supply, pulmonary artery carries blood from right ventricle through lungs for oxygenation of blood at a mean arterial pressure 20 mm of Hg and most of its capillary network and arteriole interact with airway at level of terminal bronchiole. The tissue of lung derive their oxygenated blood supply from bronchial arterial circulation which arises from proximal descending thoracic aorta. Bronchial artery circulation runs the entire length of bronchial tree and is at systemic arterial pressure. Due to higher circulatory pressure and closer proximity to airways, hemoptysis is more likely to arise from bronchial rather than from pulmonary arterial circulation. Bleeding from pulmonary vessel alone is rare except in situation of an arteriovenous malformation. In lung cancer, the tumor has to achieve a supply of oxygenated blood and thus develops connections from the systemic circulation. The vessels in a tumor are often poorly formed and thus prone to bleed. Anything that damages the tumor, e.g. endobronchial radiotherapy (brachytherapy), may cause bleeding from damaged systemic vessels. In addition, a tumor may invade large vessels such as the pulmonary artery or the aorta, leading to massive bleeding.

PATHOGENESIS OF HEMOPTYSIS IN TUBERCULOSIS

Hemoptysis is usually found in 12–30% of patients with pulmonary tuberculosis. It may occur at any stage of disease but is more likely to occur in far advanced disease. Some patient may have hemoptysis as first presenting symptom while in others it may be the terminal event. Some patient even may have recurrent bouts of hemoptysis even though they continue to be getting effective chemotherapy. Patients of pulmonary tuberculosis who have hemoptysis as first presenting symptoms are lucky because they do not delay in attending the hospital. Hemoptysis can occur in pulmonary tuberculosis either in active stage of disease or as a sequelae to healed pulmonary tuberculosis.

Hemoptysis in Active Pulmonary Tuberculosis

In active pulmonary tuberculosis bleeding can occur in following ways: From cavity due to rupture of aneurysmal dilatation (Rasmussen's aneurysm) of vessels in and around the cavity, from endobronchial lesion due to acute tuberculous ulceration of bronchial mucosa and sometimes from acute exudative lesions due to necrosis of small branches of pulmonary artery or vein. Very rarely bleeding can occur due to alteration of hemostatic mechanism like increase in prothrombin time due to pyrazinamide and thrombocytopenia due to pyrazinamide, rifampicin and thioacetazone.

Hemoptysis in Healed Pulmonary Tuberculosis

In healed pulmonary tuberculosis bleeding can occur in following ways: From calcified lesions which can erode bronchus or a blood vessel, bleeding can also occur from open healed cavities (open negative syndrome) such cavities, despite epithelialization, continue to be traversed by degenerated and dilated blood vessels, which are liable to breakdown at the slightest provocation or fungus ball, which can grow in healed cavities and erodes the blood vessels. Healed fibrotic parenchymal lesion due to the irritation of granulation tissue in the walls of bronchiectatic airways in the same areas. Scar carcinoma can develop in healed tuberculous lesions rarely and can cause hemoptysis It is important to distinguish between the hemoptysis caused by active tuberculosis and that caused by healed tuberculosis whereas the former calls for antituberculosis drugs and same is not needed for the later.

DIAGNOSIS OF HEMOPTYSIS

History, physical examination and investigations are done to establish the cause of hemoptysis and localize the site of bleeding. An episode of hemoptysis is first routinely evaluated and special evaluation is done according to results of the routine evaluation and the possible categories of the cause of hemoptysis concerned. Following evaluation can be done in patients of hemoptysis.

1. Careful examination of upper respiratory tract is important in establishing whether the bleeding has originated from sources other than the lungs and bronchi (Pseudohemoptysis). One should examine the mouth for ulcerations or tumors, dentures to look for a bleeding site. A mirror examination of larynx is indicated to rule out the pharyngeal causes of hemoptysis.
2. Investigation should begin with routine techniques like history, physical examination and chest X-ray (Tables 8.2 to 8.4). The initial laboratory evaluation of patient should include a hemogram, bleeding and coagulation time (Table 8.5).
3. Sputum smear examination for acid-fast bacilli (AFB) and malignant cells.
4. Bronchoscopy is most valuable diagnostic techniques and should be done in all patients with hemoptysis of uncertain cause. Timing of bronchoscopy remains controversial. There is high rate of localization

Table 8.2: Diagnostic clues in hemoptysis: History

Clinical clues	Suggested diagnosis
• Anticoagulant use	• Medication effect, coagulation disorder
• Association with menses	• Catamenial hemoptysis
• Dyspnea on exertion, fatigue, orthopnea, paroxysmal nocturnal dyspnea, frothy pink sputum	• Congestive heart failure, left ventricular dysfunction, mitral valve stenosis
• Fever, productive cough	• Upper respiratory infection, acute sinusitis, acute bronchitis, pneumonia, lung abscess
• History of breast, colon, or renal cancers	• Endobronchial metastatic disease of lungs
• History of chronic lung disease, recurrent lower respiratory tract infection, cough with copious purulent sputum	• Bronchiectasis, lung abscess
• HIV, immunosuppression	• Neoplasia, tuberculosis, Kaposi's sarcoma
• Nausea, vomiting, melena, alcoholism, chronic use of nonsteroidal anti-inflammatory drugs	• Gastritis, gastric or peptic ulcer, esophageal varices
• Pleuritic chest pain, calf tenderness	• Pulmonary embolism or infarction
• Tobacco use	• Acute bronchitis, chronic bronchitis, lung cancer, pneumonia
• Weight loss	• Emphysema, lung cancer, tuberculosis, bronchiectasis, lung abscess, HIV

Table 8.3: Diagnostic clues in hemoptysis: Physical examination

Clinical clues	Suggested diagnosis
• Cachexia, clubbing, voice hoarseness, Cushing's syndrome, hyperpigmentation, Horner's syndrome	• Bronchogenic carcinoma, small cell lung cancer, other primary lung cancers
• Clubbing	• Primary lung cancer, bronchiectasis, lung abscess, severe chronic lung disease, secondary lung metastases
• Dullness to percussion, fever, unilateral rales	• Pneumonia
• Facial tenderness, fever, mucopurulent nasal discharge, postnasal drainage	• Acute upper respiratory infection, acute sinusitis
• Fever, tachypnea, hypoxia, hypertrophied accessory respiratory muscles, barrel chest, intercostal retractions, pursed lip breathing, rhonchi, wheezing, tympani to percussion, distant heart sounds	• Acute exacerbation of chronic bronchitis, primary lung cancer, pneumonia
• Gingival thickening, mulberry gingivitis, saddle nose, nasal septum perforation	• Wegener's granulomatosis
• Heart murmur, pectus excavatum	• Mitral valve stenosis
• Lymph node enlargement, cachexia, violaceous tumors on skin	• Kaposi's sarcoma secondary to human immunodeficiency virus infection
• Orofacial and mucous membrane telangiectasia, epistaxis	• Osler-Weber-Rendu disease
• Tachycardia, tachypnea, hypoxia, jugulovenous distention, S3 gallop, decreased lung sounds, bilateral rales, dullness to percussion in lower lung fields	• Congestive heart failure caused by left ventricular dysfunction or severe mitral valve stenosis
• Tachypnea, tachycardia, dyspnea, fixed split S2, pleural friction rub, unilateral leg pain and edema	• Pulmonary thromboembolic disease
• Tympani to percussion over lung apices, cachexia	• Tuberculosis

of hemoptysis site[8] with early bronchoscopy but timing rarely alters the suspected cause of bleeding or overall patients management. Early bronchoscopy is recommended in the management of massive hemoptysis choice of bronchoscope whether flexible or rigid is also debated although flexible bronchoscope is the instrument of choice for nonmassive hemoptysis as it is well tolerated by patients and provide extravisual range into segmental bronchi. In massive hemoptysis choice depend upon users experience. Many surgeons advocate use of rigid bronchoscope because of better suctioning capacity, larger lumen and allow continuous airway control.[9] Bronchogenic carcinoma has been detected in 2–13% patients with hemoptysis and a normal chest X-ray. Foreign body, bronchial adenoma and other causes of bleeding can be identified and site of bleeding usually can be determined. While need

Table 8.4: Diagnostic clues in hemoptysis: Chest radiograph

Chest radiograph finding	Suggested diagnosis
• Cardiomegaly, increased pulmonary vascular distribution	• Chronic heart failure, mitral valve stenosis
• Cavitary lesions	• Lung abscess, tuberculosis, necrotizing carcinoma
• Diffuse alveolar infiltrates	• Chronic heart failure, pulmonary edema, aspiration, toxic injury
• Hilar adenopathy or mass	• Carcinoma, metastatic disease, sarcoid
• Hyperinflation	• Chronic obstructive pulmonary disease
• Lobar or segmental infiltrates	• Pneumonia, thromboembolism, obstructing carcinoma
• Mass lesion, nodules, granulomas	• Carcinoma, metastatic disease, Wegener's granulomatosis, septic embolism, vasculitides
• Normal or no change from baseline	• Bronchitis, upper respiratory infection, sinusitis, pulmonary embolism
• Patchy alveolar infiltrates (multiple bleeding sites)	• Bleeding disorders, idiopathic pulmonary hemosiderosis, Goodpasture's syndrome

Table 8.5: Diagnostic clues in hemoptysis: Laboratory tests

Test	Diagnostic findings
• White blood cell count and differential diagnosis	• Elevated cell count and differential shifts may be present in upper and lower respiratory tract infections
• Hemoglobin, hematocrit	• Decreased in anemia
• Platelet count	• Decreased in thrombocytopenia
• Prothrombin time, International normalized ratio, partial thromboplastin time	• Increased in anticoagulant use, disorders of coagulation
• Arterial blood gases	• Hypoxia, hypercarbia
• D-dimer	• Elevated in pulmonary embolism
• Sputum gram stain, culture, acid-fast bacillus smear and culture	• Pneumonia, lung abscess, tuberculosis, mycobacterial infections
• Sputum cytology	• Neoplasm
• Purified protein derivative skin test	• Positive increases risk for tuberculosis
• Human immunodeficiency virus test	• Positive increases risk for tuberculosis, Kaposi's sarcoma
• Erythrocyte sedimentation rate	• Elevated in infection, autoimmune disorders (e.g. Wegener's syndrome, systemic lupus erythematosus, sarcoid, Goodpasture's syndrome), may be elevated in neoplasia

for fiberoptic bronchoscopy in evaluating hemoptysis is clear but its timing in the face of active bleeding is somewhat controversial. Early bronchoscopy is desirable because it minimizes the likelihood that the site of bleeding will go undetected because bleeding has stopped. There is concern however that (1) cough induced by procedure may promote more bleeding and (2) blood may spread through tracheobronchial tree by the procedure and obscure the bleeding site. Most chest physician now favor early bronchoscopy in the patients with hemoptysis of unknown cause, since fiberoptic bronchoscopy with good local anesthesia rarely exacerbates bleeding and lavage can clear blood from sites not actively bleeding.

5. CT scan is a potential tool for investigating cause and site of hemoptysis if earlier investigations could not ascertain a cause. CT scan is a non-invasive investigations though carrying a radiation exposure. Chest CT scan is invaluable in patients with normal chest radiograph and hemoptysis to detect peripheral neoplasm and bronchiectasis it should precede bronchoscopy to direct bronchoscopic techniques to area of abnormality[10] HRCT has replaced bronchography for diagnosis of bronchiectasis.[11]
6. Bronchial arteriography: Its main advantage is to localize the site of bleeding to plan bronchial artery embolization.
7. Blood gas analysis may be done when patient is suspected to be in respiratory failure.
8. Perfusion and ventilation lung scan may occasionally be indicated to detect regional ventilation and perfusion alterations including those due to pulmonary embolism.

Lymph node, pleural and lung biopsy may occasionally be required in some patients. Very rarely exploratory thoracotomy may be required in few to establish the cause of hemoptysis.

For diagnosis of nonmassive hemoptysis see Flow Chart. 8.1.

TREATMENT OF HEMOPTYSIS

Treatment of hemoptysis varies according to amount of bleeding, the specific cause and the overall condition of the patient and basic objectives of treatment are to prevent asphyxiation, stop bleeding and to treat primary cause. Treatment of hemoptysis can be divided into supportive and definitive treatment.

Supportive Treatment

1. *Strict bed rest:* Complete physical and mental rest is must.
2. *Posture of patient:* Back rest is given in alert patient. Head low position is adviced in comatose or semicomatose patients. Patient should be

Flow Chart 8.1: Algorithm for evaluation of nonmassive hemoptysis

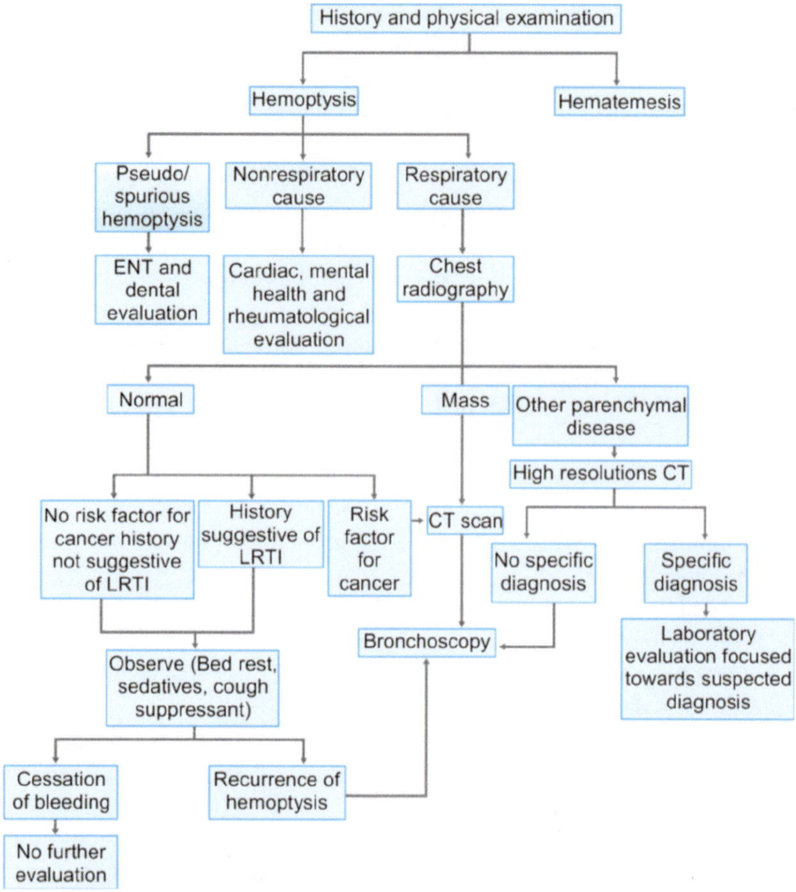

positioned with the suspected bleeding site dependent so as to minimize the aspiration of blood into contralateral lung, if bleeding site is unknown then patient is advised to lie supine.

3. *Sedation:* Small doses of sedatives are used since these drugs may depress consciousness and may allow the aspiration of blood into the contralateral lung. Usually phenobarbitone in doses of 30–60 mg three times daily is used. Diazepam 5–10 mg three times daily, chlordiazepoxide 10–25 mg/24 h oral can also be used. If adequate sedation is not achieved, pentazocine 30 mg IM, morphine 5–7.5 mg S/C or 2 mg IV, buprenorphine 0.2 mg IV are usually given. Habbit forming drugs like morphine or its derivatives or pethedine should be avoided.
4. *Suppression of cough:* Following cough suppressant are commonly used:
   i. Codeine phosphate 15–30 mg. 3 or 4 times daily (in children 1.5–2.5 mg/kg/day in divided doses).

   ii. Noscapine 15–30 mg, 3–4 times daily.
   iii. Dextromethorphan hydrobromide 15–30 mg, 3–4 times daily (in children 1 mg/kg/day in divided doses).
   iv. Chlophedianol hydrochloride 20–40 mg, 3–4 times daily
   v. Pipazethate hydrochloride 40 mg 3–4 times daily.
   vi. Peripherally acting antitussives like benzonatate (Adults and children older than 10 years: 100 mg, TID up to 600 mg/d) and levodropropizine 30 mg 3–4 times daily.

   Recently some physicians have raised controversy over the use of antitussives since cough may be necessary to clear blood from airways and to avoid asphyxiation, but antitussives are essentially used in our country to control the hemoptysis.
5. *Antibiotic:* Since blood is a good culture medium, there is every possibility of respiratory superinfection, so appropriate antibiotic is usually empirically started.
6. *Blood transfusion:* It may be required when there is marked blood loss; it is usually given when hematocrit value is less than 30% or hemoglobin is less than 8 g%.
7. *Oxygen:* It is given only if patient is dyspneic or in low general condition. If bleeding is moderate to massive and there is minimal respiratory reserve, an emergency situation exists. Arterial blood gases should be monitored and hypoxemia corrected with supplemental oxygen. An arterial oxygen tension of 50 to 60 mm of Hg with supplemental oxygen is a reasonable therapeutic goal. Patient with hypercapnia and respiratory acidemia from massive hemoptysis should ideally be intubated and treated with mechanical ventilation. Following intubation, suctioning should be done, which may partially or completely reverse the respiratory failure.
8. *Avoid:* Following thing should be avoided as far as possible when patient is actively bleeding:
   i. Detailed history taking and physical examination, frequent movement from bed to bed and bed to X-ray room.
   ii. Steam inhalations and warm saline gargles
   iii. Postural drainage and frequent chest percussion
   iv. Expectorants and mucolytic drugs
   v. Bronchodilator as it can precipitate renewed bleeding by vasodilation.
9. *Coagulants:* Do not use coagulants unless there is deficiency of clotting factor. Drugs like estrogen, snake venom, lung extract, n-butanol, aminocaproic and stylin, vitamin C and calcium, etc. have no proven efficacy in the control of hemoptysis. Unfortunately, such drugs are very frequently used in our country for the control of hemoptysis.

Definitive Treatment

Definitive treatment will depend upon cause and amount of bleeding and patient underlying lung functions.

1. *Mild to moderate hemoptysis:* Apart from supportive treatment, treatment of specific cause is carried out. Usually, bleeding is controlled in 4–7 days[13] with the help of supportive treatment. If bleeding still persists or its amount increase then patient should be treated as massive hemoptysis.
2. *Massive hemoptysis:* Definitive treatment of massive hemoptysis included treatment of specific disease and immediate control of bleeding while maintaining airways. Conservative "wait and see" management of massive hemoptysis is associated with death up to 60% while immediate surgical intervention may reduce the mortality to 20%. The method by which bleeding is stopped is also depend on underlying cause, local facilities, local expertise and lung functions. For active control of bleeding, supportive treatment may be tried for 24–48 hours, if bleeding persists then ideally bleeding site is localized by bronchoscope (rigid or fiberoptic). Bronchoscopy also helps to remove blood from airways and if bronchoscope is not available or it is contraindicated by poor clinical status of patient endotracheal intubation is recommended to allow aspiration to clear the airway of clot and blood.[12] Cold saline[9] lavage and epinephrine 1:20,000 instillation of bleeding site may be done through bronchoscope. If bleeding still persists then endobronchial balloon tamponade using fogarty balloon catheter through bronchoscope may be tried to stop the bleeding.[14]

If bleeding is not controlled by above mentioned measures then emergency surgery is indicated provided patient is fit for surgery. Choice of surgery is resection if not possible then thoracoplasty may be done and if patient is not fit for surgery then collapse measures like artificial pneumothorax (when side of bleeding is known) or pneumoperitoneum (when side of bleeding is not known and artificial pneumothorax is not possible due to presence of adhesions) may be tried. Where facilities for bronchial artery angiography and embolization are available, bronchial artery embolization using foam-based material is done. The diagnostic and therapeutic role of bronchial artery angiography and embolization are not well defined but usually indicated (i) when source of massive bleeding is not defined by other methods and (ii) therapeutically when surgery cannot be performed and bleeding is refractory to other conservative methods. This procedure is usually advised to be done in patients who are either actively bleeding or within 6–12 hours of bleeding or within 6–12 hours of bleeding and required highly skilled physicians.

REFERENCES

1. Marini JJ. Hemoptysis. In: Respiratory Medicine for the House Officer. 2nd edn. Baltimore: Williams and Wilkins. 1987:223-5.
2. Gale D. Overgrowth of Serratia marcescens in respiratory tract simulating hemoptysis. JAMA. 1957;164:1328-30.
3. Johnston RN, Lockhart W, Ritchie RT, Smith DM. Hemoptysis. Br Med J. 1960;1:592-5.
4. Winter SM, Ingbar DH. Massive hemoptysis: pathogenesis and management. J Intensive Care Med. 1988;3:171-88.
5. Israel RH, Poe RH. Hemoptysis. Clin Chest Med. 1987;8:197-205.
6. Pursal SE, Lindskog GE. Haemoptysis: a clinical evaluation of 105 patients examined consecutively on a thoracic sugery service. Am Rev Respir Dis. 1961;84:329-36.
7. Lyons HA. Diffrential diagnosis of haemoptysis and its treatment. ATS News. 1976;26-30.
8. Gong H, Salvatierra C. Clinical efficacy of early and delayed fiberoptic bronchoscopy in patients with hemoptysis. Am Rev Respir Dis. 1981;124 221-5.
9. Conlan AA, Hurwitz SS. Management of massive hemoptysis with the rigid bronchoscope and cold saline lavage. Thorax. 1980;35:901-4.
10. Millar AB, Boothroyd AE, Edwards D, Hetzel M. The role of computed tomography (CT) in the investigations of unexplained haemoptysis. Respir Med. 1992;86:39-44.
11. Naidich DP, Funt S, Ettenger NA, Arranda C. Haemoptysis CT bronchoscopic correlations in 58 cases. Radiology. 1990;177:357-62.
12. Dellinger RP. Fiberoptic bronchoscopy in adult airway management. Crit Care Med. 1990;18:882-7.
13. Prasad R, Garg R, Singhal S, Srivastava P. Lessons from patients with hemoptysis attending a chest clinic in India. ATM. 2009;4(1):10-2.
14. Hiebert CA. Balloon catheter control of life-threatening hemoptysis. Chest. 1974;66:308-9.

Chapter 9

Diagnostic Techniques in Tuberculosis

9A: DIAGNOSIS OF LATENT TUBERCULOSIS INFECTION

One-third of the world's population is infected with *Mycobacterium tuberculosis*. The only available test to detect infection was, until recently, the tuberculin skin test (TST).

TUBERCULIN SKIN TEST

The tuberculin skin test is generally used to detect infection with *M. tuberculosis* which is based on the fact that the infection with the bacillus produces sensitivity to certain components present in culture extracts called tuberculins. It is actually a glycerine extract of the tubercule bacilli. It was first described by Robert Koch in 1890. The material used by him was named as old tuberculin (OT) which was gradually replaced by purified protein derivative (PPD). It is a precipitate of nonspecies-specific molecules obtained from filtrates of sterilized, concentrated cultures. The test is named after Charles Mantoux, a French physician who facilitated the work of Koch by developing the intradermal test to be administered by injection as a measured volume. Several other techniques were also developed such as Heaf test and Tine test but variation in the dose of tuberculin has made these techniques obsolete except the Mantoux test that has been widely used in recent times. The TST measures delayed type hypersensitivity response to the purified protein derivative (PPD). Currently, only two tubeculins have been accepted as standard tuberculins by WHO, i.e. PPD-S and PPD RT 23. The International Standard tuberculins are in custody of the Laboratory of Biological Standards, Staten Serum Institute (SSI), Copenhagen, Denmark.[1] In India PPD-RT 23 is manufactured at Guindy Laboratory, Chennai. All tuberculins have been standardized for activity in tuberculin units against PPD-S. One tuberculin unit (TU) of PPD was defined as the activity contained in 0.02 microgram of PPD. A standard 5 tuberculin unit (5 TU) dose of PPD-S is defined as delayed skin activity contained in a 0.1 μg/0.1 mL dose of PPD-S. 1 TU of PPD-RT 23 is equivalent to 5 TU of PPD-S.[2] This is for maintaining uniformity and comparability of various test results all over the world. Any pharmaceutical company marketing formulations containing any other type of PPD or in any different strength from the one mentioned above are best ignored. PPD-RT 23 with Tween 80 of strength 1 TU and 2 TU are standardized tuberculins available in India supplied by BCG vaccine Laboratory, Guindy, Chennai. Other tuberculins available in the market are not standardized. Tween 80 is a detergent added to tuberculin to prevent their adsorption on glass or plastic surface. Presently, all tuberculins are manufactured and standardized with Tween 80.[3] A series of studies conducted in India demonstrated equal sensitivity for 1 TU and 2 TU in detection of true infection with TB bacillus and no change in potency of 1 TU PPD has been observed. Most countries prefer to use PPD RT23 with Tween 80 while some countries like USA use PPD-S (Siebert) of lot 49608. The tuberculins are also extracted from species of non-tuberculous mycobacteria such as PPD-B from *Mycobacterium intracellulare*, PPD-G from *Mycobacterium scrofulaceum* and PPD-A from *Mycobacterium avium*. These are used only for epidemiological surveys. Tuberculin sensitivity is a delayed type of hypersensitivity reaction in the form of induration at the test site in sensitized host. Histologically the earliest phase of reaction is seen as a perivascular cuffing of mononuclear cells followed by more extensive exudation of mononuclear and polymorphonuclear cells which later migrate to leave only mononuclear cells. When these sensitized T cells come in contact with specific antigens they secrete lymphokines, which in turn, recruit more lymphocytes at the site of inflammation and give rise to characteristic type IV response.[4]

Procedure

A standard dose of 5 Tuberculin units (0.1 mL) of PPD-S or 1 Tuberculin (0.02 μg) of PPD RT-23 in 0.1 mL of the diluents with Tween 80 is injected intradermally (between the layers of dermis) and read 48–72 hours later. A person who has been exposed to the bacteria is expected to mount an immune response in the skin containing the bacterial proteins. The reaction is read by measuring the diameter of induration (palpable raised hardened area) across the forearm (perpendicular to the long axis) in millimeters. If there is no induration, the result should be recorded as "0 mm". Erythema (redness) should not be measured. If a person has had a history of a positive tuberculin skin test, another skin test is not needed. The delayed type of hypersensitivity reaction peaks at 48–96 hours with an area of maximal erythmatous induration.

Classification of Tuberculin Reaction

The results of this test must be interpreted carefully. The person's medical risk factors determine at which increment (5 mm, 10 mm, or 15 mm) of induration the result is considered positive (Table 9.1).

Conversion is defined as the development of new delayed type hypersensitivity to mycobacteria antigens following new infection with *M. tuberculosis,* nontuberculous mycobacteria, or BCG vaccination. It is confidently stated when a previously tuberculin negative individual becomes positive after receiving BCG vaccination, following significant exposure such as during an outbreak or as a result of close contact with a highly contagious index case. An increased reaction is more likely because of new mycobacterial infection if several prior tuberculin tests were negative, particularly if baseline two-step tuberculin testing was performed.[5] In terms of size, it has been defined as a second reaction of 10+ mm and an increase of at least 6 mm.[6] This criteria has variability depending on studies in populations with high prevalence of boosting. Loss of tuberculin reactivity over time has been termed reversion and is estimated to occur at a rate of 5% per year in a healthy population. This is primarily due to a specific waning of cell-mediated immunity for tuberculin antigen. The percentage of significant reactors to tuberculin declines with age in elderly subjects and many adults.

Table 9.1: Interpretation of the tuberculin skin test

A positive result indicates TB exposure
• 5 mm or more is positive in:
– HIV-positive person
– Recent contacts of TB case
– Persons with nodular or fibrotic changes on chest X-ray consistent with old healed TB
– Patients with organ transplants and other immunosuppressed patients
• 10 mm or more is positive in:
– Recent arrivals (less than 5 years) from high-prevalence countries
– Injection drug users
– Residents and employees of high-risk congregate settings (e.g. prisons, nursing homes, hospitals, homeless shelters, etc.)
– Mycobacteriology laboratory personnel
– Persons with clinical conditions that place them at high risk (e.g. diabetes, prolonged corticosteroid therapy, leukemia, end-stage renal disease, chronic malabsorption syndromes, low body weight, etc.)
– Children less than 4 years of age, or children and adolescents exposed to adults in high-risk categories
– Cross-sensitivity induced by environmental mycobacteria
• 15 mm or more is positive in:
– Persons with no known risk factors for TB

The phenomenon of increased tuberculin reactions upon re-testing in the absence of new infection, is believed to result from recall of waned cell-mediated immunity, akin to the anamnestic serologic response. Boosting is maximal if the interval between the first and second test is between 1 and 5 weeks and is much less frequent if the interval is only 48 hours or more than 60 days, although boosting can be detected one or more years after a first negative tuberculin test.[7]

Limitations of Tuberculin Test

The tuberculin test seems attractive because it involves low technology, is inexpensive and is relatively easy to administer and read. However, the test is not useful for the diagnosis of tubercular disease and is unable to distinguish latent or dormant infection from infection associated with active disease and will often be misleading because of false-negative and false-positive results (Table 9.2). A major limitation of PPD is the fact that it is a crude mixture of several antigens, many of which are shared among *M. tuberculosis, M. bovis* BCG, and several nontuberculous mycobacteria (NTM). At the time of diagnosis, the tuberculin test is falsely negative in 10–47% patients with active tuberculosis. The likelihood of false negative reaction increases with the extent of disease and the age of individual. In the presence of co-infection with HIV a far higher proportion of patients with active disease will have a false-negative result. It may be positive in individuals who have had prior BCG vaccination and cross-reacting sensitivity to nontubercular mycobacterial antigen. If BCG is given in infancy, a reaction of more than 10 mm is rare

Table 9.2: False-positive and false-negative tuberculin skin test results

Tuberculin skin test result	Possible reasons	Individuals who are likely to have result
False-positive	BCG vaccination	History of BCG vaccination in the past, especially after infancy, or if repeated BCG vaccinations
	Nontuberculous Mycobacteria	History of exposure to nontuberculous mycobacteria or past illness of infection or disease with NTM species
False-negative	Anergy	HIV infection, certain viral infections like measles, live virus vaccinations, immunosuppressive medications such as steroids, cancer chemotherapy, malnutrition, elderly, renal failure, severe TB disease, lymphoma or leukemia
	Recent TB infection	Recent infection within past 10–12 weeks
	Very young age	Children younger than 6 months
	Technical reasons	Inadequate dose or poor quality of PPD, poor technique, faulty interpretation

after the age of 5 years. In persons vaccinated in older age 15–25% will remain positive for as long as 22–25 years. It is a common misconception that larger tuberculin reactions are more likely to indicate active disease. Beyond 5 mm the size of the reaction does not distinguish in any way between those with active tuberculosis disease, inactive tuberculosis, recent or remote infection.

INTERFERON-γ ASSAYS

The successful sequencing of *M. tuberculosis* and *M. bovis* genomes has lead to the emergence of the field of comparative genomics (i.e. analysis and comparison of genomes from different species). Recent advances in genomics, molecular biology, and immunology have led to a promising generation of alternative tests such as T cell based, in vitro, interferon-γ (IFN-γ) assays.[8-11] While early versions of IFN-γ assays employed PPD as the stimulating antigen, it became clear that such assays will have the same specificity problems seen with the PPD based TST.[11] Extensive basic science research lead to the development of newer assays that employ antigens that are highly specific to *M. tuberculosis*. These antigens include the early secretory antigenic target 6 (ESAT-6) and culture filtrate protein (CFP-10). These low molecular weight proteins, encoded within the region of difference 1 (RD1) of the *M. tuberculosis* genome, are more specific to *M. tuberculosis* than PPD, and they are not shared with the BCG substrains and most NTM species (with the exception of *M. kansasii, M. marinum* and *M. szulgai*).[8-10]

The QuantiFERON-TB® assay was the first IFN-γ assay to become commercially available. This whole blood test was approved by the US Food and Drug Administration (FDA) in 2001 and is available in many countries.[12] However, this first generation assay measures IFN-γ response to PPD and thus is susceptible to the same specificity problems as the TST.[8] This PPD-based assay is currently being replaced by an enhanced assay, the QuantiFERON-TB-Gold® test (which uses ESAT-6 and CFP-10 in place of PPD). This new assay is currently available in Europe, and was approved by the US FDA in December 2004. PPD had 100% sensitivity but 0% specificity while ESAT-6 had 100% sensitivity and 88% specificity. Other assays, including those using the enzyme-linked immunospot (ELISPOT) to detect IFN-γ response, have also been evaluated in different settings.[8-11] The T SPOT-TB® is the second assay to reach commercial development. This assay, performed using peripheral blood mononuclear cells (PBMC), employs ESAT-6 and CFP-10, and detects the number of IFN-γ producing T cells using a sensitive ELISPOT technology. This test, currently available in Europe, is awaiting US FDA approval. In India, both QuantiFERON-TB Gold and T SPOT-TB assays have been evaluated in research settings, in rural[13] and urban populations.[14] However, these assays are currently not used in clinical practice in India.

Both the QFT and the SPOT-TB assay have been evaluated for the diagnosis of active TB and detection of LTBI among TB patients and healthy controls from areas with low, medium, and high prevalence of the disease. In a meta-analysis of numerous studies on IFN-γ assays, the sensitivity was 0.76 (95% confidence interval, CI: 0.7–0.83) by QFT and 0.88 (95% CI: 0.81–0.95) by the SPOT-TB assay when active TB patients were used as the gold standard for LTBI, indicating that the sensitivity of the SPOT assay is greater than that of QFT. On the other hand, the specificity of the IFN-γ assays was very high at 0.97 (95% CI: 0.95–0.99) by QFT and 0.92 (95% CI: 0.88–0.95) by the SPOT-TB assay when healthy controls with a low risk of LTBI were used as the negative control, indicating a greater specificity with QFT than with the SPOT-TB assay. In comparison, TST showed a sensitivity of 0.71 (95% CI: 0.65–0.74) and a specificity of 0.66 (95% CI: 0.41–0.84). The results indicate that, despite the high specificity, the sensitivity of IFN-γ assays is suboptimal and may be due to immune suppression among TB patients, which was evident in patients with cavity formation. The specificity of TST was very low, largely due to BCG vaccination in the study populations. The IFN-γ assays have been employed for diagnosis of active TB and for monitoring patients undergoing chemotherapy. In addition, IFN-γ assays have been analyzed for use in monitoring TB patient progress with chemotherapy treatment while QFT failed to show a difference in values before and after chemotherapy in TB patients. In addition, QFT values decreased when individuals with LTBI were given INH for six months for chemoprophylaxis, indicating that QFT can be also be used to monitor the efficacy of prophylactic treatment of LTBI. Likewise, IFN-γ assays were employed to monitor subjects at high risk of *M. tuberculosis* infection in order to identify newly infected persons between test intervals.

More studies are needed, however, to assess the usefulness of these tests in the management of immunocompromised individuals, in children and in those with extrapulmonary TB.[15] To fully evaluate the utility of IFN-γ assays in high burden countries such as India, long-term Cohort studies are needed to determine the association between positive IFN-γ results and the subsequent risk of active TB. If these studies consistently demonstrate a strong association between positive IFN-γ results and risk of active TB, and if the effect is stronger than that of TST, this would indicate that IFN-γ assays have a better ability to identify those at higher risk for progressing to active disease.[15]

REFERENCES

1. Bleiker JA. The past, the present and future of tuberculin test in tuberculosis control. Bull Int Tuber Lung Disease. 1989;64:33-4.
2. US Department of Health, Education and Welfare, Food and Drug Administration. Skin test antigens: Proposed implementation of efficacy review. Fed Reg. 1977;42:674-723.
3. American Thoracic Society. The tuberculin skin test–official ATS statement. Am Rev Respir Dis. 1984;124:356-63.

4. Beck JS. Skin changes in tuberculin test. Tubercle. 1991;72:81-7.
5. Bass JB, Serio RA. The use of repeated skin tests to eliminate the booster phenomenon in serial tuberculin testing. Am Rev Respir Dis 1981;123:394-6.
6. Canadian Thoracic Society. Canadian Tuberculosis Standards. Canadian Lung Association, Ottawa 1996.
7. Cauthen GM, Snider DE, Onorato LM. Boosting of tuberculin sensitivity among Southeast Asian refugees. Am J Respir. Crit Care Med. 1994;149:1597-600.
8. Andersen P, Munk ME, Pollock JM, Doherty TM. Specific immune-based diagnosis of tuberculosis. Lancet. 2000;356:1099-104.
9. Barnes PF. Diagnosing latent tuberculosis infection: turning glitter to gold. Am J Respir Crit Care Med. 2004;170:5-6.
10. Lalvani A. Spotting latent infection: the path to better tuberculosis control. Thorax. 2003; 58:916-8.
11. Pai M, Riley LW, Colford JM. Interferon-γ assays in the immunodiagnosis of tuberculosis: a systematic review. Lancet Infect Dis. 2004;4:761-76.
12. Mazurek GH, Villarino ME. Guidelines for using the QuantiFERON-TB test for diagnosing latent *Mycobacterium tuberculosis* infection. Centers for Disease Control and Prevention. MMWR Recomm Rep. 2003;52:15-8.
13. Pai M, Gokhale K, Joshi R, Dogra S, Kalantri SP, Mendiratta DK, et al. *Mycobacterium tuberculosis* infection in health care workers in rural India: comparison of a whole-blood, interferon-γ assay with tuberculin skin testing. JAMA. 2005;293:2746-55.
14. Lalvani A, Nagvenkar P, Udwadia Z, Pathan AA, Wilkinson KA, Shastri JS, et al. Enumeration of T cells specific for RD1-encoded antigens suggests a high prevalence of latent *Mycobacterium tuberculosis* infection in healthy urban Indians. J Infect Dis. 2001;183: 469-77.
15. Pai M. Alternatives to the tuberculin skin test: Interferon-γ assays in the diagnosis of *Mycobacterium tuberculosis* infection. Indian J Med Microbiol. 2005;23:151-8.

9B: RADIOLOGY

The introduction of radiography as a diagnostic tool was a landmark in our knowledge of the natural history of tuberculosis and its diagnosis. It is still widely believed that pulmonary tuberculosis can be diagnosed by chest radiography alone. However, practical experience has shown that no radiographic pattern is diagnostic of tuberculosis and many diseases may mimic tuberculosis and show a similar radiographic appearance. In studies which examined the extent of over reading and under reading of chest radiograph with special attention being paid to experience of reader found average rate of under reading to be 21.8% and over reading to be 19.5% (being lower by about 6–8% among readers who had more experience).[1,2] Another study which compared reader disagreement in chest radiography and smear microscopy[3,4] found that the highest level of disagreement between microscopists was substantially lower than the lowest level of disagreement between readers of chest radiographs. Index of disagreement on chest radiographs varied from 28–60 (least for cavitations). Both inter- and intra-individual disagreement among observers were seen when radiographs were read for case detection and diagnosis and also when serial films of cases already diagnosed were compared for follow-up. In a study by the author 49.2% of doctors of modern medicine adviced chest X-ray alone for diagnosis of pulmonary tuberculosis. Nonutilization of sputum smear microscopy and continued reliance on CXR alone was associated with a significantly higher probability of prescribing antitubercular treatment in patients with nontubercular conditions.[5]

IMAGING MODALITIES

Chest X-ray, CT scan of thorax and ultrasonography are some radiological modalities used in the diagnosis of tuberculosis. Radiography can help to localize abnormalities in the lung, but further examination is required in order to establish the tuberculous etiology of an abnormality and only bacteriology can provide the ultimate proof.

In a patient suspected of having pulmonary tuberculosis, Chest X-ray PA view is usually the first modality and is generally sufficient for diagnosis and follow-up. Computed tomography (CT) thorax can give full idea about the involvement, including finer details obscured on X-ray. Ultrasonography is used for evaluating pleural pathology usually.

IMAGING IN PULMONARY TUBERCULOSIS

This can be considered under two broad headings—(i) primary tuberculosis and (ii) postprimary tuberculosis. Though they both differ in terms of nature of lesion, site of involvement, lymphadenopathy and pleural involvement, there is considerable overlap in the findings in the above two.

Primary Tuberculosis

This form is seen in pediatric patients who are usually asymptomatic at presentation. Difficulty in obtaining sputum from them makes tuberculin skin test and abnormal chest X-ray as the only clues to make diagnosis.[6]

It involves lung parenchyma, lymph nodes, tracheobronchial tree and pleura.

Parenchymal Involvement

Consolidation

The primary tubercular lesion is generally seen as an area of consolidation. The lesion can be single, homogenous with ill-defined margins or may involve the entire lobe due to endobronchial obstruction.[7] It can affect any lobe of lung;[7] however, in adults suffering with primary TB lesion is often present in lower lobe. Cavitation is uncommon in children but it can be seen in adults with primary TB.[8] Endobronchial spread is rare. Computed tomography (CT) is superior to chest X-ray in demonstrating parenchymal lesions. Consolidation is seen as a homogenous soft tissue attenuation lesion with air bronchogram or areas of breakdown within.

Tuberculoma

It is a persistent mass-like opacity seen in both primary and postprimary tuberculosis. It is a round or oval lesion, most often seen in upper lobes and in right lung. Small discrete lesions (satellite lesions) may also be seen in the immediate vicinity.[9] Cavitation can also be seen in about 10–50% of patients.[7] On CT, it usually appears as a nodule with a regular and smooth outline. Calcification may also be seen in it.

Miliary tuberculosis

Dissemination of organisms via hematogenous route leads to miliary tuberculosis in lungs and other organs.[10] It is seen in both primary as well as postprimary tuberculosis. They are seen as small 1–2 mm tiny discrete

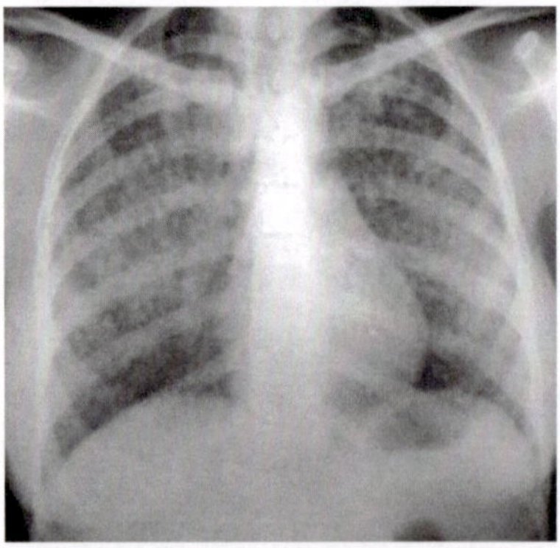

Fig. 9.1: Chest X-ray showing miliary tuberculosis

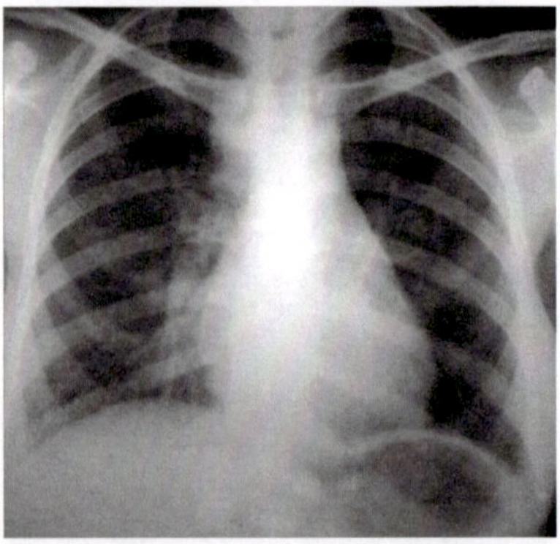

Fig. 9.2: Chest X-ray showing clearing of miliary shadows after ATT

nodules; more at lung bases due to more gravity dependent blood flow.[9] If not treated these nodules coalesce together presenting a snow storm appearance.[9] Often in a patient of miliary tuberculosis chest X-ray is normal. In such cases, HRCT is helpful in establishing miliary nodules with and without lymphadenopathy. With treatment, radiographic clearance is seen in two to six months (Figs 9.1 to 9.4).

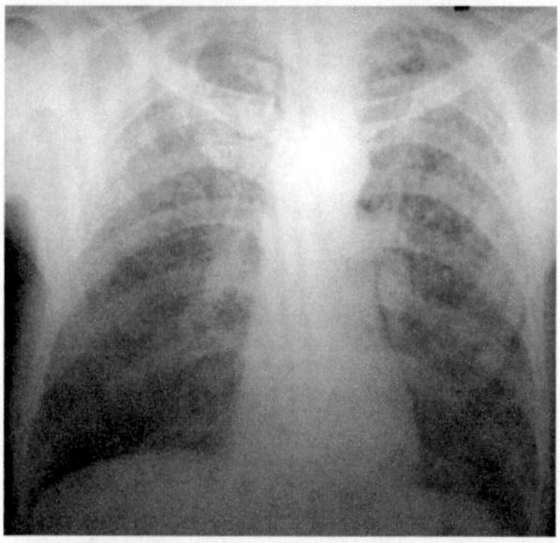

Fig. 9.3: Chest X-ray showing miliary TB

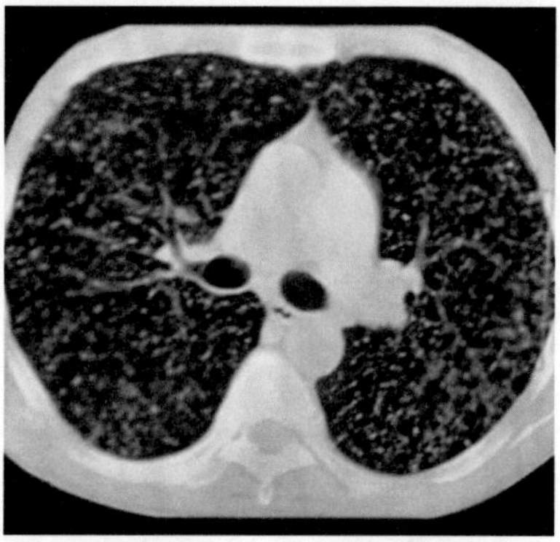

Fig. 9.4: CT thorax showing miliary TB

Lymph Node Involvement

Lymphadenopathy is a common feature of primary tuberculosis. In 96% children[11] and 10–43% adults[8] with primary TB, lymphadenopathy is seen. Right hilum and right paratracheal areas are most commonly involved areas. Bilateral adenopathy is also seen in about 31% patients.[11] Right sided predominance of lymph nodes can be due to the fact that right sided nodes drain the entire right lung along with left lower lobe. Occurrence of isolated lymphadenopathy decreases with increasing age.[6]

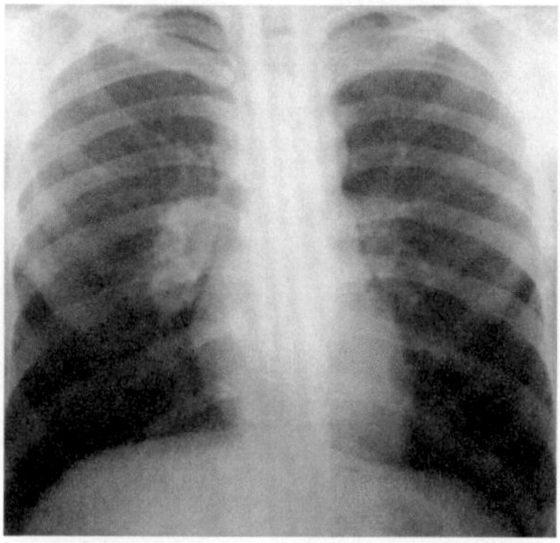

Fig. 9.5: Hilar lymphadenopathy right (Tubercular)

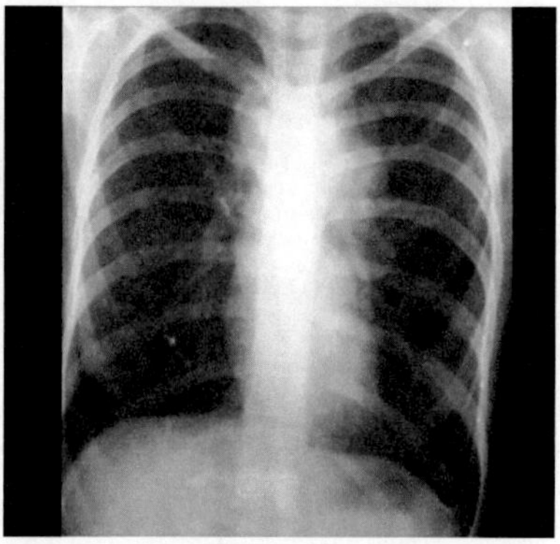

Fig. 9.6: Mediastinal lymphadenopathy (Tubercular)

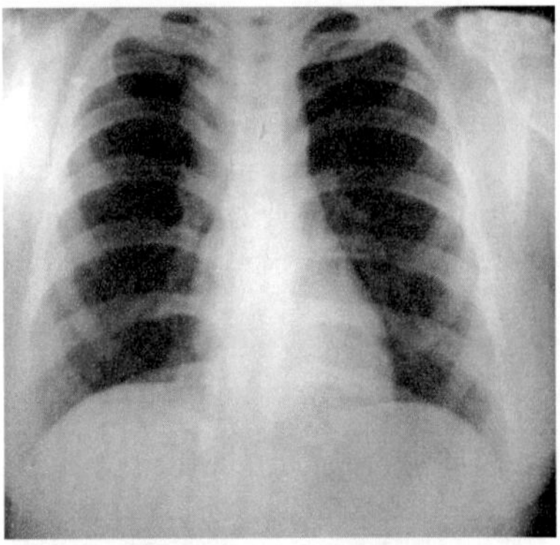

Fig. 9.7: Chest X-ray PA view showing mediastinal lympadenopathy (Tubercular)

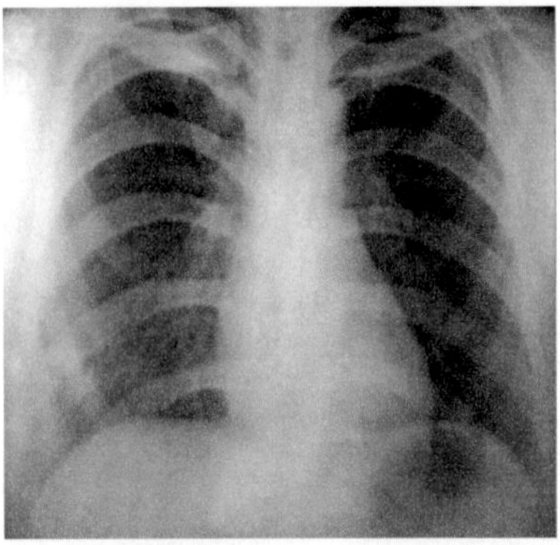

Fig. 9.8: Mediastinal lymphadenopathy disappeared after ATT

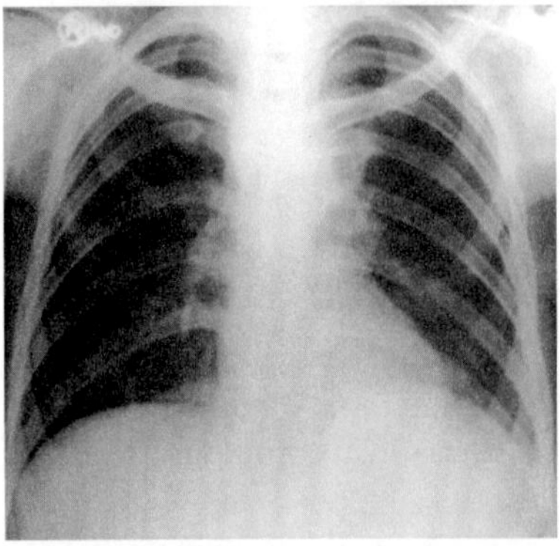

Fig. 9.9: Chest X-ray PA view showing no abnormality

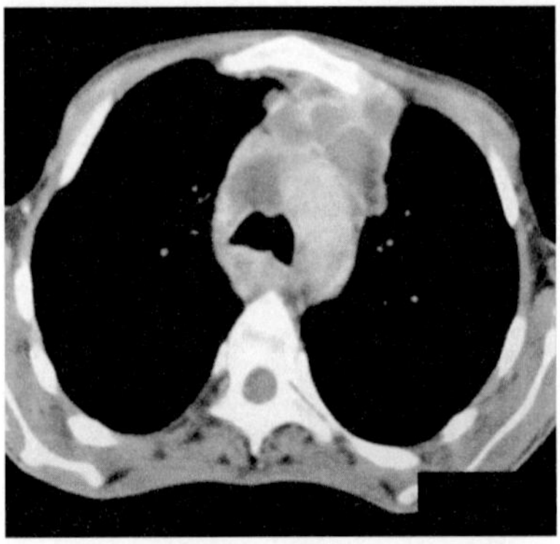

Fig. 9.10: CT thorax showing caseating enlarged mediastinal lymph nodes (Tubercular)

CT is more sensitive than a chest radiograph for detection and characterization of intrathoracic lymph nodes.[12] Peripheral rim enhancement with or without central low attenuation is the most common pattern. Rim enhancement can be uniform, thin, complete enhancing rim or thick, irregular complete or incomplete, peripheral rim or conglomerated group of lymph nodes showing peripheral and central areas of rim enhancement (Figs 9.5 to 9.10).

Airways Involvement

It is caused either due to extrinsic compression by the lymph nodes or due to endobronchial TB. The resultant narrowing leads to segmental or lobar atelectasis. Atelectasis in primary tuberculosis affects the anterior segment of upper lobe or medial segment of middle lobe. This is less commonly seen in adults.[13]

Pleural Involvement

Pleural effusion is not very common in young children with primary TB. It is commonly present in adolescents and young adults. It is most commonly present unilateral, nonloculated and moderate to large in quantity. They may also manifest as subpulmonic effusions producing an apparent elevation in ipsilateral diaphragm. Complications are usually rare but seen in the form of empyema, bronchopleural fistula, empyema necessitates or bone erosion. After healing, pleural thickening or calcification may remain. Ultrasonography is a useful investigation in the evaluation of pleural effusion, pleural thickening and empyema. CT demonstrates extent of disease, site and amount of loculations in empyema, effusion, status of underlying rib and lung pathology. On contrast enhanced CT, loculated empyema is seen as an encysted pleural collection of fluid with smooth, enhancing surrounding pleura (Figs 9.11 to 9.25).

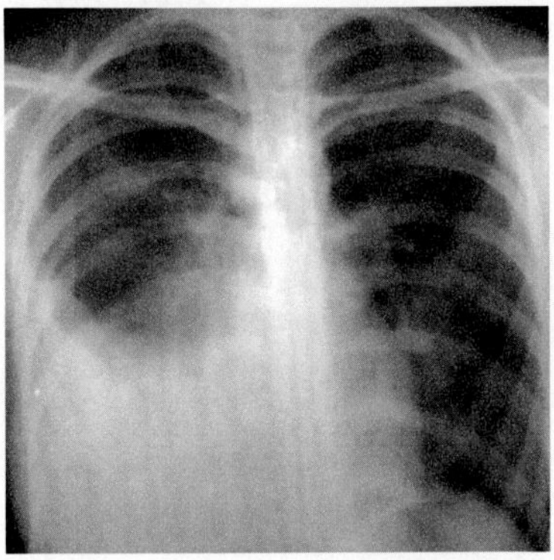

Fig. 9.11: Chest X-ray showing pleural effusion (Right)

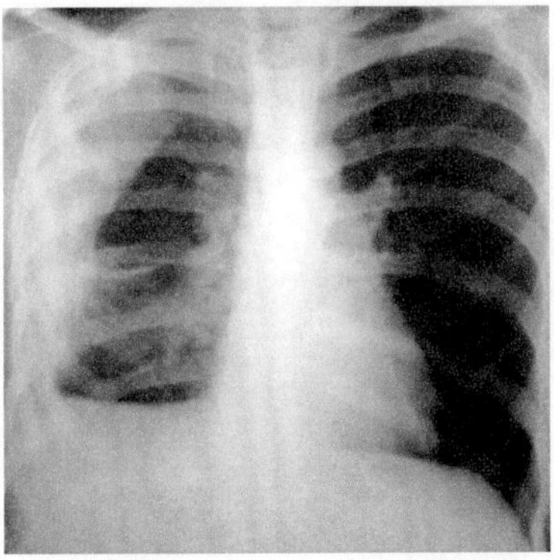

Fig. 9.12: Chest X-ray showing atypical pleural effusion (Right)

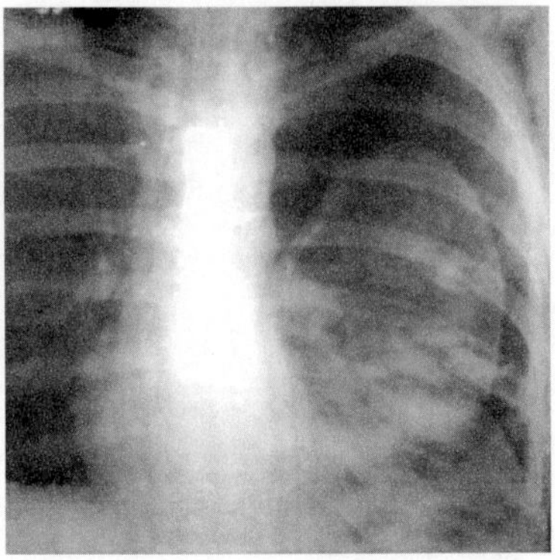

Fig. 9.13: Chest X-ray showing pneumothorax

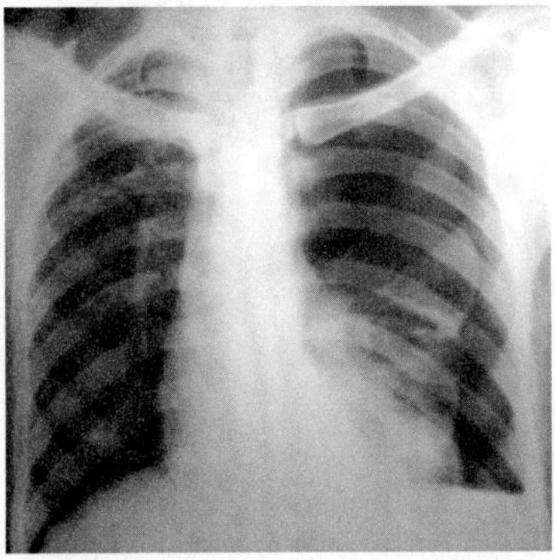

Fig. 9.14: Chest X-ray showing hydro-pneumothorax

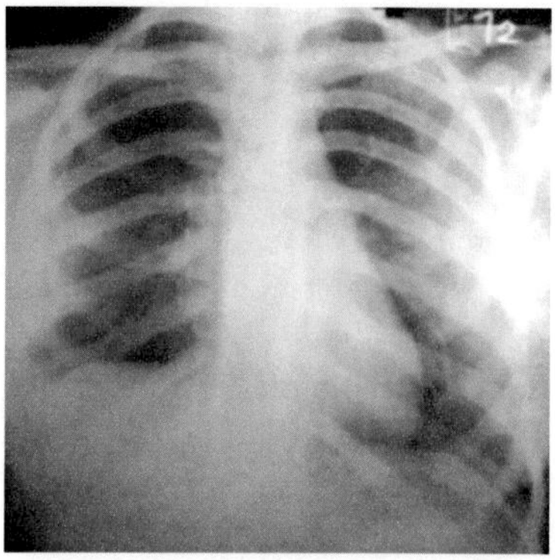

Fig. 9.15: Chest X-ray PA view showing subpulmonic effusion (Right side)

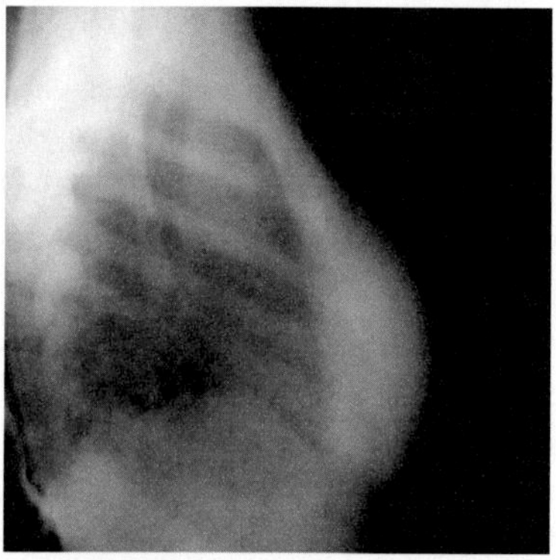

Fig. 9.16: Chest X-ray right lateral view of same patient

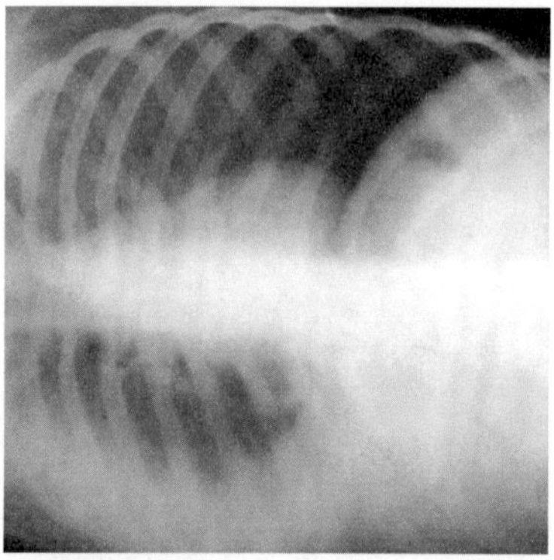

Fig. 9.17: Chest X-ray right lateral decubitus view showing pleural effusion

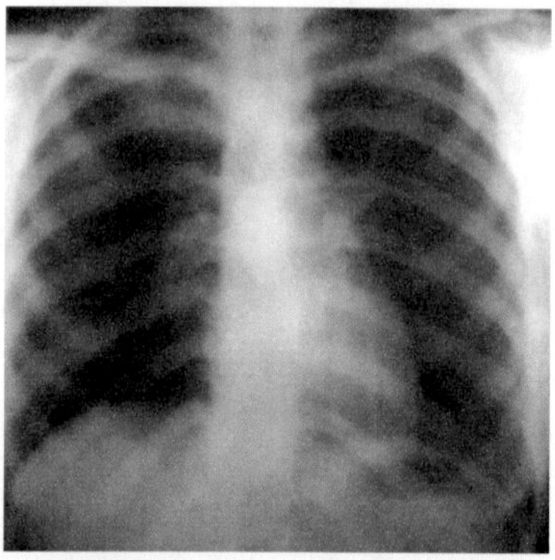

Fig. 9.18: Chest X-ray showing resolution of effusion after treatment

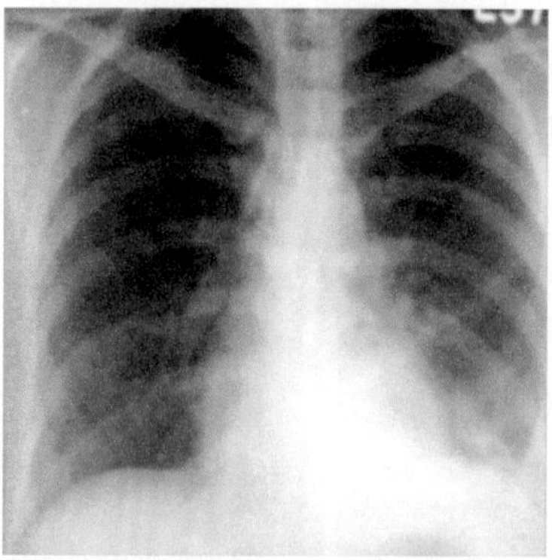

Fig. 9.19: Chest X-ray showing subpulmonic effusion (Left)

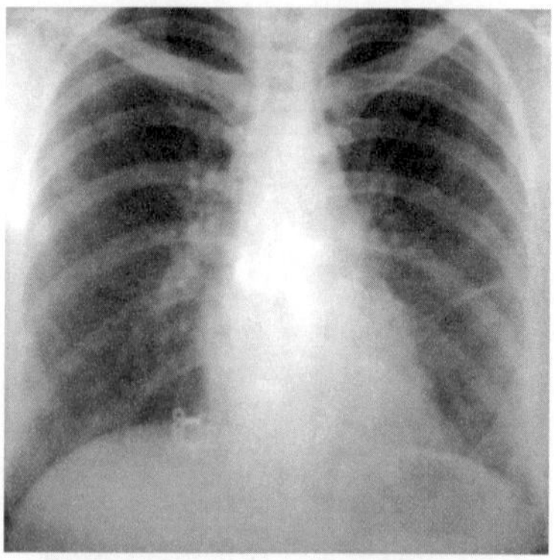

Fig. 9.20: Chest X-ray showing disappearance of subpulmonic effusion (Left) after ATT

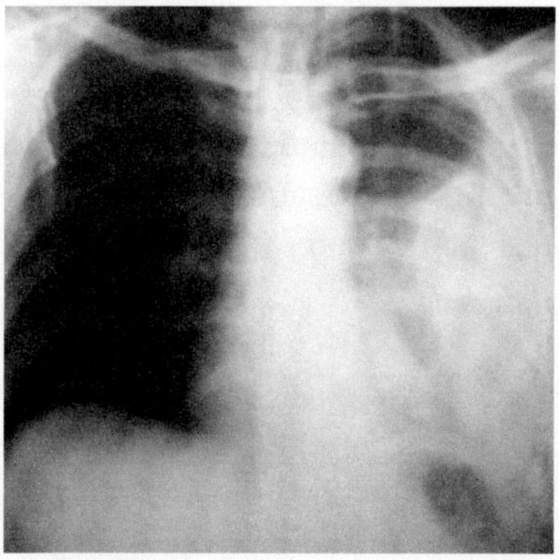

Fig. 9.21: Chest X-ray showing encysted pleural effusion (Left)

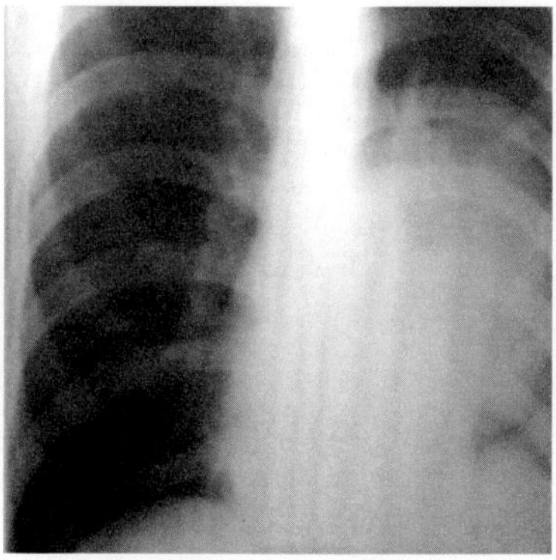

Fig 9.22: Chest X-ray showing encysted pleural effusion (Left)

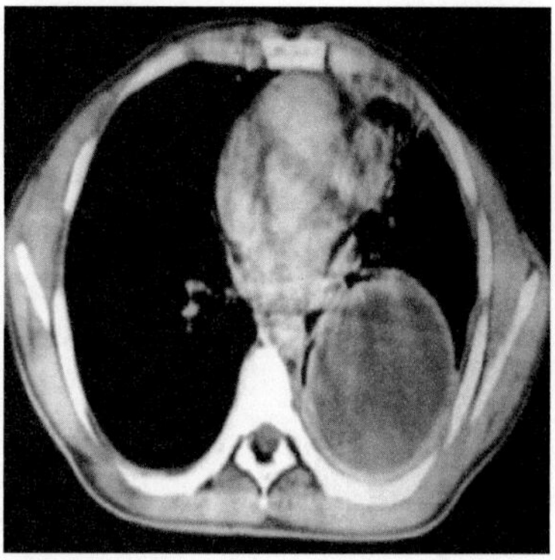

Fig. 9.23: CT thorax showing encysted pleural effusion (Left)

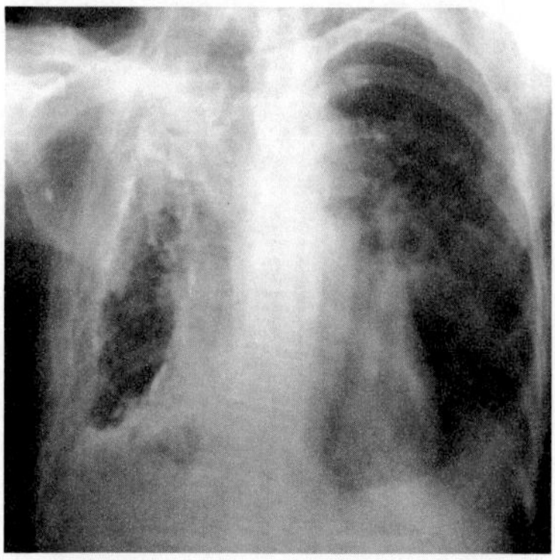

Fig. 9.24: Chest X-ray showing pleural thickening

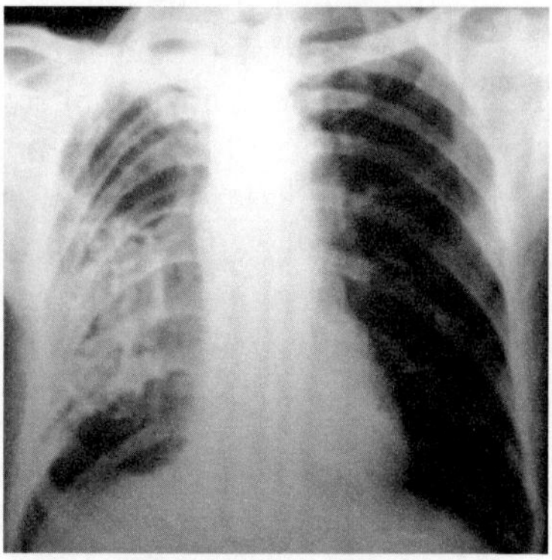

Fig. 9.25: Chest X-ray showing pleural calcification

Follow-up of Primary Tuberculosis

Two-third of patients shows complete clearance. Resolution may take six months to two years time. Associated lymphadenopathy takes more time to resolve as compared to parenchymal lesions. Paradoxical worsening of lesions radiographically can be seen within three months of treatment.[14]

Postprimary Tuberculosis

Majority of postprimary tuberculosis occurs as a result of reactivation of acquired infection. Though both primary and postprimary TB overlap on chest X-ray, they can be distinguished by the fact that latter usually have upper zone predilection, often cavitate and rarely present with lymphadenopathy.[7]

Parenchymal Involvement

Exudative lesion

Patchy or confluent heterogeneous consolidation can occur at specific location like apical and posterior segment of upper lobe or superior segment of a lower lobe. It can be even bilaterally present in nearly half of the patients. Cavitation is also seen in many patients.[14] With treatment the lesion completely resolves. If not treated properly, exudative lesion may lead to rapid destruction or conversion to fibroproductive lesion.

Fibroproductive of fibroproliferative lesion

These are more sharply defined medium to coarse reticular and nodular opacities. Healing occurs by replacement of granulation tissue by fibrous tissue resulting in a considerable loss of volume. In some cases apical opacity or apical cap develops due to pleural thickening and subpleural atelectasis.

Cavitation

When the center of tubercular lesion undergoes liquefactive necrosis, the caseous material of the center is expelled out leading to the development of a cavity. Cavitation in an area of consolidation is likely to be an active disease. Cavitatory disease is usually indicative of apical and or posterior segment of upper lobe or superior segment of lower lobe. Wall of an untreated TB cavity may be thick or thin walled and smooth or internally nodular. Healed cavities usually thin out with treatment and ultimately balloon out into a large emphysematous space or resolve with or without scarring (Figs 9.26 to 9.29).[15]

Tuberculosis bronchopneumonia

Endobronchial spread to other parts of ipsilateral and contralateral lung occurs due to spread of caseous material in cavitatory lung disease or rupture of lymph node. The nodules are distributed in the peribronchial and centrilobular regions in characteristic "tree in bud" appearance. These

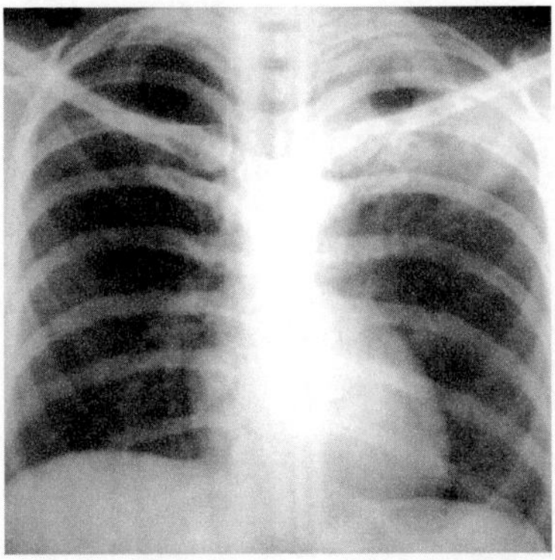

Fig. 9.26: Chest X-ray showing cavity left upper zone

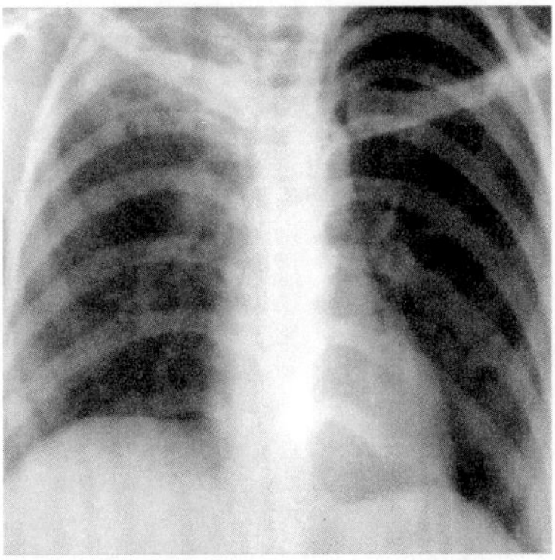

Fig. 9.27: Chest X-ray showing cavity right upper zone

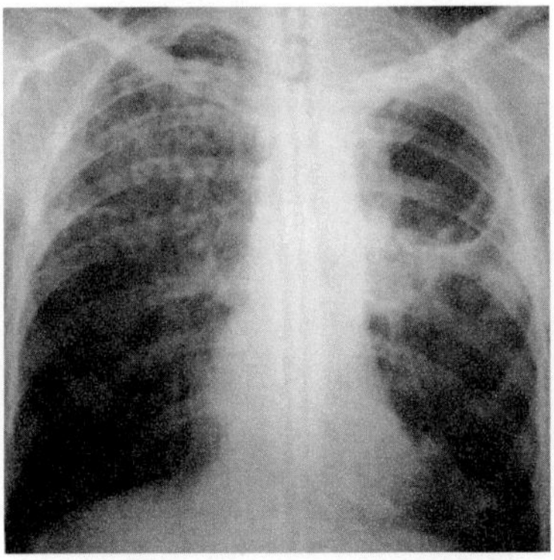

Fig. 9.28: Chest X-ray showing cavity left upper zone with bilateral lesions (Tubercular)

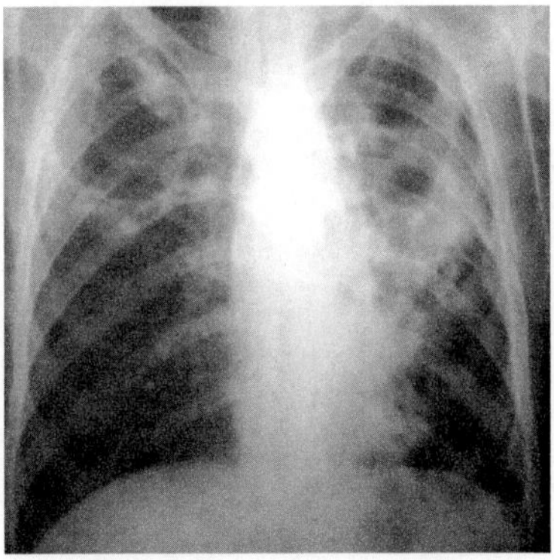

Fig. 9.29: Chest X-ray showing bilateral upper lobe healed cavities (Open negative syndrome)

lesions are an important sign of activity.[16] With treatment while majority of such lesions clear completely, about one-third of them have parenchymal scarring, calcification or residual nodules (Figs 9.30 to 9.33).[9]

Airway Involvement (Bronchostenosis)

Bronchostenosis can occur with active TB by direct extension from adjacent lymphadenitis, endobronchial spread of infection or lymphatic dissemination to airways.

Pleural Involvement

It is not a common presentation of post primary tuberculosis.[13] It is usually small; generally loculated associated with parenchymal lesion. Pneumothorax may also occur due to rupture of a cavity into the pleural space.

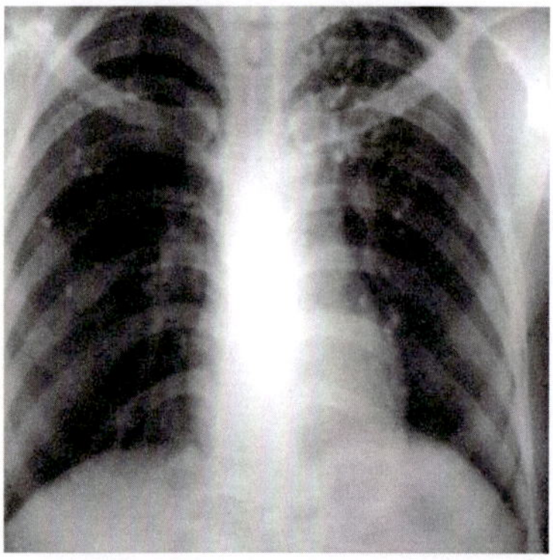

Fig. 9.30: Healed pulmonary tuberculosis (Calcified lesions left upper zone)

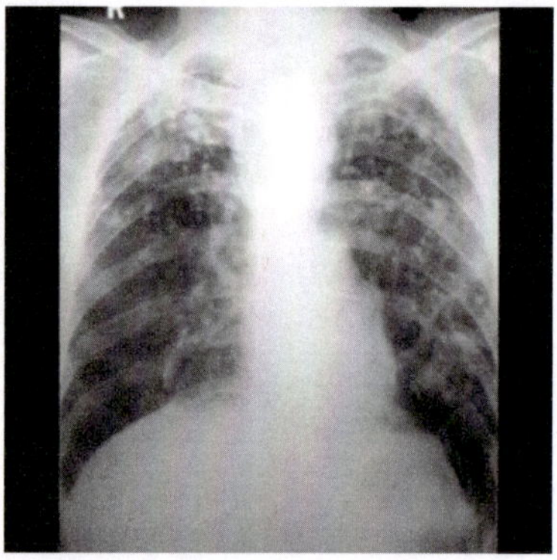

Fig. 9.31: Healed pulmonary tuberculosis (Bilateral calcified lesions)

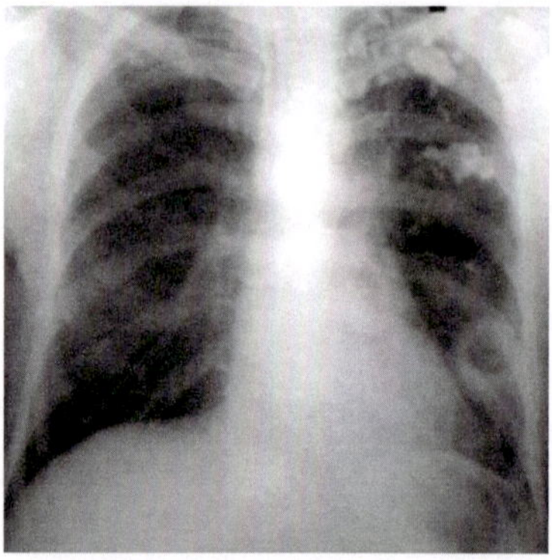

Fig. 9.32: Chest X-ray showing healed TB with lung abscess

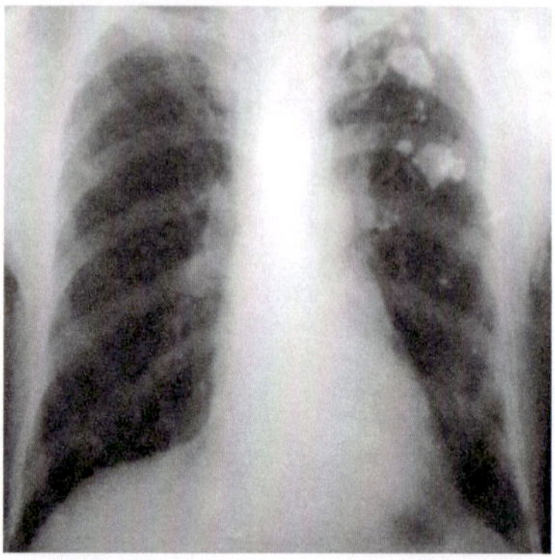

Fig. 9.33: Chest X-ray showing persistant healed lesions and lung abscess dissolved with antibiotics

SEQUELAE AND COMPLICATIONS OF TUBERCULOSIS

Parenchymal Complications[17]

They include thin-walled cavities, fibrotic bands with grooving, calcification and retraction of lung parenchyma, cicatrization, end stage lung destruction and aspergilloma.

Airway Complications[17]

They include bronchiectasis, tracheobronchial stenosis and broncholithiasis.

Pleural Complications[17]

They include chronic empyema, fibrothorax, bronchopleural fistula and pneumothorax.

Vascular Complications[17]

They include pulmonary or bronchial arteritis and thrombosis, bronchial artery dilatation and Rasmussen aneurysm.

RADIOGRAPHIC FOLLOW-UP SCHEDULE

Recommendations of the American Thoracic Society and Centers for Disease Control[18] states that in patients with negative sputum mycobacterial culture repeat chest X-ray is indicated after two months and desirable at the end of treatment. In patients with positive sputum mycobacterial cultures, repeat chest X-ray at the end of two months and at the end of treatment are considered desirable not indicated.[19] Change in size of cavities and increase in size of existing lesions and appearance of new lesions are signs of disease progression and activity. However, one should also realize that radiological worsening may be due to intercurrent pneumonia, pulmonary embolism and supervening carcinoma. Therefore, one has to keep in mind that radiological follow-up is less reliable as compared to bacteriological follow-up.

REFERENCES

1. Nakamura K, et al. Studies on the diagnostic value of 70 mm radiophotograms by mirror camera and the reading ability of physicians. Kekkaku. 1970;45:121-8.
2. WHO expert committee on tuberculosis. Ninth report. Geneva. World Health Organization, 1974 (WHO technical Report series, no. 552).
3. Springett VH. Results of the study on X-ray readings of the *adhoc* committee for the study of classification and terminology in tuberculosis. Bulletin of IUATLD. 1968;412:107-9.
4. Springett VH. Results of the international study on X-ray classification. Conclusions. Bulletin of the International union against tuberculosis. 1968;41:125-7.
5. Prasad R, Nautiyal RG, Mukerji PK, Jain A, Singh K, Ahuja RC. Diagnostic evaluation of pulmonary tuberculosis. What do doctors of modern medicine do in India? Int J Tuberc Lung Dis. 2003;7(1):52-7.
6. Lamont AC, Cremin BJ, Pelteret RM. Radiological patterns of pulmonary tuberculosis in paediatric age group. Paediatr Radiol. 1986;16:2-7.
7. McAdams HP, Erasmus J, Winter JA. Radiologic manifestations of pulmonary tuberculosis. Radiol Clin North Am. 1995;3:655-78.
8. Choyke PL, Sostman HD, Curtis AM, Ravin CE, Chen JT, Godwin JD, et al. Adult onset pulmonary tuberculosis. Radiology. 1983;148:357-62.
9. Fraser RG, Pare JA, Fraser RS, Genereux GP. In: Diagnosis of the diseases of the chest. Vol II. 3rd ed. Philadelphia: WB. Saunders and Company.1989. p. 882-933.
10. Sharma SK, Mohan A, Sharma A, Mitra DK. Miliary Tuberculosis: new insights into an old disease. Lancet Infect Dis. 2005;5:415-30.
11. Lee JY, Lee KS, Jung KJ, Han J, Kwon OJ, Kim J, et al. Pulmonary tuberculosis: CT and pathologic correlation. J Comput Assist Tomogr. 2000;24:691-8.
12. Pombo F, Rodriguez E, Mato J, Perez-Fontan J, Rivera E, Valvuena L. Patterns of contrast enhancement of tuberculous lymph nodes demonstrated by computed tomography. Clin Radiol. 1992;46:13-7.
13. Woodring JH, Vandiviere HM, Fried AM, Dillon ML, Williams TD, Melvin IG. Update: the radiographic features of pulmonary tuberculosis. AJR Am J Roentgenol. 1986;146:497-506.

14. Agrons GA, Markowitz RI, Kramer SS. Pulmonary tuberculosis in children. Semin Roentgenol 1993;28:158-72.
15. Im JG, Itoh H, Shim YS, Lee JH, Ahn J, Hans MC, et al. Pulmonary tuberculosis: CT findings-early active change and sequential change with anti-tuberculous therapy. Radiology. 1993;186:653-60.
16. Im JG, Itoh H, Lee JH, Hans MC. CT-pathology correlation of pulmonary tuberculosis. Crit Rev Diagn Imaging. 1995;36:227-85.
17. Kim HY, Song KS, Goo JM, Lee JS, Lee KS, Lim TH. Thoracic sequelae and complications of tuberculosis. Radiographics. 2001;21:839-58.
18. Abernathy RS. Tuberculosis in children and its management. Semin Respir Infect. 1989;4:232-42.
19. Blumberg HM, Burman WJ, Chaisson RE, Daley CL, Etkind SC, Friedman LN, et al. American Thoracic Society, Centers for Disease Control and Prevention and the Infectious Disease Society of America. Treatment of tuberculosis. Am J Respir Crit Care Med. 2003;167;603-62.

9C: BACTERIOLOGY

Although microscopic detection of tubercular bacilli is an age old procedure, still it is considered to be the gold standard tool even after the introduction of so many new and rapid tests for the diagnosis of tuberculosis. Definite diagnosis of tuberculosis depends on smear examination and culture of appropriate biological fluids. In case of pulmonary tuberculosis, sputum is the specimen of choice while in extrapulmonary tuberculosis relevant specimens like CSF, urine, pleural fluid, gastric lavage, etc. are considered.

DIRECT DEMONSTRATION BY STAINING TECHNIQUE

Sputum microscopy is the most efficient way of identifying sources of tuberculosis infection and also to monitor the progress of infectious patients during treatment, including confirmation of cure. Its main advantage is that it is inexpensive, simple, rapid and is relatively easy to perform. The tubercle bacilli are gram-positive. After they are stained by carbol fuchsin (Ziehl-Neelsen method), they retain their red color even after decolorization with acid-alcohol (Fig. 9.34). Hence they are called "acid fast". Sputum microscopy can also be done by fluorescence microscopy (Fig. 9.35). The major advantage of fluorescence microscopy is that it allows the same area of a smear to be scanned in a much shorter time than can by achieved by conventional microscopy. Its major limitations being relative high cost, maintenance, need of advanced technical skill and a continuous supply of electrical power.

A specimen that is consistently found to be positive would have to contain at least 100,000 AFB/mL.

Sputum smear may be graded according to WHO as:

Examination	Grading	No. of fields examined	Result
More than 10 AFB per oil immersion field	3+	20	Positive
1–10 AFB per oil immersion field	2+	50	Positive
10–99 AFB per 100 oil immersion fields	1+	100	Positive
1–9 AFB per 100 oil immersion fields	Record exact no.	200	Scanty
No AFB in 100 oil immersion fields	0	100	Negative

While a single smear of sputum has a reported sensitivity of only 22–43%, when 2–3 smears are examined over 2 days, about 50–70% of patients with active pulmonary tuberculosis will have positive smear.[1] Furthermore, to find one AFB in every 10 fields would require 1000 such bacilli to be present in the smear (10,000 fields) or 100,000 mL of sputum. Therefore, a specimen that is consistently found to be positive would have to contain at least 100,000 AFB/mL.

Another method of grading of smear for AFB is through Gaffky Scale[2] mentioned in the following table:

I	1–4 bacilli/smear
II	1 bacilli/many fields
III	1 bacilli/field
IV	2–3 bacilli/field
V	4–6 bacilli/field
VI	7–12 bacilli/field
VII	13–25 bacilli/field
VIII	50 bacilli/field
IX	100 bacilli/field
X	Countless bacilli

Sputum smear may give false-negative or false-positive results. False-positive sputum smear may result due to food particles, precipitated stains, environmental acid-fast bacilli, nontubercular *Mycobacterium*, *Nocardia*, spores of *Bacillus subtilis*, yeast, fibers, pollens, scratches on the slide, contamination through transfer of bacilli from one slide to another. False-negative smear may result due to improper sputum collection, improper storage condition (exposure to heat or sunlight), failure to select suitable sputum particles for smear preparation, improper preparation of smears or staining of slides and improper smear examination. False results may also occur due to administrative or reading errors.

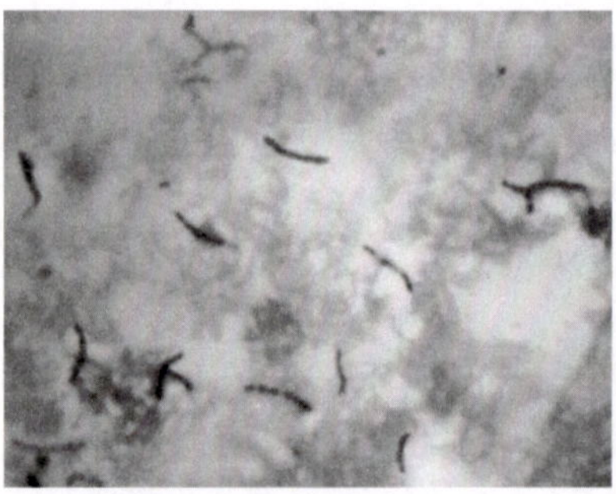

Fig. 9.34: Smear positive for acid-fast bacilli by Ziehl-Neelsen method (For color version, see Plate 2)

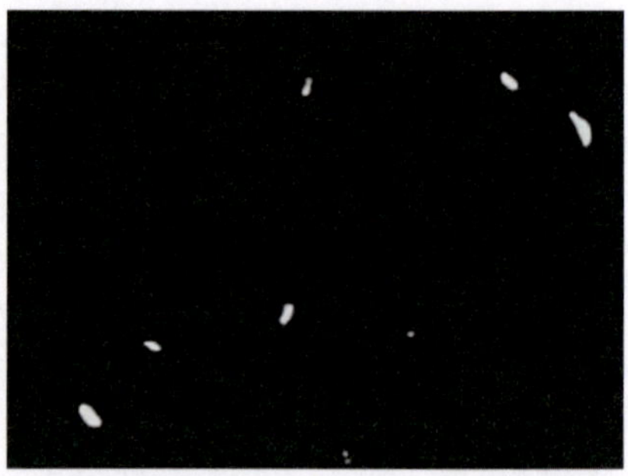

Fig. 9.35: Smear positive for MTB by fluorescence staining method (For color version, see Plate 2)

MYCOBACTERIAL CULTURE IN THE DIAGNOSIS OF TUBERCULOSIS

Isolation of *Mycobacterium* from clinical samples by culture still represents the cornerstone on which definitive diagnosis of tuberculosis relies.

The probability of finding AFB in sputum specimens by smear microscopy is directly related to the concentration of bacilli in the sputum. At concentrations below 1000 organisms per mL, the chance of observing bacilli in a smear becomes less than 10%. In comparison, mycobacterial culture can detect far lower numbers of AFB, the detection limit being around 100 organisms per mL. Moreover, culture makes it possible to identify the mycobacterial species as well as perform drug susceptibility testing (DST) where feasible. Thus for the diagnosis of tuberculosis, both the sensitivity and specificity of culture methods are far better than those of smear microscopy. A second culture increases the culture sensitivity from 63–84%.[3,4] At present, mycobacterial culture can be performed on conventional egg-based solid medium such as Lowenstein-Jensen medium and agar-based ones, such as Middlebrook 7H10 or 7H11 and liquid media such as Kirchner's or Middlebrook 7H9 broth. The major constraint of culturing *Mycobacterium* in conventional media is its slow growth which necessitates a mean incubation period of at least 4 weeks. The drug susceptibility tests to antituberculosis drugs require additional 4–6 weeks. Most of the laboratories in the developing world rely on solid media for culture of *Mycobacterium*. Although a combination of solid and liquid media is currently the gold standard for the primary isolation of *Mycobacterium*, a few modern, rapid methods are also available.

Three to six percent of smear-positive patients have negative cultures in patients receiving treatment. The organisms may have lost their ability to grow on culture media and are practically dead. In a few instances, positive smears may be caused by nontuberculous mycobacteria. In patients who have not have treatment sputum specimen may have been exposed to sunlight or heat, stored too long, dried out or contaminated, decontamination procedures before inoculation, overheating during centrifugation, inadequate culture media and deficient incubation may also result in a negative culture.

There are three methods for drugs susceptibility testing: Absolute concentration, proportion method and resistant ratio method. Proportion method is a recommended method of drug susceptibility test.

It is difficult to perform susceptibility testing accurately even when skills personal are available and laboratory facilities are of a high standard. In countries where skilled manpower and adequate facilities are scarce' accuracy is even more difficult to achieve.

Rapid Culture Methods

Rapid culture methods have an advantage over conventional methods using egg-based or agar-based media that time taken for detection of growth is shorter. In case of extrapulmonary specimens, the time taken may be even longer by conventional media. It has been proven that the combined use of both methods produced better and faster-positive mycobacterial culture yield. Various types of culture methods are mentioned below:

Bactec 460

The most widely used of the newer culture techniques is Bactec system where in C^{14} labeled palmitic acid in 7H12 medium is used (Fig. 9.36). This system detects the presence of *Mycobacterium* based on their metabolism rather than visible growth. When the C^{14} labeled substrate present in the medium is metabolized, $C^{14}O_2$ is produced and measured by the Bactec system instrument and reported in terms of growth index (GI) value. The Bactec system is also useful in the identification of *M. tuberculosis* using specific inhibitor, para-nitro-α-acetylamino-β-hydroxypropiophenone. Using the same system, drug susceptibility tests can also be performed for all the antituberculosis drugs when sufficient GI is observed. Comparison of the Bactec radiometric method with the conventional culture and drug susceptibility testing methods showed that the rate of isolation of positive cultures was significantly faster with the Bactec method, with 87% of the positives being obtained by 7 days and 96% by 14 days. There was a good correlation in drug susceptibility tests and most of these results could be obtained within 8 days by the Bactec method.[5] Thus various studies have proved that sensitivity of the Bactec is slightly higher and the time taken for detection is less than conventional methods.[6-8]

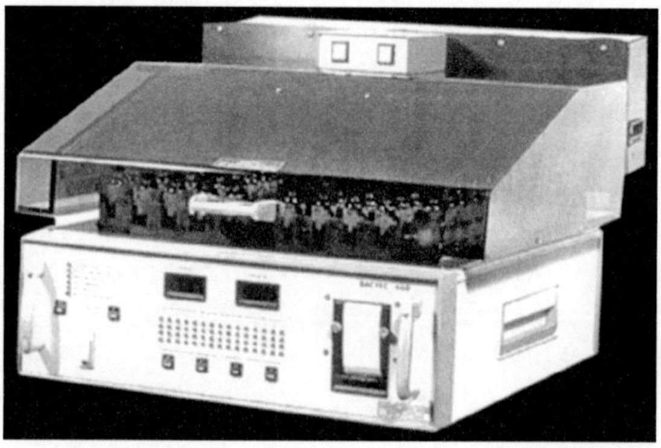

Fig. 9.36: Bactec 460 (For color version, see Plate 2)

MGIT Mycobacteria Detection System

It is an automated system for growth detection based on the metabolic O_2 utilization and subsequent intensification of an O_2 quenched fluorescent dye contained in a tube of modified MGIT. In a multicenter evaluation which compared the growth and recovery of mycobacteria to that of Bactec 460 TB and conventional culture methods[9] average time of detection for the Bactec 460 and MGIT 960 systems were 8.7 versus 8.6 days for *M. avium* complex (MAC) and 13.4 versus 15.5 days for *M. tuberculosis,* respectively. It was revealed that MGIT 960 system exhibits greater potential as a rapid, accurate and cost-effective method for a high volume mycobacteriology laboratory.

Septi-Check Method

It combines broth and solid media into a single device. Septi-check AFB contains 20 mL of Middlebrook 7H9 broth in carbon-dioxide-enriched culture bottle capped with a slide containing three solid media: a nonselective Middlebrook 7H11 agar, an egg-based media and chocolate agar. This method requires about 3 weeks of incubation. The unique advantage of this technique is the simultaneous detection of *M. tuberculosis*, nontuberculous mycobacteria (NTM), other respiratory pathogens and even contaminants. A multicentric study conducted in the USA has shown that the system gives a better culture result when compared to other methods including Bactec 460 TB system.[10]

MB/BacT System

This is a nonradiometric continuous monitoring system with a computerized database management based on colorimetric detection of CO_2. Comparison of the performance of MB/BacT system with that of Bactec 460 showed that the mean time for detection of *M. tuberculosis* by the Bactec system was 11.6 days vs 13.7 days by the MB/BacT system. It was concluded that the MB/BacT with the computerized data management system is an acceptable alternative for Bactec 460 method despite some minor disadvantages such as increased contamination and slightly longer time for detection of growth.[11]

ESP Culture System II

This is a fully automated continuous monitoring system based on the detection of pressure changes within the headspace above the broth culture medium in a sealed bottle. The system was evaluated in clinical specimens for the detection of *Mycobacterium* against Bactec 460 and 7H11 agar solid medium. The mean time for recovery of all *Mycobacterium, M. tuberculosis* complex and MAC was found to be 13.1, 15.5 and 10.9 days, respectively. Hence, the ESP II culture system seems to be a reliable nonradiometric less labor-intensive alternative to Bactec 460 system for the growth and detection of *Mycobacterium*. However, as with other liquid culture systems, ESP II should be used in combination with a solid medium, not as a stand-alone system.[12]

DRUG SUSCEPTIBILITY TESTING

Drug susceptibility testing (DST) methods include the proportion method, the absolute concentration method, and the resistance ratio method.[13] With the introduction of the Bactec radiometric system and its adaptation to perform DST of *M. tuberculosis* these four methods were considered as the gold standard.[14] The long turn around time (TAT) and laboriousness of these methods stimulated the search for alternative and faster techniques. These new methods can be differentiated into genotypic and phenotypic methods.

Genotypic Methods

These methods search for the genetic determinants of resistance rather than the resistance phenotype. In general, they have two basic steps: a molecular nucleic acid amplification step, such as PCR to amplify sections of the *M. tuberculosis* genome, known to be altered in resistant strains and a second step of assessing the amplified products for specific mutations correlating with resistance. These methods have several advantages: a faster turn around time (days instead of weeks), no need for growth of the organism, the possibility for direct application to clinical specimens, reduction of biohazard risks, and feasibility for automation. Unfortunately, they also have disadvantages, including problems with inhibitors when applying these methods directly to clinical samples. DNA sequencing of PCR-amplified products has been the most widely used method, becoming the gold standard. It has been performed by both manual and automated procedures although the latter has been the most commonly used.[15] It has been thoroughly used for characterizing mutations in the rpoB gene in rifampicin-resistant strains and to detect mutations responsible for resistance to other anti-TB drugs.[16] Several other genotypic methods have been proposed to detect resistance to antibiotics, such as PCR-single strand conformation polymorphism,[15] PCR-heteroduplex formation,[17] and solid-phase hybridization assays. Moreover, the Line Probe Assay (LiPARif) based on the hybridization of amplified DNA from cultured strains or clinical samples to ten probes encompassing the core region of the rpoB gene of *M. tuberculosis*, immobilized on a nitrocellulose strip,[18] and the genotype *M. tuberculosis* test (MTB) DR (Hain, Germany), a commercial system for the detection of the *M. tuberculosis* complex and its resistance to rifampicin and isoniazid from culture samples based on the detection of the most common mutations in the rpoB and katG genes, respectively. DNA microarrays and real-time PCR (RT-PCR) techniques have also been proposed as alternative methods for drug resistance detection; the former still beyond the reach of clinical diagnostic laboratories, and the latter being increasingly evaluated with promising results.[19]

Phenotypic Methods

New phenotypic methods assess inhibition of *M. tuberculosis* in the presence of antibiotics by detecting earlier signs of growth using various technologies, for example, the measurement of metabolism with the aid of color indicators, or oxygen consumption by early visualization of micro-colonies, and by the use of phages.

The MGIT system, in its manual or automated version and based on the measurement of oxygen consumption, has been thoroughly evaluated for DST of *M. tuberculosis* to first- and second-line drugs showing a good concordance with the gold standard proportion method.[20]

The E-test based on strips with impregnated gradients of antibiotics for the determination of drug susceptibility allows the reading of minimal inhibitory concentrations directly on agar plates. Several studies have evaluated this test in comparison with the proportion method finding an agreement of 90%.[21]

Two other commercial and automated methods for DST are the MB/BacT system and the ESP culture system II. Both systems rely on heavy equipment and have also been evaluated in several studies.[22] Among the in-house methods of recent application for DST of *M. tuberculosis*, three types of methods deserve a mention: (1) phage-based assays; (2) colorimetric methods; and (3) the nitrate reduction assay.

Application of phage-based assays for DST is being applied for detecting rifampicin resistance of *M. tuberculosis* both in culture samples and directly from sputum. Results are available, on average, in 2 days with a concordance of 95% when compared with the gold standard proportion method.[23] Colorimetric methods are based on the reduction of a colored indicator added to the culture medium after *M. tuberculosis* has been exposed in vitro to different antibiotics. Resistance is detected by a change in the color of the indicator, which is directly proportional to the number of viable mycobacteria in the medium.[24] The nitrate reduction assay is a very simple technique based on the capacity of *M. tuberculosis* to reduce nitrate to nitrite, which is detected by adding a chemical reagent to the culture medium. *M. tuberculosis* is cultivated in the presence of the antibiotic and its ability to reduce nitrate is measured after 10 days of incubation. Resistant strains will reduce the nitrate revealed by a pink-red color in the medium, while susceptible strains will loose this capacity as they are inhibited by the antibiotic, leaving the medium colorless.[25] It has the added advantage of using the same format and culture medium as used in the standard proportion method. In their current format, colorimetric methods seem more appropriate for reference laboratories with the facilities and biosafety conditions to manipulate small volumes of liquid cultures in a microplate format. The phage-based assay can be implemented in mycobacteriology diagnostic laboratories with the appropriate trained personnel, while the nitrate reduction assay is ideal for implementation in the TB diagnostic laboratories routinely performing DST.[25]

NEWER TOOLS UNDER DEVELOPMENT[26]

LED Fluorescence Microscopy

The use of fluorescence microscopy (FM) could potentially increase the sensitivity of smear microscopy and improve the efficiency of facilities. These microscopes allow a much larger area of the smear to be seen, resulting in more rapid examination of the specimen (up to four times faster) and making it easier to count bacilli. Light-emitting diodes (LEDs) are more sustainable and user friendly than the quartz-halogen lamps or high-pressure mercury vapor lamps typically used in FM: powered correctly, they have an extremely long life-expectancy (10,000 hours versus 200 for a conventional mercury lamp). Unlike the light emitted by mercury vapor lamps, LEDs do not produce ultraviolet (UV) light (a cause of concern to many users). LEDs significantly decrease the instrument's power consumption, allowing long-lasting battery operation. LED technology allows FM at a much lower cost than conventional FM. In some countries, it may be difficult to find the LED lamps required. Also, the Royal Blue color LED lamp which works best for FM was only very recently developed and may not be widely available. Some issues with the stability of reagents under field conditions, and the stability of stained smears for blinded rechecking, have been reported. These need further investigation. Proper training is critical; it must be carefully considered and carried out properly. The sensitivity, specificity, cost-effectiveness and cost-benefit of this approach have not yet been adequately established. International guidance on quality assurance for FM does not currently exist (Figs 9.37 to 9.38).

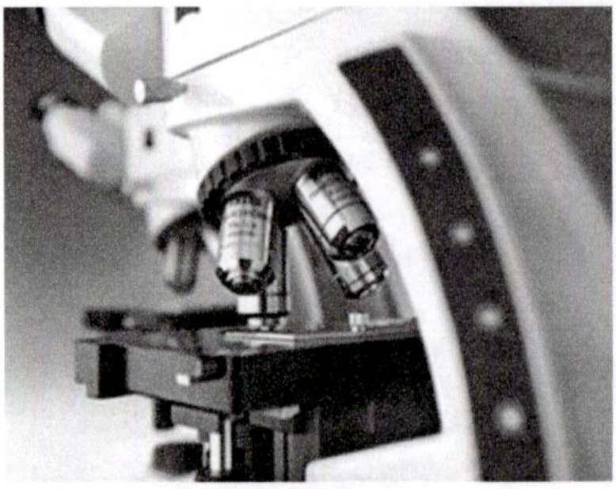

Fig. 9.37: LED microscope (For color version, see Plate 3)

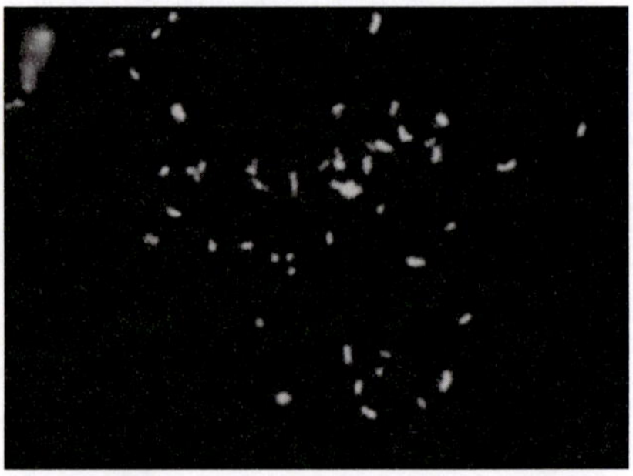

Fig. 9.38: Smear positive for MTB by flourescence staining (done with LED microscope) (For color version, see Plate 3)

Microscopic Observation Drug Susceptibility

Microscopic observation drug susceptibility (MODS) is a manual liquid culture technique that uses basic laboratory equipment (including an inverted light microscope) and microscopy skills to detect TB bacteria. Microscopic colonies (micro-colonies) of *M. tuberculosis* are observed in the culture media using an inverted microscope, through the bottom of a sealed plastic container. The characteristic pattern of growth of *M. tuberculosis* complex allows ready identification. Concurrent culture of sputum in drug-free and drug-containing media facilitates direct rifampicin and isoniazid DST.

Thin Layer Agar Culture (TLA)

The technique uses a standard microscope to simultaneously detect TB bacteria and indicate isoniazid and rifampicin resistance. Plates with a thin layer of agar medium are incubated and examined microscopically on alternate days for the first two weeks and less frequently thereafter. Inexpensive compared to other culture techniques. Test can be done with a standard light microscope. At least one study has demonstrated that this technique provides results faster (in about 11 days) than traditional solid culture using Löwenstein-Jensen medium (26.5 days). Sensitivity obtained with thin layer agar is slightly better than with Löwenstein-Jensen. TB bacteria can be detected in as little as 7 days, with results for DST between 10–15 days. Uses solid media, which may be safer than liquid media. Simpler to manage large numbers of samples than for manual liquid culture. The contamination rate is slightly higher than when using Löwenstein-Jensen medium. Although reportedly faster than traditional solid culture techniques, it is not as fast or as sensitive as liquid culture. Further studies are required to adequately validate this technique.

Lipoarabinomannan (LAM) Detection in Urine

M. tuberculosis LAM has been shown to be excreted in the urine of TB patients. Urine is an easier specimen to collect than sputum, and may be less variable in quality and safer to handle. There are several versions of this assay in development, including in-tube ELISA and dipstick methods. Urinary antigen detection may be of particular value in diagnosing TB in HIV co-infected patients. It may prove valuable for rapid and simple diagnosis of TB in particular in developing countries at peripheral levels.

REFERENCES

1. American thoracic society and center for control and prevention. Diagnostic standard and classification of tuberculosis in adults and children. American Journal of Respiratory and Critical Care Medicine. 2000;161:1376-95.
2. Gaffky GTA. Ein Beitrag zum Verhalten der Tuberkelbacillen im sputum. Mittheilungen aus dem Kaiserlichen Gesundheitsamte.1884;2:126–30.
3. Nagpaul DR, Naganathan N, Prakash M, Diagnostic photofluorograph and sputum microscopy in tuberculosis case-findings. Proceedings of the 9th eastern region tuberculosis conference and 29th National conference on tuberculosis and chest diseases Delhi November 1974. Delhi, Tuberculosis association of India, 1975.
4. Nair SA, et al. Precision of estimate of prevalence of bacteriologically confirmed pulmonary tuberculosis in general population. Indian Journal Tuberculosis. 1976;23:152-9.
5. Venkataraman P, Herbert D, Paramasivan CN. Comparison of BACTEC radiometric method with conventional method for drug susceptibility testing. Indian J Med Res. 1998;108:20.
6. Robert GD, Goodman NL, Heifets L, et al. Evaluation of BACTEC radiometric method for recovery of mycobacteria and drug susceptibility testing of *Mycobacterium tuberculosis* from acid-fast smear-positive specimen. J Clin Microbiol. 1983;18:689-96.
7. Morgan MA, Horstmeier CD, De Young DR, et al. Comparison of a radiometric method (BACTEC) and conventional culture media for recovery of mycobacteria from smear-negative specimen. J Clin Microbiol 1963;18:384-8.
8. Stager LE, Libonati JP, Siddiqui SH, et al. Role of solid media when used in conjunction with BACTEC system for mycobacterial isolation and identification. J Clin Microbiol. 1991;29:154-7.

9. Tortoli E, Mandler F, Tronci M, Penati V, Sbaraglia G, Costa D, et al. Multicenter evaluation of mycobacteria growth indicator tube (MGIT) compared with the BACTEC radiometric method, BBL biphasic growth medium and Lowenstein-Jensen medium. Clin Microbiol Infect. 1997;3:468.
10. Isenberg HD, D' Amato R, Heifets L, Murray PR, Scardamaglia M, Jacobs MC, et al. Collaborative feasibility study of a biphasic system (Roche Septi-Check AB) for rapid detection and isolation of mycobacteria. J Clin Microbiol. 1991;29:1719.
11. Rohner P, Ninet B, Metral C, Emler S. Auckenthaler R. Evaluation of the MB/BacT system and comparison with BACTEC 460 system and solid media for isolation of mycobacteria from clinical specimens. J Clin Microbiol. 1997;35:3127.
12. Woods GL, Fish G, Plaunt M, Murphy T. Clinical evaluation of Difco ESP culture system II for growth and detection of mycobacteria. J Clin Microbiol. 1997;35:121.
13. Canetti G, Fox W, Khomenko A, et al. Advances in techniques of testing mycobacterial drug sensitivity, and the use of sensitivity tests in tuberculosis control programmes. Bull World Health Organ. 1969;41:21-43.
14. Heifets LB, Cangelosi GA. Drug susceptibility testing of *Mycobacterium tuberculosis*: a neglected problem at the turn of the century. Int J Tuberc Lung Dis. 1999;3 564-81.
15. Telenti A, Imboden P, Marchesi F, et al. Detection of rifampicin-resistance mutations in *Mycobacterium tuberculosis*. Lancet. 1993;341:647-50.
16. Takiff HE, Salazar L, Guerrero C, et al. Cloning and nucleotide sequence of *Mycobacterium tuberculosis* gyrA and gyrB genes and detection of quinolone resistance mutations. Antimicrob Agents Chemother. 1994;38:773-80.
17. Williams DL, Waguespack C, Eisenach K, et al. Characterization of rifampin-resistance in pathogenic mycobacteria. Antimicrob Agents Chemother. 1994;38:2380-6.
18. De Beenhouwer H, Lhiang Z, Jannes G, et al. Rapid detection of rifampicin resistance in sputum and biopsy specimens from tuberculosis patients by PCR and line probe assay. Tuberc Lung Dis. 1995;76:425-30.
19. Sougakoff W, Rodriguez M, Truffot-Pernot C, et al. Use of a high-density DNA probe array for detecting mutations involved in rifampicin resistance in *Mycobacterium tuberculosis*. Clin Microbiol Infect. 2004;10:289-94.
20. Sanders CA, Nieda RR, Desmond EP. Validation of the use of Middlebrook 7H10 agar, BACTEC MGIT 960, and BACTEC 460 12B media for testing the susceptibility of *Mycobacterium tuberculosis* to levofloxacin. J Clin Microbiol. 2004;42:5225-8.
21. Hausdorfer J, Sompek E, Allerberger F, Dierich MP, Rusch-Gerdes S. E-test for susceptibility testing of *Mycobacterium tuberculosis*. Int J Tuberc Lung Dis. 1998;2:751-5.
22. Ruiz P, Zerolo FJ, Casal MJ. Comparison of susceptibility testing of *Mycobacterium tuberculosis* using the ESP culture system II with that using the BACTEC method. J Clin Microbiol. 2000;38:4663-4.
23. Albert H, Trollip A, Seaman T, Mole RJ. Simple, phagebased (FASTPplaque) technology to determine rifampicin resistance of *Mycobacterium tuberculosis* directly from sputum. Int J Tuberc Lung Dis. 2004;8:1114-9.
24. Abate G, Mshana RN, Miorner H. Evaluation of a colorimetric assay based on 3-(4,5-dimethylthiazol-2-yl)-2,5-diphenyl tetrazolium bromide (MTT) for rapid detection of rifampicin resistance in *Mycobacterium tuberculosis*. Int J Tuberc Lung Dis. 1998;2:1011-6.
25. Montoro E, Lemus D, Echemendia M, Martin A, Portaels F, Palomino JC. Comparative evaluation of the nitrate reduction assay, the MTT test, and the resazurin microtitre assay for drug susceptibility testing of clinical isolates of *Mycobacterium tuberculosis*. J Antimicrob Chemother. 2005;55:500-5.
26. Stop TB Partnership and World Health Organization. New Laboratory Diagnostic Tools for TB Control. Geneva, World Health Organization, 2008. www.stoptb.org.

9D: HISTOPATHOLOGY

Pulmonary tuberculosis is diagnosed by clinical findings, radiography, and sputum examination for acid-fast bacilli (AFB). Whereas clinical findings and radiographic findings are only suggestive of pulmonary tuberculosis, diagnosis is confirmed by demonstration of mycobacteria in sputum by direct smear examination or by culture. Many patients having clinical and radiological features suggestive of pulmonary tuberculosis do not raise sputum or their sputum is negative for *Mycobacterium tuberculosis* by smear and culture. In patients with HIV positive, radiographic findings of pulmonary tuberculosis disease are often atypical and sputum is often negative. Therefore, a presumptive diagnosis of tuberculosis may be more speculative in these patients. In these situations, histopathology is a great diagnostic tool for diagnosis.

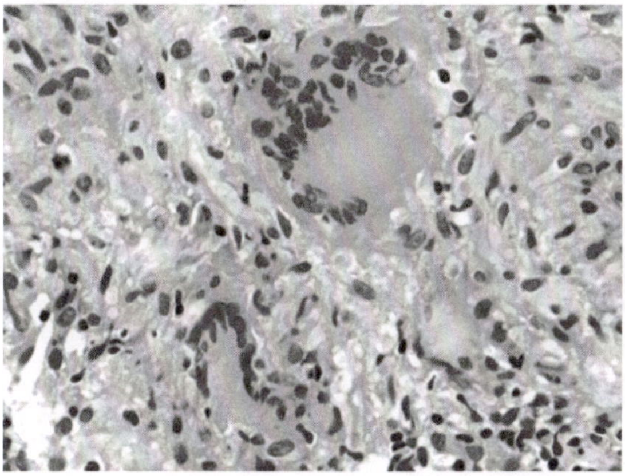

Fig. 9.39: TB granuloma (For color version, see Plate 3)

The histopathological hallmark of TB is granuloma (Fig. 9.39). A granuloma[1] is a focal area of granulomatous inflammation. It consists of a microscopic aggregation of macrophages that are transformed into epithelium-like cells surrounded by a collar of mononuclear leukocytes, principally lymphocytes and occasionally plasma cells. In the usual hematoxylin and eosin preparations, the epithelioid cells have a pale pink granular cytoplasm with indistinct cell boundaries, often appearing to merge into one another. The nucleus is less dense than that of a lymphocyte, is oval or elongate, and may show folding of the nuclear membrane. Older granulomas develop an enclosing rim of fibroblasts and connective tissue. Frequently, but not invariably, epithelioid cells fuse to form giant cells in the periphery or sometimes in the center of granulomas. These giant cells may attain diameters of 40–50 microns. They comprise a large mass of cytoplasm containing 20 or more small nuclei arranged either peripherally (Langhans-type giant cell) or haphazardly (foreign body-type giant cell). There are two types of granulomas—foreign body granulomas and immune granulomas.

The prototype for the immune granuloma is that caused by the bacillus of tuberculosis. In this disease, the granuloma is referred to as a tubercle and is classically characterized by the presence of central caseous necrosis. In contrast, caseating necrosis is rare in other granulomatous diseases.

Definitive diagnosis of extrapulmonary tuberculosis is established by visualizing mycobacteria on histopathology sections or on smears stained for acid-fast bacilli or by mycobacterial culture. As the mycobacteria are not documented in every case, certain histopathological changes have been accepted as suggestive of TB. These include granulomatous inflamation with necrosis, however, it must be clarified that, although highly suggestive these changes are by no means specific and may sometimes be seen in other diseases also.

FNAC is a reliable procedure for the diagnosis of tuberculosis[2] (Figs 9.40 to 9.41). The characteristic cytopathological changes include epitheloid cell granulomas with or without multinucleate giant cells and caseation necrosis. Diagnostic yield can be improved by doing culture of aspirated material in addition to cytological analysis.

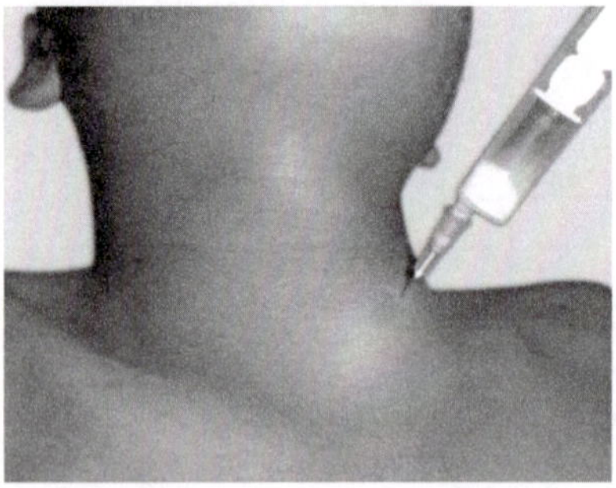

Fig. 9.40: FNAC of lymph node in the neck (For color version, see Plate 3)

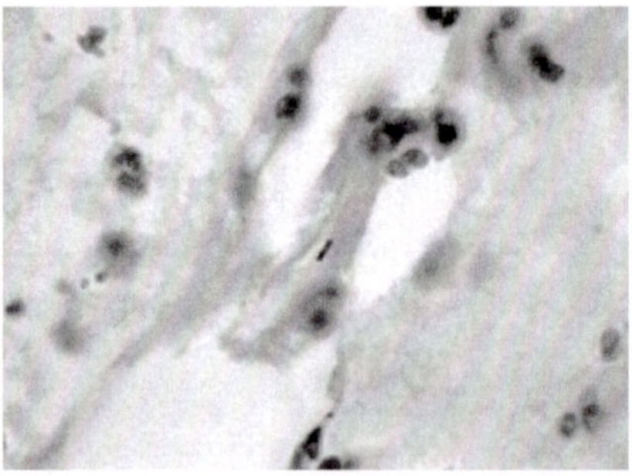

Fig. 9.41: FNAC lymphnode showing AFB (For color version, see Plate 3)

REFERENCES

1. Robbins and Cotran. Pathologic Basis of Disease. Elsevier Saunders, 7th edition:83-4.
2. Beg M, Ahmad Z, Bhargava R, Sharma DK, Akthar N. Role of Transthoracic Needle Aspiration in Diagnosis of Pulmonary Tuberculosis. JIACM. 2002;3:159-63.

9E: POLYMERASE CHAIN REACTION (PCR)

It is a recent method in the diagnosis of tuberculosis using molecular genetics. It involves process of DNA extraction, PCR amplification and visualization of amplified products by ethidium bromide stained acrylamide gel (Fig. 9.42). Results are available in 48 hours. It is a costly test and requires technical expertise. The test is highly sensitive (able to detect 10 AFB/mL) and specific.[1-3] Many different mycobacterial genes have been processed as target for the diagnosis of *M. tuberculosis* in clinical samples. It can also detect nonviable organism. Recently, real-time PCR methods have been proposed for the detection of various microorganisms including *M. tuberculosis.*[4] Real-time PCR methods are based on hybridization of amplified nucleic acids with fluorescent-labeled probes spanning DNA regions of interest and monitored inside thermal cyclers.[5] The fluorescent signal increases in direct proportion to the amount of amplified product inside the reaction tube. This technology has been evaluated in several studies in cultures and more recently in clinical samples. The sensitivity has ranged from 71–98% with specificity close to 100%.[6] Due to the irregular distribution of bacilli in the clinical specimens, however, sensitivity of the test could be affected by the initial volume of DNA present. This was addressed in a recent study by Burggraf,[7] et al. using a new MTBC Light Cycler assay with higher volumes of template DNA. A sensitivity of 100% and specificity of 98.6% was obtained. The main advantage of real-time PCR methods is its speed in giving results, 1.5–2.0 hours after DNA extraction, and lower risks of contamination since both reaction and detection occurs in a single tube.

PCR in diagnosis of tuberculosis: The polymerase chain reaction (PCR) has been evaluated for the detection of *M. tuberculosis* from a range of specimens and seems to have sensitivity equal to or greater than that of the culture method. Initially developed PCR could detect as low as 10 bacilli in the specimen. Recent modifications have enabled DNA extracted from a fraction of a bacilli to be detected after suitable amplification.[8]

Role of PCR in sputum smear-positive pulmonary TB: A recent systematic review showed that pooled sensitivity and specificity were 96% and 85%, respectively.[9] Considering high sensitivity and relatively low specificity, a positive PCR in sputum smear-positive patients does not help in distinguishing tuberculosis from other diagnosis but this test can be confidently used to exclude TB in patients with smear-positive samples when PCR is negative.

Role of PCR in sputum smear-negative pulmonary TB: A recent systematic review showed that pooled sensitivity and specificity were 66% and 98%, respectively. Considering low sensitivity and relatively high specificity PCR can be used to confirm TB in a proportion of smear-negative cases.[9] However,

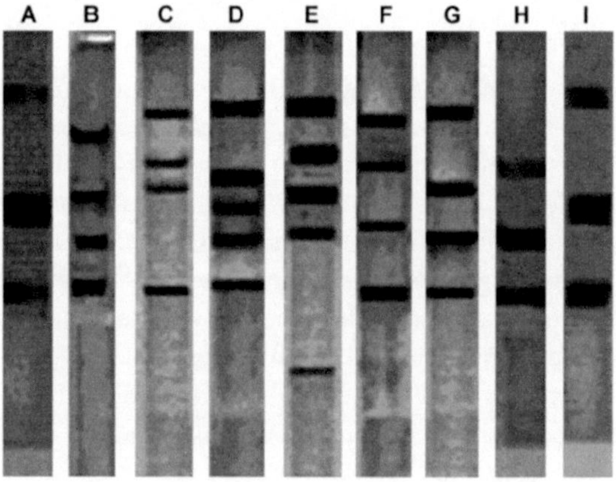

Fig. 9.42: Polymerase chain reaction (PCR)

meta-analysis of PCR for diagnosis of smear-negative pulmonary tuberculosis showed that sensitivity varied from 9–100% and specificity varied from 25–100%. It concluded that PCR is not consistently accurate enough to be routinely recommended for the diagnosis of smear-negative pulmonary TB. However, PCR of bronchial specimens could be useful in highly suspicious smear-negative pulmonary tuberculosis cases.[10]

Role of PCR in diagnosis of drug resistance: Real-time PCR techniques have also been introduced for rapid detection of drug resistance. The main advantages of real-time PCR techniques are the speed of the test and a lower risk of contamination. The main disadvantages would be the requirement for expensive equipment and reagents, and the need for skilled technical personnel. Real-time PCR was initially applied to *M. tuberculosis* strains[11] but more recently it has been successfully applied directly in clinical samples.[12] Results could be obtained in an average of 1.5–2.0 hours after DNA extraction. Real-time PCR could eventually be implemented in reference laboratories with the required capacity to properly set up the technique and in settings where it can contribute to the management of TB patients.

Role of PCR in extrapulmonary TB: In suspected cases of extrapulmonary TB rapid and accurate laboratory diagnosis is of prime importance since the traditional techniques for detecting AFB have limitations (Extrapulmonary TB is usually paucibacillary) and delayed chemotherapeutic interventions is associated with poor prognosis. PCR can give rapid and accurate results in samples from pus and tissue biopsies but it is inferior to culture in samples of BAL and pleural fluid. In the mean time when a rapid diagnosis is required, other tissue should be obtained for testing. One study found that the specificity of PCR in nonpulmonary specimens for detection of tuberculosis is 85%. In TB meningitis sensitivity of PCR in CSF sample is 48%, compared to nine percent in CSF AFB smear.[13] PCR can be applied to the CSF obtained after initiation of ATT. Role of PCR from blood in diagnosis of tuberculosis is not clear.

REFERENCES

1. Shanker P, Manjunath N, Lakshmi R, Aditi B, Seth P, Shriniwas. Identification of mycobacterial tuberculosis by polymerase chain reaction. Lancet. 1990;335:423.
2. Shanker P, Manjunath N, Mohan KE, et al. Rapid diagnosis of tubercular meningitis by polymerase chain reaction. Lancet. 1991;337:5-7.
3. Manjunath N, Shanker P, Rajan L, Bhargava A, Saluja S, Sriniwas. Evaluation of polymerase chain reaction for the diagnosis of tuberculosis. Tubercle. 1991;72:21-7.
4. Lemaitre N, Armand S, Vachee A, et al. Comparison of the real-time PCR method and the Gen-Probe amplified *Mycobacterium tuberculosis* direct test for detection of *Mycobacterium tuberculosis* in pulmonary and nonpulmonary specimens. J Clin Microbiol. 2004;42:4307-9.
5. Shamputa IC, Rigouts L, Portaels F. Molecular genetic methods for diagnosis and antibiotic resistance detection of mycobacteria from clinical specimens. APMIS. 2004;112:728-52.
6. Broccolo F, Scarpellini P, Locatelli G, et al. Rapid diagnosis of mycobacterial infections and quantitation of *Mycobacterium tuberculosis* load by two real-time calibrated PCR assays. J Clin Microbiol. 2003;41:4565-72.
7. Burggraf S, Reischl U, Malik N, et al. Comparison of an internally controlled, large-volume Light Cycler assay for detection of *Mycobacterium tuberculosis* in clinical samples with the COBAS AMPLICOR assay. J Clin Microbiol. 2005;43:1564-9.
8. Rodrigues LC, Smith PG. Tuberculosis in developing countries and methods for its control. Trans R Soc Trop Med Hyg. 1990;84:739-44.
9. Greco S, Girardi E, Navarra A, Saltini C. Current evidence on diagnostic accuracy of commercially based nucleic acid amplification tests for the diagnosis of pulmonary tuberculosis. Thorax. 2006;61:783-90.
10. Sarmiento OL, Weigle KA, Alexander J, Weber DJ, Miller WC. Aseessment by meta-analysis of PCR for diagnosis of smear-negative pulmonary tuberculosis J Clin Microbiol. 2003;41:3233-40.
11. Sajduda A, Brzostek A, Poplawska M, et al. Molecular characterization of rifampin- and isoniazid-resistant *Mycobacterium tuberculosis* strains isolated in Poland. J Clin Microbiol. 2004;42:2425-31.
12. Ruiz M, Torres MJ, Llanos AC, et al. Direct detection of rifampin- and isoniazid-resistant *Mycobacterium tuberculosis* in auramine-rhodamine-positive sputum specimens by real-time PCR. J Clin Microbiol. 2004;42:1585-9.
13. Kox LF, Kuijper S, Kolk AH. Early diagnosis of tuberculous meningitis by PCR. Neurology. 1995;45:2228-32.

9F: SEROLOGY

Tuberculosis is a major public health problem in India. Approximately, one-third of the world's population is infected with *Mycobacterium tuberculosis*, and it is estimated that 9.4 million new cases and 1.8 million deaths occur every year.[1] The standard diagnosis of tuberculosis (TB) is still made by clinical examination, direct sputum microscopy and mycobacterial culture.[2] However, only up to 50% of pulmonary and 25% extrapulmonary tuberculosis are diagnosed by smear examination. Traditional culture methods take around 6 weeks and if diagnosis of tuberculosis is delayed, it leads to increased morbidity and in some cases, mortality. It is, therefore, important to correctly diagnose TB before the onset of therapy. To improve the diagnosis of TB, more rapid diagnostic techniques have been investigated in recent years. The development of an easy and inexpensive diagnostic tool for TB is an important goal, particularly in view of a global increase in the number of cases of active TB, which primarily affects developing countries.[3,4] The demand for a more rapid diagnostic procedure has focused on the possibility of demonstrating the presence of specific antibodies. Detection of antibodies is relatively simple and cheap, hence serodiagnosis of TB has been extensively investigated.[5]

Test manufacturers and distributors are marketing dozens of different antibody detection diagnostic commercial kits. The extent of their use is largely unknown; however, companies report sales volumes between 3,000 and 300,000 tests per year.[6] The question is "do they work in making the diagnosis of tuberculosis?" These tests differ in a number of their features, including antigen composition, antigen source (e.g. native or recombinant), chemical composition (e.g. protein, carbohydrate, or lipid), extent and manner of purification of the antigen(s), class of immunoglobulin detected (e.g. IgG, IgM, or IgA) and number of formats depending on the membrane, antigen(s) coating, and incubation technique (viz. ELISA, immunochromatographic tests).

The serological tests used for the diagnosis of tuberculosis are further divided into three types–antibody based, antigen based and immune complex mediated.

ANTIBODY-BASED TESTS

The available antibody-based tests are of various types like radio-immunoassays, enzyme-linked immunosorbent assay (ELISA), agglutination tests, immuno-precipitation tests, serum antibody competition test (SACT), serum antibody fluorescent testing (SAFA). The antibodies were tested against antigens. Antigens can be classified into five categories according to the type of compound: (i) recombinant proteins, (ii) native proteins, (iii) lipids,

Table: 9.3: Sensitivity and specificity of various tests

Antigen type	Sputum positive HIV status	Specificity	Sensitivity
1. Recombinant proteins			
A. Recombinant 38 kDa (Rv0934)	Sp positive	94% (95% CI, 86–98)	47% (95% CI, 39–55)
B. Recombinant malate synthase (Rv1837c)	Sp positive	98% (95% CI, 95–100)	73% (95% CI, 58–85)
C. Recombinant MPT51 (Rv3803c)	Sp positive HIV negative Sp positive HIV positive	94% 97%	59%; 95% (CI,38–76) 58%; (95% CI, 30–82);
D. Recombinant CFP-10 (Rv3874)	Sp positive	96% (95% CI, 83–99)	48% (95% CI, 29–68)
E. Recombinant TbF6	Sp positive	93% (95% CI, 69–99)	70% (95% CI, 37–90)
2. Native antigens			
A. Native 38 kDa (Rv0934)	Sp positive Sp negative	97% 97%	49% (95% CI, 37–61) 31% (95% CI, 15–52)
B. Native Ag85B (Rv1886c)	HIV negative HIV positive	95% 95%	53% (95% CI, 20–83) 62% (95% CI, 19–92)
C. Native-crystallin (2031c)	Sp positive	96% (95% CI, 83–99)	48% (95% CI, 29–68)
3. Lipids			
A. DAT	-	81% (95% CI, 50–96)	63% (95% CI, 45–78)
B. TAT	-	59% (95% CI, 8–96)	80% (95% CI, 56–93)
C. SL-I	-	59% (95% CI, 8–96)	80% (95% CI, 56–93)
D. Cord Factor	-	91% (95% CI, 78–97)	69% (95% CI, 28–94)
E. TbF6 plus DPEP	HIV negative	94% (95% CI, 86–99)	75% (95% CI, 50–91)
4. Combination antigens			
A. Malate synthase + MPT51	HIV negative HIV positive	97% 97%	80% (95% CI, 73–87) 77% (95% CI, 56–91)
B. TbF6 plus DPEP plus malate synthase		97% (95% CI, 83–100)	85%

(iv) multiple antigens (protein-protein or lipid-lipid additive reactivity) and (v) protein-lipid antigens. The detail of each of the above antigens is described below, while sensitivity and specificity are presented in the tabulated form (Table 9.3).

Recombinant Proteins

Recombinant 38 kDa (Rv0934)

38 kDa, a major protein present in culture filtrates of *M. tuberculosis*, has been studied extensively.[7,8] Several studies have shown an association between the presence of anti-38 kDa antibodies and advanced cavitary TB.[8]

Recombinant Malate Synthase (Rv1837c)

Malate synthase (81 kDa), present in *M. tuberculosis* culture filtrates, the cell wall, and cytoplasmic subcellular fractions, is an enzyme of the glyoxylate pathway used by *M. tuberculosis* during intracellular replication in macrophages and functions as an adhesin that enhances bacterial adherence to host cells.[9] The likelihood positive ratio (40:78) was considerably higher for malate synthase than for other antigens. Antimalate synthase antibodies are usually seen to be elicited earlier during the progression of TB, being present in patients who have not yet developed cavities.[10]

Recombinant MPT51 (Rv3803c)

The 27-kDa protein MPT51, a culture filtrate protein, is closely related to the antigen 85 (Ag85) complex, which comprises Ag85A, Ag85B, and Ag85C. MPT51 is an adhesion reported to be a fibronectin-binding protein of *M. tuberculosis*. A sufficient number of studies evaluating the performance of MPT51 were available to stratify the results by HIV infection status. In sputum smear-positive patients, MPT51 provided equivalent sensitivities in both HIV-negative TB patients (59%; 95% CI, 38–76%) and HIV-positive TB patients (58%; 95% CI, 30–82%); the specificities were 94% and 97%, respectively.[11]

Recombinant CFP-10 (Rv3874)

Culture filtrate protein 10 (CFP-10), a culture filtrate and cell wall protein, has been identified as one of the earliest proteins expressed by *M. tuberculosis* during culture in bacteriological media.[12]

Recombinant TbF6

TbF6 is a single antigen combining four distinct antigens (CFP-10, MTB8, MTB48 and 38 kDa) as a genetically fused polyprotein.[13] The high sensitivity obtained with TbF6 is likely due to the fact that it comprises immunogenic domains from multiple antigens.

Native Proteins

Native 38 kDa (Rv0934)[14]

Native Ag85B (Rv1886c)

Ag85B, present in *M. tuberculosis* culture filtrates and cell walls, is a major component of the Ag85 complex. Like MPT51, Ag85B is a fibronectin-binding protein.[15]

Native-crystallin (2031c) B Material

Crystallin is a 14/16-kDa cell wall protein shown to be induced in bacteria under hypoxia.[15]

Lipids

A variety of lipid-containing antigens are common to mycobacterial species. Several lipid moieties have been purified and intensely studied for their serological potential for TB diagnosis.

DAT

2, 3-diacyl trehalose (DAT), a component of the *M. tuberculosis* cell wall, has been postulated to play a role in modulating host immune responses.[16]

TAT

2,3,6-triacyl-trehalose (TAT) is an antigenic glycolipid compound found in the *M. tuberculosis* cell wall.[16]

SL-I

2, 3, 6-Tetraacyl-trehalose 2-sulfate [sulfolipid I (SL-I)], a compound found abundantly in the *M. tuberculosis* cell wall, may affect the human immune system and play a role in the pathogenesis of TB.[16]

Cord Factor

Cord factor (trehalose 6,6_-dimycolate), a major component of *M. tuberculosis* cell walls, is named for its central role in aggregating mycobacteria into cord structures. Cord factor may contribute to the virulence of *M. tuberculosis* by facilitating cavity formation.[16]

TbF6 plus DPEP

TbF6 polyprotein plus DPEP was the multiple-antigen combination most frequently evaluated. As described above, TbF6 is a polyprotein. DPEP, also known as MPT32, is a proline-rich 45/47-kDa antigen suggested to have a role in the cross-linking of molecules produced by or bordering *M. tuberculosis*. Earlier studies with native MPT32 have demonstrated that it is a highly immunogenic protein that provided higher sensitivity than the 38-kDa protein when it was tested in the same patient cohort.[13]

Performance of Tests with Multiple Antigens

Assays based on multiple antigens provided higher sensitivities [median, 76%; range, 16–96% (57 studies)] than assays based on single antigens [median, 53%; range, 2–100% (197 studies)], while they maintained high specificities (median, 96%; range, 79–100%). The combination of malate synthase plus MPT51 was evaluated in three studies, two studies involving HIV-negative TB patients and one study involving HIV-infected TB patients.[9] The combination of TbF6 plus DPEP plus malate synthase achieved a sensitivity of approximately 85% with both HIV negative and HIV-infected TB patients.[13]

Performance of Serological Test Based on Types of Immunoglobins Tested

Stratification by immunoglobulin class showed that in comparison with the results of studies that detected antibodies to IgG (median sensitivity, 61%; range, 8–100%) or IgA (median sensitivity, 40%; range 10–90%), studies that detected antibodies to IgM had considerably lower sensitivities (median, 11%; range, 2–71%). The median specificities were similar: 96%, 96%, and 98%, respectively (Table 9.4). In addition, compared with the results of tests that detected only anti-IgG or anti-IgA antibodies, tests that detected IgG plus IgA showed higher sensitivities (median,71%; range, 43–97%). However, the inclusion of IgM (IgG plus IgA plus IgM) did not further enhance the sensitivity (median, 71%; range, 60–83%). Immunoglobulin G holds the great promise in diagnosing an active disease in both children as well as adults, as compared to IgM or IgA class.[17,18] IgG antibodies are found to be significantly useful for monitoring of treatment.[17,18] The levels decrease with treatment. In general IgG levels have been found to be increased in active TB increased IgM levels have also revealed no significant change.[17,18] IgA levels have also been reported to be increased in several studies[18] but more or less in extensive, advanced diseases which are unlikely to be missed on clinical examination.[18]

ANTIGEN-BASED TESTS

Unlike antibody detection, *M. tuberculosis*-specific antigen detection provides direct evidence of current *M. tuberculosis* infection, thus warranting immediate chemotherapy against TB. Limitation of antigen detection is the low sensitivity due to the scarcity of *M. tuberculosis* antigens in body fluids such as cerebrospinal fluid (CSF), pleural fluid, blood and urine. Antigen detection formats include sandwich ELISA (sELISA) and dot-ELISA.

Target antigens vary markedly depending on the nature of the clinical samples and the test format. Lipoarabinomannan (LAM). has been most frequently used as the target antigen, and its monoclonal and polyclonal antibodies have been used to detect antigen in sputum samples. It is actually a nonspecific antigen due to the presence in other mycobacterial species.

Table 9.4: Sensitivity and specificity of in-house antibody detection tests by Ig class[19]

Ig class	Sensitivity [Median (range)%]	Specificity [Median (range)%]
IgG	61 (8–100)	96 (26–100)
IgA	40 (10–90)	96 (48–100)
IgM	11 (2–71)	98 (89–100)
IgG and IgA	71 (43–97)	97 (85–100)
IgG and IgM	36 (32–52)	98 (98–99)
IgG, IgA and IgM	71 (60–83)	93 (90–93)

Other antigens, such as whole cells, PPD, culture filtrate protein (CFP), 65 kDa, 14 kDa, among others, have been used as target antigens for antigen detection in CSF and sputum samples.

Sensitivity and specificity of antigen detection varies depending on the clinical specimens and the target antigen. In CSF samples, the sensitivity ranged from 50[20]-90%[21] with the specificity ranging from 80[21]-100%[22] Interestingly, LAM antigen was detectable in 74-93% of urine samples from TB patients and in 4-13% of those from healthy controls in the study areas. In sputum samples, the sensitivity of antigen detection varied from 71-91% with a specificity ranging from 91-100%. Due to the complexity of sELISA and sputum processing steps, however, further studies are necessary to develop simple and highly specific antigen detection methods. In order to overcome the limitation of nonspecificity, analytical tools, such as liquid chromatography-mass spectrometry, MRI, and NMR, among others, needs to be explored to determine if they can directly detect mycobacterial antigens in clinical samples.[23]

The results from a meta-analysis by Steingart, et al. demonstrated that (i) in sputum smear-positive patients, sensitivities significantly >50% were provided for recombinant malate synthase (73%; 95% CI, 58-85%) and TbF6 plus DPEP (75%; 95% CI, 50-91%); (ii) protein antigens achieved high specificities; (iii) among the lipid antigens, cord factor had the best overall performance [sensitivity, 69% (95% CI, 28-94%); specificity, 91% (95% CI, 78-97%)]; (iv) compared with the sensitivities achieved with single antigens (median sensitivity, 53%; range, 2-100%), multiple antigens yielded higher sensitivities (median sensitivity, 76%; range, 16-96%).[19]

SEROLOGY IN DIAGNOSING PULMONARY TB IN PATIENTS WITH HIV INFECTION

It is a rapidly evolving field. While newer methods are being developed, the clinical utility remains to be established. Thirty studies evaluating antigens (all proteins) in HIV-infected TB patients were observed; all studies involving sputum smear-positive patients. Of the total, 23 (77%) studies evaluated assays for the detection of IgG[26] and/or IgA antibodies,[24] four studies evaluated assays for the detection of IgM antibodies[25] and three studies evaluated assays for the detection of IgG, IgA and IgM antibodies.

Antibodies to all five single antigens (38 kDa, malate synthase, Ag85B, alpha-crystallin, and recombinant MPT51) evaluated in these studies were detected in the patients of HIV too. With assays for the detection of IgG and/or IgA antibodies, the sensitivities reported for 38 kDa (range, 35-68%) and alpha-crystallin (range, 15-58%) were similar to those provided for MPT51 and Ag85B. Malate synthase achieved higher sensitivities (range 73-92%). Compared with tests for the detection of only IgG and/or IgA antibodies, tests for the detection of IgM antibodies provided considerably lower sensitivities (range, 4-5%). The inclusion of tests for the detection of IgM (IgG plus IgA plus IgM) did not appreciably increase the sensitivity. The specificities provided by all of the above antigens were high (range, 89-100%).[19] According to a meta-analysis by Steingart, et al. potential candidate antigens for an antibody detection test for pulmonary tuberculosis in HIV-infected and -uninfected patients have been identified, although no antigen achieves sufficient sensitivity to replace sputum smear microscopy. Combinations of select antigens provide higher sensitivities than single antigens. Efforts are needed to improve the methodological quality of tuberculosis diagnostic studies.[19]

ROLE OF SEROLOGY IN DIAGNOSING TUBERCULOSIS IN CHILDREN

There is limited data regarding study of serological tests in children for the diagnosis of tuberculosis. Children with sputum positive pulmonary tuberculosis mount a significant response in serology too. However, in children with sputum negative for AFB and undergoing diagnostic dilemma the antibody response too is inconsistent.[19]

ROLE OF SEROLOGY IN DIAGNOSING EXTRAPULMONARY TB

Through various studies, it has been found that serology is found to be useful in chronic forms of tuberculosis like bone and joint tuberculosis, renal and gastrointestinal tuberculosis but less useful in acute forms of extrapulmonary tuberculosis like miliary tuberculosis, tubercular meningitis and tubercular pleural effusion (Table 9.5).[26-32] The results from a recently published systematic review on extrapulmonary tuberculosis showed that (1) all commercial tests provided highly variable estimates of sensitivity (range 0.00-1.00) and specificity (range 0.59-1.00) for all extrapulmonary sites combined; (2) the Anda-TB IgG kit showed highly variable sensitivity (range 0.26-1.00) and specificity (range 0.59-1.00) for all extrapulmonary sites combined; (3) for all tests combined, sensitivity estimates for both lymph

Table 9.5: Sensitivity and specificity of various serology test in extrapulmonary tuberculosis

Type of tuberculosis	Antigen/Antibody	Sensitivity (%)	Specificity (%)
TBM[29]	–	35–62	75–90
Pleural[29] effusion	IgG26 BCG28 Anti-PPD28	34–72 12 23	93–100 100 95
Intestinal	H37 RA M5E H37RA	100 83	85 91
Miliary	30 kDa IgG32 IgM32	22 85–99 20–46	95 69–82 91–98
Lymph node		58–90	71–97

node tuberculosis (range 0.23–1.00) and pleural tuberculosis (range 0.26–0.59) were poor and inconsistent; and (4) there were no data to determine the accuracy of the tests in children or in patients with HIV infection, the two groups for which the test would be most useful. At present, commercial antibody detection tests for extrapulmonary tuberculosis have no role in clinical care or case detection.[32]

CONCLUSION

After going through the exhaustive list of available types of serologic testing and their specificity and sensitivity, one may get confused. Thousands of tests are present in the market with strong boasting from manufacturers; clinicians should weigh their relevance before ordering them. Although commercial serological tests—by virtue of being rapid, simple to use and noninvasive—are appealing, sufficient evidence to justify their use for the diagnosis of both pulmonary and extrapulmonary tuberculosis is lacking. Lack of methodological rigor in these studies was identified as a concern. Another area of concern is that though potential candidate antigens are identified for diagnosing pulmonary TB in both HIV infected and non-HIV infected individuals, none of the antigens achieves sufficient sensitivity to replace sputum smear microscopy. A focus on antigen discovery for the serodiagnosis of TB in smear-negative, HIV seropsitive and pediatric patients should be encouraged. Hence serological tests cannot be, as of now, taken as confirmatory tool; they can only be used as a supportive tool to clinical diagnosis. No serodiagnostic approach to diagnosis of tuberculosis is currently of widespread clinical utility and is still not recommended for routine diagnostic purposes for tuberculosis. Findings from systematic review on the diagnostic accuracy of serological test for both pulmonary and extra-pulmonary TB suggest that these tests are inaccurate and imprecise. After considering all available evidence, the WHO issued a strong recommendation against the use of currently available commercial serological test for the diagnosis of TB. The recent ban on import or sale of TB serological test by the Indian Health Ministry is a welcome step in the right direction.[33]

REFERENCES

1. World Health Organization. (2009) Global tuberculosis control: a short update to the 2009 report. Geneva: World Health Organization. who.int/tb/publications/global_report/2009/update.
2. Demkow U, Ziokowski J, Filewska M, et al. Diagnostic value of different serological tests for tuberculosis in Poland. J Physiol Pharmacol. 2004;55 (Suppl. 3):57-66.
3. Julian E, Matas L, Hernandez A, Alcaide J, Luquin M. Evaluation of a new serodiagnostic tuberculosis test based on immunoglobulin A detection against Kp-90 antigen. Int J Tuberc Lung Dis. 2000;4:1082-5.
4. Wilkins EG, Ivanyi J. Potential value of serology for diagnosis of extrapulmonary tuberculosis. Lancet. 1990;336:641-4.

5. Silva VMC, Kanaujia G, Gennaro ML, Menzies D. Factors associated with humoral response to ESAT-6, 38 kDa and 14 kDa in patients with a spectrum of tuberculosis. Int J Tuberc Lung Dis. 2003;7:478-84.
6. Special Programme for Research and Training in Tropical Diseases, Foundation for Innovative New Diagnostics Current TB diagnostics market. Diagnostics for tuberculosis: Global demand and market potential. Geneva: World Health Organization. 2006;pp.49-72.
7. Chan ED, Heifets L, Iseman MD. Immunologic diagnosis of tuberculosis: a review. Tuber Lung Dis. 2000;80:131-40.
8. Daniel TM, Debanne SM. The serodiagnosis of tuberculosis and other mycobacterial diseases by enzyme-linked immunosorbent assay. Am Rev Respir Dis. 1987;135:1137-51.
9. Wanchu A, Dong Y, Sethi S, Myneedu VP, Nadas A, Liu Z, et al. Biomarkers for clinical and incipient tuberculosis: performance in a TB-endemic country. PLoS One 3. 2008:e2071.
10. Samanich K, Belisle JT, Laal S. Homogeneity of antibody responses in tuberculosis patients. Infect. Immun. 2001.69:4600-9.
11. Ramalingam B, Uma Devi KR, Raja A. Isotype specific anti-38 and 27 kDa (MPT 51) response in pulmonary tuberculosis with human immunodeficiency virus co-infection. Scand J Infect Dis. 2003;35:234-9.
12. Zhang H, Wang J, Lei J, Zhang M, Yang Y, Chen Y, et al. PPE protein (Rv3425) from DNA segment RD11 of *Mycobacterium tuberculosis*: a potential B-cell antigen used for serological diagnosis to distinguish vaccinated controls from tuberculosis patients. Clin Microbiol Infect. 2007;13:139-45.
13. Houghton RL, Lodes MJ, Dillon DC, Reynolds LD, Day CH, McNeill PD, et al. Use of multiepitope polyproteins in serodiagnosis of active tuberculosis. Clin Diagn Lab. Immunol. 2002;9:883-91.
14. Kumar S, Uma Devi KR, Alamelu R. Isolation and evaluation of diagnostic value of two major secreted proteins of *Mycobacterium tuberculosis*. Indian J Chest Dis Allied Sci. 2002;44: 225-32.
15. Uma Devi KR, Ramalingam B, Raja A. Antibody response to *Mycobacterium tuberculosis* 30 and 16kDa antigens in pulmonary tuberculosis with human immunodeficiency virus coinfection. Diagn Microbiol Infect Dis. 2003;46:205-9.
16. Julian E, Matas L, Alcaide J, Luquin M. Comparison of antibody responses to a potential combination of specific glycolipids and proteins for test sensitivity improvement in tuberculosis serodiagnosis. Clin Diagn Lab Immunol. 2004;11:70-6.
17. Wong CT, Saha N. Changes in serum proteins (albumin, immunoglobulins and acute phase proteins) in pulmonary tuberculosis during therapy. Tubercle. 1990;71:193-7.
18. Faulkner JB, Carpenter RL, Patnode RA. Serum protein and immunoglobulin levels in tuberculosis. Am J Clin Pathol. 1967;48:556-60.
19. Steingart KR, Dendukuri N, Henry M, Schiller I, Nahid P, Hopewell PC, et al. Performance of purified antigens for serodiagnosis of pulmonary tuberculosis: a meta-analysis. Clinical and Vaccine Immunology. 2009;16:260-76.
20. Bera S, Shende N, Kumar S, Harinath BC. Detection of antigen and antibody in childhood tuberculous meningitis. Indian J Pediatr. 2006;73:675-9.
21. Venkatesh K, Parija SC, Mahadevan S, Negi VS. Reverse passive haemagglutination (RPHA) test for detection of mycobacterial antigen in the cerebrospinal fluid for diagnosis of tubercular meningitis. Indian J Tuberc. 2007;54:41-8.
22. Sumi MG, Mathai A, Reuben S, Sarada C, Radhakrishnan VV, Indulakshmi R, et al. A comparative evaluation of dot immunobinding assay (Dot-Iba) and polymerase chain reaction (PCR) for the laboratory diagnosis of tuberculous meningitis. Diagn Microbiol Infect Dis. 2002;42:35-8.
23. Sang-Nae Cho. Current issues on molecular and immunological diagnosis of tuberculosis. Yonsei Med J. 2007;48:347-59.

24. Uma Devi KR, Ramalingam B, Raja A. Diagn Microbiol Infect Dis. 2003;46:205-9.
25. Ramalingam B, Uma Devi KR, Raja A. Scand J Infect. Dis. 2003;35:234-9.
26. Caminero JA, deCastro FP, Carrila T, et al. Diagnosis of pleural tuberculosis by detection of specific IgG anti-antigen 60 in serum and pleural fluid. Respiration 1993;60:58-61.
27. Banchuin N, Wongurajana S, Pumprueg U, et al. Value of an ELISA for mycobacterial antigen detection as a routine diagnostic test of pulmonary tuberculosis. Asian Pac J Allergy Immunol. 1990;8:5-11.
28. Murate T, Mizoguchi K, Amano H, et al. Antipuified protein derivative antibody in tuberculous pleural effusions. Chest. 1990;97:670-3.
29. Gopi A, Madhavan SM, Sharma SK, Sahn SA. Diagnosis and treatment of tuberculous pleural effusion in 2006. Chest. 2007;131:880-9.
30. Steingart KR, Henry M, Laal S, Hopewell PC, Ramsay A, Menzies D, et al. A systematic review of commercial serological antibody detection tests for the diagnosis of extrapulmonary tuberculosis. Thorax. 2007;62:911-8.
31. McConkey SJ, Youssef FG, Azem E, et al. Evaluation of a rapid format antibody test and the tuberculin skin test for diagnosis of tuberculosis in two contrasting endemic settings. Int J Tuberc Lung Dis. 2002;6:246-52.
32. Gevaudan MJ, Bollet C, Charpin D, et al. Serological response of tuberculosis patients to antigen 60 of BCG. Eur J Epidemiol. 1992;8:666-76.
33. Steingart KR, Ramsay A, Dowdy D, Pai M, et al. Serological tests for the diagnosis of active tuberculosis: relevance for India. Indian J Med Res. 2012;135:695-702.

9G: FIBEROPTIC BRONCHOSCOPY

Since the discovery of fiberoptic bronchoscope in 1967 by Dr Shigeto Ikeda.[1] Its use is increasing day-by-day for diagnosing pulmonary infections especially in immunocompromised host and in suspected cases of pulmonary tuberculosis whose sputum smear is negative or not producing sputum. Flexible fiberoptic bronchoscopy is a tool which gives access to diseased area and better bacteriological and histological yield, leading to definitive diagnosis.

INDICATIONS

i. Definitive diagnosis of pulmonary tuberculosis if:
   a. Sputum smear negative
   b. Lack of sputum production
ii. Early diagnosis of pulmonary tuberculosis
iii. Pulmonary tuberculosis in immunocompromised hosts
iv. Childhood tuberculosis
v. Miliary tuberculosis
vi. Endobronchial tuberculosis
vii. Exclude any other pathology.

SPECIMEN COLLECTED

i. Bronchial washing
ii. Bronchoalveolar lavage
iii. Brush biopsy
iv. Endobronchial/transbronchial biopsy
v. Postbronchoscopy sputum.

The specimens are obtained from the lung segment with a new infiltrate based on chest X-ray or the segment that upon inspection has purulent secretion. In patients without radiographic densities, the right middle lobe or the lingula is to be chosen as the sampling area.

Bronchial Washing

5–10 mL of 0.9% saline is instilled with each wash and about 25–50% of this can be aspirated into the trap. A yield of 5–10 mL aspirate is usually sufficient.

Bronchoalveolar Lavage

Bronchoalveolar lavage (BAL) should be performed in an affected segment preferably other than from which selective culture and brush biopsy have been taken. Sterile buffer saline is infused in 50 mL aliquots to a cumulative amount of 200–300 mL. The fluid is aspirated with low-pressure suction (50–100 mm Hg) after each aliquots of fluid inserted.

Brush Biopsy

The ordinary single sheathed brush is adequate for taking specimens for *M. tuberculosis*. No suction should apply before taking specimens. After obtaining specimen, smear should be prepared on glass slide immediately to avoid drying. The brush can also be agitated in 1 mL of sterile Ringer lactate solution and this fluid is used for direct plating on to Löwenstein-Jensen media.

Endobronchial/Transbronchial Biopsy

Endobronchial biopsy is an effective way to obtain specimen from directly visualized lesion and a histopathological diagnosis can be made immediately. When the lesion is in a segmental or subsegmental bronchus or distal to a bronchial stenosis it can be biopsied with a curette.

Transbronchial biopsy is performed with fluoroscopic control and should always be confined to one lung because of the risk of inducing bilateral pneumothorax. If disease appears to be unilateral on chest X-ray, the segment with highest density of shadowing is chosen for the site of biopsy. With bilateral extensive disease, the lateral segment of the right middle lobe is selected. Usually 4–6 specimens are taken. The specimens obtained is fixed in 10% formalin solution and it should be 2 mm in diameter and float in the fixative indicating that they include alveolar tissue. Transbronchial needle aspiration can be done to sample mediastinal lymph node.

RESULT

The fiberoptic bronchoscopy (FOB) facilitates the rapid diagnosis and offers the additional advantage of the diagnosis of several conditions that may mimick pulmonary tuberculosis.[2] In various studies[3-10] conducted for diagnosing pulmonary tuberculosis by bronchoscopy, the immediate yield by examination (Ziehl-Neelsen/Auramine Rhodamine) and histopathological examination are 28–73% and a definite diagnosis of tuberculosis by culture of bronchial washings, lavage, transbronchial biopsy and postbronchoscopic sputum can be made in 73–93% cases. Exclusive diagnosis can be made by culture of BAL in 9–41% of cases, culture of bronchial washing in 12–44%, brush biopsy smear in 20% of cases and transbronchial biopsy in 9–37% of cases. Yield can be increased by obtaining a combination of specimens. FOB in combination with transbronchial biopsy provided diagnosis (60–85%) in smear-negative pulmonary tuberculosis in different studies. Wallace, et al.[11] and Danek and Bower[5] have reported 95% culture positivity of specimens obtained by FOB and therefore negative culture provided strong evidence against tuberculosis. Bronchoscopy is also very useful in diagnosing pulmonary tuberculosis in children.[12] N somu, et al. found that the diagnostic yield of bronchoalveolar lavage and gastric lavage was 34%.[13]

Transbronchial biopsy specimens show granulomatous inflammation in miliary tuberculosis in 45–75% of cases.[14] In another study, it was found that bronchoscopy with transbronchial lung biopsy was valuable for the early diagnosis of pulmonary tuberculosis.[15] Bronchoalveolar lavage in miliary tuberculosis shows increase in CD8 count and the number of CD8 count correlates strongly to the radiological clearing of the disease.[16] Atypical mycobacteria can also be diagnosed reliably by staining and culture of BAL specimen. KS Dasgupta, et al. suggested that in areas with high prevalence of tuberculosis, bronchoscopy should be perfomed for early dignosis and initiation of therapy in sputum smear negative pulmonary tuberculosis.[17]

PRECAUTIONS

It is very essential to follow strict cleansing, sterilization and universal precautions to prevent cross-infection to other patients and health care personals:

Cleansing

It should be done using a detergent antiseptic solution, clean water and 50–70% alcohol as usual.

Sterilization

All bronchoscope, biopsy forceps and other instruments should be totally immersible and following routine cleansing, they should be sterilized by 30 minutes immersion in 2% glutaraldehyde or ethylene oxide to decontaminate a fiberoptic bronchoscope that has been contaminated by *M. tuberculosis*. The instrument subsequently must be washed and irrigated in sterile water before use.

Precautions During Procedure

It has been suggested that all patients should be assumed to be potential cases so following precautions should be taken routinely in all bronchoscopes to limit potential infection to staff and other patients.

1. The bronchoscopist and assistant should wear disposable gloves and eye protection in the form of close fitting spectacle or goggles. Operator must wear a surgical mask to prevent contamination by droplet infection to mouth.
2. All detritus including swabs collected during bronchoscopy should be disposed off properly, taking it to be potentially infective.
3. All contaminated surfaces should be cleaned with a 10% solution of household bleach (sodium hypochlorite).
4. Specimens obtained at bronchoscopy should be packed carefully and labeled “high risk of AIDS” if a done in immunocompromised host.
5. Lignocaine should be used sparingly as it may inhibit growth of some bacteria but probably not *M. tuberculosis*.[18]
6. It is desirable to use the totally immersible newer generation instruments for proper sterilization.

DRAWBACK

Peculiar problems encountered in bronchoscopy for suspected tuberculosis include the inhibitory effect of local anesthetic agents on *M. tuberculosis*[18] and transfer of infection from one patient to another.[19] Anderson, et al.[20]

concluded in their study that sputum induction is well tolerated, low cost and provides the same, if not better, diagnostic yield compared with bronchoscopy in the diagnosis of smear-negative pulmonary tuberculosis.

CONCLUSION

Finally, it can be concluded that fiberoptic bronchoscopy can provide excellent material with good yield for diagnosis of suspected cases of pulmonary tuberculosis from whom smears of expectorated sputum do not reveal *Mycobacterium* or from whom no sputum can be obtained. Besides, it is also useful for the diagnosis of miliary tuberculosis, endobronchial tuberculosis and childhood tuberculosis.

REFERENCES

1. Ikeda S. Flexible bronchofiberscope. Ann otol Rhinol Laryngol. 1970;79:916-9.
2. Mohan A, Sharma SK. Indian J Chest Dis and Allied Scei. 2008;50(1):67-8.
3. Rousell MD, Torrington KG, Teholder MF. A ten year experience with iberoptic bronchoscopy for mycobacterial isolation. Am Rev Resp Dis. 1986;133:1069-71.
4. Burk JR, Viroslav J, Bynum KLJ. Miliary tuberculosis diagnosed by fiberoptic bronchoscopy and transbronchial biopsy. Tubercle. 1978;59:107-9.
5. Danek SJ, Bower JS. Diagnosis of pulmonary TB by flexible bronchoscopy. Am Rev Resp Dis. 1979;119:677-9.
6. Sarkar SK, Sharma GS, Gupta PR, Sharma RK. Fiberoptic bronchoscopy in the diagnosis of pulmonary tuberculosis. Tubercle. 1980;61:97-9.
7. Jaiswal AK, Kulpati DD, Jain NK, Singh MM. Ind J Tub. 1989;36:233-6.
8. Kulpati DDS, Heera HS. Diagnosis of sputum negative pulmonary tuberculosis with flexible bronchoscopy. Ind J Tub. 1986;33:179-82.
9. Uddenfeldt M, Lundgren GH. Role of fiberoptic bronchoscopy in diagnosis of pulmonary tuberculosis. Tubercle. 1981;62:197-9.
10. Funashashi A, Lohaus GH. Role of fiberoptic bronchoscopy in the diagnosis of mycobacterial disease. Thorax 1983;38:267-70.
11. Wallace JM, Harell MD, Moser KM. Bronchocopy and transbronchial biopsy in evaluation of patients with suspected active TB. Am Rev J Med. 1991;70:1189-94.
12. De Blic J, Azevedo I, Burren CP, Le Bourgeous M, Lallemand D, Scheimann P. The value of flexible bronchoscopy in childhood pulmonary tuberculosis. Chest. 1991;100:688-92.
13. Somu N, Swaminathan S, Paramasivan CM, Vijayasekaran D. Value of bronchoalveolar lavage and gastric lavage in the diagnosis of pulmonary tuberculosis in children. Tubercle. 1995;76:295-9.
14. Wilcoy PA, Potgieter PD, Bateman ED et al. Rapid diagnosis of sputum negative miliary tuberculosis using flexible fiberoptic bronchoscope. Thorax, 1986;41:681.
15. Noriaki T, Nobuko U, Tomohiro U, Hiroshi A, Tomoko K, Chiharu O, et al. Clinical value of bronchoscopy for diagnosis of pulmonary tuberculosis. Journal of the Japan Society for Bronchology. 2001;23:332-5.
16. Aisle GM, Soloman JA, Bateman ED. Lymphocyte and lymphocyte subset numbers in blood and in BAL and pleural fluid in various forms of human pulmonary tuberculosis at presentation and during recovery. Thorax. 1992;47:513.
17. Dasgupta KS, Mundada PS, Soni N. Diagnostic role of fibreoptic bronchoscopy in pulmonary tuberculosis. Indian Journal of Otolaryngology and Head & Neck Surgery. 2000;4:347-9.
18. Conte BA, Laforet EG. The role of topical anaesthetic agent in modifying bacteriological dataobtained by bronchoscopy. New Eng J Med. 1962; 267:957-60.
19. Nelson KE. Transmission of tuberculosis of flexible fiberoptic bronchoscope. Am Rev Resp Dis. 1983;127:97-100.
20. Anderson C, Inhaber N. Comparision of sputum induction with fiberoptic bronchoscopy in the diagnosis of pulmonary tuberculosis. Am J Resp Crit Care Med. 1995;152:1570-4.

9H: OTHERS

FINE NEEDLE ASPIRATION CYTOLOGY

Fine needle aspiration cytology (FNAC) of lymph nodes and some times of intrathoracic lesion is quite reliable, safe, rapid and economical diagnostic tool for diagnosis of tuberculosis. An accuracy of 91.5% in diagnosis of tuberculous lymphadenitis by FNAC has been reported.[1-3]

RADIOACTIVE BROMIDE PARTICLES TEST

It has been useful in the diagnosis of tuberculous meningitis. It has a sensitivity of 86–94% and specificity of 88–96% and requires around 48 hours.[4]

ADENOSINE DEAMINASE ASSAY

Adenosine deaminase assay (ADA) is a lymphocytic enzyme that increases in tuberculosis. Its estimation in various body fluids and serum has been done and elevated ADA levels point towards the diagnosis of tuberculosis. Levels more than 70 U/L in pleural fluid strongly suggest tuberculous etiology, while levels <40 U/L rules out tuberculous etiology.[5] Author's assessment of ADA levels in pleural fluid showed that a cut-off level of 30 U/L had a sensitivity and specificity of 100%.[6] It also has useful role in diagnosis of tuberculous meningitis.[7] ADA activity is found in pathologic conditions other than TB.[8] Nevertheless, high levels of the enzyme are more strongly associated with pleural TB.[9] A recent meta-analysis indicated sensitivity of 0.92, specificity 0.90, positive predictive value of 0.93 and negative predictive value of 0.10.[11]

TUBERCULOSTEARIC ACID ESTIMATION

Tuberculostearic acid estimation (TBSA) is found in cell walls of *Mycobacterium*. It is identified by gas chromatography or mass spectrometry. However, due to complex technique and costly equipment, its estimation is seldom used in the diagnosis of tuberculosis. The test has a sensitivity of 95% and specificity of 90% in diagnosis of tuberculous meningitis.[10]

REFERENCES

1. Prasad R, Garg SK, Mukerji PK, Agarwal PK. Role of fine needle aspiration cytology in the diagnosis of lymphadenopathy. Indian J Chest Dis. Allied Sci. 1993;35:27-9.
2. Narag RK, Pradhan S, Singh RP, Chaturvedi S. Place of FNAC in the diagnosis of lymphadenopathy. Indian J Tuber. 1990;37:29.
3. Malankar D, Jajoo UN, Swarup K, Gupta OP, Jain AP, Poflee VW. A clinical evaluation of FNAC in the diagnosis of lymphadenopathy. Indian J Tuber. 1991;38:17.
4. Mandal BK, Evans DIK, Ironside AG, Pullan BR. Radioactive bromide particle test in differential diagnosis of tuberculous meningitis. BMJ. 1972;4:413-5.

5. Valder L, et al. Diagnosis of tuberculous pleurisy using biological parameter ADA, lysosome and interferon gamma. Chest. 1991;103:458-65.
6. Prasad R, Tripathi RP, Mukerji PK, Srivastava VML. Adenosine deaminase activity in pleural fluid: A diagnostic test of tuberculous pleural effusion. Ind J Chest Dis Allied Sci. 1992;34:123.
7. Prasad R, Kumar A, Khanna BK, et al. Adenosine deaminase activity in cerebrospinal fluid for diagnosis of tubercular meningitis. Ind J Tub. 1991;38:99.
8. Burgess LI, Maritz FJ, Le Roux I, et al. Use of adenosine deaminase as a diagnostic tool for tuberculous pleurisy. Thorax. 1995;50:672-4.
9. Shibagaki T, Hasegawa Y, Saito H, et al. Adenosine deaminase isoenzymes in tuberculous pleural effusion. J Lab Clin Med. 1996;127:348-52.
10. French GL, Teoh R, Chan CY, et al. Diagnosis of tuberculous meningitis by detection of tuberculostearic acid in cerebrospinal fluid. Lancet. 1987;2:117-9.
11. Liang QL, Shi HZ, Wang K, Qin SM, Qin XJ. Diagnostic accuracy of adenosine deaminase in tuberculous pleurisy: a meta-analysis. Respir Med. 2008;102:744-54.

Chapter 10

Differential Diagnosis of Pulmonary Tuberculosis

INTRODUCTION

There are a number of conditions which simulate pulmonary tuberculosis and it is very essential to differentiate these conditions from pulmonary tuberculosis for the proper management of the patient. Aim of this chapter is to review the list of the diseases, which are included in the differential diagnosis of pulmonary tuberculosis.

PNEUMONIA

The term pneumonia refers to a syndrome caused by acute infection, usually bacterial, characterized by clinical and/or radiographic signs of consolidation of one or both lungs. The common etiologic agents of pneumonia include *Streptococcus pneumoniae, Haemophilus influenzae, Staphylococcus aureus, Escherichia coli, Klebsiella, Pseudomonas aeruginosa,* etc. A segmental pneumonia with upper zone opacities may mimick pulmonary tuberculosis. In contrast to tuberculosis where symptoms may be absent or prolonged, the acute pneumonia patient usually has symptoms of fairly recent onset. If the patient is symptomatic, oral antibiotics should be prescribed and if the radiologic opacities have not cleared or improved in 2 to 3 weeks then tuberculosis is more likely. With pneumonia refractory to standard treatment, especially if the white cell count is normal, repeated sputum specimens should be examined for acid-fast bacilli. X-ray of the patient shows unilateral or bilateral infiltrates in the form of bronchopneumonia or lobar pneumonia. In some cases, cavitation may be present. The condition is usually differentiated from mycobacterial infection by sputum examination by Gram's stain and Ziehl-Neelsen staining, sputum culture and tuberculin testing. Other tests include blood culture and serological testing. If the sputum examination is noncontributory, bronchoalveolar lavage (BAL) fluid examination for *M. tuberculosis* and *Pneumocystis carinii* cysts is indicated.[1,2]

FUNGAL DISEASES

Fungi of medical importance infecting the lungs are of the class zygomycetes, ascomycetes, basidiomycetes, hypomycetes and blastomycetes. X-ray chest shows a variety of features from bilateral nodular infiltrates to diffuse consolidation and fibrosis. Cavitation may also be present. Diagnostic tests include sputum examination, histopathological examination of tissue specimens and serological tests (Figs 10.1 to 10.7).

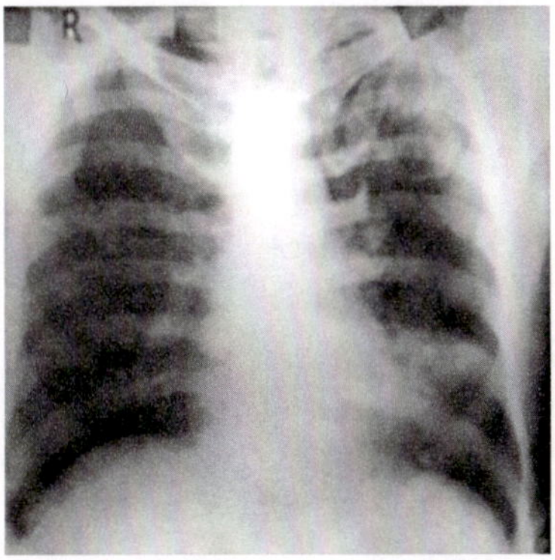

Fig. 10.1: Chest X-ray showing cavity in left upper zone

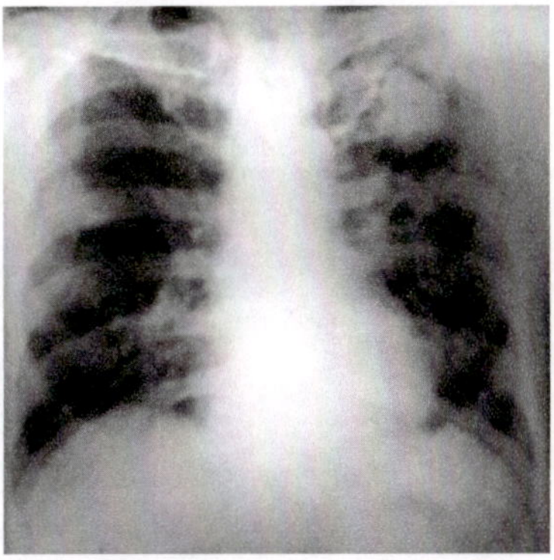

Fig. 10.2: Chest X-ray showing semi-invasive aspergillosis under progression

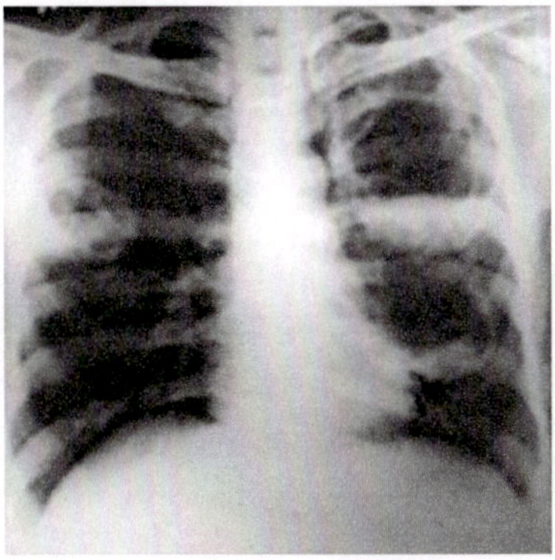

Fig. 10.3: Chest X-ray showing semi-invasive aspergillosis under progression

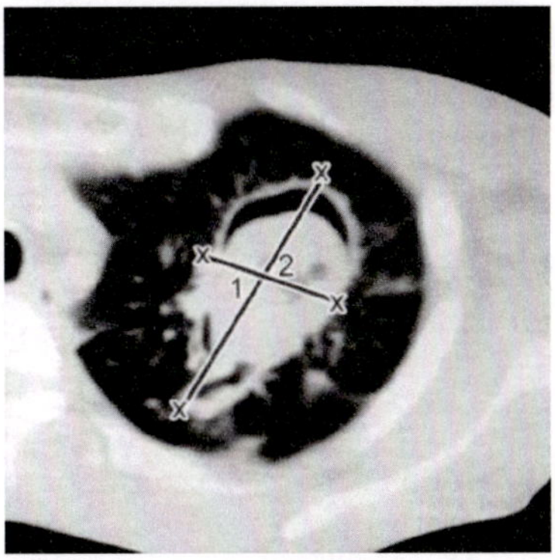

Fig. 10.4: CT thorax showing semi-invasive aspergillosis

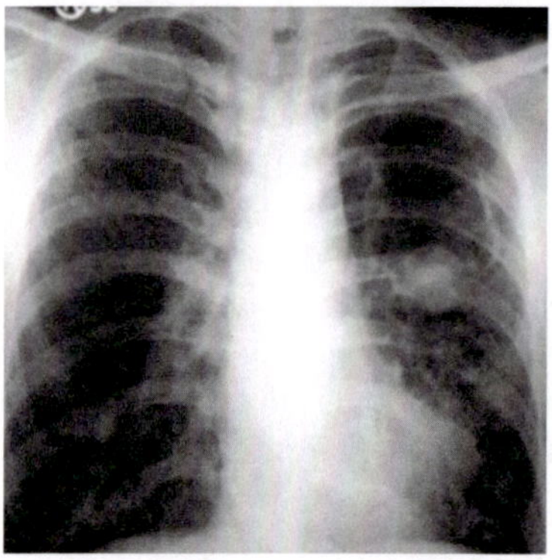

Fig. 10.5: Chest X-ray PA view showing healed cavity with aspergilloma

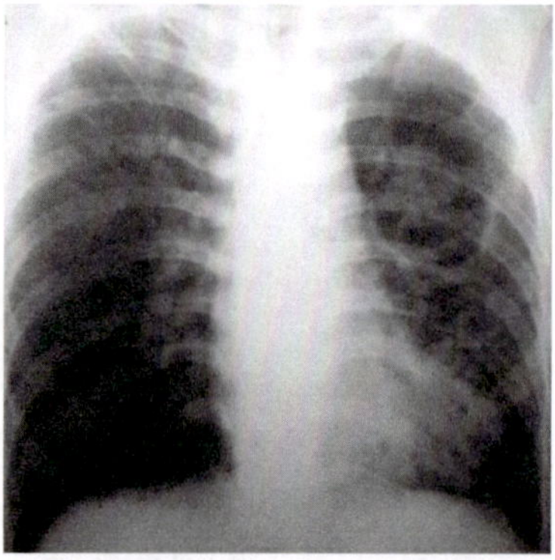

Fig. 10.6: Chest X-ray Trendelenburg view showing movement of aspergilloma

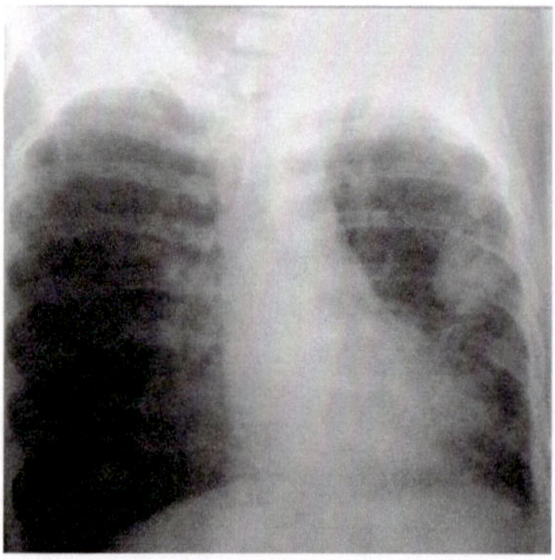

Fig. 10.7: Chest X-ray left lateral decubitus view showing movement of aspergilloma

PARASITIC DISEASE

Eosinophilic pneumonia, e.g. Loefflers syndrome caused by ascaris infection as it passes through the lung may present with a radiological picture suggestive of pulmonary tuberculosis. Tropical pulmonary eosinophilia may produce a military pattern on chest X-ray. Similarly, hydatid infection of the lung may produce a radiological picture resembling pulmonary tuberculosis especially when the cyst begins to leak and collapses. The conditions are usually differentiated from pulmonary tuberculosis by sputum smear examination (Figs 10.8, 10.9).

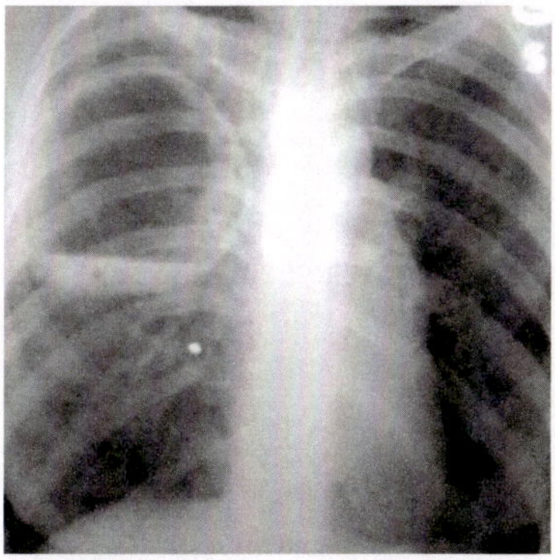

Fig. 10.8: Chest X-ray PA view showing ruptured hydatid cyst in right lung misdiagnosed as pulmonary tuberculosis

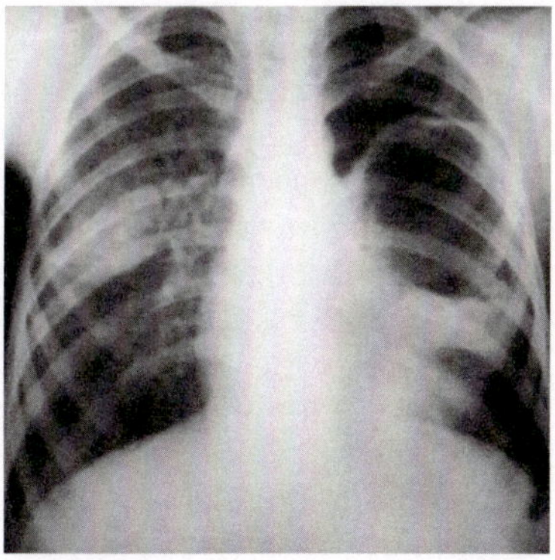

Fig. 10.9: Chest X-ray showing hydatid cyst bilateral (ruptured in left lung and another in right lung)

BRONCHIECTASIS

It is a condition in which the bronchi are permanently and abnormally dilated. It may be due to developmental defects, infection, inhalation/aspiration injury, immunodeficiency syndromes or autoimmune disease. Cough is the most common symptoms of bronchiectasis which is persistent and productive of mucopurulent sputum. Dyspnea is usually a late symptoms. The patient has coarse crepts. Clubbing of the fingers and/or toes may be present. It may be associated with patchy fibrosis and consolidation, which may mimick pulmonary tuberculosis. X-ray of the patient may show ring shadows, parallel lines and solid tubular opacities. HRCT thorax is the investigation of choice for differentiating this condition from pulmonary tuberculosis (Figs 10.10, 10.11).

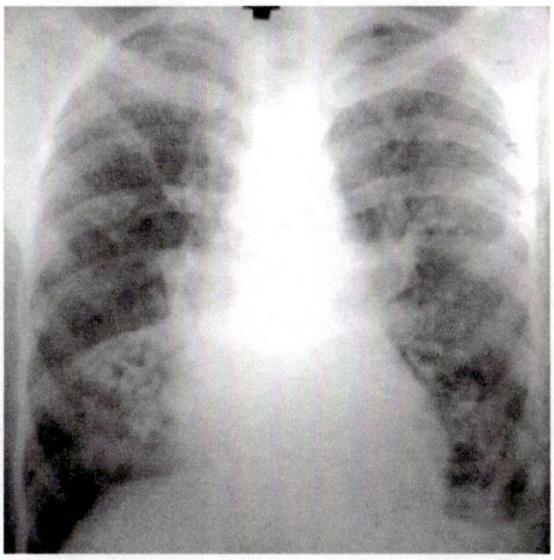

Fig. 10.10: Chest X-ray showing bilateral bronchiectasis

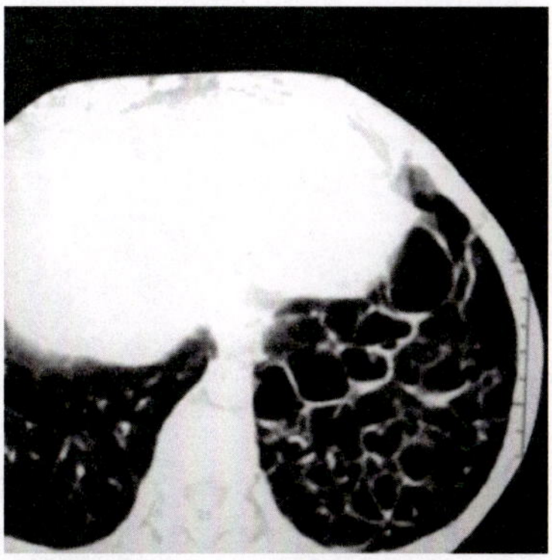

Fig. 10.11: Chest X-ray showing bilateral bronchiectasis

LUNG ABSCESS

Lung abscess is a localized area of destruction of lung parenchyma in which infection by pyogenic organisms results in tissue necrosis and suppuration. They frequently contain air fluid levels. When multiple and small (< 2 cm in diameter) they are sometimes referred to as necrotizing or suppurative pneumonia. Apart from pyogenic organisms, these lung abscess are also caused by tuberculosis, fungi and protozoa. The predominant symptoms are cough with purulent sputum, fever, dyspnea and chest pain. Digital clubbing may develop in some patients. Lung abscess due to *Staphylococcus aureus* or *Klebsiella pneumoniae* is usually an acute severe illness with marked leukocytosis and the organism is readily isolated from blood or sputum. With cavitatory tuberculosis, the sputum is usually but not always positive on direct smear. X-ray chest may initially show a pneumonic infiltrate followed by the development of one or more spherical areas of more homogenous density in which air-fluid levels often arise. The other investigations include sputum examination, blood cultures, CT scan thorax and bronchoscopy in some cases as a possible method of microbiological sampling (Figs 10.12 to 10.19).

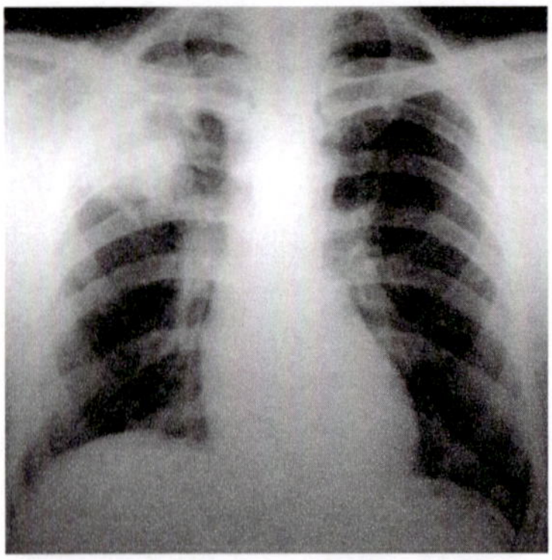

Fig. 10.12: Chest X-ray showing right sided lung abscess

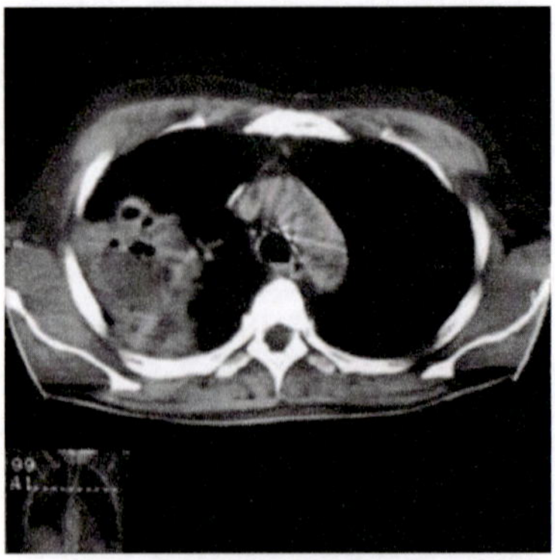

Fig. 10.13: CT thorax showing right sided lung abscess

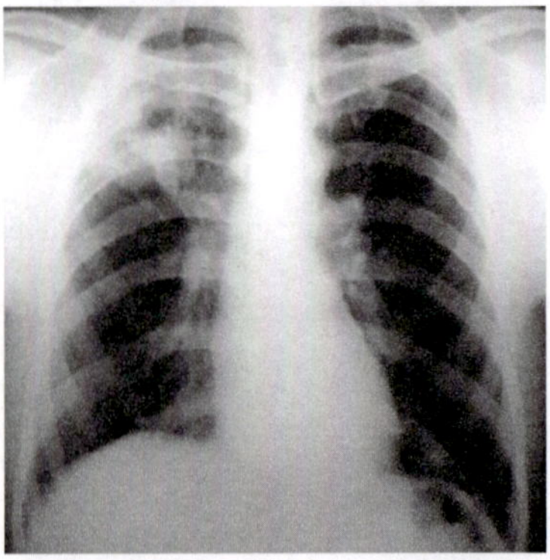

Fig. 10.14: Chest X-ray showing resolution of lung abscess after two weeks of treatment

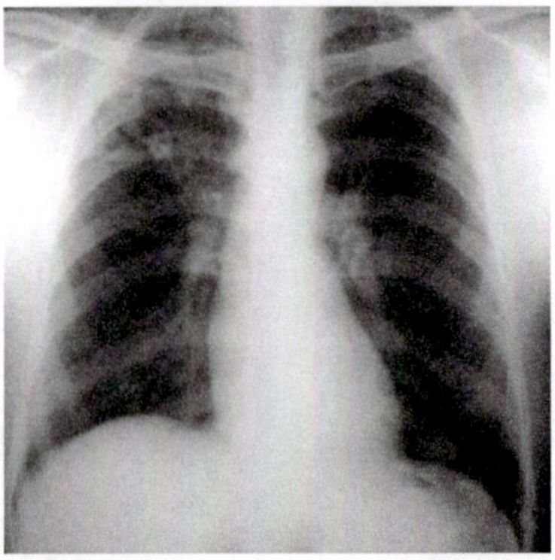

Fig. 10.15: Chest X-ray showing resolution of lung abscess after one month of treatment

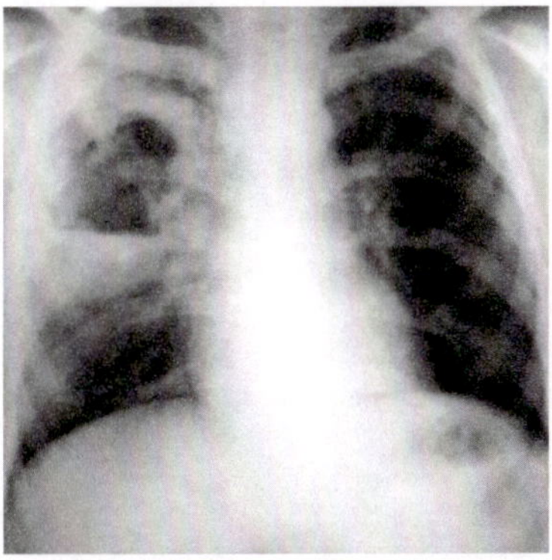

Fig. 10.16: Chest X-ray showing right sided lung abscess

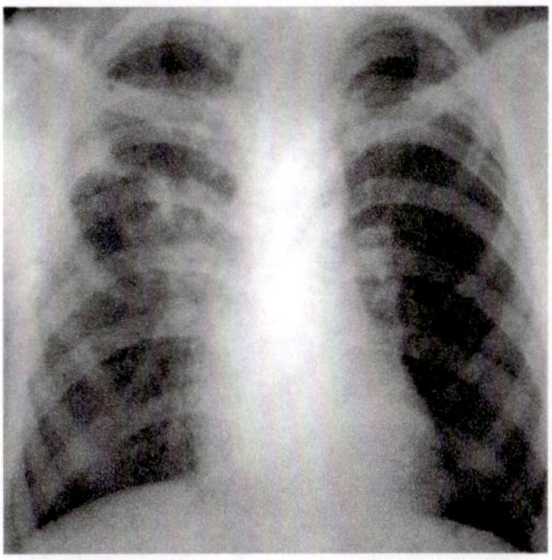

Fig. 10.17: Chest X-ray showing resolution of lung abscess after 10 days of antibiotics

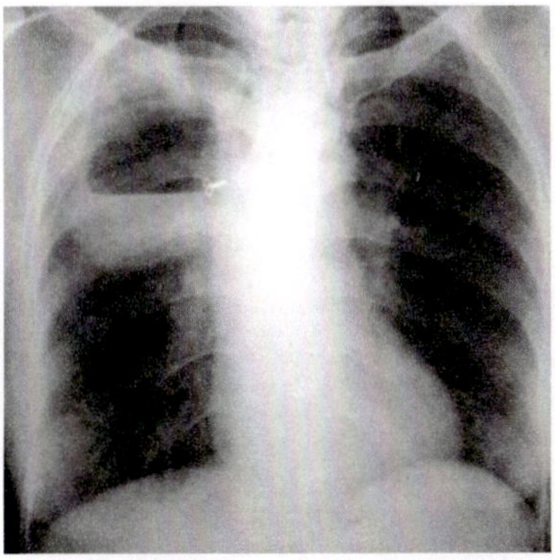

Fig. 10.18: Chest X-ray showing right side apical lung abscess

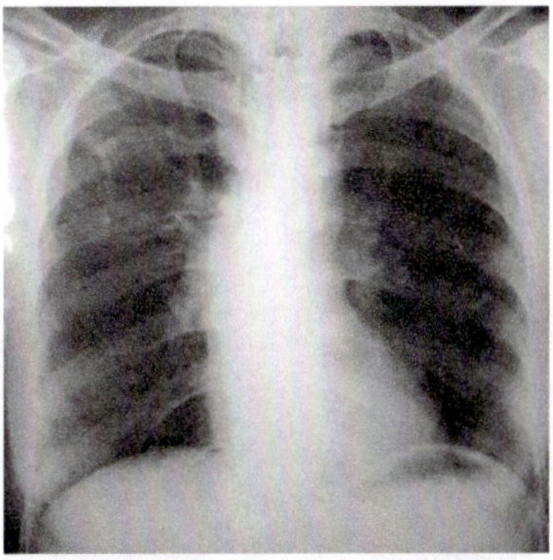

Fig. 10.19: Chest X-ray showing resolution of lung abscess after antibiotics

ALLERGIC BRONCHOPULMONARY ASPERGILLOSIS

Allergic bronchopulmonary aspergillosis (ABPA) is an inflammatory lung disease characterized by an allergic inflammatory response to *Aspergillus* or other fungi in the lung. It is characterized by asthmatic symptoms, recurrent shadows on the chest radiograph and blood eosinophilia. The expectoration of inspissated mucus in the form of bronchial casts is relatively common. These infiltrates when present in the upper zone on X-ray chest may mimick pulmonary tuberculosis. The condition is differentiated from mycobacterial infection by the presence of pulmonary eosinophilia, positive skin test to *Aspergillus*, serum precipitins to *Aspergillus*, elevated total serum IgE, culture of *Aspergillus* from sputum, elevated *Aspergillus* fumigates specific IgE and IgG and a history suggestive of bronchial asthma. ABPA very commonly mimicks pulmonary tuberculosis as author himself reported that 90.5% patients of ABPA were already prescribed antitubercular drug[4] (Figs 10.20 to 10.25).

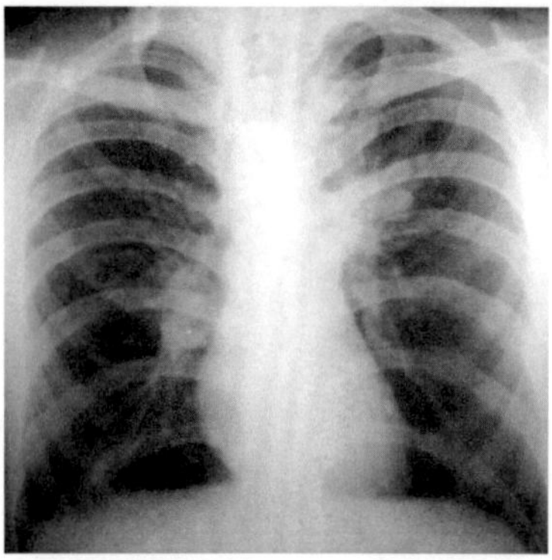

Fig. 10.20: Chest X-ray of a patient of asthma presented with hemoptysis and was misdiagnosed as pulmonary tuberculosis

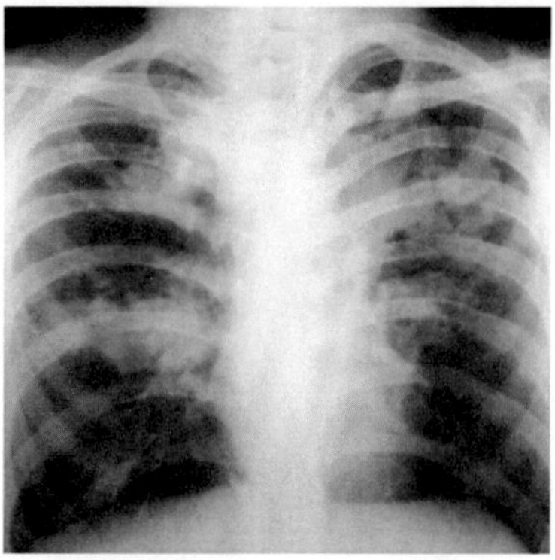

Fig. 10.21: Chest X-ray showing increase of lesion after 6 months of ATT

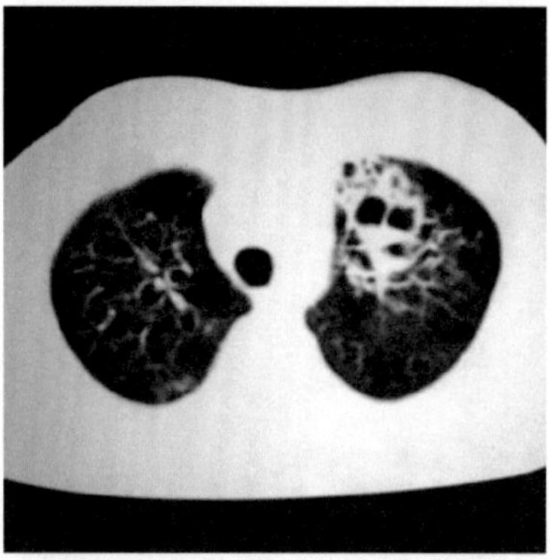

Fig. 10.22: CT thorax showing bilateral central bronchiectasis

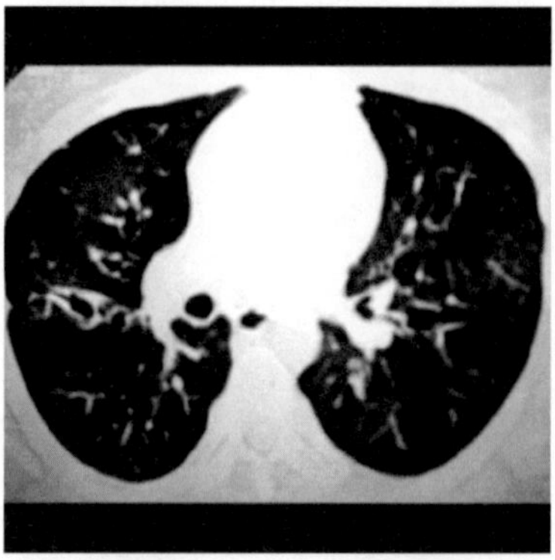

Fig. 10.23: CT thorax showing bilateral central bronchiectasis

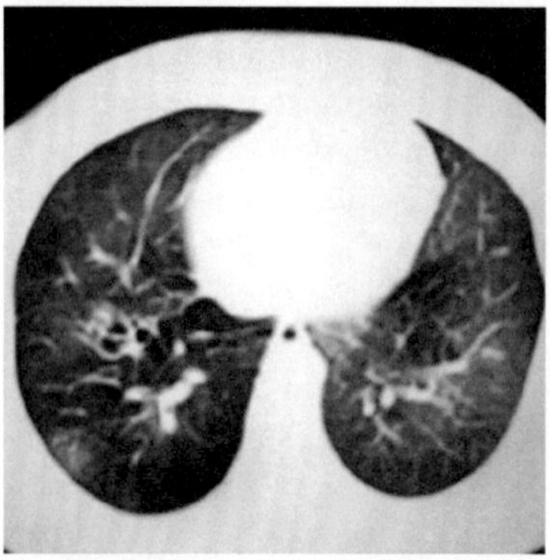

Fig. 10.24: CT thorax showing bilateral central bronchiectasis

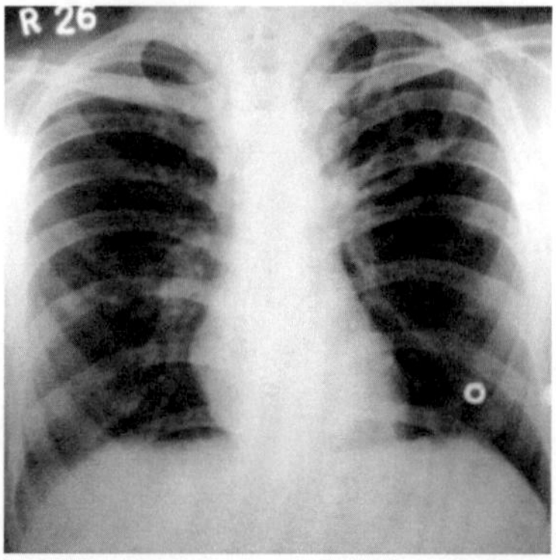

Fig. 10.25: Chest X-ray showing resolution of shadows after treatment of allergic bron-chopulmonary aspergillosis

PULMONARY EDEMA

Pulmonary edema is defined as an excess of extravascular water within the lungs. This fluid may accumulate within the interstitial tissues, in alveolar walls and around vessels (Interstitial edema), within alveoli (alveolar edema) or commonly both. X-ray chest initially shows features of interstitial edema followed by diffuse pulmonary clouding and the presence of Kerley A and B lines. As the edema increases, nodular opacities and ultimately signs of alveolar consolidation appear.

LUNG CANCER

Consolidation distal to a proximal carcinoma, particularly in the upper zone, may be cavitated and closely mimic tuberculosis. Occasionally, primary tuberculosis in the elderly presents with a peripheral lesions and enlarged hilar nodes may closely mimick carcinoma. Isolated solid pulmonary opacities, the presence of satellite lesions or calcification, suggests tuberculosis. Isolated malignant cavity may also mimic tuberculosis. Irregularity of the wall or polypoid protrusions into the interior suggest carcinoma. A malignant cavity is usually thick walled, eccentric with irregular inner wall of cavity. Bilateral shadows suggest tuberculosis. Lung cancer is more common in men than women. Lung cancer usually presents as chest pain, cough, breathlessness, hemoptysis, hoarseness of voice, neurological symptoms due to CNS metastasis, metastasis to liver or cervical, axillary or supraclavicular lymphadenopathy. X-ray chest may show areas of heterogenous opacity, unresolving consolidation or lung collapse. In some cases, cavitation may be evident. The condition is usually differentiated from pulmonary tuberculosis by CT scan thorax, bronchoscopy (Figs 10.26 to 10.43).

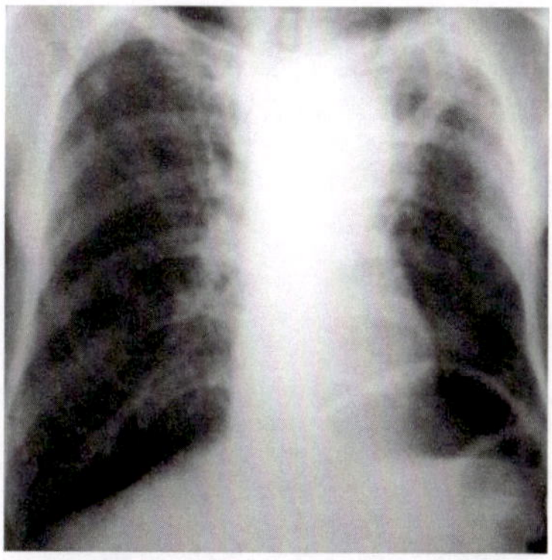

Fig. 10.26: Chest X-ray showing thick-walled cavity in left upper zone and misdiagnosed as pulmonary tuberculosis

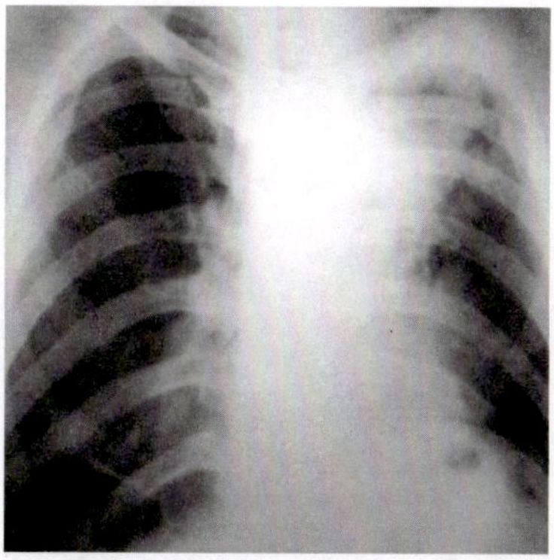

Fig. 10.27: Chest X-ray showing progression of lesion after 2 months of ATT

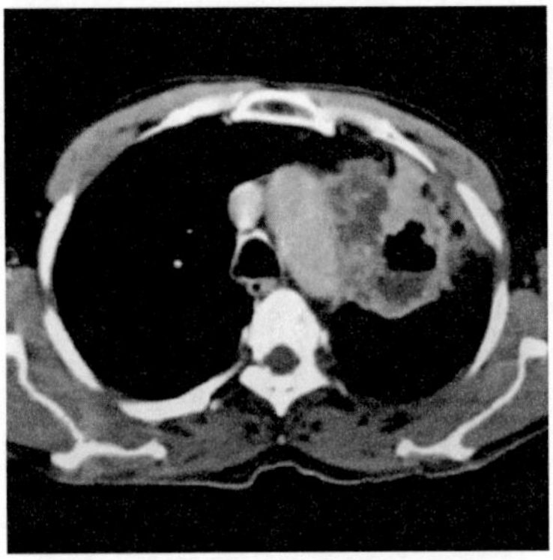

Fig. 10.28: CT thorax showing thick-walled cavity

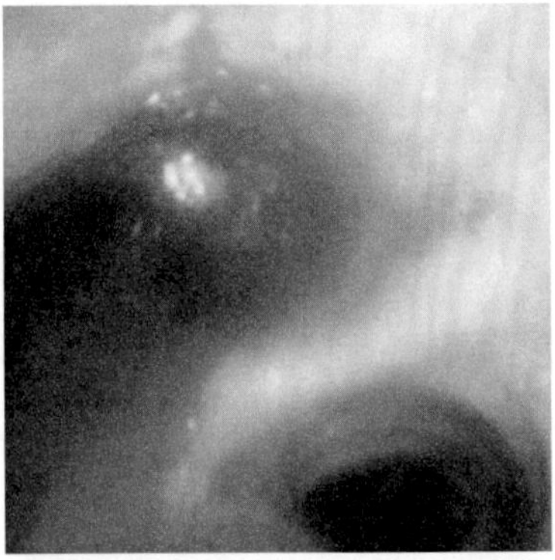

Fig. 10.29: FOB showing growth proven to be squamous cell carcinoma in the left main bronchus (For color version, see Plate 4)

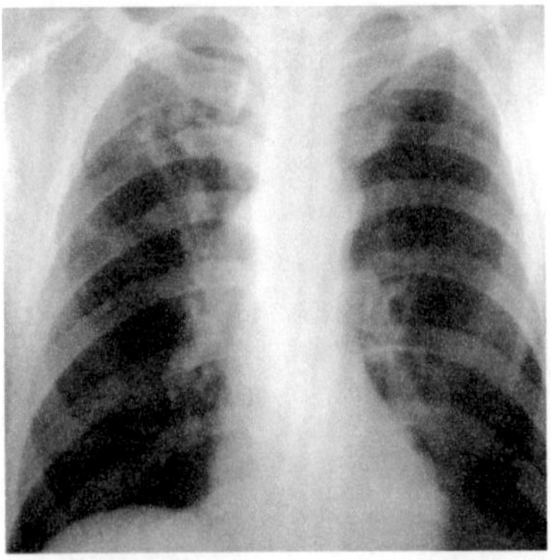

Fig. 10.30: Chest X-ray showing infiltrative lesion right upper zone misdiagnosed as pulmonary tuberculosis

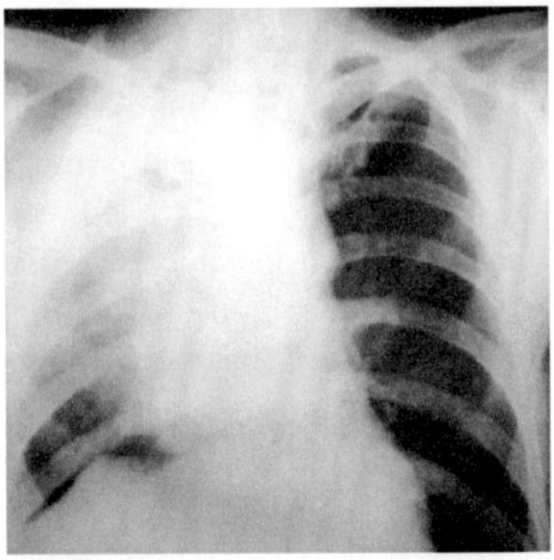

Fig. 10.31: Chest X-ray showing progression of lesion after 6 months of ATT

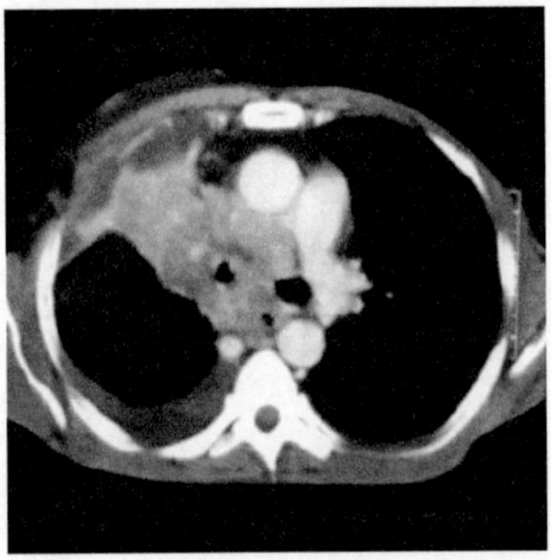

Fig. 10.32: CT thorax showing growth in the right lung

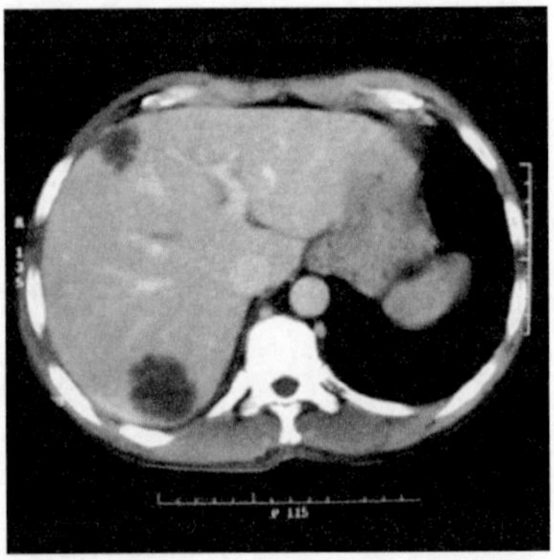

Fig. 10.33: CT thorax showing secondaries in liver diagnosed as BACA Stage IV

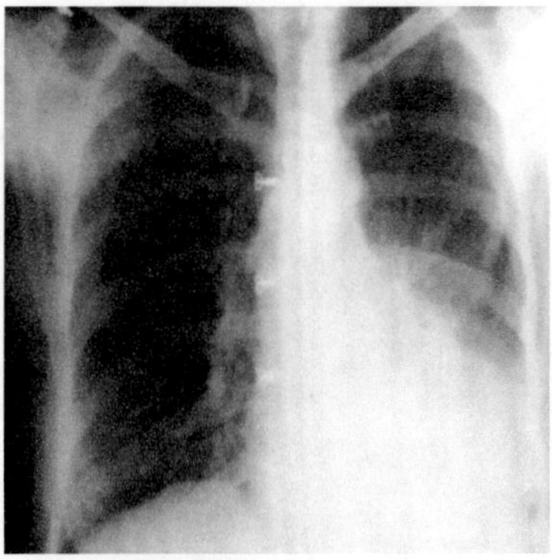

Fig. 10.34: Chest X-ray showing mass in the parahilar area of left lung

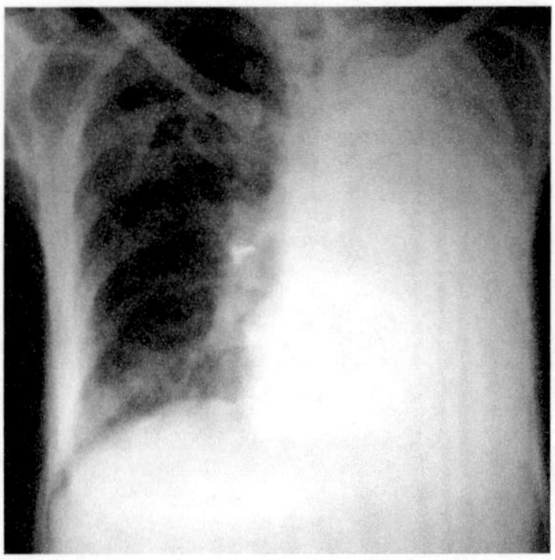

Fig. 10.35: Chest X-ray showing collapse with effusion on left side

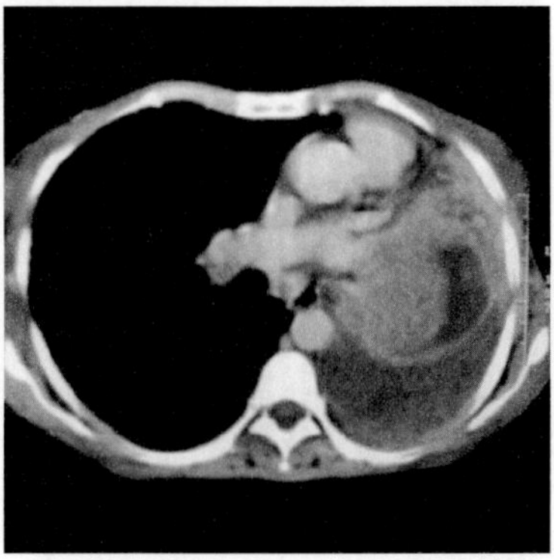

Fig. 10.36: CT thorax showing mass with necrosis with pleural effusion

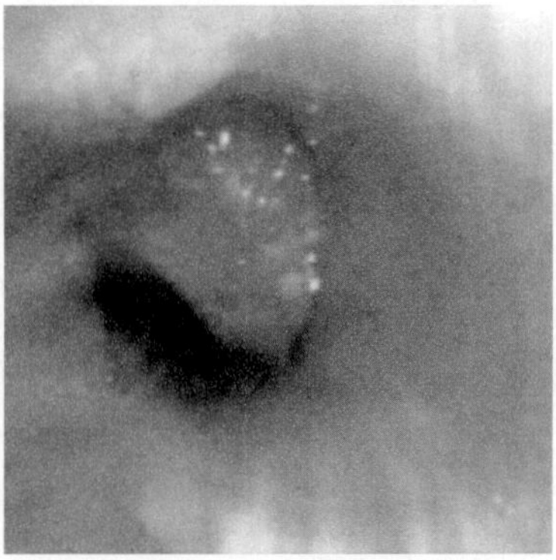

Fig. 10.37: FOB showing irregular growth in left main bronchus just before its bifurcation (For color version, see Plate 4)

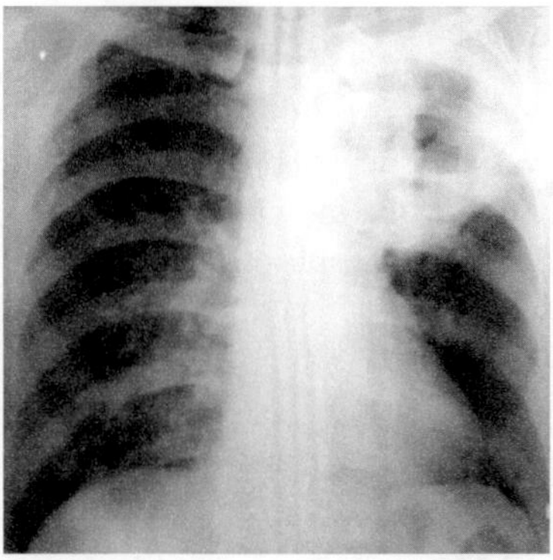

Fig. 10.38: Chest X-ray showing thick-walled left upper zone cavity with air fluid level misdiagnosed as pulmonary tuberculosis

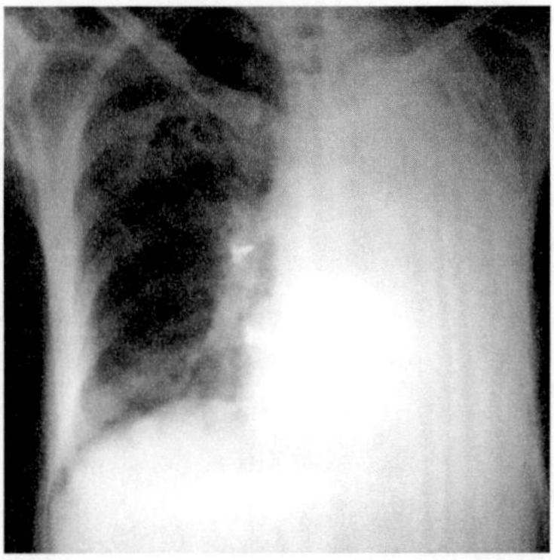

Fig. 10.39: Chest X-ray showing progression of lesions after 3 months of ATT

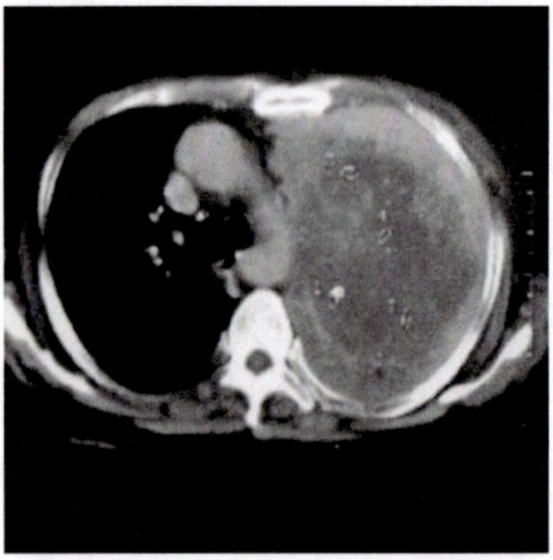

Fig. 10.40: CT thorax showing growth in left lung

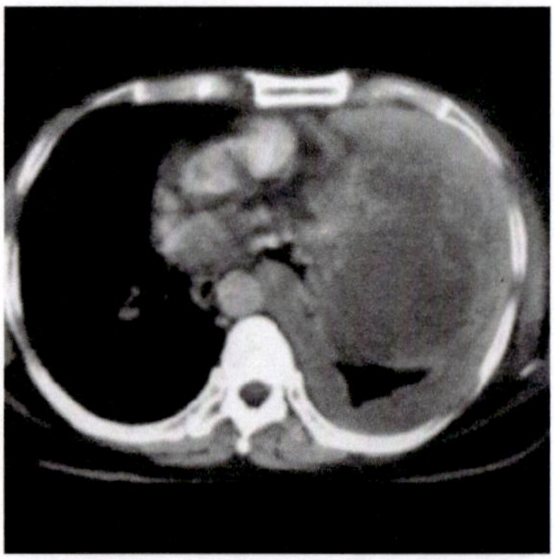

Fig. 10.41: CT thorax showing growth in left lung

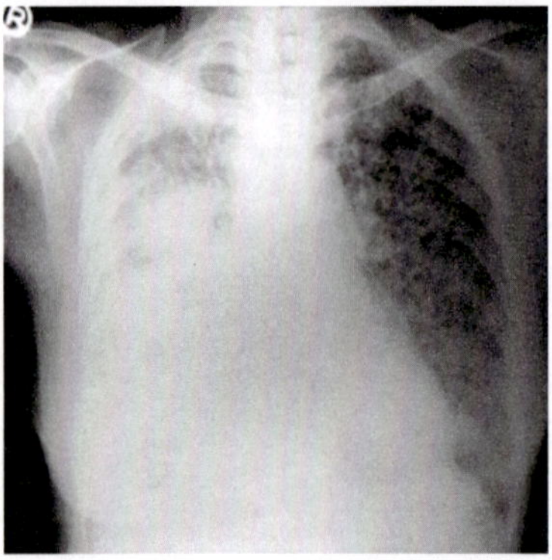

Fig. 10.42: Chest X-ray showing right-sided mass with pleural effusion with diffuse lung shadow misdiagnosed as pulmonary tuberculosis

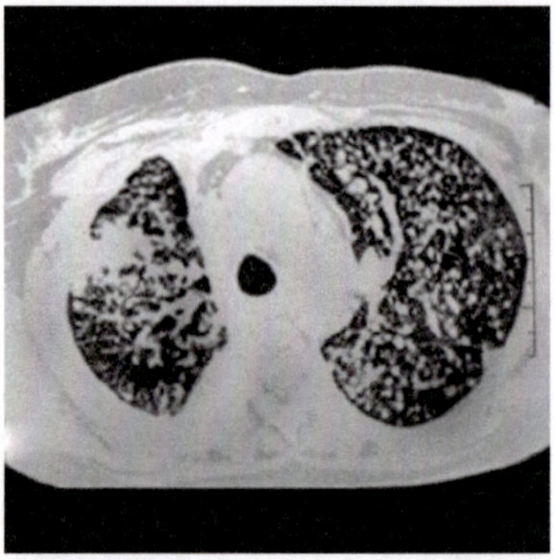

Fig. 10.43: CT thorax showing mass on the right side and diffuse lung shadow in the left suggestive of lymphangitis carcinomatosis

INTERSTITIAL LUNG DISEASE

Interstitial lung disease is a collection of non-neoplastic lung disorders, both is it acute and chronic, that present with variable degrees of inflammation and fibrosis. It is also known as diffuse parenchymal lung disease (DPLD). idiopathic interstitial pneumonia (IIP) includes the subset of DPLD that are of unknown etiology. Each of these diseases is associated with a distinct pathological pattern. IPF is associated with the UIP pattern. X-ray shows reticulonodular pattern. If this reticulonodular pattern is predominant in the upper lobes then it may mimic pulmonary tuberculosis. The condition is differentiated from mycobacterial infection by HRCT thorax, sputum examination and blood investigation (Figs 10.44 to 10.50).

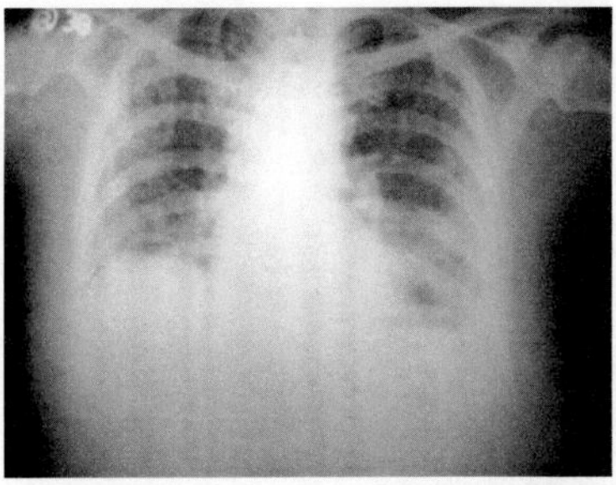

Fig. 10.44: Chest X-ray showing bilateral infiltrates misdiagnosed as pulmonary tuberculosis

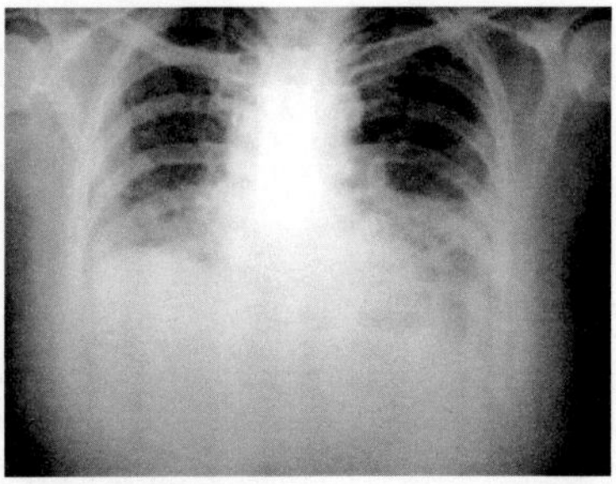

Fig. 10.45: Chest X-ray showing progression of lesion after 8 months of ATT

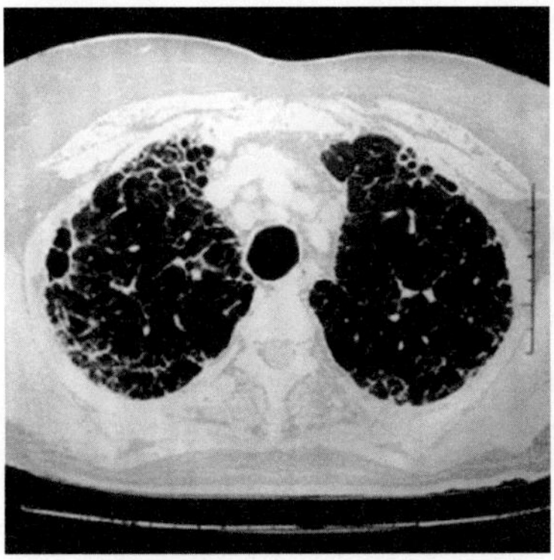

Fig. 10.46: CT thorax showing interstitial lung diseases

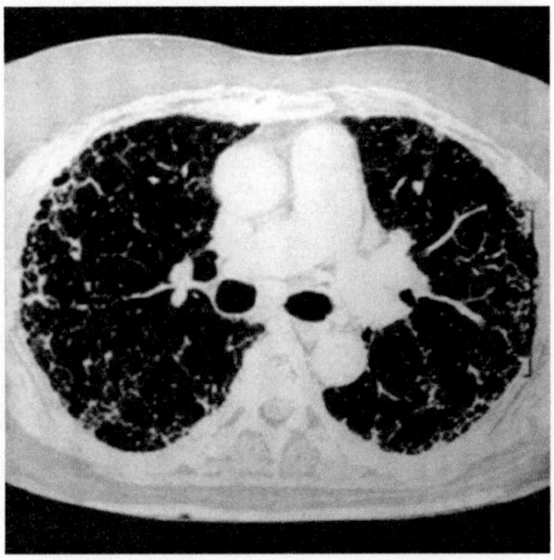

Fig. 10.47: CT thorax showing interstitial lung diseases

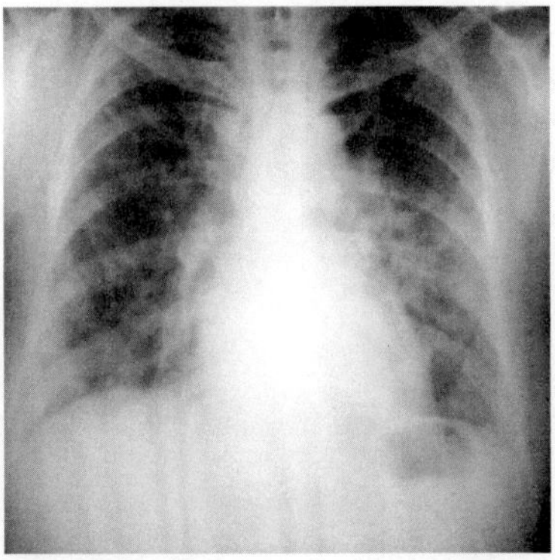

Fig. 10.48: Chest X-ray showing bilateral infiltrates misdiagnosed as pulmonary tuberculosis

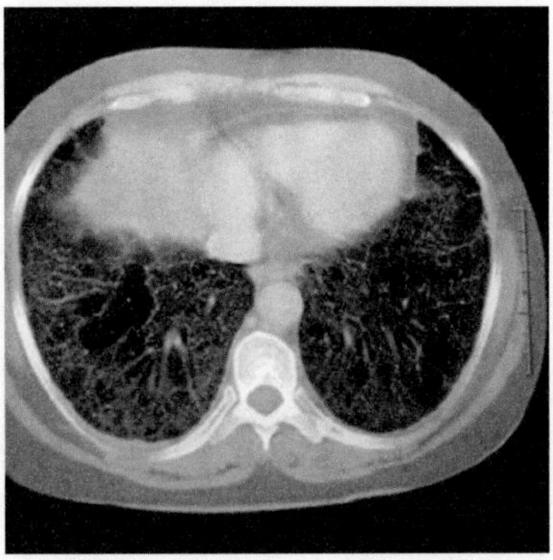

Fig. 10.49: CT thorax showing interstitial lung diseases

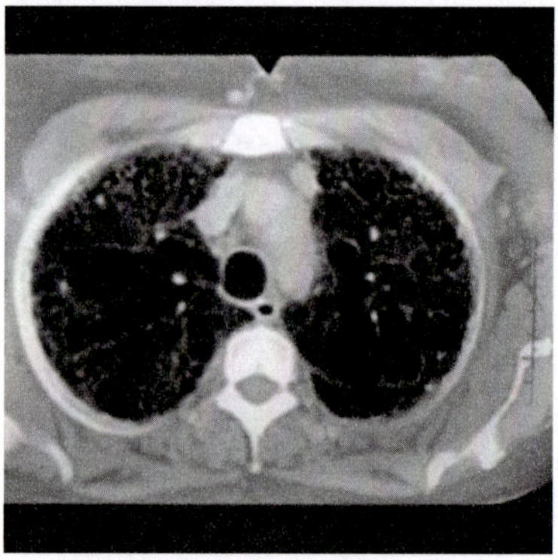

Fig. 10.50: CT thorax showing interstitial lung diseases

SARCOIDOSIS

Sarcoidosis is a multisystem granulomatous disorder of unknown etiology most commonly affecting young adults and presenting most frequently with bilateral hilar lymphadenopathy, pulmonary infiltration and skin or eye lesions. Histologically, widespread noncaseating epitheloid granulomas may be present. X-ray chest and CT scan thorax may show ground glassing, reticular abnormalities, nodular shadows and mediastinal and hilar lymphadenopathy. These radiological abnormalities if present in the upper lobe also may mimic pulmonary tuberculosis (Figs 10.51 to 10.58). These patients have negative tuberculin test and the sputum is negative for *M. tuberculosis*.[3] It is differentiated from pulmonary tuberculosis by serum angiotensin converting enzyme test, bronchoscopy (BAL), serum calcium and 24 hours urinary calcium. Lung biopsy is required in rare cases.

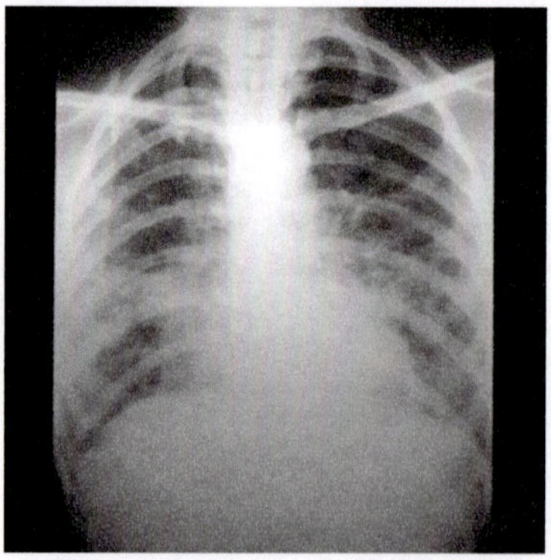

Fig. 10.51: Chest X-ray showing bilateral lesion misdiagnosed as pulmonary tuberculosis

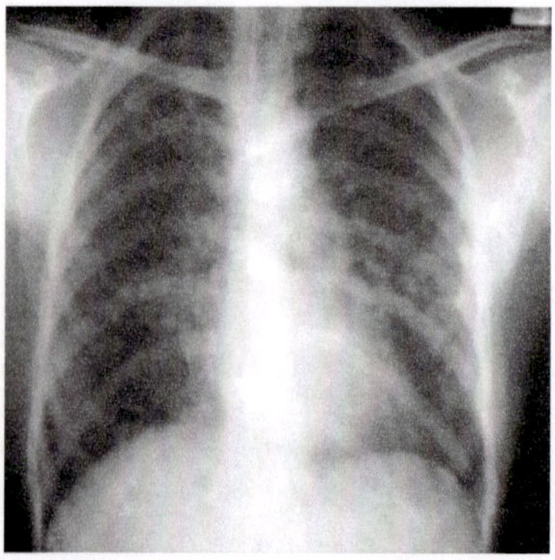

Fig. 10.52: Chest X-ray showing no response after 10 months of ATT

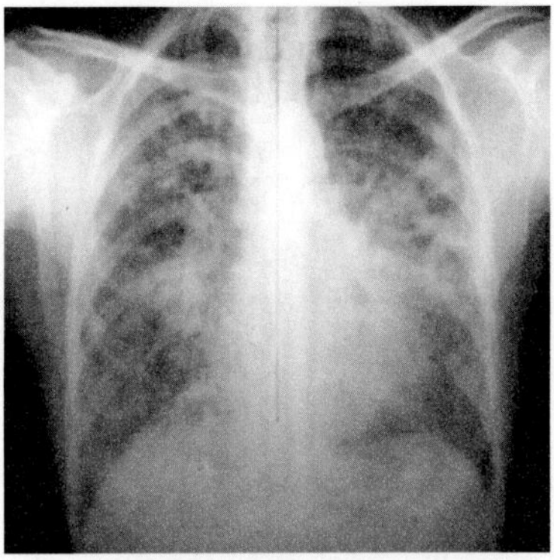

Fig. 10.53: Chest X-ray showing progression of lesions

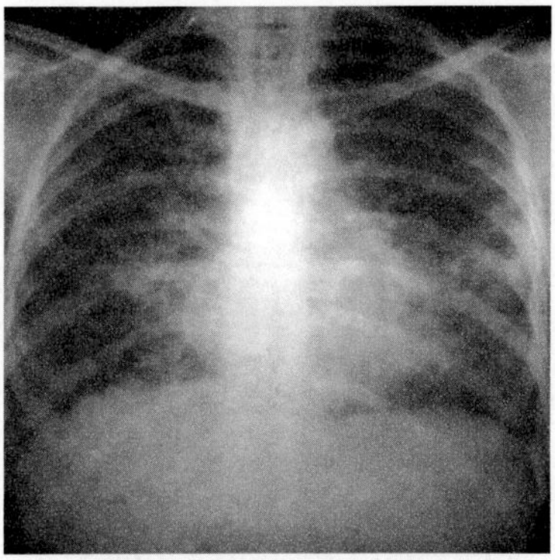

Fig. 10.54: Chest X-ray showing progression of lesions

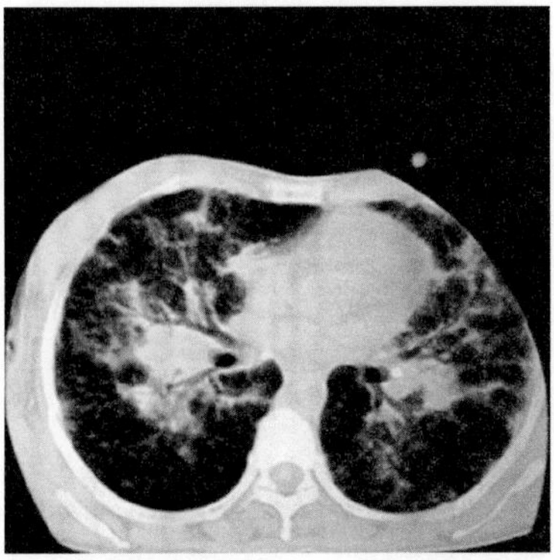

Fig. 10.55: CT thorax showing bilateral hilar lymphadenitis with parenchymal involvement

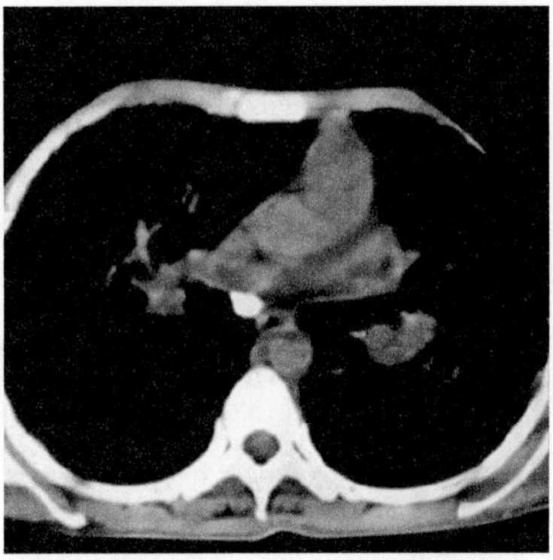

Fig. 10.56: CT thorax showing hilar adenopathy due to sarcoidosis

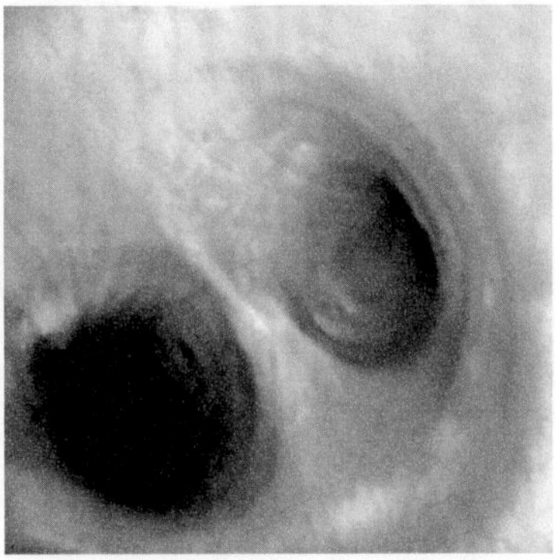

Fig. 10.57: Fiberoptic bronchoscopy showing hyperemic mucosa and endobronchial biopsy from main carina revealed non-caseating granuloma (For color version, see Plate 4)

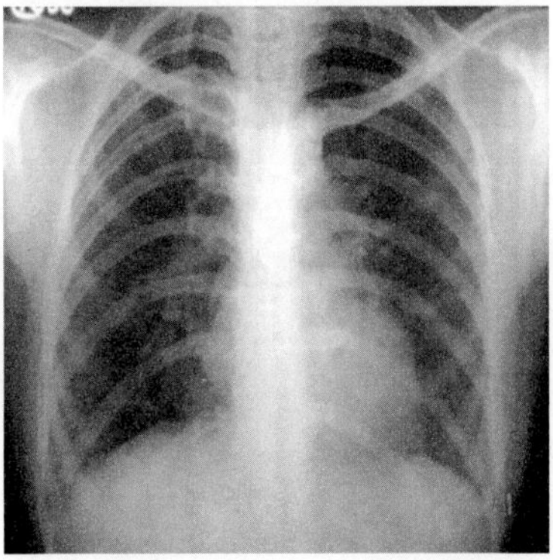

Fig. 10.58: Chest X-ray showing resolution of lesions after treatment for sarcoidosis

OCCUPATIONAL LUNG DISEASES

These include diseases like asbestosis, coal workers pneumoconiosis, silicosis, etc. The X-ray picture in these patients will show nodular opacities resembling miliary tuberculosis. In occupational lung disease, signs and symptoms of infection will usually be absent. The condition is usually differentiated from pulmonary tuberculosis by a careful occupational history and sputum smear examination.

PULMONARY INFARCTION

Upper zone pulmonary infarcts, especially if bilateral and/or cavitating may cause difficulty in diagnosis. Routine investigations, evidence of deep vein thrombosis and serial chest films that show rapid change in pulmonary infarction usually differentiate it from pulmonary tuberculosis.

CONGENITAL CONDITIONS

Congenital conditions of the lung, e.g. lung sequestration, lung cysts, cavernous hemangiomas and hamartomas may also present a radiological picture resembling pulmonary tuberculosis. In these congenital conditions, clinical features of infection will usually be absent and sputum smear examination will be negative for *M. tuberculosis* (Figs 10.59, 10.60).

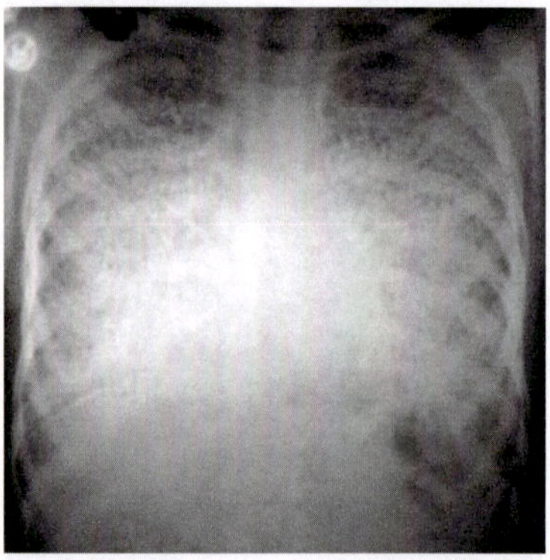

Fig. 10.59: Chest X-ray showing bilateral diffuse lung shadows without any symptoms

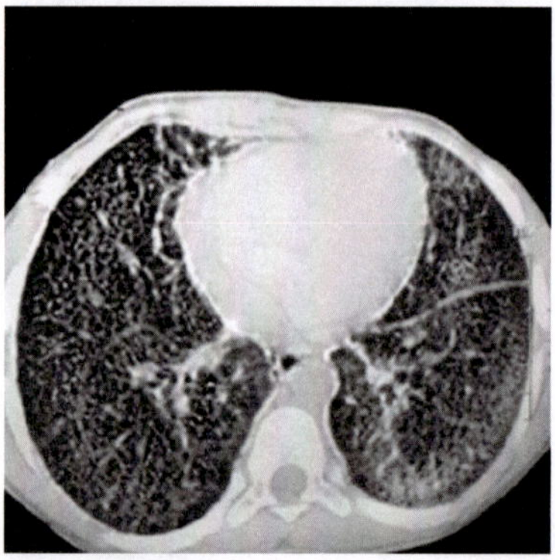

Fig. 10.60: CT thorax showing dense diffuse lung shadows diagnosed as alveolar microlithiasis

CARDIOVASCULAR DISEASES

Some cardiac disease, e.g. mitral stenosis may present with hemoptysis. Further cardiac evaluation by echocardiography may help in differentiating the cardiac condition from pulmonary tuberculosis.

REFERENCES

1. Mohan A, Pande JN, Sharma SK, Rattan A, Guleria R, Khilanani GC. Bronchoalveolar lavage in pulmonary tuberculosis. A decision analysis approach. QJM. 1995;88:269-76.
2. Sharma SK, Pande JN. Fiberoptic bronchoscopy (editorial). Indian J Chest Dis Allied Sci. 1988;36:163-5.
3. Sharma SK, Mohan A, Guleria R, Padhy AK. Diagnostic dilemma: Tuberculosis? Or sarcoidosis? Indian J Chest Dis Allied Sci. 1997;39:119-23.
4. Prasad R, Garg R, Sanjay, Shukla AD. Allergic bronchopulmonary aspergillosis: A review of 42 patients from a tertiary care centre in India. Lung India. 2009;26:38-40.

Chapter 11

Complications of Tuberculosis

INTRODUCTION

Although pulmonary tuberculosis is curable, it can lead to serious complications especially in the infants, elderly, in the immunocompromised and in those who do not get prompt medical treatment. The complications of pulmonary tuberculosis contribute significantly to the morbidity and mortality of the patients. Aim of this chapter is to describe the various complications of pulmonary tuberculosis.

The complications of pulmonary tuberculosis are as follows:

- Hemoptysis
- Post-tubercular bronchiectasis
- Fungal ball (Aspergilloma)
- Tuberculosis endobronchitis and tracheitis
- Spontaneous pneumothorax
- Scar carcinoma
- Disseminated calcification of the lungs
- Pulmonary function changes, obstructive airway disease
- Secondary pyogenic infections
- Secondary amyloidosis
- Chronic respiratory failure
- Chronic cor pulmonale.

HEMOPTYSIS

It is a common, potentially serious complication of pulmonary tuberculosis.[1-4] The incidence of hemoptysis in patients with pulmonary tuberculosis is 30–35%. Hemoptysis may occur as the initial manifestation of active tuberculosis, during the course of therapy or even after the disease is apparently cured. Hemoptysis can be streaky or massive and life-threatening.

Causes of hemoptysis in pulmonary tuberculosis:

- Bleeding from cavity wall
- Rupture of Rasmussens aneurysm
- Direct erosion of capillaries/arteries by granulomatous inflammation
- Tuberculous endobronchitis
- Post-tubercular bronchiectasis
- Aspergilloma
- Broncholith, cavernolith
- Scar carcinoma.

Walls of a tuberculosis cavity may be affected by inflammation and necrosis. Increased pressure can lead to weakening of the walls, dilatation of blood vessels and formation of Rasmussen's aneurysm.[5-10] The vessels can also rupture due to increased pressure during strenuous exercise or coughing. The vessel walls can also be eroded directly either because of endarteritis or vasculitis secondary to tuberculosis. Sometimes, an intense allergic response to antigens of *Mycobacterium tuberculosis* damages the vessel wall and gives rise to hemoptysis. Bleeding from tuberculosis granulomas in the bronchi can result in hemoptysis. Blood vessels with aneurysmal dilatation and accentuated bronchopulmonary communications are present surrounding these granulomas. In this case, the bronchial blood vessels which are under systemic pressure can be the source of bleeding.

FUNGUS BALL

Infection of inactive tuberculosis cavity by *Aspergillus fumigatus* gives rise to solid mass-like lesions inside the cavity. Majority of these lesions are due to *Aspergillus* species, although *Mucor* species have occasionally been implicated. The overall incidence of aspergilloma in the general population has been estimated to be 0.01% in Great Britain and 0.017% in the USA.[11,12] Apart from tuberculosis, aspergillomas have been identified in cavities associated with histoplasmosis, sarcoidosis, bronchial cysts, asbestosis, ankylosing spondylitis, bronchiectasis and malignant disease.[13,14] Of these, TB is the most frequently associated condition.[15] Occasionally, they are described in cavities due to other fungal infections.[16,17] In a large multicentric study by the British Thoracic and Tuberculosis Association which surveyed patients with healed tubercular cavities on chest radiograph measuring 2.5 cm or greater in diameter, 25% had precipitins against *Aspergillus fumigatus* in the serum and 11% had radiological evidence of aspergilloma.

Aspergilloma starts as a subacute suppurative process and continues into the more chronic form. The most common predisposing factor for the formation of aspergilloma appears to be the presence of a pre-existing cavity in the lung. The mycelia grow in the cavity wall but tissue invasion is most unusual. Rarely, such growth may lead to invasive life-threatening infection. The fungus ball may be present for a long period without any clinical symptoms and may be found incidentally. Eventually, most of the patients with aspergilloma become symptomatic. Hemoptysis is the most common presentation and has been reported to occur in 5–90% of the patients. Hemoptysis in aspergilloma may be due to mechanical friction due to the fungus ball, an endotoxin with hemolytic properties, an anticoagulant factor derived from *Aspergillus*, local vasculitis and direct vascular invasion of the blood vessels in the wall of the cavity. The amount may be very minimal to severe particularly in patients with associated tuberculosis.[19] Other features include chronic cough, weight loss and rarely fever and dyspnea.[20-23] In approximately 10% of the cases, it may increase in size or resolve spontaneously without treatment.[18] Risk factors associated with poor prognosis of aspergilloma include severe underlying disease, immunocompromised state, increasing *Aspergillus* specific IgG titers, recurrent large volume hemoptysis and underlying sarcoidosis or HIV infection.[24]

The typical radiographic appearance of aspergilloma is a bell-like image with the fungus ball appearing as a clapper inside the bell. A semicircular, crescentic air shadow appears around the radiopaque fungus ball located in the upper lobe lung cavity (air-crescent sign).[25] The fungus ball changes its position as the patient moves.[26] This is best appreciated on fluoroscopy or by taking chest radiographs in different positions. The radiological differential diagnosis includes organized hematoma or pus inside a cavity, neoplasm and a hydatid cyst. The natural history of an aspergilloma is highly variable. It may remain stable, increase in size or resolve spontaneously. In the early phase of its evolution, the fungus ball grows inside a cavity and consists of both living and dead fungi. If death occurs due to local conditions, the fungus ball will be expectorated. Calcification occurs less frequently.

Sputum culture may confirm the presence of fungus but may be negative in some cases.[27] The serum precipitins against *Aspergillus* species are positive in almost all patients. Skin testing is less helpful.[27] On bronchoscopy, the fungus ball may be visualized in direct continuity with the bronchial lumen. Bronchial washings, brushings and forceps biopsy may be carried out to isolate the fungus.

Despite several published series from various parts of the country, this disease is still under recognized and misdiagnosed as pulmonary tuberculosis. This has serious clinical implications as patients with aspergilloma often receive antitubercular therapy for a long time while lung damage continues to progress relentlessly.[28] Treatment of aspergilloma is controversial. Systemic antifungal treatment is ineffective in treating these lesions. The antifungal agents do not penetrate into the intracavitary fungi.[29] Instilling antifungal agents (Amphotericin B, nystatin, sodium iodide) into the cavity with a fiberoptic bronchoscope has been attempted with varied success.[30-32] Systemic antifungal therapy using intravenous Amphotericin B has no effect.[33] Itraconazole has been tried with varying success.[34] Bronchial artery embolization rarely controls hemoptysis because of extensive collateral blood vessels. This procedure may, however, be used as a temporary measure to control massive hemoptysis.[35] Surgery is indicated when the hemoptysis is repetitive and severe and the patient has adequate pulmonary reserve.[36-40] The surgical treatment of aspergilloma is associated with a relatively high mortality rate that ranges between 7% and 23%.[36,37] In younger patients with adequate lung reserve, the morbidity and mortality are lower.[38,39] Patients with mild, infrequent hemoptysis or those without symptoms should be carefully followed up. Pulmonary mycetomas have also been documented in HIV seropositive individuals.[41-43] In HIV positive patients with a $CD4^+$ count of less than or equal to 100 cells/μL, the disease progressed despite treatment.

BRONCHIECTASIS

The pathogenesis of bronchiectasis in tuberculosis is multifactorial.[44] In it there is caseation necrosis and granulomatous inflammation in the wall of the dilated and destroyed bronchi. Scarring that follows tuberculous inflammation produces bronchial stenosis. This may be followed by mixed bacterial infection and retention of purulent bacterial secretions leading to destruction and dilatation of the bronchi. Compression of the bronchial lumen by enlarged lymph nodes produces consequences similar to those of an intraluminal obstruction. It is more common in young children and adolescents in whom tuberculous hilar lymphadenitis is common. In both the conditions, inflammatory destruction of the bronchial wall is usually the sequelae of secondary bacterial infection rather than the direct effect of *M. tuberculosis*. Another rare, but important cause of bronchial obstruction is penetration of the airway by a calcified tuberculous lymph node and the formation of broncholith. Some or all of the bronchiectatic cavities may represent healed or healing tuberculous cavities that have been re-lined with ciliated columnar epithelium. Recently, it has been found that *Mycobacterium avium*-intracellulare infection of the lungs is associated with bronchiectasis. Post-tuberculosis bronchiectasis is commonly seen in the upper lobes since the disease is more common at this site. It is a "dry" or "sicca" type of bronchiectasis because of the effective drainage of the upper lobes by gravity. The usual presentation is with hemoptysis or repeated episodes of secondary bacterial infection. Bronchography performed with a radiopaque, iodinated lipid dye, provides excellent visualization of the dilated airways. However, in the recent years computerized tomography of the chest has replaced bronchography. Treatment of bronchiectasis includes antibiotics or antitubercular drugs and postural drainage.

TUBERCULOSIS ENDOBRONCHITIS AND TRACHEITIS

Tuberculosis endobronchitis and tracheitis are observed in about one-third of the patients with pulmonary tuberculosis.[45] These structures can be infected by direct implantation of *M. tuberculosis*, through submucosal lymphatics, hematogenous spread or from the lymph nodes. Clinical features include cough, breathlessness, hemoptysis and constriction in the substernal region. Healing can lead to bronchostenosis. Bronchoscopy may be essential for the early diagnosis of this condition. Treatment includes antitubercular drugs with or without steroids. Patients who develop significant degree of bronchial stenosis may be treated with balloon dilatation with carbon dioxide laser. More recently, self-expanding metallic stents have also been reported to be useful.

SPONTANEOUS PNEUMOTHORAX

Spontaneous pneumothorax has been reported in 5–15% of patients with pulmonary tuberculosis.[46,47] In countries where tuberculosis is a common problem, it is an important cause of pneumothorax. Spontaneous pneumothorax may develop due to rupture of a subpleural tuberculous cavity into the pleural space. Other causes of pneumothorax include rupture of an open healed cavity or rupture of a bleb or bulla secondary to fibrosis and destruction of the lung.[48]

CALCIFICATION

Tuberculous lung lesions may heal by calcification. In fact localized or extensive calcification of the lungs is seen in healed primary tuberculosis. Calcification can be microscopic or macroscopic. Most often these calcifications present as discrete radiopaque shadows in patients with parenchymal disease and sheet-like calcification in patients with pleural disease. Occasionally, however, these calcified concretions may get detached from the lung tissue and erode through a bronchial wall or blood vessel and result in massive hemoptysis. The patient may also give history of coughing out calcified stones in the sputum (broncholiths or pneumoliths). Extensive calcification may result in respiratory failure or chronic cor pulmonale.

TUBERCULOUS LARYNGITIS

Involvement of larynx during the course of pulmonary tuberculosis occurs in about 4–40% of cases.[49] The incidence increases with extensive involvement of the lungs and presence of cavitary disease. The usual mode of infection is by direct implantation or through lymphatics and blood vessels. The symptoms include soreness or pain in the throat, dry, hacking cough and hoarseness of voice. Laryngoscopy may reveal an ulcer, granuloma, paresis or paralysis, destruction of cords or stenosis of the vocal cords. The vocal cords, arytenoids and the interarytenoid space are most commonly affected. The sputum is usually positive for *M. tuberculosis*. Treatment mainly includes antitubercular drugs with surgical intervention needed in selective cases.

TUBERCULOUS ENTERITIS

Tuberculous enteritis seldom occurs as a complication of pulmonary tuberculosis in the present era. Abdominal tuberculosis is defined as tuberculosis infection of the abdomen including gastrointestinal tract, peritoneum, omentum, mesentery and its nodes and other solid intra-abdominal organs like liver, spleen and pancreas. It is one of the most common forms of extrapulmonary tuberculosis. *Mycobacterium tuberculosis, Mycobacterium bovis* and atypical mycobacteria can cause abdominal tuberculosis. Abdominal pain is the most common symptom and is present in almost all the patients. Investigations like abdominal ultrasonography, abdominal computed tomography, barium studies, colonoscopy, peritoneal biopsy and laparoscopy may be required for diagnosis. Treatment includes antitubercular drugs and elective surgery may be performed after 4 to 6 weeks of antituberculosis treatment. Surgical options include bypass surgery such as entero-enterostomy, stricturoplasty or a limited right hemicolectomy with end-to-end anastomosis.

OPEN NEGATIVE SYNDROME

Patients with open negative syndrome have thin-walled cavities with epithelialization extending from bronchioles down to the inner lining of the cavity.[50-52] Although they are known as "isoniazid cavities", they can also occur with other antituberculosis drugs. Complete epithelialization prevents these cavities to collapse but renders them innocuous. From a clinical point of view they are regarded as inactive cavities. On chest X-ray they appear as ring shadows with thin walls. Although the cavities themselves will not produce any symptoms, they are associated with hemoptysis, secondary infection, colonization with fungi producing fungal balls, scar carcinoma, spontaneous pneumothorax and loss of effective volume of the lungs (Figs 11.1, 11.2).

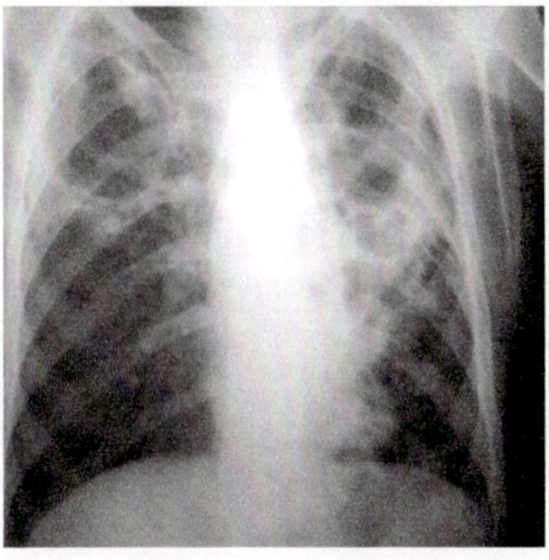

Fig. 11.1: Bilateral healed cavities (Open negative syndrome)

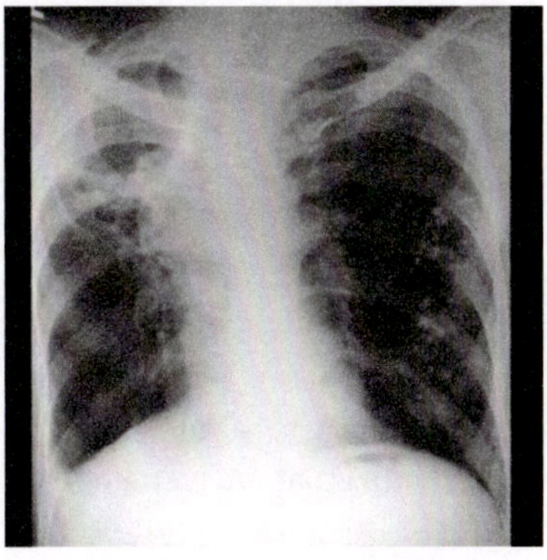

Fig. 11.2: Right sides healed cavity (Open negative syndrome)

SCAR CARCINOMA

In the series reported by Auerbach, et al.[53] scar cancer was observed in 82 of the 1186 autopsied cases (1%); 23% of these had originated from TB scars. A similar association between scars of TB and lung cancer has been documented in several reports.[54,55] However, other reports indicate that the association between TB and lung cancer was merely coincidental.[56,57] A receptor with sensitivity for oxygen and carbon dioxide which produce a number of autocrine growth factors is considered to be crucial in the malignant transformation.[58-60] CT thorax and lung biopsy will help in the diagnosis.

PHYSIOLOGICAL CHANGES

Thirty to sixty percent of cases with pulmonary tuberculosis suffer from diffuse airways obstruction.[61,62] Further, because of diffuse parenchymal fibrosis, pleural effusion, pleural thickening and fibrothorax, a restrictive type of pulmonary function defect may also occur. Thus, in patients with pulmonary tuberculosis an obstructive, restrictive or a mixed type of lung function abnormality is possible depending upon the type and extent of involvement or residual damage.[63] Several studies have observed that early and partially treated tuberculosis results in airways obstruction. In one study 68% of 71 subjects had evidence of airway obstruction after 5.6 years of follow-up from diagnosis of tuberculosis. Impairment of airflow was related to the extent of tuberculosis determined radiologically and to the amount of sputum produced at the end of follow-up, which also correlated with the extent of disease. The residual damage to the lung tissue after completion of tuberculosis treatment includes varying degrees of fibrosis, bronchovascular distortion, emphysema and bronchiectasis. Increased sputum production was also observed several years after tuberculosis treatment that correlated with the initial extent of tuberculosis. The increased number of episodes of tuberculosis corresponded with increasing loss of lung function. This loss was highest in the first six months after diagnosis of tuberculosis and became stable in 13-18 months. The estimated decrease in FEV1 in one episode of tuberculosis was 326 mL after 6 months, 247 mL after 1 year, and stabilized at an average residual loss 153 mL over the total follow-up period, for subjects with two episodes of tuberculosis, the temporal loss of FEV1 was 499 mL after six month 419 mL after 12 months, and stabilized at an average residual loss of 326 mL from 12 months onwards while for subject with three episodes of tuberculosis, the temporal loss of FEV1 was 583 mL after six months, and stabilized at an average residual loss of 410 mL. For FVC the estimated decrease in subjects with one episode of tuberculosis was 305 mL after six months, 213 mL after one year and stabilized at an average residual loss of 96 mL after the total follow-up period, for subjects with two episodes of temporal loss of FVC was 495 mL after six months, 403 mL after 12 months and stabilized at an average residual loss of 286 mL from 12 months onwards, and for subjects with three episodes of tuberculosis, the temporal loss of FVC was 554 mL after six months, 462 mL after 12 months and stabilized at an average residual loss of 345 mL. The effect of pneumoconiosis on loss of lung function was similar to that of one episode of tuberculosis. Thus, tuberculosis can cause chronic lung function impairment which increases with the number of episodes of tuberculosis, affecting approximately 18% of subjects with one episode, 27% of subjects with two episodes and 35% of subjects with three episodes of tuberculosis (Fig. 11.3).

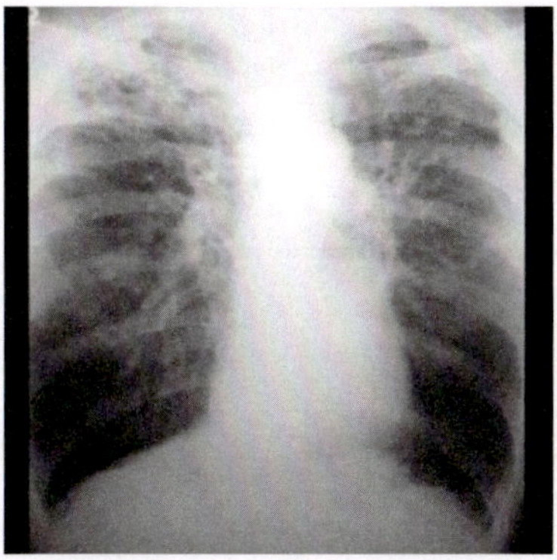

Fig. 11.3: Post-tubercular obstructive airway disease proven with spirometry

AMYLOIDOSIS

Amyloidosis is characterized by the deposition of an extracellular eosinophilic substance in various organs. Although the name suggests carbohydrate deposition, the substance deposited is predominantly protein in origin.[72] The incidence of renal amyloidosis in pulmonary tuberculosis has been reported to range from 8–33%.[73-77] Tuberculosis of various organs was the most common predisposing cause accounting for 59.1% of secondary amyloidosis, followed by chronic suppurative lung diseases. Amongst tuberculosis, pulmonary tuberculosis was the leading cause in 81.6% cases followed by glandular and abdominal tuberculosis. The interval between the onset of predisposing disease and the first evidence of secondary renal amyloidosis varied from 1 to 30 years with a mean of 6.9 years. The interval was greater than 5 years in 67% of the patients; however, the interval may be as short as 6 months or as long as 43 years. Secondary amyloidosis is now a rare complication of pulmonary tuberculosis because of the use of modern chemotherapy. However, tuberculosis is still the most common cause of secondary amyloidosis in Indian patients.[76] Abdominal fat pad, rectal, mucosal, liver or kidney biopsy specimens are useful in confirming the diagnosis of secondary amyloidosis.

CHRONIC RESPIRATORY FAILURE

Chronic respiratory failure may complicate pulmonary tuberculosis especially if the disease had been extensive and the patient survived because of adequate treatment. Respiratory failure develops due to extensive destruction of pulmonary parenchyma and the resultant ventilation-perfusion (V/Q) mismatch. Associated pleural thickening and fibrothorax result in thoracic wall malfunction and lead to further compromise of the lung function.[64-66] Atrophy or disuse of the respiratory muscles can also contribute to chronic respiratory failure. Tachypnea, hypoxia and hypercapnea develop ultimately which may even lead to the patients death. Treatment includes oxygen supplementation, treatment of the underlying disease, bipap ventilation and in severe cases invasive ventilation may be required.

CHRONIC COR PULMONALE

Cor pulmonale is defined as enlargement (dilatation and/or hypertrophy) of the right ventricle due to increased right ventricular overload from intrinsic pulmonary diseases including those of pulmonary circulation, of inadequate function of chest bellows or inadequate ventilatory drive from the respiratory centers and when right heart abnormalities secondary to left heart failure or congenital heart disease are excluded. Right heart failure need not be present although this is a clinical manifestation of the overloaded right ventricle that precedes the clinically unrecognizable cor pulmonale. Cor pulmonale is usually chronic except when the disease is complicated by massive pulmonary thromboembolism. The possible causes of chronic cor pulmonale in pulmonary tuberculosis include abnormalities of the pulmonary parenchyma or thoracic wall. The basic pathophysiology of chronic cor pulmonale is an increase in the pulmonary artery vascular resistance and pulmonary hypertension. Mechanisms causing these changes include occlusion or destruction of vascular bed due to lung parenchymal destruction, vasculitis and endarteritis with diminished cross-sectional area of the pulmonary circulation. Other less important causes include hypoxia, acidosis with hypercapnia and increased blood viscosity due to polycythemia. These causes are also important in the causation of chronic cor pulmonale in patients with chronic obstructive pulmonary disease.

Normal mean pulmonary artery pressure is 13 to 14 mm Hg in a young adult and is less than 18 mm Hg in 80% of all subjects. Pulmonary artery pressure of greater than 20 mm Hg signifies pulmonary artery hypertension. The normal pulmonary vascular resistance is 10 to 20 times less than systemic vascular resistance. The effective cross-sectional area of the pulmonary vascular bed must be reduced by more than 50% before any change in pulmonary artery pressure can be detected at rest, although exercise will increase the pressure at lower levels of increased blood flow. Experiments in dogs have shown that more than two-thirds of the lungs had to be ablated before pulmonary artery pressures approach hypertensive levels.[67,68] Obliterative vascular diseases increase pulmonary vascular resistance by vascular occlusion while diffuse interstitial and parenchymal diseases act primarily by compressing and obliterating small vessels. The diagnosis of chronic cor pulmonale is often not made until significant right ventricular hypertrophy or overt right ventricular failure is present. Heart failure occurs insidiously causing further impairment of lung function and is frequently misinterpreted as worsening of the underlying lung disease. Episodes of leg edema, atypical chest pain, exertional dyspnea, exercise induced cyanosis in the periphery, prior respiratory failure and excessive day time sleepiness are important historical clues suggesting the possibility of cor pulmonale.

General physical examination reveals distended neck veins, peripheral edema and cyanosis. Signs and symptoms suggestive of heart failure like dyspnea, orthopnea, edema, hepatomegaly and raised jugular venous pressure can also occur due to chronic obstructive airways disease without right heart failure. However, the raised jugular venous pressure (JVP) is present in both phases of respiration in right heart failure. The apical impulse and the right ventricular lift are often not palpable. The second heart sound may be palpable in the pulmonary area. The earliest sign of pulmonary hypertension is an accentuated pulmonic component of second heart sound. A right ventricular S3 gallop is heard in the epigastrium along the sternum. With advanced pulmonary artery hypertension, characteristic diastolic murmur of pulmonary regurgitation and pansystolic murmur of tricuspid regurgitation, which accentuates during inspiration can be heard along with a systolic ejection sound. Cor pulmonale due to restricted vascular bed is manifested by a strikingly high pulmonary arterial pressure associated with a low cardiac output. Tachypnea which persists even during sleep is the rule, particularly with multiple pulmonary emboli. Chest pain is common. Enlargement of right ventricle occurs in these disorders. Prominent "a" and "v" waves appear in the jugular veins. The classic radiographic evidence of right ventricular enlargement (crossing the right vertebral border) will be present. The suggestive indices of pulmonary hypertension include right atrial and ventricular enlargement which is suggested on the ECG by P pulmonale in leads II, III, aVF. S1Q3 OR S1-S2-S3 patterns, right axis deviation, R:S ratio in V6 of 1.0 rSR pattern in the right precordial leads and partial or complete right bundle branch block.[69-71] Dominant R or R′ in lead V1 or V3R in association with inverted T waves in the right precordial leads are more suggestive indices.

REFERENCES

1. Bidwell JL, Pachner RW. Hemoptysis: diagnosis and management. Am Fam Physician. 2005;72:1253-60.
2. Pamra SP, Goyal SS, Raj B, Mathur GP. Epidemiology of haemoptysis. Indian J Tuberc. 1970;17:111-8.

3. Sharma SK, Mohan A. Pulmonary tuberculosis: typical and atypical cases. Case track series 1. Mumbai: Merind, 1997.
4. Reechaipichitkul W, Latong S. Etiology and treatment outcomes of massive hemoptysis. Southeast Asian J Trop Med Public Health. 2005;36:474-80.
5. Van den Heuvel MM, Van Rensburg JJ. Images in clinical medicine. Rasmussen's aneurysm. N Engl J Med. 2006;355:e17.
6. Keeling AN, Costello R, Lee MJ. Rasmussen's aneurysm: a forgotten entity? Cardiovasc Intervent Radiol. 2007;30:1234-7. Epub 2007 Sep5.
7. Kato A, Kudo S, Matsumoto K, Fukahori T, Shimizu T, Uchino A, et al. Bronchial artery embolization for hemoptysis due to benign diseases: immediate and long-term results. Cardiovasc Intervent Radiol. 2000;23:351-7.
8. Lee JH, Kwon SY, Yoon HI, Yoon CJ, Lee KW, Kang SG, et al. Haemoptysis due to chronic tuberculosis vs. bronchiectasis: comparison of long-term outcome of arterial embolisation. Int J Tuberc Lung Dis. 2007;11:781-7.
9. Metin M, Sayar A, Turna A, Solak O, Erkan L, Dincer SI, et al. Emergency surgery for massive haemoptysis. Acta Chir Belg. 2005;105:639-43.
10. Naidoo R. Active pulmonary tuberculosis: Experience with resection in 106 cases. Asian Cardiovasc Thorac Ann. 2007;15:134-8.
11. British Tuberculosis Association. Aspergillus in persistent lung cavities after tuberculosis. A report from the Research Committee of the British Tuberculosis Association. Tubercle. 1968;49:1-11.
12. British Thoracic and Tuberculosis Association. Aspergilloma and residual tuberculous cavities—the results of a resurvey. Tubercle. 1970;51:227-45.
13. Kauffman CA. Quandry about treatment of aspergillomas persists. Lancet. 1996;347:1640.
14. Zizzo G, Castriota-Scanderbeg A, Zarrelli N, Nardella G, Daly J, Cammisa M. Pulmonary aspergillosis complicating ankylosing spondylitis. Radiol Med (Torino). 1996;91:817-8.
15. Kawamura S, Maesaki S, Tomono K, Tashiro T, Kohno S. Clinical evaluation of 61 patients with pulmonary aspergilloma. Intern Med. 2000;39:209-12.
16. Rosenheim SH, Schwartz J. Cavitary pulmonary cryptococosis complicated by aspergilloma. Am Rev Respir Dis. 1975;111:549-53.
17. Sarosi GA, Silberfarb PM, Saliba NA, Huggin PM, Tosh FE. Aspergillomas occurring in blastomycotic cavities. Am Rev Respir Dis. 1971;104:581-4.
18. Gefter WB. The spectrum of pulmonary aspergillosis. J Thoracic Imaging. 1992;7:56-74.
19. Faulkner SL, Vernon R, Brown PP, Fisher RD, Bender HW Jr. Hemoptysis and pulmonary aspergilloma: operative versus nonoperative treatment. Ann Thorac Surg. 1978;25:389-92.
20. Tomee JF, Van der Werf TS, Latge JP, Koeter GH, Dubois AE, Kauffman HF. Serologic monitoring of disease and treatment in patient with pulmonary aspergilloma. Am J Respir Crit Care Med. 1995;151:199-204.
21. Addrizzo-Harris DJ, Harkin TJ, McGuinness G, Naidich DP, Rom WN. Pulmonary aspergilloma and AIDS. A comparison of HIV-infected and HIV-negative individuals. Chest. 1997;111: 612-8.
22. Wallac JM, Lim R, Browdy BL, et al. Pulmonary complications of HIV infection study group. Risk factors and outcomes associated with identification of Aspergillus in respiratory specimens from persons with HIV disease. Chest. 1998;114:131-7.
23. Aslam PA, Eastridge CE, Hughes FA Jr. Aspergillosis of the lung. An eighteen year experience. Chest. 1971;59:28-32.
24. Stevens DA, Kan VL, Judson MA, et al. Practice guidelines for disease caused by Aspergillus. Infectious Diseases Society of America. Clin Infect Dis. 2000;30:696-709.
25. Tuncel E. Pulmonary air meniscus sign. Respiration. 1984;46:139-44.
26. Roberts CM, Citron KM, Strickland B. Intrathoracic aspergilloma. Role of CT in diagnosis and treatment. Radiology. 1987;165:123-8.

27. McCarthy DS, Pepys J. Pulmonary aspergilloma: clinical immunology. Clin Allergy. 1973;3: 57-70.
28. Rafferty P, Biggs BA, Crompton GK, Grant IW. What happens to patients with pulmonary aspergilloma? Analysis of 23 cases. Thorax. 1983;38:579-83.
29. Pennington JE. Aspergillus lung disease. Med Clin North Am. 1980;64:475-90.
30. Jewkes J, Kay PH, Paneth M, Citron KM. Pulmonary aspergilloma: analysis of prognosis in relation to haemoptysis and survey of treatment. Thorax. 1983;38:572-8.
31. Yamada H, Kohno S, Koga H, Maesaki S, Kaku M. Topical treatment of pulmonary aspergilloma by antifungals. Relationship between duration of the disease and efficacy of therapy. Chest. 1993;103:1421-5.
32. Munk PL, Vellet AD, Rankin RN, Muller NL, Ahmad D. Intracavitary aspergilloma: transthoracic percutaneous injection of amphotericin gelatin solution. Radiology. 1993;188:821-3.
33. Hammermann KJ, Sarosi GA, Tosh FE. Amphotericin B in the treatment of saprophytic forms of pulmonary aspergillosis. Am Rev Respir Dis. 1974;109:57-62.
34. Campbell JH, Winter JH, Richardson MD, Shankland GS, Banham SW. Treatment of pulmonary aspergilloma with itraconazole. Thorax. 1991;46:839-41.
35. Uflacker R, Kaemmerer A, Picon PD, et al. Bronchial artery embolization in the management of hemoptysis: technical aspects and long-term results. Radiology. 1985;157:637-44.
36. Okubo K, Kobayashi M, Morikawa H, Hayatsu E, Ueno Y. Favorable acute and long-term outcomes after the resection of pulmonary aspergillomas. Thorac Cardiovas Surg. 2007;55: 108-11.
37. Pratap H, Dewan RK, Singh L, Gill S, Vaddadi S. Surgical treatment of pulmonary aspergilloma: A series of 72 cases. Indian J Chest Dis Allied Sci. 2007;49:23-7.
38. Chen JC, Chang YL, Luh SP, Lee JM, Lee YC. Surgical treatment for pulmonary aspergilloma: a 28 year experience. Thorax. 1997;52:810-3.
39. Regnard JF, Icard P, Nicolosi M, Spagiarri L, Magdeleinat P, Jauffret B, et al. Aspergilloma: a series of 89 surgical cases. Ann Thorac Surg. 2000;69:898-903.
40. Glimp RA, Bayer As. Pulmonary aspergilloma: Diagnostic and therapeutic considerations. Ann Intern Med. 1983;143:303-8.
41. Lombardo GT, Anandarao N, Lin CS, Abbate A, Becker WH. Fatal hemoptysis in a patient with AIDS-related complex and pulmonary aspergilloma. NY State J Med. 1987;87:306-8.
42. Hohler T, Schnutgen M, Mayet WJ, Meyer zum Buschenfelde KH. Pulmonary aspergilloma in a patient with AIDS. Thorax. 1995;50:312-3.
43. Greenberg AK, Knapp J, Rom WN, Addrizzo-Harris DJ. Clinical presentation of pulmonary mycetoma in HIV-infected patients. Chest. 2002;122:886-92.
44. Rosenzweig DY, Stead WW. The role of tuberculosis and other forms of bronchopulmonary necrosis in the pathogenesis of bronchiectasis. Am Rev Respir Dis. 1966;93:769-85.
45. Rikimaru T. Endobronchial tuberculosis. Expert Rev Anti Infect Ther. 2004;2:245-51.
46. Kim HY, Song KS, Goo JM, Lee JS, et al. Thoracic sequelae and complications of tuberculosis. Radiographics. 2001;21:839-58.
47. Hussain SF, Aziz A, Fatima H. Pneumothorax: a review of 146 adult cases admitted at a university teaching hospital in Pakistan. J Pak Med Assoc. 1999;49:243-6.
48. Borrego Galan JC, Rivas Lopez P, Remacha Esteras MA. Recurrent tuberculous pneumothorax and tuberculous empyema: an association of two rare complications. Arch Bronconeumol. 2003;39:478-9.
49. Lim JY, Kim KM, Choi EC, Kim YH, Kim HS, Choi HS. Current clinical propensity of laryngeal tuberculosis: Review of 60 cases. Eur Arch Otorhinolaryngol. 2006;263:838-42. Epub 2006 Jul 12.
50. Elemanov MG, Kharcheva KA, Vavillin GI. Evaluation of the 'Open-negative' syndrome in the clinical course of tuberculosis. Probl Tuberk. 1974;52:19-23.
51. Miyagi Y. "Open-negative' syndrome. Clinical course of its development and subsequent destiny. Jpn J Tuberc. 1966;13(Suppl):54-9.

52. Breuer J, Abeles H, Chaves AD, Robins AB. Observations on ambulatory tuberculous patients with pulmonary cavities and noninfectious sputum (the open-negative syndrome). Am Rev Tuberc. 1958;78:725-34.
53. Auerbach O, Garfinkel L, Parks VR. Scar cancer of the lung: increase over a 21 year period. Cancer. 1979;43:636-42.
54. Gao YT. Risk factors for lung cancer among nonsmokers with emphasis on lifestyle factors. Lung Cancer. 1996;14 Suppl (1):S39-45.
55. Wu-Williams AH, Dai XD, Blot W, Xu ZY, Sun XW, Xiao HP, et al. Lung cancer among women in north-east China. Br J Cancer. 1990;62:982-7.
56. Jindal SK, Malik SK, Bedi RS, Gupta SK. Risk of lung cancer in patients with old tuberculosis—a prospective study. Lung India. 1986;4:59-61.
57. Hinds MW, Cohen HI, Kolonel LN. Tuberculosis and cancer risk in nonsmoking women. AM Rev Respir Dis. 1982;125:776-8.
58. Johnson DE, Geogieff MK. Pulmonary perspective: Neuroendocrine cells in health and disease. Am Rev Respir Dis. 1989;140:1807-12.
59. Youngson C, Nurse C, Yeger H, Cutz E. Oxygen sensing in airway chemoreceptors. Nature. 1993;365:153-5.
60. Schuller HM, Miller M, Park PD, Orloff MS. Promoting mechanisms of CO_2 on neuroendocrine cell proliferation mediated by nicotine receptor stimulation. Significance for lung cancer risk in individuals with chronic lung disease. Chest. 1996;109:20S-21S.
61. Hallet WY, Martin CJ. The diffuse obstructive pulmonary syndrome in a tuberculosis sanatorium. I. Etiologic factors. Ann Intern Med. 1961;54:1146-55.
62. Snider GL, Doctor L, Demas TA, Shaw AR. Obstructive airway disease in patients with treated pulmonary tuberculosis. Am Rev Respir Dis. 1971;103:625-40.
63. Lee JH, Chang JH. Lung function in patients with chronic airflow obstruction due to tuberculous destroyed lung. Respir Med. 2003;97:1237-42.
64. Macklem PT. Respiratory muscles: the vital pump. Chest. 1980;78:753-8.
65. Park JH, Na JO, Kim EK, Lim CM, Shim TS, Lee SD, et al. The prognosis of respiratory failure in patients with tuberculous destroyed lung. Int J Tuberc Lung Dis. 2001;5:963-7.
66. Bone RC. Treatment of respiratory failure due to advanced chronic obstructive lung disease. Arch Intern Med. 1980;140:1018-21.
67. Ferrer MI. Cor pulmonale (pulmonary heart disease): Present day status. Am heart J. 1975;89:657-64.
68. Fishman AP. State of the art: Chronic cor pulmonale. Am Rev Respir Dis. 1976;114:775-94.
69. Kleiger RE, Senior Rm. Long-term electrocardiographic monitoring of ambulatory patients with chronic airway obstruction. Chest. 1974;65:483.
70. Padmavati S, Raizada V. Electrocardiogram in chronic cor pulmonale. Br Heart J. 1975;34:648.
71. Prabhaker R. Laboratory aspects of tuberculosis. Indian J tuberc. 1987;34:67-80.
72. Glenner GG, Terry WD, Isersky C. Amyloidosis: its nature and pathogenesis. Semin Hematol. 1973;10:65-86.
73. Shah PKD, Jain MK, Mangal HN, Singhvi NM. Kidney changes in pulmonary tuberculosis—a study by kidney biopsy. Indian J Tuberc. 1975;1:23-7.
74. Mittal OP, Sharma GS, Singh SK, Agarwala MC. Renal biopsy in pulmonary tuberculosis. Indian J Chest Dis. 1966;8:20-4.
75. Abdulpurkar AG, Desai MG, Shankar PS. Renal changes in pulmonary tuberculosis. Lung India. 1987;5:82-5.
76. Chugh KS, Singhal PC, Sakhuja V, Datta BN, Jain SK, Dash SC. Pattern of renal amyloidosis in Indian patients. Postgrad Med J. 1981;57:31-5.
77. Kennedy AC, Burton JA, Allison ME. Tuberculosis as a continuing cause of renal amyloidosis. Br Med J. 1974;3:795-7.

Chapter 12

Post-tubercular Obstructive Airway Impairment

INTRODUCTION

Pulmonary impairment after tuberculosis refers to chronic pulmonary function loss that occurs in persons who have achieved microbiologic cure of pulmonary tuberculosis. Previous infection of tuberculosis is an independent risk factor for obstructive lung disease even if the lesion is minimal and tuberculosis can be an important cause of obstructive lung disease in never smokers especially among high tuberculosis endemic areas. Effort on prevention and control of tuberculosis is important in reduction of obstructive lung disease, especially in countries with more than intermediate burden of tuberculosis. This chapter aims to describe the pathophysiology, diagnosis and treatment of post-tubercular obstructive airway disease.

PATHOPHYSIOLOGY

Tuberculosis, a disease of great antiquity has become the most important communicable disease in the world. Nearly, two million new cases of tuberculosis occur every year in India.[1] Obstructive airway disease can be due to many causes. Tuberculosis can also be a cause of obstructive airway disease but it has not been studied in detail. For many patients of tuberculosis, microbiological cure does not protect the patient from the sequelae of the illness. Post-tubercular pulmonary impairment has emerged as a distinct clinical entity, which is almost indistinguishable from other forms.[2,3] Cavitation, extensive fibrosis, bulla formation and bronchiectasis have been implicated in the genesis of COPD caused by the destroyed lung due to pulmonary tuberculosis.[4-6] Chronic bronchitis or bronchiolitis and emphysema often occur as complications of pulmonary tuberculosis.

Some workers have found association of history of smoking in post-tubercular patients who have developed obstructive airway disease.[7,8] Additional exposure to cigarette smoke and other environmental risk factors leads to an increase in such occurrences.[9-11] The degree of obstructive airway changes in subjects treated for pulmonary tuberculosis increases with age, the number of cigarettes smoked and the extent of initial disease.

The average duration of onset of obstructive airway disease has been found to be variable. Hnizdo, et al.[12] found that the average time between the diagnosis of the last episode of tuberculosis and the impairment of lung function test was 4.6 years (range one month to 31 years). The loss of lung function was highest within six months of the diagnosis of tuberculosis and stabilized after 12 months when the loss was considered to be chronic.

The most common complex clinicophysiological manifestations of pulmonary dysfunctions are functional changes in lung tissue characterized by hyperinflation and restriction of the lungs and rise or decline of their elasticity. Disorders of bronchial patency and pulmonary gas exchange were second in their detection rate, most commonly manifested by impaired flow rate and decline in lung capacity.[13]

Rajasekharan, et al.[14] concluded that patients with moderate and far advanced healed lesions on chest skiagram had more persistent symptoms and low peak expiratory flow rate. Pathological changes such as "emphysematous change" on the radiograph could be considered as an important cause of obstructive ventilator impairment.[15] Plit, et al. found that the extent of lung infiltration (radiographic score) both at the outset and after chemotherapy was significantly and inversely related to forced expiratory volume in one second (FEV1).[16]

Patients of post-pulmonary tuberculosis had variable presentation in lung function testing. Lee and Chang, in 2003[17] compared lung function in patients with chronic airflow limitation due to tuberculous destroyed lung and COPD patients and concluded that forced vital capacity (FVC) and post-bronchodilator forced expiratory volume in 1st second (FEV1) of post-tuberculous patients were lower compared to those of COPD. Here bronchodilator therapy could be useful for treating chronic airflow limitation in post-tubercular cases especially those presenting with wheezing. Similarly in another study by Pasipanodya JG, et al.[18] found that after adjusting for risk, it was found that survivors of tuberculosis were 5.4 times more likely to have abnormal PFTs than latent tuberculosis infection patients. Pulmonary impairment was found in 59% of tuberculosis patients and 20% of latent tuberculosis infection patients.

De Valliere and Barker in a study to find out the residual lung damage after completion of treatment for multidrug resistant tuberculosis showed that restrictive and combined obstructive and restrictive lung function patterns were the predominant abnormalities.[6] A study undertaken by

Hnizdo, et al.[12] found that the estimated average chronic deficit in forced expiratory volume in one second [FEV (1)] after one, two, and three or more episodes of tuberculosis was 153 mL, 326 mL, and 410 mL, respectively. The corresponding deficits for forced vital capacity (FVC) were 96 mL, 286 mL, and 345 mL. The percentage of subjects with chronic airflow impairment (FEV1 < 80% predicted) was 18.4% in those with one episode, 27.1% in those with two, and 35.2% in those with three or more episodes of tuberculosis.[15] Even lung diffusion capacity of pulmonary tuberculosis patients was changed in post-pulmonary tuberculosis impairment. Study by Nefedov, et al.[19] in 159 patients with focal, infiltrative, disseminated and fibrocavitatory tuberculosis showed a decrease in DLCO in half of the patients with disseminated and fibrocavitatory tuberculosis and in less than one/fifth of the patients with focal and infiltrative tuberculosis.

It has also been observed that effective chemotherapy decreases the likelihood of development of obstructive lung disease. Deterioration of lung function was seen mainly during ineffective chemotherapy, while rarely during successful chemotherapy.[20] Majority of the studies observed that, most common abnormality on spirometry was restrictive lung disease, followed by irreversible obstructive airway disease. Nefedov and Smirnova[13] showed that among 100 patients with destructive pulmonary tuberculosis, majority had restrictive lung pathology. Yasuda et al.,[15] found that out of 102 patients selected, 38 patients had FEV1% of 55% or lower and 64 patients had FEV1% of above 55%. It is postulated that the leading factor of a decrease in DLCO in the patients with disseminated and fibrocavitatory tuberculosis was the reduction of the lung respiratory surface resulting from a decrease in the effective alveolar volume and the leading factor in infiltrative tuberculosis was a decrease in alveolocapillary membrane permeability.[20]

DIAGNOSIS

Diagnosis is based on chest X-ray and spirometry.[21,22] Pulmonary function tests objectively quantify lung function and impairment and are used to evaluate persons with chronic lung disease. On spirometry, air flow limitation is defined as post-bronchodilator FEV_1/FVC < 70% predicted or lower limit of normal. Levels of pulmonary impairment are determined via spirometry using ATS/ERS Guidelines 2005.[23] Impairment is scaled on the basis of FEV1% as mild > 70%, moderate 60–69%, moderately severe 50–59%, severe 35–49%, very severe < 35% of predicted FEV1. On chest X-ray TB lesion is defined as the presence of discrete linear or reticular fibrotic scars or dense nodules with discrete margins, with or without calcification, within the upper lobes.[21] Treated pulmonary tuberculosis is a significant cause of obstructive airway disease with an inverse relationship between FEV1 and the extent of the disease on the original chest radiograph.[24]

TREATMENT

Treatment consists of patient education, smoking cessation, long-term oxygen therapy if required and drug therapy which includes bronchodilators (beta 2 agonists, anticholinergics, theophyllines), corticosteroids (inhaled or systemic) and antibiotics in case of secondary infection. Patients with pulmonary impairment after tuberculosis may benefit from the methods used to ameliorate other respiratory illness such as immunization against respiratory illness, pulmonary rehabilitation and surgical intervention.

CONCLUSION

There is an important contribution of tuberculosis to airflow obstruction, linking two of the most common ailments in the world. For many persons with tuberculosis, microbiological cure is just the beginning of their illness. It must be kept in mind that the chronic impairment of lung function caused by tuberculosis increases incrementally with the number of episodes of tuberculosis. Thus, it is necessary to prevent and adequate treat tuberculosis, so as to reduce the burden of airflow obstruction in all countries especially the developing countries. However, the exact abnormality that results from tuberculosis infection has to be considered in detail with future studies and a better understanding of the pathophysiology of airflow limitation may point the way to therapeutic strategies for control of symptoms in these patients.

REFERENCES

1. Global tuberculosis control: surveillance, planning, financing. WHO report 2010. Geneva, World Health Organization.
2. Macnee W. Chronic Bronchitis and Emphysema. In: Seaton A, Seaton D, Leitch AG (Eds). Crofton and Douglas's Respiratory Disease, United Kingdom: Blackwell Science. 2002, pp 616-7.
3. Leitch AG. Pulmonary tuberculosis: Clinical features. In: Seaton A, Seaton D, Leitch AG, (Eds). Crofton and Douglass's Respiratory Disease, United Kingdom: Blackwell Science. 2002, p 523.
4. Hassan IS, Al-Jahdali HH. Obstructive airways disease in patients with significant post-tuberculous lung scarring. Saudi Med J. 2005;26:1155-7.
5. Willcox PA, Ferguson AD. Chronic obstructive airways disease following treated pulmonary tuberculosis. Respir Med. 1989;83:195-8.
6. De valliere S, Barker RD. Residual lung damage after completion of treatment for multidrug-resistant tuberculosis. Int J Tuberc Lung Dis. 2004;8:767-71.
7. Snider GL, Doctor L, Demas TA, Shaw AR. Obstructive airway disease in patients with treated pulmonary tuberculosis. Am Rev Respir Dis. 1971;103:625-40.
8. Lowe CR. An association between smoking and respiratory tuberculosis. BMJ. 1956;2: 1081-6.
9. McKenna MT, Hutton M, Cauthen G, Onorato IM. The association between occupation and tuberculosis. A population-based survey. Am J Respir Crit Care Med. 1996;154:587-93.
10. Mishra VK, Retherford RD, Smith KR. Biomass cooking fuels and prevalence of tuberculosis in India. Int J Infect Dis. 1999;3:119-29.

11. Perez-Padilla R, Perez-Guzman C, Baez-Saldana R, Torres- Cruz A. Cooking with biomass stoves and tuberculosis: a case control study. Int J Tuberc Lung Dis. 2001;5:441-7.
12. Hnizdo E, Singh T, Churchyard GJ. Chronic pulmonary function impairment caused by initial and recurrent pulmonary tuberculosis following treatment. Thorax. 2000;55:32-8.
13. Nefedov VB, Smirnova DG. Disorders of the pulmonary function in patients with destructive tuberculosis. Probl Tuberk. 1991;11:51-4.
14. Rajasekharan S, Savitri S, Jeyaganesh D. Post-tuberculosis bronchial asthma. Ind J Tub. 2001; 48:139.
15. Yasuda J, Okada O, Kuriyama T, Nagao K, Yamagishi F, Hashizume I, et al. Investigation of pulmonary hemodynamics and chest X-ray findings in patients with pulmonary tuberculosis sequelae and obstructive ventilator impairment. Kekkaku. 1999;74:5-18.
16. Plit ML, Anderson R, Van Rensburg CEJ, Page-Shipp L, Blott JA, Fresen JL, et al. Influence of antimicrobial chemotherapy on spirometric parameters and pro-inflammatory indices in severe pulmonary tuberculosis. Eur Respir J. 1998;12:351-6.
17. Lee JH, Chang JH. Lung function in patients with chronic airflow limitations due to tuberculous destroyed lung. Respir Med. 2003;97:1237-42.
18. Pasipanodya JG, Miller TL, Vecino M, Munguia G, Garmon R, Bae S, et al. Post-tuberculosis pulmonary impairment. Chest. 2007;131:1817-24.
19. Nefedov VB, Shergina EA, Popova LA. Pulmonary function in patients with disseminated pulmonary tuberculosis: Probl Tuberk Bolezn Legk. 2007;9:27-30.
20. Nefedov VB, Izmailova ZF, Dzhenzhera En. Lung diffusion capacity of pulmonary tuberculosis patients: Ter Arkh. 1987;59:65-9.
21. Lee Sei Won, et al. The risk of obstructive lung disease by previous pulmonary tuberculosis in a country with intermediate burden of tuberculosis. JKMS. 2011;26(2):268-73.
22. Pasipanodya Jotam G, et al. Pulmonary impairment after tuberculosis and its contribution to TB burden. BMC Public Health. 2010;10:259.
23. Pellegrino R, Viegi G, Brusasco V, Crapo RO, Burgos F, Casaburi R, et al. Interpretative strategies for lung function tests. Eur Respir J. 2005;26:948-68.
24. Verma SK, Narayan KV, Kumar S. A study on prevalence of obstructive airway disease among post-pulmonary tuberculosis patients. Pulmon. 2009;11:4-7.

Chapter 13

Antitubercular Drugs Used in Newly Diagnosed Patients of Tuberculosis and their Adverse Effect

ISONIAZID

Isoniazid is the hydrazide of isonicotinic acid, a chemical compound first synthesized in Prague in 1912 but its effectiveness in treating tuberculosis was recognized in 1952.[1] It is the most powerful antitubercular drug amongst all other agents. Isoniazid is effective only against the tubercle bacillus, not against any other bacteria. It is bactericidal for rapidly dividing microorganism. It is readily absorbed from gastrointestinal tract when administered orally/ parentally, with peak plasma concentration of approximately 3 to 5 μg/mL in about 1–2 hours after administration. Most strains of *M. tuberculosis* are inhibited in vitro by concentration of 0.025 to 0.05 μg/mL. The mechanism of action is by inhibiting *Mycobacterium* cell wall. Resistance to it develops by mutation in at least 5 of different genes (katG, inhA, ahpC, kasA, ndb); more likely to inhA. Exposure to isoniazid leads to loss of acid fastness and decrease the quantity of methanol extractable lipid of microorganism. It penetrates all body tissue, tubercular cavity, placenta and meninges.[2,3] It is extensively metabolized in liver; most important pathway being acetylation including fast and slow acetylators. The rate of isoniazid acetylation shows genetic variation and proportion of fast and slow acetylators differ in different parts of world. 75–95% of the dose of isoniazid is excreted within 24 hours, mostly as inactive metabolites.

Preparation and Dose

Isoniazid is supplied in 50 mg, 100 mg and 300 mg tablets or as an elixir containing 50 mg/5 mL. Combined preparations with rifampicin, ethambutol, and pyrazinamide are available. The dose for daily therapy is 5 (4–6) mg/kg, i.e. 300 mg. In twice weekly regimen dosage is 15 (13–17) mg/kg/day and in thrice weekly regimen dosage is 10 (8–12) mg/kg/day.[2,3]

Drug Interactions

Isoniazid inhibits metabolism of phenytoin, carbamazepine, diazepam and warfarin; may raise their blood levels. Aluminum hydroxide inhibits isoniazid absorption. PAS competes with the acetylation of isoniazid and prolongs half life.

Contraindications

Isoniazid should not be given in known hypersensitivity and active liver disease.

Effect in Pregnancy

Isoniazid is safer in pregnancy.

Overdosage

Overdosage of isoniazid produce nausea, vomiting, dizziness, blurring of vision and slurring of speech within 30 minute to 3 hours. Massive dosage results in unconsciousness followed by respiratory depression and stupor. Severe intractable seizure may occur. Gastric lavage, activated charcoal, antiepileptic and IV sodium bicarbonate, may be of value if undertaken within few hours of ingestion. Hemodialysis may be of value. Administration of large dosage of pyridoxine is necessary to prevent seizures.

Adverse Effects

Isoniazid is well tolerated by most patients. Peripheral neuritis in the form of paresthesias[4] and numbness is a major dose dependent side effect. Tuberculosis patients infected with HIV are at higher risk of peripheral neuritis. The frequency of peripheral neuritis increases with dosage and more common in slow acylators, patients with diabetes mellitus, uremia, malnourished patients and daily users of alcohol. Rarely, it may precipitate convulsion in patients with seizure disorder. A number of mental abnormalities like euphoria, transient impairment of memory, separation of ideas and reality, loss of self-control and florid psychosis may appear during the use. Isoniazid-induced neurotoxicity can be prevented by pyridoxine 10 mg daily.

Hepatitis is another side effect produced by INH, is rare in children but more in adults above 35 years of age and in alcoholics.[5,6] Characteristic pathological process is bridging and multilobular necrosis, mechanism responsible for this toxicity is unknown but believed that acetyl hydrazine, a metabolite of INH causes hepatic damage. Isoniazid induced hepatotoxicity is reversible if the drug is stopped early. Skin rash, generalized hypersensitivity, pellagra in nicotinamide deficient patients, hemolytic anemia in G6PD deficiency, arthralgia, lupoid reactions, dryness of mouth, epigastric distress, tinnitus, urinary retention, methemoglobinemia, optic neuritis are rarely observed untoward effects (Table 13.1).

Table 13.1: Adverse drug reactions in first-line antitubercular treatment (ATT)

Sl. No	Drug	Common adverse effect	Rare adverse effect
1.	Isoniazid	Peripheral neuritis Hepatotoxicity Skin rash	Anemia Arthralgia Dysarthria Irritability Seizure Dysphoria Lupoid reaction Pellagra Vasculitis Thrombocytopenia
2.	Rifampicin	Gastrointestinal reactions Hepatitis	Osteomalacia Thrombocytopenia Hemolytic anemia Acute renal failure Pseudomembranous colitis Pseudoadrenal crisis
3.	Ethambutol	Retrobulbar neuritis	Skin reactions Arthralgia Peripheral neuritis
4.	Pyrazinamide	Arthralgia Hepatotoxicity	Gastrointestinal reaction Cutaneous reaction Sideroblastic anemia
5.	Streptomycin	Vestibular and auditory nerve damage Nephrotoxicity Cutaneous reaction Pain, induration at site of injection	Hypersensitivity reaction Anaphylactic shock Hemolytic anemia Aplastic anemia Agranulocytosis Thrombocytopenia
6.	Thioacetazone	Cutaneous reaction, nausea, vomiting, abdominal discomfort	Anemia, acute hepatic failure Agranulocytosis Thrombocytopenia

Management of Adverse Effects

Isoniazid is well tolerated drug in most of the patients. Peripheral neuritis is the most common toxic manifestation of isoniazid which can be prevented by giving vitamin B_6 (pyridoxine), 10 mg daily. For established peripheral neuropathy, pyridoxine should be given at larger dosage of 50–75 mg daily. Pyridoxine in higher dosage may reduce the bactericidal activity of isoniazid.[4] In isoniazid induced psychosis, patient needs consultation by psychiatric physician.

For rash or other form of hypersensitivity and hepatitis—see management of common adverse effects (Tables 13.2 and 13.3).

Table 13.2: Symptoms based approach to minor adverse reactions not requiring stoppage of treatment

Abdominal pain, nausea	Related to rifampicin	Reassures the patients
Burning of the feet	Related to isoniazid Peripheral neuropathy	Continue isoniazid, and give pyridoxine 50–75 mg daily; Large dose of pyridoxine, may interfere the action of isoniazid
Drowsiness	Related to isoniazid	Reassures the patients
Gastrointestinal upset	Any oral medications	Reassure patients; give drugs with less water; give drugs over longer period of time (e.g. 20 minutes), give drugs with small amount of food; if these measure fails, provide antiemetic
Joint pains	Related to pyrazinamide	Continue pyrazinamide; use aspirin or nonsteroidal anti-inflammatory drugs. Use intermittent directly observed treatment if possible
Red urine	Related to rifampicin	Reassures the patients
Women on rifampicin	Rifampicin may reduce the effectiveness of oral contraceptive pills	Alternative method of contraception should be provided

Table 13.3: Symptoms-based approach to major adverse effects requiring stoppage of treatment

Symptoms	Drug	Management
Loss of hearing	Related to streptomycin	Otoscopy to rule out wax Stop streptomycin if no other explanation
Dizziness	If true vertigo and nystagmus, related to streptomycin	Stop streptomycin; if just dizziness with no nystagmus, try dose reduction for one week; if there is no improvement stop streptomycin
Generalized reactions including shock and purpura	May be due to rifampicin, pyrazinamide and/or streptomycin, thioacetazone	Stop all medications; use different combination of drugs
Jaundice	May be due to drug induced hepatitis	Stop all antituberculosis drugs until jaundice resolves and liver enzyme revert to base levels Reintroduce same regimen either gradually or all at once If hepatitis has been life-threatening and was not of viral origin, It is safer to use regimen like streptomycin, ethambutol and isoniazid, fluroquinolones
Moderate to severe skin rash	Related to all antituberculosis drugs	Stop all antituberculosis drugs Reintroduce drug one by one once the rash has subsided
Visual impairment	Related to ethambutol	Visual examination Stop ethambutol
Vomiting/ Confusion	Suspect drug induced hepatitis	Urgent liver enzyme test. If liver enzyme test unavailable, stop antituberculosis drugs and observe

RIFAMPICIN

Rifampicin is a semisynthetic antibiotic,[7] and bactericidal in action. It was discovered in 1966. Rifampicin is produced by *Streptomyces mediterranei*. In addition to its antituberculosis activity, it has a wide range of activity against other bacteria, including *Staphylococcus, Streptococcus, Clostridium, Pseudomonas, E. coli, Proteus, Salmonella, Shigella, Bacteroides* and *Legionella*. It acts by inhibiting DNA dependent RNA polymerase of *Mycobacterium*. Rifampicin is readily absorbed when administered orally and peak plasma levels of 6–7 μg/mL are reached in 3 hours. Most strains of *M. tuberculosis* are inhibited in vitro by concentration of 0.5 μg/mL. It penetrates all body tissue, tubercular cavity, placenta and meninges. It is extensively metabolized in liver to an active deacylated metabolite which is excreted mainly in bile, some in urine also. Rifampicin should be given preferably 30 minutes before meal[8] since absorption is reduced when the drug is taken with food.

Preparation and Dose

Rifampicin is available as capsule or tablets of 150 mg, 300 mg, 450 mg, and 600 mg and as syrup containing 100 mg/5 mL. Combined preparations with isoniazid, and with isoniazid plus pyrazinamide are also available.

The dose for daily therapy being 10 (8–12) mg/kg/day (maximum 600 mg) and it is same in twice or thrice weekly regimen.[2, 3]

Drug Interactions

Rifampicin being inducer of hepatic p450 microsomal enzyme enhances its own metabolism and that of many other drugs including, warfarin, oral contraceptive, corticosteroids, sulfonylureas and digitoxin and antifungal drugs. Rifampicin also reduces the levels of protease inhibitor and non-nucleoside reverse transcriptase inhibitors used to treat HIV. Newer derivatives of rifampicin like rifabutin and rifapentene with longer half-life has less effect on the pharmacokinetics of antiretroviral drugs. Rifampicin reduces the effectiveness of oral contraceptive so contraceptive failures have occurred and patients should be advised to switch over to an oral contraceptive containing higher dose (50 μg) of estrogen or use alternative method of contraception.

Contraindications

Rifampicin should not be given in known hypersensitivity and hepatic dysfunction.

Effect in Pregnancy

Rifampicin is safer in pregnancy.

Overdosage

Overdosage of rifampicin can be reverted by gastric lavage if undertaken with in few hours of ingestion. Very large dosage may depress central nervous system. There is no specific antidote and treatment is supportive.

Adverse Effects

Rifampicin is well tolerated by most patients at currently recommended dosage. Unlike other drugs, rifampicin produces some adverse reactions more frequently with intermittent therapy than with daily regimens. Moreover, the risk of adverse effect increases with the interval between doses. Hepatitis in the form of asymptomatic elevation in serum transaminase levels is the common adverse effect by this drug and generally resolves spontaneously, more likely in patients with pre-existing liver impairment and in alcoholics. Rarely serious hepatotoxicity generally with cholestatic pattern may occur. Rifampicin cause orange-red discoloration of body secretions such as urine-feces, tears, and sweat and may results in permanent discoloration of soft contact lenses. Gastrointestinal disturbance (epigastric distress, nausea, vomiting, abdominal cramps, diarrhea) are other common adverse effects by this drugs. Less common adverse effects are fever, influenza-like syndrome and thrombocytopenia.[9] Exfoliative dermatitis is more common in HIV-positive tuberculosis patients.

Reactions more frequently observed with intermittent regimens are as follows: (1) a cutaneous syndrome consisting of flushing/pruritis, with or without rash involving face and scalp, often with redness and watering of the eyes (2) an abdominal syndrome consisting of nausea, vomiting less commonly diarrhea (3) a flu syndrome consisting of fever, chills, headache, bone pain; (4) purpura and other rare reactions such as acute hemolytic anemia, shock, renal damage (5) a respiratory syndrome characterized by breathlessness, rarely associated with collapse and shock, (6) elevated serum levels of transaminase are quite common and transient hepatotoxicity may also occur (see Table 13.1).

Management of Adverse Effects

For gastrointestinal reactions the patients should be reassured. If gastro-intestinal intolerance is severe enough to risk interruption of treatment, suspension of rifampicin for 3 or 4 doses, use of medications that provide symptomatic relief (e.g. metoclopramide to counteract vomiting or as a last resort giving rifampicin either with small amount of food or 30 minutes of breakfast) may allow continued use of the drug in almost of patients. Although concomitant ingestion of food reduces absorption of rifampicin slightly, but this is preferable to complete discontinuation of rifampicin.

In case of thrombocytopenia, shock, acute renal failure, hemolytic[10] anemia, the drug should be stopped immediately and should never be used again.

For hepatitis and skin reaction, other form of hypersensitivity—see management of common adverse effects (Table 13.2 and 13.3).

ETHAMBUTOL

Ethambutol is a water-soluble and heat-stable antibiotic and bacteriostatic in action. It was discovered in 1961, acts by blocking arabinosyl transferase enzyme being involved in cell wall biosynthesis of *Mycobacterium*. About 75-80% of orally administered ethambutol is absorbed from gut. Peak plasma concentration of 4 µg/mL reached 2 to 4 hours after a dose of 15 mg/kg. Ethambutol in concentration of 0.005 to 0.2 µg/mL inhibits growth of *M. tuberculosis* in vitro. Nearly all strains of *M. tuberculosis* are sensitive to ethambutol.[11] Bacterial resistance to drug develops in vivo via single amino acid change in *embA* genes when given in absence of another effective agent. It is widely distributed but penetrates meninges incompletely. Seventy-five percent of ingested drug is excreated unchanged in urine and major reduction in daily ehambutol dosage is recommended in patients with renal failure.

Preparation and Dose

Ethambutol is supplied in 400 mg, 600 mg, 800 mg and 1000 mg tablets. Combined preparations with isoniazid are available.

The dosage for daily therapy being 15 (15–20) mg/kg/day and in twice weekly regimen dosage is 45 (40–50) /mg/kg/day and in thrice weekly regimen dosage is 30 (25–35) mg/kg/day.[2,3]

Contraindications

Ethambutol should not be given in known hypersensitivity and previously existing visual disorder and renal failure.

Effect in Pregnancy

Ethambutol is safer in pregnancy.

Overdosage

Overdosage of ethambutol can be reverted by gastric lavage and emesis if undertaken with in few hours of ingestion. Subsequently, dialysis may be of value. There is no specific antidote and treatment is supportive.

Adverse Effects

Ethambutol may produce retrobulbar neuritis. Three types of neuritis are reported with ethambutol.[6] These include the axial, periaxial and mixed type.

Both eyes are usually involved and visual loss may vary from mild to severe form. Color (red, green) vision is also variably affected. Ethambutol related ocular toxicity is strongly dose related.[12-23] In a study reported by Carr and Hen kind[12] showed incidence of ocular toxicity in 45% in patients receiving 60 to 100 mg/kg/day. Another report showed incidence of ocular toxicity to be 18.6% in patients receiving 53 mg/kg/day of ethambutol. With 25 mg/kg/day, the reported incidence of ethambutol related optic neuritis was 1.5-15%.[22] Toxicity occurs rarely if no more than 15 mg/kg is given daily.[12-22]

Guideline have been proposed by British Joint Tuberculosis Committee with respect to ethambutol related ocular toxicity.[22] These include: (1) Avoid ethambutol in patients with impaired renal function; (2) Do not exceed the recommended ethambutol dosage and duration; (3) Record of any previous and present ocular disease must be maintained; (4) Patients must be informed about the possibility of ethambutol affecting vision and drug should be stopped if vision becomes impaired; (5) Routine visual test during treatment are not recommended; (6) It is best to avoid ethambutol in children and adults in whom assessment of visual acuity is difficult to perform; (7) When a patients on treatment presents with visual impairment, he or she should be referred to ophthalmologist. Rarely observed side effects during treatment with ethambutol are skin rash, joints pain, peripheral neuropathy and thrombocytopenia (see Table 13.1).[24]

Management of Adverse Effects

If patients are taking ethambutol he/she should be warned that ocular examination is must by ophthalmologist if visual symptom occurs during treatment. Vision returns to normal if drug is stopped early but permanent optic nerve damage occurs if drug is continued. In case of patients with renal failure major reduction in ethambutol dosage is recommended. Recommended dosage in renal failure varies from 5 to 10 mg/kg/day by various workers (see Table 13.2).

PYRAZINAMIDE

Pyrazinamide is the synthetic pyrazine analog of nicotinamide and exhibiting bactericidal activity in vitro only at a slightly acidic pH.[25] Activity at acid pH is ideal, since *M. tuberculosis* reside in an acidic phagosome within macrophage. It acts by inhibiting *Mycobacterium* fatty acid synthase I gene involved in mycolic acid biosynthesis. It is well absorbed from gastrointestinal tract, with peak plasma levels 50 μg/mL occurring 1.5–2 hours of ingestion. Pyrazinamide in concentration of 12.5 μg/mL inhibits growth of *M. tuberculosis* in vitro. Pyrazinamide is well absorbed from gut and is cleared primarily by liver but its metabolites are also excreted in the urine and distributed widely throughout the body tissue, with good penetration in cerebrospinal fluid (CSF).

Preparation and Dose

The drug is available in 500 mg, 1000 mg and 1500 mg or combined preparation with rifampicin plus isoniazid. The dose for daily patients being 25 (20–30) mg/kg and in twice weekly regimen dosage is 50 (40–60)/mg/kg/day and in thrice weekly regimen dosage is 35 (30–40) mg/kg/day.[2,3]

Contraindications

Pyrazinamide should not be given in known hypersensitivity and hepatic dysfunction.

Effect in Pregnancy

Pyrazinamide is safer in pregnancy.

Overdosage

Overdosage of pyrazinamide may results into acute liver damage and hyperuricemia and reverted by gastric lavage and emesis if undertaken within few hours of ingestion. There is no specific antidote and treatment is supportive.

Adverse Effects

Injury to liver is a major side effect of pyrazinamide. When a dose of 40 mg/kg/day is administered orally, sign and symptom appears in only 15% of patients, with jaundice in 2–3% and death due to hepatic necrosis in rare instances. Elevation of serum aminotransferase is earliest abnormality produced by the drug. Nausea and vomiting are common at standard dosage, more severe at higher dosages. Severe hepatotoxicity has been observed when regimens containing rifampicin and pyrazinamide are used. Polyarthalgia may occur in up to 40% of patients receiving daily dosage of pyrazinamide. It is due to inhibition of renal tubular secretion of uric acid by pyrazinoic acid, the main metabolite of pyrazinamide but this rarely requires discontinuation of treatment. Acute gout is rare except in patients with pre-existing gout. Pyrazinamide may cause photosensitivity. Hypersensitivity including fever, rash and other cutaneous reactions and sideroblastic anemia and gastrointestinal reactions may occasionally occur (see Table 13.1).

Management of Adverse Effects

For arthralgia, simple treatment with analgesics usually minimize symptoms. Indomethacin may be used for more severe joint involvement, if frank gout occurs, treatment with colchicines is required. Arthalgia is much less common with thrice weekly treatment. Asymptomatic elevation of serum uric acid levels is expected and does not require either a change in medication or administration of other medications.

For hepatitis—see management of common adverse effects (Table 13.3).

STREPTOMYCIN

Streptomycin is an aminoglycoside antibiotic and was discovered in 1944 and bactericidal in an alkaline environment. It is derived from *Streptomyces griseus*.[26] It acts by inhibiting protein synthesis process in multi step process.[27,28] It is given parenterally and peak plasma levels in range of 40 µg/mL are achieved 1 hour after injection. Most strains of *M. tuberculosis* are inhibited in vitro by concentration of 8 µg/mL. Streptomycin does not penetrate cell walls or normal biological membranes such as the meninges or the pleura, unless inflammatory changes have taken place. It crosses the placenta and fetal serum levels are about half those in maternal blood. The drug is excreted entirely by glomerular filtration. Streptomycin is administered by deep intramuscular (IM) injection. Injections are often painful with hot, tender masses developing at the site of injection.

Preparation and Dose

Streptomycin sulfate for intramuscular injection is supplied as a powder in vials and should be reconstituted immediately before use. The dose for daily therapy being 15 (range 12–18) mg/kg/day and same in twice or thrice weekly regimen.[2,3] Patients aged over 60 years may not be able to tolerate more than 500–750 mg daily.

Contraindications

Streptomycin should not be given in known hypersensitivity, auditory nerve impairment, myasthenia gravis and renal failure.

Effect in Pregnancy

Streptomycin should not be given in pregnancy because it crosses the placental barrier producing auditory nerve impairment in fetus and renal impairment.

Overdosage

In streptomycin over dosage, hemodialysis can be beneficial. There is no specific antidote and treatment is supportive.

Adverse Effects

Most important adverse drug reaction caused by streptomycin is ototoxicity, with vestibular damage more common than hearing impairment. Toxicity is manifested as vertigo, ataxia, tinnitus and loss of hearing. The patients usually complain of giddiness. Damage to vestibular apparatus is best shown by caloric test but it is a crude test. The simplest way of demonstrating ataxia is to ask the patients to walk along straightline with closed eyes. If the patient walks more unsteady than open eyes, ataxia is present. The risk increases with age or concomitant use of loop diuretics (frusemide, ethacrynic acid) and thioacetazone. Streptomycin commonly causes circumoral paresthesias immediately after the injection. Streptomycin induced nephrotoxicity occur less commonly than with amikacin, kanamycin or capreomycin. Streptomycin is contraindicated in pregnancy because of risk of fetal hearing loss. Streptomycin should be used cautiously in patients with renal impairment because clearance is almost exclusively by kidneys. Less common side effects are hypersensitivity reactions and anaphylactic shock and blood dyscrasias including hemolytic and aplastic anemia, thrombocytopenia and agranulocytosis (see Table 13.1).

Management of Adverse Effects

For vestibular auditory and renal damage the risk increases with dose and age. The dose should not exceed 15–20 mg/kg and should be reduced in patients aged 45 years or more. Damage to the vestibular and auditory system usually occurs in the first 2 months and is manifested by ringing in ears, giddiness, ataxia, and/or deafness. The condition is reversible if the drug dose is reduced or the drug is stopped. Intermittent dosages are less likely to cause serious toxicity.

In renal failure dose reductions is needed and follow-up with serum creatinine and blood urea nitrogen every one to two month regularly.

THIOACETAZONE

Thioacetazone is a thiosemicarbazol antibiotic and bacteriostatic in activity. When it was introduced in the late 1940s, there was good evidence of its efficacy, but the relatively high dosage used in those days meant that adverse effects and toxicity were frequent. Thus with the advent of isoniazid a few years later, thioacetazone was forgotten. In the early 1960s, thioacetazone was reinvestigated as a companion drug to isoniazid. The aim was to find an alternative to PAS that would prevent the development of resistance to isoniazid well and less bulky. The result was introduction of regimen containing 150 mg of thioacetazone and 300 mg of isoniazid, given in one dose only daily, proved to be effective as PAS-isoniazid combination. There may be cross-resistance between thioacetazone and ethionamide. The drug should not be used in liver disease.

Preparation and Dose

The dosage recommended is 2.5 mg/kg body weight daily; it is not effective when given intermittently.

Contraindications

In HIV-positive patients, the risk of major, potentially fatal cutaneous reactions caused by thioacetazone is unacceptably high. It should never be used in patients who may be HIV-positive or in areas where HIV infection is common.

Adverse Effects

Most common adverse drug reaction caused by thioacetazone is cutaneous reactions. A cutaneous reaction may present, first as itching; may be followed by a skin rash that may quickly develop into toxic epidermal necrolysis, with case fatality of 20–30%. Other common adverse effects are nausea, vomiting and abdominal discomfort. Less common adverse effects are anemia, acute hepatic failure, agranulocytosis, thrombocytopenia, cerebral edema, conjunctivitis, blurred vision and jaundice (see Table 13.1).

Management of Adverse Effects

If rash or other sign of hypersensitivity develops, all the treatment should be stopped and thioacetazone should not be used again. If there is itching with mild rash then symptomatic treatment with antihistaminic may be tried and if severe rash or there is mucosal involvement with hypotension then oral prednisolone, 40–60 mg, should be given daily until there is response; dose should be reduced gradually in following days according to the patients response.

Because HIV serology is not routinely being performed in most setting where TB and HIV are more prevalent, so thioacetazone should not be administered in areas where HIV prevalence is high. The closest alternative is ethambutol and isoniazid combination, as they are well tolerated and have higher efficacy. But main drawback is that it may increase rifampicin and ethambutol resistance.

MANAGEMENT OF COMMON ADVERSE EFFECT

Hepatitis

Transient, asymptomatic increase in serum liver transaminases occur during the early week of treatment. Three of the first-line antituberculosis drugs, INH, RIF and PZA, can cause drug induced liver injury (AST level three or more times the upper limit of normal in the presence of symptoms, or five or more times the upper limit of normal in the absence of symptoms). If the AST level is less than 5 times the upper limit of normal, toxicity can be considered mild, and AST level 5–10 times normal (i.e. greater than 500 IU) is severe. In addition to AST elevation, occasionally there are disproportionate increase in bilirubin and alkaline phosphatase. This pattern is more consistent with rifampin hepatotoxicity. There is no need to interrupt or change treatment unless there is anorexia, malaise, vomiting or clinically evident jaundice. Clinical features of concern include protracted vomiting, mental changes, and signs of bleeding—all of which suggest impending acute liver failure and require immediate discontinuation of antituberculosis medications.

If jaundice or any of the clinical features suggestive of acute liver failure develop, all drugs must be stopped until the jaundice or hepatic symptoms have resolved and the liver enzymes have returned to baseline levels. If liver enzyme cannot be measured, it is advisable to wait 2 weeks after the jaundice disappeared before starting tuberculosis treatment.

Reintroduction of Antituberculosis Drugs

Once hepatitis has resolved, the same drug regimen can be reintroduced either gradually or all at once. However, if hepatitis has been life-threatening and was not of viral origin, it is probably safer to use the regimen of streptomycin, isoniazid and ethambutol.

Cutaneous and Generalized Hypersensitivity Reaction

Skin Rashes

Any antituberculosis drug may produce a generalized hypersensitivity reaction but this is rarely seen with current short course chemotherapy than it was on treatment with PAS, streptomycin and isoniazid. Occasionally patients is sensitized to more than one drugs, such type of reactions are rarely observed during the first week of treatment and being commonest in second to four week and very rarely in later weeks of therapy. Hypersensitivity reactions are clinically manifested earliest by fever followed by rash within few days. The rash is erythematous, macular, or papular and associated with itching, more prominent over face, neck, and extremities. In severe cases, manifestations are periorbital swelling, generalized lymphadenopathy, hepatosplenomegaly, encephalitis, rigors and high-grade fever, exfoliative dermatitis and Steven-Johnson syndrome and rarely resulting into death.

Itching with no Rash or with Mild Rash

If the patients (not receiving thiacetazone) complains of itching without a rash or itching with a mild rash, symptomatic treatment with antihistamines may be tried and tuberculosis treatment continued and the patients must be monitored with each subsequent dose of antituberculosis drugs. If patients are receiving thioacetazone, it should be withdrawn and should never be used again.

Itching with Moderate/Severe Rash

If a moderate or severe rash developed, all treatment should be stopped and treatment with corticosteroids should be instituted. Oral prednisolone, 40–60 mg should be given daily until there is a response, the dose should be reduced gradually in the following days according to the patients response. Tuberculosis treatment should be withheld until the reaction has completely subsided. Isoniazid and rifampicin are the least likely to cause such reaction and should be re-introduced first. Subsequently pyrazinamide and ethambutol may be reintroduced. If the initial cutaneous reaction was severe, initial challenge doses should be given. If the patients is restarted on the adequate tuberculosis treatment regimens (e.g. isoniazid, rifampicin, pyrazinamide), re-challenging with the rest of implicated drugs is not advisable.

REFERENCES

1. Byrd RB, Horn Soloman DA, Grieg GW. Toxic effects of isoniazid in tuberculosis chemoprophylaxis. Role of biochemical monitoring in 1000 patients. JAMA. 1979;241;1239-41.
2. Jhonston RN, et al. Prolonged streptomycin and isoniazid for pulmonary tuberculosis. BMJ. 1964;1:1679-83.
3. Peloquin CA, et al. Pharmacokinetics of isoniazid under fasting condition, with food and antacids. Int J Tub and Lung Dis. 1999;3:703-10.
4. McCune R, Deuschle K, et al. The delayed appearance of isoniazid antagonism by pyridoxine in vivo. American Review of Tuberculosis and Pulmonary Diseases. 1957;76:1100-5.
5. Ormerold LP. Hepatotoxicity of antituberculosis drugs. Thorax. 1996;51:111-3.
6. World Health Organization collaborating centre for international drug monitoring: Adverse drug reaction terminology (ART) 1979.http://www.WHO-UMC.org.
7. Furesz S. Chemical and biological properties of rifampicin. Antibiot; Chemotherapy. 1970;16: 316-51.
8. Accocela G. Clinical pharmacokinetics of rifampicin. Clinical pharmacokinetics. 1978;3:108-27.
9. Prasad R, Mukherji PK. Rifampicin induced thrombocytopenia. Ind J Tub. 1989;36:44-5.
10. Steele MA, Burk RF, DesPrez RM. Toxic hepatitis with isoniazid and rifampicin: A meta-analysis. Chest. 1991;99:465-71.
11. Belanger AE, Bersa GS, Ford ME, et al. The embAB genes of *Mycobacterium avium* encode an arabinosyl transferase in cell wall biosynthesis that is the target for drug ethambutol. Proc Natl Acad Sci USA. 1996;93:11919-24.
12. Carr RE, Henkind P. Ocular manifestation of ethambutol toxicity. Thorax. 1996;51:111-3.
13. Place VA, Perts EA, et al. Metabolic and special study of ethambutol in healthy volunteers and tuberculosis patients. Ann NY Acad Sci. 1966;135:775-95.
14. Leibold JE. The ocular toxicity of ethambutol and its relation to dose. Ann NY Acad Sci. 1966; 135:904-9.
15. Bobrowitz ID. Ethambutol in retreatment of tuberculosis. Ann NY Acad Sci. 1966;135:796-822.
16. Ciffron KM. Ethambutol: A review with special reference to ocular toxicity. Tubercle. 1969;5: 32-6.
17. Barron GJ, Tepper L, et al. Ocular toxicity from ethambutol. Am J Opthalmol. 1974;77:256-60.
18. Donomae I, Yamamoto K. Clinical evaluation of ethambutol in primary tuberculosis. Ann NY Acad Sci. 1966;135:849-81.
19. Fledelius HC, Petrera JE, et al. Ocular ethambutol toxicity. Acta Ophthalmol. 1987;65:251-5.
20. Gomez-Pimienta JL, Shibayama Hernandez H, et al. Retreatment of pulmonary tuberculosis with ethambutol. Ann NY Acad Sci. 1966;135:882-9.
21. Pyle MM. Ethambutol in retreatment of pulmonary tuberculosis: four year clinical investigation. Ann NY Acad Sci. 1966;135:835-48.
22. Chaterjee VKK, Buchanan DR, et al. Ocular toxicity following ethambutol in standard dosage. Br J Dis Chest. 1986;80:288-91.
23. Ciffron KM, Thomas GO, et al. Ocular toxicity from ethambutol (editorial). Thorax. 1986; 41:787-9.
24. Prasad R, Mukherji PK. Ethambutol induced thrombocytopenia. Tubercle. 1989;70:211-2.
25. Ziersky M. Pharmacology, toxicology and clinical use of pyrazinamide. Praxis und Klink der Pneumogie. 1981;35:1075-105.

26. Barclay, ML Kirppatrick, et al. Once daily aminoglycoside therapy. Is it less toxic than multiple daily dosage and how should it be monitored? Clinical Pharmacokinet. 1999;36:89-98.
27. Barza M, Ioannidis JP, et al. Single or multiple daily dosage of aminoglycosides. BMJ. 1996;312 338-45.
28. Busse HJ, Wostmann C, Bakkar, et al. The bactericidal action of streptomycin. J. Gen Microbio. 1992;138:551-61.

Chapter 14

Antitubercular Drugs Used in Previously Treated Patients of Tuberculosis and their Adverse Effects

KANAMYCIN

Drug Class

Aminoglycoside.

Activity Against TB, Mechanism of Action and Metabolism

Bactericidal, Aminoglycosides

It is used as reserve drugs in multidrug-resistant (MDR) tuberculosis not responding to primary antitubercular drugs.[1] It was second systemically used aminoglycoside, after streptomycin, in tuberculosis.[2,3] Inhibit protein synthesis by irreversibly binding to 30S ribosomal subunit; aminoglycosides are not metabolized in the liver, they are excreted unchanged in the urine. Most strains of tuberculosis is inhibited in vitro at the concentrations of 10 μg/mL.[4]

Distribution

0.2–0.4 L/kg; distributed in extracellular fluid, abscesses, ascitic fluid, pericardial fluid, pleural fluid, synovial fluid, lymphatic fluid and peritoneal fluid. Not well distributed into bile, aqueous humor, bronchial secretions, sputum and cerebrospinal fluid (CSF).

Preparation and Dose

Kanamycin sulfate, sterile powder for intramuscular injection in sealed vials. The powder needs to be dissolved in 2 mL of 0.9% sodium chloride or water for injections before use. The optimal dose is 15 (12–18) mg/kg body weight, usually 750 mg to 1 g given daily or 5–6 days per week, by deep intramuscular injection. Rotation of injection sites avoids local discomfort. When necessary, it is possible to give the drug at the same total dose 2 or 3 times weekly during the continuation phase, under close monitoring for adverse effects.

Storage

Powder stable at room temperature (15-25°C), diluted solution should be used the same day.

Oral Absorption

There is no significant oral absorption.

CSF Penetration

Penetrates inflamed meninges only.

Special Circumstances

Pregnancy/Breastfeeding

Safety class D. Eighth cranial nerve damage has been reported following in utero exposure to kanamycin. Excreted in breast milk. The American Academy of Pediatrics considers kanamycin to be compatible with breastfeeding.

Renal Disease

Use with caution. Levels should be monitored for patients with impaired renal function. Interval adjustment (12-15 mg/kg—2 or 3 times per week) is recommended for creatinine clearance < 30 mL/min or hemodialysis.

Hepatic Disease

Drug levels not affected by hepatic disease (except a larger volume of distribution for alcoholic cirrhotic patients with ascites). Presumed to be safe in severe liver disease; however, use with caution as—some patients with severe liver disease may progress rapidly to hepatorenal syndrome.

Adverse Effects (Table 14.1)

Frequent

- Pain at injection site
- Renal failure (usually reversible).

Occasional

- Vestibular and auditory damage (usually irreversible)
- Nephrotoxicity (dose-related to cumulative and peak concentrations)
- Increased risk with renal insufficiency (often irreversible)
- Peripheral neuropathy
- Rash.

Ototoxicity potentiated by certain diuretics (especially loop diuretics), advanced age, and prolonged use. The effect of nondepolarizing muscle relaxants may be increased.

Table 14.1: Adverse effects of antitubercular drugs used in retreatment cases

Drug	Frequent	Occasional	Rare
Amikacin	Pain injection site Proteinuria Electrolyte disturbances (hypokalemia and hypomagnesemia)	Cochlear ototoxicity Vestibular toxicity Nephrotoxicity Peripheral neuropathy Rash Eosinophilia	Fever
Capreomycin	Nephrotoxicity Tubular dysfunction Urticaria Maculopapular rash	Cochlear ototoxicity Vestibular toxicity Electrolyte disturbances (hypokalemia, hypomagnesemia and hypocalcemia) Pain at injection site induration and sterile abscesses at site of injection Neurotoxicity	Rash
Clofazimine	Ichthyosis Dry skin Pink to brown black discoloration of skin, cornea, retina and urine Anorexia Abdominal pain	Hepatitis Hypersensitivity Nephrotoxicity Acneform eruption	Phototoxicity
Cycloserine	Neurological disturbances (headache and tremors) Psychiatric disturbances (sleep disturbances, anxiety, depression, irritability, confusion, drowsiness) Inflammation of gums Pale skin	Visual changes and eye pain Skin rash Jaundice (hepatitis) Burning, tingling and numbness in hands and feet	Seizures Suicidal thoughts Impaired hearing in fetus Hypersensitivity
Ethionamide and prothionamide	Severe gastrointestinal intolerance (including nausea, vomiting, diarrhea, abdominal pain, excessive salivation metallic taste)-dose related Headache Anorexia and weight loss Stomatitis	Neurological disturbances Psychiatric disturbances (depression, restlessness, drowsiness) Allergic reactions Postural hypotension Reversible hepatitis (transient increase in serum bilirubin) Hypothyroidism (especially when combined with PAS) Menstrual irregularity Gynecomastia Arthralgias Leukopenia	Peripheral neuritis Optic neuritis Pellagra like syndrome Rash Photosensitivity Thrombocytopenia Alopecia Impotence Purpura

Contd...

Contd...

Drug	Frequent	Occasional	Rare
Kanamycin	Pain at injection site Renal damage (usually reversible)	Cochlear and vestibular otoxicity (usually irreversible) Peripheral neuropathy Rash Nephrotoxicity (dose related to cumulative and peak concenteration, often irreversible)	Fever
Levofloxacin	Generally well tolerated	Gastrointestinal intolerance (diarrhea) Neurological disturbances (insomnia, restlessness, dizziness) Allergic reactions Photosensitivity	QT prolongation Peripheral neuropathy Tendon rupture Rash
Moxifloxacin	Generally well tolerated	Gastrointestinal intolerance (diarrhea) Neurological disturbances (insomnia, restlessness, dizziness) Allergic reactions Photosensitivity	QT prolongation (in isolated cases) Rash
Ofloxacin	Generally well tolerated	Gastrointestinal intolerance (diarrhea) Neurological disturbances (headache, insomnia, restlessness)	Allergic reactions Photosensitivity Peripheral neuropathy Tendon rupture Increased liver function tests
Para-aminosalicylic acid (PAS)	Gastrointestinal intolerance (including metallic taste, anorexia, diarrhea) Hypothyroidism especially when combined with ethionamide	Hepatitis Thyroid enlargement Allergic reactions Fever Increased prothrombin time Malabsorption syndrome (e.g. steatorrhea and low serum folate level)	
Linezolid	Gastrointestinal intolerance Rash Headache	Myelosuppression Peripheral neuropathy Optic neuropathy	
Clarithromycin	Gastrointestinal intolerance (abdominal pain, nausea, vomiting, diarrhea) Hepatitis Ventricular arrhythmias		Hypersensitivity reaction Pseudomembranous colitis Fever Rash

Contd...

Contd...

Drug	Frequent	Occasional	Rare
Imipenem/ Cilastatin	Gastrointestinal intolerance Hypersensitivity reaction Palpitation Tachycardia	Seizure Hypotension Anemia Thrombophlebitis	Renal failure Hemorrhagic colitis Pseudomembranous colitis
Thiacetazone	Gastrointestinal intolerance Rash Anemia	Hepatitis Exfoliative dermatitis Stevens-Johnson syndrome	Bone marrow depression Ototoxicity
Amoxicillin/ Clavulanate	Diarrhea Rash Hypersensitivity reaction	*Candida stomatitis* Vaginitis	Hepatic injury

Drug Interactions

Loop diuretics (bumetanide, furosemide, ethacrynic acid, torsemide).

Coadministration of aminoglycosides with loop diuretics may have an additive or synergistic auditory ototoxicity. Ototoxicity appears to be dose-dependent and may be increased with renal dysfunction. Irreversible ototoxicity has been reported.

Avoid concomitant administration; if used together, careful dose adjustments in patients with renal failure and close monitoring for ototoxicity are required.

Nondepolarizing muscle relaxants (atracurium, pancuronium, tubocurarine, gallamine triethiodide): possible enhanced action of nondepolarizing muscle relaxant resulting in possible respiratory depression. Avoid coadministration; if concurrent administration is needed, titrate the nondepolarizing muscle relaxant slowly and monitor neuromuscular function closely.

Nephrotoxic agents (amphotericin B, foscarnet, cidofovir): additive nephrotoxicity. Avoid coadministration; if used together, monitor renal function closely and discontinue if warranted.

Penicillins: In vitro inactivation (possible). Do not mix together before administration.

Contraindications

- Pregnancy (congenital deafness seen with streptomycin and kanamycin use in pregnancy)
- Hypersensitivity to aminoglycosides
- Caution with renal, hepatic, vestibular or auditory impairment.

Monitoring

Monthly creatinine and serum potassium in low-risk patients (young with no comorbidities), more frequently in high-risk patients (elderly, diabetic, or HIV-positive patients, or patients with renal insufficiency). If potassium is low, check magnesium and calcium. Baseline audiometry and monthly monitoring in high-risk patients. For problems with balance, consider increasing dosing interval.

Alerting Symptoms

- Problems with hearing; dizziness
- Rash
- Trouble breathing
- Decreased urination
- Swelling, pain or redness at injection site
- Muscle twitching or weakness.

Management of Adverse Effects (Table 14.2)

Hearing loss can be prevented by:

1. Changing injectable to capreomycin if patient has documented susceptibility to capreomycin.
2. Discontinue suspected agents without compromising the regimen.
3. Lower dose of suspected agents without compromising the regimen.

In renal failure, dose reduction is needed and follow up with serum creatinine and blood urea is required every one to two months regularly. If renal profile is uncontrolled despite of decreased dosage, then discontinue suspected agent and consider using capreomycin.

AMIKACIN

Drug Class

Aminoglycoside.

Activity Against TB, Mechanism of Action and Metabolism

Bactericidal, inhibit protein synthesis through disruption of ribosomal function; less effective in acidic pH, aminoglycosides are not metabolized in the liver, they are excreted unchanged in the urine.

Preparation and Dose

Amikacin sulfate, colorless solution. 250 mg/mL (2 or 4 mL vials) and 50 mg/mL (2 mL vial). The optimal dose is 15–20 mg/kg body weight, usually 750 mg to 1 g given daily or 5–6 days per week by deep intramuscular injection. Rotation of injection sites avoids local discomfort. When necessary, it is

Table 14.2: Common adverse effects, suspected agent(s) and management strategies of antituberculous drugs used in retreatment patients of TB

Adverse effects	Suspected agent	Suggested management strategies
Seizures	**Cs** H Fq	• Suspend suspected agent pending resolution of seizures • Initiate anticonvulsant therapy (e.g. phenytoin, valproic acid) • Increase pyridoxine to maximum daily dose (200 mg per day) • Restart suspected agent or reinitiate suspected agent at lower dose, if essential to the regimen • Discontinue suspected agent if this can be done without compromising regimen • Anticonvulsant is generally continued until MDR-TB treatment is completed or suspected agent discontinued • History of previous seizure disorder is not a contraindication to the use of agents listed here if a patient's seizures are well controlled and/or the patient is receiving anticonvulsant • Patients with history of previous seizures may be at increased risk for development of seizures during MDR-TB
Peripheral neuropathy	**Cs** **Lzd** **H** S Km Am Cm Eto/Pto Fq	• Increase pyridoxine to maximum daily dose (200 mg per day) • Change injectable to capreomycin if patient has documented susceptibility to capreomycin • Initiate therapy with tricyclic antidepressants such as amitriptyline. Nonsteroidal anti-inflammatory drugs or acetaminophen may help alleviate symptoms • Lower dose of suspected agent, if this can be done without compromising regimen • Discontinue suspected agent, if this can be done without compromising regimen • Patients with comorbid disease (e.g. diabetes, HIV, alcohol neuropathy (dependence) may be more likely to develop peripheral neuropathy, but these conditions are not contraindications to the use of the agents listed here • Neuropathy may be irreversible; however, some patients may experience improvement when offending agents are suspended
Hearing loss	**S** **Km** **Am** **Cm** Clr	• Document hearing loss and compare with baseline audiometry, if available • Change parenteral treatment to capreomycin if patient has documented susceptibility to capreomycin • Decrease frequency and/or lower dose of suspected agent if this can be done without compromising the regimen (consider administration three times per week) • Discontinue suspected agent if this can be done without compromising the regimen • Patients with previous exposure to aminoglycosides may have baseline hearing loss. In such patients, audiometry may be helpful at the start of MDR-TB therapy • Hearing loss is generally not reversible • The risk of further hearing loss must be weighed against the risks of stopping the injectable in the treatment regimen • While the benefit of hearing aids is minimal to moderate in auditory toxicity, consider a trial use to determine if a patient with hearing loss can benefit from their use

Contd...

Contd...

Adverse effects	Suspected agent	Suggested management strategies
Psychotic symptoms	**Cs** **H** Fq Eto/Pto	• Stop suspected agent for a short period of time (1–4 weeks) while psychotic symptoms are brought under control • Initiate antipsychotic therapy • Lower dose of suspected agent if this can be done without compromising regimen • Discontinue suspected agent if this can be done without compromising regimen • Some patients will need to continue antipsychotic treatment throughout MDR-TB therapy • Previous history of psychiatric disease is not a contraindication to the use of agents listed here but may increase the likelihood of psychotic symptoms developing during treatment • Psychotic symptoms are generally reversible upon completion of MDR-TB treatment or cessation of the offending agent
Depression	**Cs** Fq Eto/Pto H	• Offer group or individual counseling • Initiate antidepressant therapy • Lower dose of suspected agent if this can be done without compromising regimen • Discontinue suspected agent if this can be done without compromising regimen • Socioeconomic conditions and chronic illness should not be underestimated as contributing factors to depression • Depressive symptoms may fluctuate during therapy and may improve as illness is successfully treated • History of previous depression is not a contraindication to the use of the agents listed but may increase the likelihood of depression developing during treatment
Hypothyroidism	**PAS** **Eto/Pto**	• Initiate thyroxine therapy • Completely reversible upon discontinuation of PAS or ethionamide/prothionamide • The combination of ethionamide/prothionamide with PAS is more frequently associated with hypothyroidism than the individual use of each drug
Nausea and vomiting	**Eto/Pto** **PAS** H E Z	• Assess for dehydration; initiate rehydration if indicated • Initiate antiemetic therapy • Lower dose of suspected agent if this can be done without compromising regimen • Discontinue suspected agent if this can be done without compromising regimen rarely necessary • Nausea and vomiting universal in early weeks of therapy and usually abate with time on treatment and adjunctive therapy • Electrolytes should be monitored if vomiting is severe • Reversible upon discontinuation of suspected agent • Severe abdominal distress and acute abdomen have been reported with the use of clofazimine. Although these reports are rare, if this effect occurs, clofazimine should be suspended
Gastritis	**PAS** **Eto/Pto**	• H_2-blockers, proton-pump inhibitors, or antacids • Stop suspected agent(s) for short periods of time (e.g. 1–7 days) • Lower dose of suspected agent, if this can be done without compromising regimen • Discontinue suspected agent if this can be done without compromising regimen

Contd...

Contd...

Adverse effects	Suspected agent	Suggested management strategies
		• Severe gastritis, as manifested by hematemesis, melena or hematochezia, is rare • Dosing of antacids should be carefully timed so as to not interfere with the absorption of antituberculosis drugs (take 2 hours before or 3 hours after antituberculosis medications) • Reversible upon discontinuation of suspected agent(s)
Hepatitis	**Z** **H** **R** Eto/Pto, PAS Fq	• Stop all therapy pending resolution of hepatitis • Eliminate other potential causes of hepatitis • Consider suspending most likely agent permanently • Reintroduce remaining drugs, one at a time while monitoring liver function • History of previous hepatitis should be carefully analyzed to determine most likely causative agent(s); these should be avoided in future regimens. • Generally reversible upon discontinuation of suspected agent
Renal toxicity	**S** **Km** **Am** **Cm**	• Discontinue suspected agent • Consider using capreomycin if an aminoglycoside had been the prior injectable in regimen • Consider dosing 2–3 times a week if drug is essential to the regimen and patient can tolerate (close monitoring of creatinine) • Adjust all antituberculosis medications according to the creatinine clearance • History of diabetes or renal disease is not a contraindication to the use of the agents listed here, although patients with these comorbidities may be at increased risk for developing renal failure • Renal impairment may be permanent
Electrolyte disturbances (hypokalemia and hypomagnesemia)	**Cm** **Km** **Am** S	• Check potassium. • If potassium is low, also check magnesium (and calcium if hypocalcemia is suspected) • Replace electrolytes as needed • If severe hypokalemia is present, consider hospitalization • Amiloride 5–10 mg QD or spironolactone 25 mg QD may decrease potassium and magnesium wasting and is useful in refractory cases • Oral potassium replacements can cause significant nausea and vomiting. Oral magnesium may cause diarrhea
Optic neuritis	**E** Eto/Pto	• Stop E • Refer patient to an ophthalmologist • Usually reverses with cessation of E • Rare case reports of optic neuritis have been attributed to streptomycin
Arthralgias	**Z** Fq	• Initiate therapy with nonsteroidal anti-inflammatory drugs • Lower dose of suspected agent if this can be done without compromising regimen • Discontinue suspected agent if this can be done without compromising regimen • Uric acid levels may be elevated in patients on pyrazinamide. Allopurinol appears not to correct the uric acid levels in such cases • Symptoms of arthralgia generally diminish overtime, even without intervention

Isoniazid (H), Rifampicin (R), Ethambutol (E), Pyrazinamide (Z), Streptomycin (S), Kanamycin (Km), Amikacin (Am), Capreomycin (Cm), Fluoroquinolones (Fq), Ethionamide (Eto), Prothionamide (Pto), Para-aminosalicylic acid (PAS), Cycloserine (Cs), Clofazimine (Cfz), Linezolid (Lzd), Clarithromycin (Clr).
Drugs that the strongly associated with adverse effects shown in bold.

possible to give the drug at the same total dose 2 or 3 times weekly during the continuation phase under close monitoring for adverse effects.

Storage

Solution is stable at room temperature (15–25°C); diluted solution is stable at room temperature for at least 3 days or in the refrigerator for at least 60 days.

Oral Absorption

There is no significant oral absorption. Intramuscular absorption may be delayed if the same site is used consistently.

CSF Penetration

Penetrates inflamed meninges only.

Special Circumstances

Pregnancy/Breastfeeding

Safety class D. No reports linking the use of amikacin to congenital defects have been reported.

Ototoxicity has not been reported as an effect of in utero exposure to amikacin; however, eighth cranial nerve toxicity in the fetus is well known following exposure to other aminoglycosides (kanamycin and streptomycin) and could potentially occur with amikacin. Only a trace amount of amikacin was found in some nursing infants. Given the poor absorption of aminoglycosides, systemic toxicity should not occur, but alteration in normal bowel flora may occur in nursing infants.

Renal Disease

Use with caution. Levels should be monitored for patients with impaired renal function. Interval adjustment (12–15 mg/kg—2 or 3 times per week) is recommended for creatinine clearance < 30 mL/min or hemodialysis.

Hepatic Disease

Drug levels not affected by hepatic disease (except a larger volume of distribution for alcoholic cirrhotic patients with ascites). Presumed to be safe in severe liver disease; however, some patients with severe liver disease may progress rapidly to hepatorenal syndrome.

Adverse Effects

Frequent

- Pain at injection site
- Proteinuria
- Serum electrolyte disturbances including hypokalemia and hypomagnesemia.

Occasional

- Cochlear ototoxicity (may be irreversible)
- Nephrotoxicity (often irreversible)
- Peripheral neuropathy
- Rash
- Vestibular toxicity (nausea, vomiting, vertigo, ataxia, nystagmus)
- Eosinophilia.

Ototoxicity potentiated by certain diuretics (especially loop diuretics), advanced age, and prolonged use. The effect of nondepolarizing muscle relaxants may be increased. Penicillins: in vitro antagonism.

Drug Interactions

Loop diuretics (bumetanide, furosemide, ethacrynic acid, torsemide).

Coadministration of aminoglycosides with loop diuretics may have an additive or synergistic auditory ototoxicity.

Ototoxicity appears to be dose-dependent and may be increased with renal dysfunction. Irreversible ototoxicity has been reported.

Avoid concomitant administration; if used together, careful dose adjustments in patients with renal failure and close monitoring for ototoxicity are required.

Nondepolarizing muscle relaxants (atracurium, pancuronium, tubocurarine, gallamine triethiodide): possible enhanced action of nondepolarizing muscle relaxants resulting in possible respiratory depression. Nephrotoxic agents (amphotericin B, foscarnet, cidofovir): additive nephrotoxicity.

Penicillins: In vitro inactivation (possible). Do not mix together before administration.

Contraindications

- Pregnancy (congenital deafness seen with streptomycin and kanamycin use in pregnancy).
- Hypersensitivity to aminoglycosides.
- Caution with renal, hepatic, vestibular, or auditory impairment.

Monitoring

Monthly creatinine and serum potassium in low-risk patients (young with no comorbidities), more frequently in high-risk patients (elderly, diabetic, or HIV-positive patients, or patients with renal insufficiency). If potassium is low, check magnesium and calcium. Baseline audiometry and monthly monitoring in high-risk patients. For problems with balance, consider increasing dosing interval.

Alerting Symptoms

- Problems with hearing, dizziness or balance
- Rash or swelling of the face
- Trouble breathing
- Decreased urination
- Swelling, pain or redness at IM site
- Muscle twitching or weakness.

Management of Adverse Effects

Hearing loss can be prevented by:

1. Changing injectable to capreomycin if patient has documented susceptibility to capreomycin
2. Discontinue suspected agents without compromising the regimen
3. Lower dose of suspected agents without compromising the regimen.

In renal failure, dose reduction is needed and follow up with serum creatinine and blood urea nitrogen is required every one to two months regularly. If renal profile is uncontrolled despite of decreased dosage, then discontinue suspected agent and consider using capreomycin.

CAPREOMYCIN

Drug Class

Cyclic polypeptide.

Activity Against Tuberculosis, Mechanism of Action and Metabolism

Bactericidal, polypeptides appear to inhibit translocation of the peptidyl-tRNA and the initiation of protein synthesis. No cross-resistance with the aminoglycosides. 50–60% excreted via glomerulofiltration. Small amount by biliary excretion.

It is obtained from *Streptomyces capreolus*.[5]

Preparation

Capreomycin sulfate is supplied as a sterile white powder for intramuscular injection in sealed vials each containing 1000 units, approximately equivalent to 1 g capreomycin base. This should be dissolved in 2 mL of 0.9% sodium chloride in water; 2–3 minutes should be allowed for complete solution.

Dose

15–20 mg/kg daily. The usual dose is 1 g in a single dose daily. When necessary, it is possible to give the drug at the same dose 2 or 3 times weekly during the continuation phase, under close monitoring for adverse effects.

Storage

Reconstituted capreomycin can be stored in the refrigerator for up to 24 hours before use.

Oral Absorption

There is no significant oral absorption. Intramuscular absorption may be delayed if the same site is used consistently.

CSF Penetration

Penetrates inflamed meninges only.

Special Circumstances

Pregnancy/Breastfeeding

Less ototoxicity reported in adults with capreomycin than with aminoglycosides. Category C animal studies show teratogenic effect ("wavy ribs" when given 3.5 times the human dose). Avoid in pregnancy. Concentrations in breast milk unknown.

Renal Disease

Use with caution. Levels should be monitored for patients with impaired renal function. Interval adjustment (12–15 mg/kg—2 or 3 times per week) is recommended for creatinine clearance < 30 mL/min or hemodialysis.

Adverse Effects

Frequent

Nephrotoxicity (20–25%), tubular dysfunction, azotemia, proteinuria, urticaria or maculopapular rash.

Occasional

Ototoxicity (vestibular > auditory); electrolyte abnormalities (decreased blood levels of calcium, magnesium, and potassium); pain, induration and sterile abscesses at injection sites.

Drug Interactions

Avoid coadministration of nondepolarizing muscle relaxants. If concurrent administration is needed, titrate the nondepolarizing muscle relaxant slowly and monitor neuromuscular function closely. Though not reported with capreomycin, neuromuscular blockade has been reported with other polypeptide antibiotics when administered with nondepolarizing muscle relaxants.

Avoid use with other nephro- or ototoxic agents because of the additive effect.

Contraindications

Patients with hypersensitivity to capreomycin and patients having myasthenia gravis. Great caution must be exercised in patients with renal insufficiency or pre-existing auditory impairment.

Monitoring

Monthly creatinine and serum potassium in low-risk patients (young with no comorbidities), more frequently in high-risk patients (elderly, diabetic, or HIV-positive patients, or patients with renal insufficiency). If potassium is low, check magnesium and calcium. Electrolyte disturbances are more common with capreomycin than other injectable agents. Baseline audiometry and monthly monitoring in high-risk patients. For problems with balance, consider increasing dosing interval.

Alerting Symptoms

- Rash
- Decreased urination
- Fever or chills
- Trouble breathing
- Bleeding or bruising
- Muscle weakness
- Problems with hearing, dizziness or balance
- Bleeding or lump at IM injection site.

Management of Adverse Effects

Hearing loss can be prevented by lowering the dose of drug, if this can be done without compromising the regimen and discontinuing the drug.

In renal failure, dose reduction is needed and follow up with serum creatinine and blood urea nitrogen is required every one to two months regularly. If renal profile is uncontrolled despite decreased dosage, then discontinue suspected agent.

ETHIONAMIDE AND PROTHIONAMIDE

Drug Class

Carbothionamides group, derivatives of isonicotinic acid.

Activity Against TB, Mechanism of Action and Metabolism

Bactericidal, ethionamide and prothionamide are bactericidal agents from the thioamide class.[6] The mechanism of action of thionamides has not been fully elucidated, but they appear to inhibit mycolic acid synthesis. Resistance develops rapidly if used alone and there is complete cross-resistance between ethionamide and prothionamide (partial cross-resistance with thioacetazone). Ethionamide is extensively metabolized, probably in the liver, to the active sulfoxide and other inactive metabolites and less than 1% of a dose appears in the urine as unchanged drug.

Most strains of *M. tuberculosis* are inhibited in vitro by concentration of 0.6 to 2.4 mcg/mL. A concentration of 10 mcg/mL or less will inhibit approximately 75% of photochromogenic mycobacteria, scotochromogen are more resistant.

Preparation and Dose

Ethionamide and prothionamide are normally administered in the form of tablets containing 125 mg or 250 mg of active drug. The maximum optimum daily dose is 15–20 mg/kg/day (max 1 g/day), usually 500–750 mg. Patients who are unable to tolerate a single dose, it may be divided into two doses.

Storage

Room temperature (15–25°C) in airtight containers.

Oral Absorption

Hundred percent absorbed but sometimes erratic absorption caused by gastrointestinal disturbances associated with the medication.

Distribution

Rapidly and widely distributed into body tissues and fluids, with concentrations in plasma and various organs being approximately equal. Significant concentrations also are present in CSF.

Special Circumstances

Pregnancy/Breastfeeding

Safety class C. Animal studies have shown ethionamide to be teratogenic. Hence, it should not be given in pregnancy. Newborns who are breastfed by mothers who are taking ethionamide should be monitored for adverse effects.

Renal Disease

Doses of the thionamides are only slightly modified for patients with severe renal impairment. When the creatinine clearance is less than 30 mL/min, the recommended dosing is 250–500 mg daily.

Hepatic Disease

Thionamides should not be used in severe hepatic impairment.

Porphyria

Ethionamide is considered to be unsafe in patients with porphyria because it has been shown to be porphyrinogenic in animals and in vitro systems.

Adverse Effects

Frequent

Severe gastrointestinal intolerance (nausea, vomiting, diarrhea, abdominal pain, excessive salivation, metallic taste, stomatitis, anorexia and weight loss). Adverse gastrointestinal effects appear to be dose-related, with approximately 50% of patients unable to tolerate 1 g as a single dose. Gastrointestinal effects may be minimized by decreasing dosage, by changing the time of drug administration, or by the concurrent administration of an antiemetic agent. Gastric tolerance is better with prothionamide as compared to ethionamide.

Occasional

- Allergic reactions
- Psychotic disturbances (including depression), drowsiness, dizziness, restlessness, headache, postural hypotension
- Neurotoxicity (administration of pyridoxine has been recommended to prevent or relieve neurotoxic effects)
- Increases in serum bilirubin; reversible hepatitis (2%) with jaundice (1–3%)
- Gynecomastia; menstrual irregularity
- Arthralgias
- Leukopenia
- Hypothyroidism especially when combined with PAS.

Rare

- Peripheral neuritis
- Optic neuritis, diplopia, blurred vision
- Pellagra-like syndrome, reactions including rash, photosensitivity
- Thrombocytopenia and purpura.

Drug Interactions

Cycloserine—potential increase incidence of neurotoxicity.

Ethionamide—has been found to temporarily raise serum concentrations of isoniazid. Thionamides may potentiate the adverse effects of other antituberculosis drugs administered concomitantly. In particular, convulsions have been reported when ethionamide is administered with cycloserine. Excessive ethanol ingestion should be avoided because of possible psychotic reaction.

PAS—possible increase in liver toxicity, monitor liver enzymes; hypothyroidism in case of combined administration.

Contraindications

Thionamides are contraindicated in patients with severe hepatic impairment and in patients who are hypersensitive to these drugs.

Monitoring

Ophthalmological examinations should be performed before and periodically during therapy. Periodic monitoring of blood glucose and thyroid function is desirable. Diabetic patients should be particularly alert for episodes of hypoglycemia. Liver function tests should be carried out before and during treatment with ethionamide.

Alerting Symptoms

- Any problems with eyes—eye pain, blurred vision, color blindness, or trouble seeing
- Numbness, tingling, or pain in hands and feet
- Unusual bruising or bleeding
- Personality changes such as depression, confusion or aggression
- Yellowing of skin
- Dark-colored urine
- Nausea and vomiting
- Dizziness.

Management of Adverse Effects

Gastrointestinal symptoms should be prevented by altering the timing of the drug administration and by prescribing antacids, antiemetics, withholding drugs for short periods, lowering dose of drug and discontinuing drug. An important factor that can influence tolerance of ethionamide is patient's determination not to give up treatment. Drug induced neurotoxicity can be prevented by pyridoxine 10 mg daily. Sometimes protionamide is better tolerated than ethionamide.

CYCLOSERINE

Drug Class

Analog of D-alanine.

Activity Against Tuberculosis, Mechanism of Action and Metabolism

Bacteriostatic, competitively blocks the enzyme that incorporates alanine into an alanyl-alanine dipeptide, an essential component of the mycobacterial cell wall. No cross-resistance with other antituberculosis drugs. 60–70% excreted unchanged in the urine via glomerular filtration; small amount excreted in feces; small amount metabolized. Cycloserine was valuable in preventing resistance to ethionamide in the re-treatment cases. Most strains are inhibited in vitro by concentrations of 20 mcg/mL. Terizidone is a combination of two molecules of cycloserine.[7]

Preparation and Dose

Cycloserine is supplied in the form of tablets of 250 mg. The dose for daily therapy being 15–20 mg/kg[8], i.e. 0.5 to 1.0 g daily and divided into two or three dose (Some producers of terizidone make 300 mg capsule preparations, while others make 250 mg).

Storage

Room temperature (15–25°C) in airtight containers.

Oral Absorption

Modestly decreased by food (best to take on an empty stomach); 70–90% absorbed.

Distribution

Widely distributed into body tissue and fluids such as lung, bile, ascitic fluid, pleural fluid, synovial fluid, lymph, sputum.

Very good CSF penetration (80–100% of serum concentration attained in the CSF, higher level with inflamed meninges).

Special Circumstances

Pregnancy/Breastfeeding

Safety class C. Cycloserine crosses the placental barrier. There are limited data on safety of drug in pregnancy. Breastfeeding with B_6 supplement to the infant.

Renal Disease

Doses of cycloserine should be reduced in patients with severe renal impairment. When the creatinine clearance is less than 30 mL/min, the recommended dosing is 250 mg/day, or 500 mg/dose 3 times per week. The appropriateness of 250 mg/day doses has not been established. There should be careful monitoring for evidence of neurotoxicity; if possible, measure serum concentrations and adjust regimen accordingly.

Adverse Effects

Frequent

- Neurological and psychiatric disturbances (headaches, irritability, sleep disturbances, aggression, and tremors)
- Gum inflammation

- Pale skin
- Depression, confusion, dizziness, restlessness, anxiety, nightmares, severe headache, drowsiness.

Occasional

Visual changes, skin rash, numbness, tingling or burning in hands and feet, jaundice, eye pain.

Rare

Seizures, suicidal thoughts.

Drug Interactions

Ethionamide

Additive nervous system side-effects.

Isoniazid

Additive nervous system side-effects.

Phenytoin

May increase phenytoin levels.
Toxic effect if combined with alcohol, increases risk of seizures.
Vitamin B_6 decreases CNS effect.

Contraindications

- Hypersensitivity to cycloserine
- Epilepsy
- Depression, severe anxiety or psychosis
- Severe renal insufficiency
- Excessive concurrent use of alcohol.

Monitoring

When available, serum drug monitoring to establish optimal dosing (not higher than 30 μg/mL).

Alerting Symptoms

- Seizures
- Shakiness or trouble talking
- Depression or thoughts of intentional self-harm
- Anxiety, confusion or loss of memory
- Personality changes, such as aggressive behavior
- Rash or hives
- Headache.

Management of Adverse Effects

- For headache rule out other causes of headache like meningitis, migraine and cluster headache. Treatment includes analgesics-acetaminophen, ibuprofen, aspirin and increasing pyridoxine to 300 mg/day
- Psychosocial support to relieve emotional components
- Amitryptiline 100–150 mg at night. In psychosis, patient needs consultation by a psychiatrist.
- In case of seizure, it is necessary to rule out other causes (previous history of seizure or epilepsy, meningitis, encephalitis, alcohol abuse, metabolic disorder like diabetes mellitus, hyper/hypocalcemia, cerebrovascular accident, malignancy with space occupying lesions). Pyridoxine may be given in a dose of 100–200 mg/day to prevent and treat neurotoxic side effects.

PARA-AMINOSALICYLIC ACID (PAS)

Drug Class

Salicylic acid; anti-folate. It was first used in 1944.[9]

Activity Against Tuberculosis, Mechanism of Action and Metabolism

Bacteriostatic, disrupts folic acid metabolism. Acetylated in the liver to N-acetyl-p-aminosalicylic acid and p-aminosalicylic acid, which are excreted via glomerular filtration and tubular secretion. Over 80% of drug is excreted in urine. Most strains of *M. tuberculosis* are sensitive to a concentration of 1 mcg/mL. PAS prevents the emergence of isoniazid resistance when used in combination.

Preparation and Dose

Tablets, sugar-coated, containing sodium salt: sodium p-aminosalicylate, 0.5 g of PAS.

Granules of PAS with an acid-resistant outer coating rapidly dissolved in neutral media, 4 g per packet.

150 mg/kg or 10–12 g daily in 2 divided doses.

Children: 200–300 mg/kg daily in 2–4 divided doses.

Storage

Packets should be kept in the refrigerator or freezer. Other formulations may not require refrigeration (consult manufacturer's recommendations).

Oral Absorption

Incomplete absorption (usually 60–65%): sometimes requires increased doses to achieve therapeutic levels.

Distribution

Distributed in peritoneal fluid, pleural fluid, synovial fluid. Not well distributed in CSF (10–15%) and bile.

Special Circumstances

Pregnancy/Breastfeeding

Safety class C. Congenital defects in babies have been reported with exposure to PAS in the first trimester. PAS is secreted into human breast milk (1/70th of maternal plasma concentration).

Renal Disease

No dose adjustment is recommended. However, PAS can exacerbate acidosis associated with renal insufficiency and if possible should be avoided in patients with severe renal impairment due to crystalluria. Sodium PAS should also be avoided in patients with severe renal impairment.

Adverse Effects

Frequent

- Gastrointestinal intolerance (anorexia and diarrhea)
- Hypothyroidism (increased risk with concomitant use of ethionamide).

Occasional

- Hepatitis (0.3–0.5%)
- Allergic reactions
- Thyroid enlargement
- Malabsorption syndrome
- Increased prothrombin time
- Fever.

Careful use in patients with glucose-6-phosphate dehydrogenase (G6PD) deficiency.

Drug Interactions

Digoxin: Possible decrease in digoxin absorption; monitor digoxin level—may need to be increased.

Ethionamide: Possible increase in liver toxicity, monitor liver enzymes; hypothyroidism in case of combined administration.

Isoniazid: Decreased acetylation of isoniazid resulting in increased isoniazid level. Dose may need to be decreased.

Contraindications

Allergy to aspirin; severe renal disease; hypersensitivity to the drug.

Monitoring

Monitor TSH, electrolytes, blood counts and liver function tests.

Alerting Symptoms

- Skin rash, severe itching, or hives
- Severe abdominal pain, nausea or vomiting
- Unusual tiredness or loss of appetite
- Black stools as a result of intestinal bleeding.

Management of Adverse Effects

Gastrointestinal symptoms should be prevented by altering the timing of drug administration and by prescribing antacids, antiemetics, withholding drug for short periods, lowering dose of drug and discontinuing drug. Hypothyroidism can be prevented by initiating thyroxine therapy.

LEVOFLOXACIN

Drug Class

Fluoroquinolone

Activity Against TB, Mechanism of Action and Metabolism

Bactericidal, the bactericidal action of fluroquinolone involves their interaction with DNA gyrase (Topoisomerase II), and its inhibition prevents replication and transcription process. Levofloxacin is generally considered to be about twice as active as its isomer, ofloxacin.[10–12]

Minimal hepatic metabolism; 87% of dose excreted unchanged in the urine within 48 hours via glomerular filtration and tubular secretion.

Preparation and Dose

Tablets (250, 500, 750 mg).

Aqueous solution or solution in 5% dextrose for IV administration vials (20, 30 mL) 500 or 750 mg and flexible containers (50, 100, 150 mL) 250; 500 or 750 mg.

Usual dose: 750 mg/day.

Storage

Tablets—room temperature (15–25°C), airtight containers protected from light.

Oral Absorption

Levofloxacin is rapidly and essentially completely absorbed after oral administration. Orally, should not be administered within 4 hours of other medications containing divalent cations (iron, magnesium, zinc, vitamins, didanosine, sucralfate).

No interaction with milk or calcium.

Distribution

Distributes well in blister fluid and lung tissues, also widely distributed (kidneys, gallbladder, gynecological tissues, liver, lung, prostatic tissue, phagocytic cells, urine, sputum and bile).

30–50% of serum concentration is attained in CSF with inflamed meninges.

Special Circumstances

Pregnancy/Breastfeeding

Safety class C. There are no adequate and well-controlled studies in pregnant women. Levofloxacin should be used during pregnancy only if the potential benefit justifies the potential risk to the fetus. Animal data demonstrated arthropathy in immature animals, with erosions in joint cartilage.

Because of the potential for serious adverse effects from levofloxacin in nursing infants, a decision should be made whether to discontinue nursing or to discontinue the drug, taking into account the importance of the drug to the mother.

Renal Disease

Doses of levofloxacin should be reduced in patients with severe renal impairment. When the creatinine clearance is less than 30 mL/min, the recommended dosing is 750–1000 mg 3 times per week.

Hepatic Disease

Given the limited extent of levofloxacin metabolism, the pharmacokinetics of levofloxacin are not expected to be affected by hepatic impairment.

Adverse Effects

Generally well tolerated.

Occasional

- Gastrointestinal intolerance
- CNS-headache, malaise, insomnia, restlessness, dizziness
- Allergic reactions
- Diarrhea
- Photosensitivity.

Rare

- QT prolongation
- Tendon rupture
- Peripheral neuropathy.

Drug Interactions

Should not be given to patients receiving Class Ia antiarrhythmic drugs (such as quinidine and procainamide) or Class III antiarrhythmics (such as amiodarone and sotalol).

Sucralfate: Decreased absorption of fluoroquinolones caused by the chelation by aluminum ions contained in the sucralfate.

Antacids (magnesium, aluminum, calcium, Al-Mg buffer found in didanosine): antacid binding to fluoroquinolone antibiotics resulting in decreased absorption and loss of therapeutic efficacy.

Probenecid: Probenecid interferes with renal tubular secretion of fluoroquinolones, which may result in 50% increase in serum level of levofloxacin.

Vitamins and minerals containing divalent and trivalent cations such as zinc and iron. Formation of fluoroquinolone-ion complex results in decreased absorption of fluoroquinolones.

Mexiletine: Fluoroquinolones may inhibit cytochrome P450 resulting in increased mexiletine concentration.

Contraindications

- Pregnancy
- Hypersensitivity to fluoroquinolones
- Prolonged QT.

Monitoring

No specific laboratory monitoring requirements.

Alerting Symptoms

- Pain, swelling or tearing of a tendon or muscle or joint pain
- Rashes, hives, bruising or blistering, trouble breathing
- Diarrhea
- Yellow skin or eyes
- Anxiety, confusion or dizziness.

Management of Adverse Effects

Gastrointestinal symptom should be prevented by altering timing of drug administration and by prescribing antacids, antiemetics, withholding drug for short periods, lowering dose of drug and discontinuing drug. In case of headache, it is important to rule out other causes of headache including meningitis, migraine and cluster headache. Treatment includes supportive treatment only.

MOXIFLOXACIN

Drug Class

Fluoroquinolone

Activity Against TB, Mechanism of Action and Metabolism

Bactericidal, the bactericidal action of fluoroquinolone involves their interaction with DNA gyrase (Topoisomerase II),[10-12] and its inhibition prevents replication and transcription process. The cytochrome P450 system is not involved in moxifloxacin metabolism, and is not affected by moxifloxacin. Approximately 45% of an oral or intravenous dose of moxifloxacin is excreted as unchanged drug (~20% in urine and ~25% in feces).

Preparation and Dose

Tablets 400 mg and intravenous solution 250 mL containg 400 mg in 0.8% saline.

Usual dose: 400 mg/day.

Storage

Tablets—room temperature (15-25°C), airtight containers protected from light.

Oral Absorption

Moxifloxacin, given as an oral tablet, is well absorbed from the gastrointestinal tract. The absolute bioavailability of moxifloxacin is approximately 90%. Co-administration with a high fat meal (e.g. 500 calories from fat) does not affect the absorption of moxifloxacin.

Distribution

Moxifloxacin has been detected in the saliva, nasal and bronchial secretions, mucosa of the sinuses, skin blister fluid, and subcutaneous tissue, and skeletal muscle following oral or intravenous administration of 400 mg.

Special Circumstances

Pregnancy/Breastfeeding

Safety class C. Since there are no adequate or well-controlled studies in pregnant women, moxifloxacin should be used during pregnancy only if the potential benefit justifies the potential risk to the fetus. Because of the potential for serious adverse effects in infants nursing from mothers taking moxifloxacin, a decision should be made whether to discontinue nursing or to discontinue the drug, taking into account the importance of the drug to the mother.

Renal Disease

No dosage adjustment is required in renally impaired patients, including those on either hemodialysis or continuous ambulatory peritoneal dialysis.

Hepatic Disease

No dosage adjustment is required in patients with mild or moderate hepatic insufficiency.

Adverse Effects

Generally well tolerated.

Occasional

- Gastrointestinal intolerance
- CNS—headache; malaise; insomnia; restlessness; dizziness
- Allergic reactions;
- Diarrhea;
- Photosensitivity.

Moxifloxacin has been found in isolated cases to prolong the QT interval.

Drug Interactions

Should not be given to patients receiving class Ia antiarrhythmic drugs (such as quinidine and procainamide) or Class III antiarrhythmics (such as amiodarone and sotalol).

Sucralfate: Decreased absorption of fluoroquinolones caused by the chelation by aluminium ions contained in the sucralfate.

Antacids (magnesium, aluminum, calcium, Al-Mg buffer found in didanosine): antacid binding to fluoroquinolone antibiotics resulting in decreased absorption and loss of therapeutic efficacy.

Vitamins and minerals containing divalent and trivalent cations such as zinc and iron: formation of fluoroquinolone-ion complex results in decreased absorption of fluoroquinolones.

Contraindications

- Pregnancy
- Hypersensitivity to fluoroquinolones
- Prolonged QT.

Monitoring

No specific laboratory monitoring requirements.

Alerting Symptoms

- Pain, swelling or tearing of a tendon or muscle or joint pain
- Rashes, hives, bruising or blistering, trouble breathing
- Diarrhea
- Yellow skin or eyes
- Anxiety, confusion or dizziness.

Management of Adverse Effects

Gastrointestinal symptom should be prevented by altering timing of drug administration and by prescribing antacids, antiemetics, withholding drug for short periods, lowering dose of drug and discontinuing drug. In case of headache, it is important to rule out other causes of headache including meningitis, migraine and cluster headache. Treatment includes supportive treatment only.

OFLOXACIN

Drug Class

Fluoroquinolones

Activity Against TB, Mechanism of Action and Metabolism

Bactericidal, the bactericidal action of fluoroquinolone involves their interaction with DNA gyrase (Topoisomerase II),[10-12] and its inhibition prevents replication and transcription process.

There is no cross-resistance with other antituberculosis agents, but complete cross-resistance between ofloxacin and ciprofloxacin.

There is limited metabolism to desmethyl and N-oxide metabolites; desmethylofloxacin has moderate antibacterial activity.

Ofloxacin is eliminated mainly by the kidneys. Excretion is by tubular secretion and glomerular filtration and 65–80% of a dose is excreted unchanged in the urine over 24–48 hours, resulting in high urinary concentrations.

Preparation and Dose

Tablets (200, 300 or 400 mg). Vials (10 mL) or flexible containers (50 and 100 mL) with aqueous or 5% dextrose IV solutions equivalent to 200 and 400 mg.

Usual dose: 400 mg twice daily.

Storage

Room temperature (15–25°C), airtight containers protected from light.

Oral absorption: 90–98% oral absorption.

Distribution

About 25% is bound to plasma proteins. Ofloxacin is widely distributed in body fluids, including the CSF, and tissue penetration is good. It crosses the placenta and is distributed into breast milk. It also appears in the bile.

Special Circumstances

Pregnancy/Breastfeeding

Usually compatible with breastfeeding.

Renal Disease

Doses of ofloxacin should be reduced in patients with severe renal impairment. When the creatinine clearance is less than 30 mL/min, the recommended dosing is 600–800 mg 3 times per week.

Adverse Effects

Generally well tolerated.

Occasional

- Gastrointestinal intolerance
- CNS-headache, malaise, insomnia, restlessness, and dizziness.

Rare

- Allergic reactions
- Diarrhea
- Photosensitivity
- Increased LFTs
- Tendon rupture
- Peripheral neuropathy.

Drug Interactions

Fluoroquinolones are known to inhibit hepatic drug metabolism and may interfere with the clearance of drugs such as theophylline and caffeine that are metabolized by the liver. Cations such as aluminum, magnesium or iron reduce the absorption of ofloxacin and related drugs when given concomitantly. Changes in the pharmacokinetics of fluoroquinolones have been reported when given with histamine H2 antagonists, possibly due to changes in gastric pH, but do not seem to be of much clinical significance. The urinary excretion of ofloxacin and some other fluoroquinolones is reduced by probenecid; plasma concentrations are not necessarily increased.

Contraindications

Pregnancy, intolerance of fluoroquinolones.

Monitoring

- No specific laboratory monitoring requirements.

Alerting Symptoms

- Pain, swelling or tearing of a tendon or muscle or joint pain
- Rashes, hives, bruising or blistering, trouble breathing
- Diarrhea
- Yellow skin or eyes
- Anxiety, confusion or dizziness.

Management of Adverse Effects

Gastrointestinal symptom should be prevented by altering timing of drug administration and by prescribing antacids, antiemetics, withholding drug for short periods, lowering dose of drug and discontinuing drug. In case of headache, it is important to rule out other causes of headache including meningitis, migraine and cluster headache. Treatment includes supportive treatment only.

CLOFAZIMINE

Drug Class

Phenazine derivative, Clofazimine is a phenazinine dye.[13]

Activity Against Tuberculosis, Mechanism of Action and Metabolism

Bacteriostatic against *M. leprae*, active in vitro against *M. tuberculosis*. Clinical effectiveness against *M. tuberculosis* is not well established. It is bacteriostatic drug and acts by binding with GC-rich *Mycobacterium* DNA and causing inhibition of transcription.[14]

Excreted in feces as unabsorbed drug and via biliary elimination. Little urinary excretion.

Preparation and Dose

Capsules (50 and 100 mg).

Storage

Store below 30°C, in airtight containers.

Oral Absorption

20–70% absorbed from gastrointestinal tract.

Distribution

Widely distributed principally to fatty tissue, reticuloendothelial system and macrophages. High concentrations found in mesenteric lymph nodes, adipose tissue, adrenals, liver, lungs, gallbladder, bile and spleen.

Special Circumstances

Pregnancy/Breastfeeding

Safety class C. Animal studies demonstrated teratogenicity (retardation of fetal skull ossification). Crosses placenta and is excreted in milk. Not recommended during breastfeeding.

Renal Disease

Usual dose.

Hepatic Disease

Dose adjustments should be considered in patients with severe hepatic insufficiency.

Adverse Effects

- Frequent
- Ichthyosis and dry skin
- Pink to brownish-black discoloration of skin, cornea, retina and urine
- Anorexia
- Abdominal pain.

Drug Interactions

May decrease absorption rate of rifampicin. Isoniazid increases clofazimine serum and urine concentrations and decreases skin concentrations.

Ingestion of clofazimine with orange juice resulted in a modest reduction in clofazimine bioavailability.

Contraindications

Pregnancy, severe hepatic insufficiency, hypersensitivity to clofazimine.

Monitoring

- No specific laboratory monitoring requirements.

Alerting Symptoms

- Nausea and vomiting
- Abdominal pain/distress (caused by crystal depositions and can present as an acute abdomen).

Management of Adverse Effects

Gastrointestinal symptom should be prevented by altering timing of drug administration and by prescribing antacids, antiemetics, withholding drug for short periods, lowering dose of drug and discontinuing drug. For skin discoloration, reassure the patients about reversal of effect after discontinuation of drug.

THIACETAZONE

Drug Class

It is a thiosemicarbazone.

Activity against Tuberculosis, Mechanism of Action and Metabolism

It is a **bacteriostatic** drug of low efficacy. It delays resistance to other antitubercular drugs like streptomycin, isoniazid and ethambutol. It is orally active and primarily excreted unchanged in urine.

Preparation and Dose

The daily dosage recommended is 2.5 mg/kg body weight daily; it is not effective when given intermittently.

Contraindications

In HIV positive patients, the risk of major potentially fatal cutaneous reaction caused by thioacetazone is very high. It should never be used in patients who may be HIV-positive or in areas where HIV infection is common.

Adverse Effects

Frequent

Cutaneous reactions, gastrointestinal intolerance (nausea, vomiting, abdominal discomfort) and anemia.

Occasional

Hepatitis, exfoliative dermatitis and Stevens-Johnson syndrome.

Rare

Bone marrow depression, ototoxicity, acute hepatic failure, cerebral edema, conjunctivitis, blurred vision.

Special Circumstances

Renal Disease

It should be avoided when renal impairment is present.

Pregnancy/Breastfeeding

Studies on the effects of thiacetazone in pregnancy and breastfeeding have not been done in humans or animals.

Monitoring

No specific laboratory monitoring requirements

Management of Adverse Effect

If rash or other sign of hypersensitivity develops, all the treatment should be stopped and thioacetazone should not be used again. If there is itching with mild rash then symptomatic treatment with antihistaminic may be tried. If there is severe rash or there is mucosal involvement with hypotension then oral prednisolone 40–60 mg/day should be given until there is response, dose should be reduced gradually according to patient's response. Thioacetazone should not be administered in areas where HIV prevalence is high.

CLARITHROMYCIN

Drug Class

It is a macrolide antibiotic.

Clarithromycin is a semi-synthetic derivative of erythromycin and is bacteriostatic in nature.[15]

It is usually active against nontubercular *Mycobacterium* particularly MAC.[12]

Mechanism of Action, Distribution, Excretion

It inhibits protein synthesis by binding reversibly to 50S ribosomal subunits.

Distribution

It is widely distributed and achieves high intracellular concentrations.

It is metabolized in liver and excreted via urine.

Adverse Effects

Frequent

Abdominal pain, nausea, vomiting and occasionally diarrhea.

Rare

- Hypersensitivity reaction
- Pseudomembranous colitis.

Drug Interactions

Several cases of QT prolongation, serious ventricular arrhythmias and death have been reported due to inhibition of CYP 3A4 resulting in high blood levels of concurrently administered terfinadine/astemizole/cisapride.

Special Circumstances

Renal and Hepatic Disease

Although the pharmacokinetics of clarithromycin are altered in patients with either hepatic or renal dysfunction, dose adjustment is not necessary until the creatinine clearance is < 30 mL/min.

Pregnancy/Breastfeeding

It is not recommended for routine use in patients with pregnancy. It should be used during pregnancy only when benefit outweighs risk. It should be used with caution in nursing mothers.

Monitoring

No specific laboratory monitoring requirements.

Management of Adverse Effects

Symptomatic management of the adverse effects. Concurrent administration of drugs, namely, terfinadine, astemizole and cisapride which are more prone to ventricular arrhythmias should be avoided.

LINEZOLID

Drug Class

Linezolid is a synthetic antimicrobial agent of oxazolidinone class.[16,17]

Mechanism of Action, Distribution, Excretion

It inhibits protein synthesis by binding to the P site of the 50S ribosomal subunit and preventing formation of the larger ribosomal-fMet-tRNA complex that initiates protein synthesis. It is 30% protein bound and distributed widely.

Approximately, 80% of the dose of linezolid appears in the urine.

Adverse Effects

Frequent

- Gastrointestinal upset
- Rash.

Rare

- Myelosuppression
- Peripheral neuropathy
- Optic neuropathy.

Preparation and Dose

Linezolid is supplied as 600 mg tablets. The dosage for daily therapy is 600 mg 12 hourly.

Special Circumstances

Renal Disease

No modification in dosage in patients with renal insufficiency.

Hepatic Disease

No modification in dosage required in patients with mild to moderate hepatic disease.

Pregnancy/Breastfeeding

It is not recommended for routine use in patients with pregnancy. It should be used during pregnancy only when benefit outweighs risk. It should be used with caution in nursing mothers.

Monitoring

No specific laboratory monitoring requirements

Management of Adverse Effects

Gastrointestinal symptom should be prevented by altering timing of drug administration and by prescribing antacids, antiemetics, withholding drug for short periods, lowering dose of drug and discontinuing drug. In case of headache, it is important to rule out other causes of headache including meningitis, migraine and cluster headache. Treatment includes supportive treatment only.

IMIPENEM/CILASTATIN

Drug Class

Imipenem belongs to the Carbapenem group of drugs. Carbapenems are beta-lactam antibiotics that have a broader spectrum of activity. Imipenem is derived from *Streptomyces cattleya*.

Mechanism of Action

Beta-lactam antibiotics interfere with the synthesis of bacterial cell wall. The beta-lactam antibiotics inhibit the transpeptidases so that cross linking of the adjacent peptide chains does not take place.

Imipenem is very resistant to hydrolysis by most beta lactamases. Activity of imipenem is excellent in vitro for a wide variety of aerobic and anaerobic microorganisms.

Pharmacokinetics

Imipenem is not absorbed orally. Imipenem is rapidly hydrolyzed by the enzyme dehydropeptidase I located on the brush border of renal tubular cells. Hence, imipenem is combined with cilastatin which is a reversible inhibitor of dehydropeptidase and thus imipenem is protected from hydrolysis.

Adverse Effects

Frequent

- Gastrointestinal upset
- Hypersensitivity reactions
- Palpitation and tachycardia.

Occasional

- Hypotension
- Thrombophlebitis
- Seizures
- Anemia.

Special Circumstances

Renal Disease

Dosage should be modified for patients with renal insufficiency.

Hepatic Disease

No modification in dosage required in patients with hepatic disease.

Pregnancy/Breastfeeding

It should be used with caution in patients with pregnancy and breast-feeding.

Monitoring

No specific laboratory monitoring requirements.

AMOXICILLIN CLAVULANATE

Drug Class

Amoxicillin is an extended spectrum semi-synthetic penicillin which is penicillinase susceptible. It is an aminopenicillin.

Mechanism of Action

Beta-lactam antibiotics interfere with the synthesis of bacterial cell wall. The beta-lactam antibiotics inhibit the transpeptidases so that cross linking of the adjacent peptide chains does not take place.

Pharmacokinetics

It is not degraded by gastric acid. Primary channel of excretion is kidney.

Adverse Effects

- Diarrhea
- Rash
- Hypersensitivity reaction.

Drug Class

Clavulanate is a beta lactamase inhibitor. It is obtained from *Streptomyces clavuligerus*.

It has a beta-lactam ring but no antibacterial activity of its own.

Pharmacokinetics

It is eliminated mainly by glomerular filtration. Its elimination and tissue distribution matches amoxicillin with which it is used.

Adverse Effects

Frequent

- Diarrhea
- Rash
- Hypersensitivity reaction.

Occasional

- Candida stomatitis and vaginitis.

Special Circumstances

Renal Disease

Dosage should be modified for patients with renal insufficiency.

Hepatic Disease

No modification in dosage required in patients with hepatic disease.

Pregnancy/Breastfeeding

It should be used with caution in patients with pregnancy and breastfeeding.

Monitoring

No specific laboratory monitoring requirements.

REFERENCES

1. Grosset J.18 National congres de la Tuberculose et des Maladaise Respiratoires, Clermont-Ferrand. Pris, Masson,1974.
2. Kucer A, Bennet NM, et al. The use of antibiotics: a comprehensive review with clinical emphasis. Philadelphia:Lippincott;1988;pp.585-1436.
3. United States Pharmacopeil Dispencing Information for health care professional. Vol.I. Englewood, CO; Micro-medex; 1999;pp.69-1419.
4. Meyer RD. Amikacin. Ann Intern Med 1981;95:328-32.
5. Sutton WB, Gordee RS, et al. In vitro and In vivo laboratory study on the antitubercular activity of capreomycin. Ann N Y Sci. 1966;135:947-59.
6. Davidson PJ, Le HQ. Drug treatment of tuberculosis-1992. Drugs.1992;43:651-73.
7. Chopra I, Brennam P. Molecular action of antimycobacterial agents. Tubercle Lung Dis. 1998;78:89-98.
8 Freidman TR, Sherman LF, Maw KL, Fujiwara, Craford JT. A multi-institutional outbreak of highly drug resistant tuberculosis: epidemiology and clinical outcome. JAMA. 1996;276:1229-35.
9. Lehman J. Paraaminosalicylic acid in treatment of tuberculosis. Lancet. 1946;1:15-6.
10. Pan X-S, Amber J, et al. Involvement of topoisomerase and DNA gyrase as ciprofloxacin targets. Antimicrob Agent Chemother. 1996;40:2321-6.
11. Tsukamura M, Nakamura E, et al. Therapeutic effect of new anti-bacterial substance ofloxacin. Am Rev Respir Dis. 1987;136:1339-42.
12. Hong Kong Chest Service/BMRC. A controlled of ofloxacin in the treatment of pulmonary tuberculosis resistant to streptomycin, rifampicin, isoniazid. Tubercle Lung Dis. 1998;78:89-98.
13. Jagannath C, Venkta Reddy M, et al. Chemotherapeutic activity of clofazimine and its analog against *M. tuberculosis* in vitro and in vivo. Am J Respir Crit Care Med. 1995;151:1083-6.
14. Hong Kong Chest Service/BMRC. Five year follow-up of a controlled trial of five 6 month regimen for chemotherapy for pulmonary tuberculosis. Am Rev Respir Dis. 1987;136:1339-42.
15. Casal M, Gutierrez J, Gonzalez J, et al. In vitro susceptibility of Mycobacterium tuberculosis to a new macrolide. Am J Respir Crit Care Med. 1995;151:1083-6.
16. Cynamon MH, Klemens SP. et al. Activity of several novel oxazolidinones against *mycobacterium tuberculosis* in a murine model. Antimicrob. Agents Chemother. 1999;43:1189-91.
17. Jones RN, Jhonson DM, et al. In vitro antimicrobial activity and spectra of U-100592 and U100766, the two novel fluorinated oxazolidine group. Antimicrob Agents Chemother. 1996;40:720-6.

Chapter 15

How Does Tuberculosis Treatment Work?

INTRODUCTION

Before the discovery of antitubercular drugs, tuberculosis treatment consisted of attempts to strengthen the patient's resistance to the disease. This included altering local and general host factors through traditional measures such as the avoidance of physical and mental strain, prolonged bed rest, a rich diet and collapse techniques. With the advent of chemotherapy, host factors are considered to be less relevant for cure, and the action of drugs on the tubercle bacillus has assumed overwhelming importance. In other words, treatment is strictly antimicrobial. The goal of tuberculosis treatment is to ensure relapse-free cure while preventing the emergence of drug resistance. The effect of treatment should therefore be judged not by the anatomical healing of lesions but by their sterilization, or at least by the elimination of bacilli from the sputum. *M. tuberculosis* is a slow-growing aerobic organism that can remain dormant for a prolonged period. Consequently, prolonged treatment with multiple drugs is required to ensure relapse-free cure and to prevent the emergence of resistance. The effect of treatment is determined mainly by bacteriological, environmental (anatomical and biochemical), and pharmacological factors. This chapter aims to describe how does tuberculosis treatment work.

BACTERIOLOGICAL FACTORS

The Numerical Factor

The number of tubercle bacilli varies widely with the type of lesion. The number of bacilli in medium-sized cavity communicating with the bronchi is about 10^8 (100 million), whereas in an encapsulated nodular lesion of the same size with no bronchial communication, the number can be as low as 100.[1] (The numbers are also rather low in extra pulmonary lesions of the skin, lymph glands, meninges, and bones). The larger the bacterial population, the higher is the probability that resistant mutant strains are present even before treatment is started. Thus in a population of one million tubercle bacilli, the number of resistant mutants resistant too .05 mcg/mL isoniazid ranges from 20,000 to 40,000; in a population of 100, the number of resistant organisms is proportionally smaller (only 0–4 at the same drug concentration). This quantative or numerical dependence is a factor of great practical importance.

The Metabolic Factor

Mycobacterium tuberculosis is an aerobic organism. In unfavorable conditions, it grows only intermittently or remains dormant for prolonged periods. Several subpopulations of bacilli, each with a distinctive metabolic state, could exist in an infected patient, e.g. rapidly growing with high bacillary load as in the wall of a cavitary lesion where oxygen tension is high and pH is neutral. These bacilli are highly susceptible to isoniazid and to a lesser extent to rifampicin, ethambutol, and streptomycin. Slow growing bacilli are located intracellularly in macrophages and at inflamed sites where pH is low. They are vulnerable to pyrazinamide, while isoniazid, rifampicin and ethambutol are less active. Spurters are present within caseous material where oxygen tension is low but pH is neutral and the bacilli grow intermittently with occasional spurts of active metabolism; rifampicin is most active on this subpopulation. Dormant bacilli remain totally inactive for prolonged periods. No antitubercular drug is active against them. Only rifampicin or pyrazinamide may attack them effectively under certain conditions. They survive even in the presence of such potent drugs as isoniazid and streptomycin and despite their susceptibility to these drugs. These organisms are also called "persisters". This phenomenon explains to some extent why not all bacilli are killed during treatment and why drug susceptible bacilli are coughed up for some time thereafter. Relapse with drug susceptible organism after the end-of-treatment or endogenous activation may be due to bacilli that have persisted for a long time in a dormant state in residual lesions.

ENVIRONMENTAL FACTORS

The Anatomical Factor

The type of tissue harboring the bacilli may affect drug action because not all drugs are able to penetrate into all tissues and cells or permeate biological membranes, including the normal blood-brain barrier. Isoniazid, rifampicin, and pyrazinamide readily cross biological membranes, whereas streptomycin fails to enter many cells and is much less effective against intracellular than extracellullar bacilli.[2,3] In humans, bacilli, particularly those in cavitary lesions, are mostly extracellular.[4]

Biochemical Factors

Environmental pH and partial oxygen pressure (PO_2) are important biochemical factors that influence the antimicrobial effect of a drug. At a neutral pH, as in cavity walls, all the bactericidal antitubercular drugs are highly effective; streptomycin, however, is most active in a slightly alkaline (extracellular) environment, whereas pyrazinamide acts largely in an acidic medium such as that found inside cells. Little is known about the factors causing dormancy in bacilli, but it is suggested that dormant organisms survive within cells or in necrotic areas of old encapsulated lesions that do not communicate with a bronchus. There, the pH is usually on the acidic side and the PO_2 is decreased. That the PO_2 is an important factor is shown by the small numbers of bacilli found in closed extrapulmonary lesions.

PHARMACOLOGICAL FACTORS

Dosage

Drugs must be given in doses large enough to produce an inhibitory concentration at the sites where bacilli are found, but it is not necessary to keep this concentration at a constant level. In fact, studies on the role of dosage and serum levels of isoniazid[4] showed that it was the peak level that was important for the response to the drug. Thus, 400 mg of isoniazid given once daily was therapeutically superior to the dose divided into two parts and administered at 12-hour intervals.[4]

Combinations of Drugs

Regimens should contain a combination of three or more drugs, particularly in the initial phase of treatment. In patients whose lesions contain large numbers of bacilli, the regimen should include at least two drugs to which the bacilli are susceptible, otherwise treatment failure due to the emergence of resistance is the likely consequence. In the early days of treatment, patients were given one drug; if that failed, further drugs were successively substituted or added, one at a time, with the result that these people eventually became chronic patients with organisms resistant to all the drugs they had received. Thus, treatment of tuberculosis disease should never be attempted with a single drug, nor should a single drug be added to a failing regimen.

The "lag period" Factor

In vitro experiments have shown that, when tubercle bacilli are exposed to a drug for a short time (6–24 hours) and after careful removal of the drug, are transferred to a drug-free medium, the surviving bacilli start to grow again after an interval of several days. This interval is called the "lag period" and varies with the type and concentration of the drug and with the length of exposure. All tuberculosis drugs have been tested for their ability to produce a lag period, in order to determine whether they are suitable for intermittent regimens. However, certain drugs are incapable of inducing this phenomenon, and the bacilli start to grow again immediately after removal of the drug. Such drugs seem to have only a bacteriostatic effect and are not suitable for intermittent use.

REFERENCES

1. Canetti G. The tubercle bacillus in pulmonary lesion of man; histobacteriology and its bearing on the therapy of pulmonary tuberculosis. New York, Springer, 1955.
2. Furesz S, et al. Rifampicin: a new rifamycin. 3. Absorption, distribution, and elimination in man. Arzneimittelforschung. 1967;17:534-7.
3. Mitchison Da. Bacteriological mechanisms in recent controlled chemotherapy studies. Bulletin of the International Union against Tuberculosis. 1970;43:322-31.
4. Tuberculosis chemotherapy Centre, Madras. A concurrent comparison of isoniazid plus PAS with three regimens of isoniazid alone in the domiciliary treatment of pulmonary tuberculosis in South India. Bulletin of the World Health Organization. 1960;23:535-85.

Chapter 16

Basic Concepts in Treatment of Tuberculosis

INTRODUCTION

Despite the discovery of the bacilli more than a hundred years ago and all the advances in our knowledge of the disease made since then, tuberculosis still remains one of the major health problems facing mankind, particularly in developing countries. In the prechemotherapy era, treatment of tuberculosis was necessarily directed towards strengthening the host's resistance.[1,2] With the advent of chemotherapy there has been a change in the understanding in the management of tuberculosis. Therefore, it is very important to know and follow certain basic concepts in the treatment of tuberculosis. This chapter deals with basic concepts in the treatment of tuberculosis.

ROLE OF SPECIAL DIET AND REST

Special diets and rest were believed to improve the patient's immune response. By imposing strict bed rest and using collapse techniques, clinicians attempted to restrict disease progression and promote healing. In controlled clinical trials, the effect of treatment was compared in two groups—one group treated with rich diet[3], good accommodation, nursing care and prolonged bed rest in a sanatorium, the other with poor diet, much less rest and often very long working hours in overcrowded homes. The results in the sanatorium patients with rich diet and rest were not superior to those in patients given domiciliary treatment and did not increase the likelihood of cure or reduce the likelihood of relapse. Thus, chemotherapy is the most important component of tuberculosis treatment and the diet which is sufficient for normal living is also sufficient for a tuberculous patient. Special diets and rest have no role in the treatment of tuberculosis. Main factors influencing the response of treatment is shown in Table 16.1.

Table 16.1: Factors influencing the response of treatment

Unimportant	Important	Relatively unimportant
• Rest, accommodation, diet	• Adequate chemotherapy	• Severity of disease
• Nursing, climate, sanatorium	• Regular drug intake	
• Psychological factors		

ROLE OF HOSPITALIZATION

In a study designed to assess the relative merits of home and sanatorium treatment found similar rates of cure and relapse[4,5] among both groups. Domiciliary treatment did not entail any special danger to the contacts that might have been prevented by sanatorium treatment.[6,7] Above all, the study also showed that treatment in a sanatorium was no safeguard against irregularity of drug intake. The sanatorium treatment also lead to disruption of the social life of the patient. This study brought about the dramatic shift from institutional to ambulatory treatment as a general policy. Thus, there is no role of hospitalization except when tuberculosis is associated with emergencies (Hemoptysis, pneumothorax, tubercular meningitis and cor pulmonale), with empyema and uncontrolled diabetes mellitus, difficult resistant and multi-drug and extensively drug resistant cases and in patients where there is a diagnostic dilemma.

SINGLE DRUG THERAPY VERSUS MULTIPLE DRUGS

There are ample experimental and clinical evidences that the initial administration of more than one drug, particularly a three or four drug regimen greatly improves the efficacy of treatment. Early work by Mitchison[8] and Canetti[9] and others showed that at least 2 drugs given concurrently were required for the treatment of active tuberculosis and field trials had shown that monotherapy led to high treatment failure and relapse rates. This led to the concept that multidrug treatment would be required to eradicate the tubercle bacilli in patients with active disease. Therefore single drug should not be used and multiple drugs are needed (2–4 drugs) to prevent resistant mutants. It has been observed that many clinicians add a single drug to a failing regimen which is equivalent to monotherapy and should be avoided.

SINGLE VERSUS DIVIDED DOSES

Many clinicians give antitubercular drugs in divided doses. Drugs should be administered in single dose and should not be given in divided doses. It has been shown that a high peak concentration in the serum is more important than a continuously minimum inhibitory concentration.[10] However, in certain circumstances where there is intolerance to a drug, it may be given in divided doses. Other drugs like PAS where large bulk of drug is required is usually given in two divided doses.

OPTIMUM DURATION OF TREATMENT

In general optimal duration of treatment for various short course regimes is 6–9 months and for standard conventional long-term regimes (without rifampicin) is 1–2 years. Sputum positive pulmonary tuberculosis: treatment of newly diagnosed smear-positive patients containing rifampicin throughout and pyrazinamide in the intensive phase (Initial 2–3 months) daily[11-21] or intermittent[11,15,16,25] should be for 6 months. Treatment should be for 8 months if rifampicin is not used in continuation phase (2RHEZ/6HT or HE).[1I,,22-24] If pyrazinamide is not used in initial intensive phase then the treatment duration is for 9 months.

Sputum smear-negative pulmonary tuberculosis: Various studies have shown that duration of regimens containing streptomycin, rifampicin, isoniazid and pyrazinamide given daily or intermittently[27-30] in smear-negative patients is at least for 4 months; however WHO recommends at least 6 months regimen for smear-negative pulmonary tuberculosis.

Standard conventional long-term non-rifampicin containing regimen: Before rifampicin and pyrazinamide become available, patients were treated for prolonged period. Standard conventional long-term regimen containing streptomycin for initial 8 weeks with isoniazid and thioacetazone (STH) practically achieve bacteriological quiescence within 6 months but about a quarter of patients relapsed in next five years.[31] There is evidence that more than 18 months of good standard conventional treatment produces no additional benefits in terms of treatment success or prevention of relapse.[32] The optimum duration of streptomycin in conventional long-term regimens is 8 weeks.[33]

FIXED DOSE COMBINATIONS (FDCs) VERSUS SEPARATE DRUGS

Drugs may be given either as fixed dose combinations or separately. WHO recommends the use of FDCs in the treatment of tuberculosis. Potential advantages of FDCs are:

Drug resistance may be less likely to emerge since multiple drugs are incorporated into the FDC.[34-36] The use of FDCs prevents treatment of tuberculosis with a single drug (monotherapy). Further, if treatment is interrupted (through default or because of inadequate drug supply), all drugs will be stopped, which should prevent resistant organisms being selected.

The use of FDCs involves fewer products and will result in more accurate prescribing practices by clinicians. This might be especially helpful for clinicians less familiar with national tuberculosis treatment guidelines. Moreover, because the amount of each drug in an FDC is invariable, there may be fewer dosage errors. Procurement, management, and distribution of drugs are simplified by the use of FDCs. Fewer tablets need to be ordered and managed, and distribution and storage at the local level may be easier. Thus, the use of FDCs may result in increased efficiency.

A treatment regimen using FDCs is simpler for the patient (fewer tablets result in increased adherence to treatment.[37,38] Rifampicin is often used to treat other infections and is sold without prescription in many countries. The use of rifampicin in FDCs may reduce inappropriate use of the drug for other infections, thus preserving its effectiveness for treating tuberculosis.

Nevertheless, the use of FDCs guarantees neither that a patient will ingest the correct number of tablets, nor that a patient will complete treatment. Effective management is still essential, including directly observed treatment.[39,40] Potential disadvantages of FDCs include:[39-41]

Bioavailability (the amount of an ingested drug absorbed into the blood) of rifampicin may decrease when it is combined with other drugs in the FDCs. Use of FDCs, particularly in three- and four-drug combinations, could therefore result in lower plasma levels of rifampicin, with consequent treatment relapses, and/or emergence of rifampicin-resistant strains of *M. tuberculosis*.[42] However, if FDCs are produced according to good manufacturing practices (GMP), they will be equivalent to administration of the constituent drugs as single-drug preparations.[43-45] Only FDCs for which bioavailability have been undertaken in human subjects should be used.[46] Demonstrating bioavailability should be a requirement for national registration.[47] However, there is often no systematic mechanism to ensure that all subsequent FDCs also have adequate bioavailability. The regulatory structure required to adequately monitor GMP and ensure bioavailability standards for FDCs (imported or domestically manufactured) is inadequate in most countries of the world.[48] In addition, few laboratories in the world have been officially certified to perform bioavailability testing.[49]

The optimal operational efficiency from using FDCs may not be achieved because the doses required for treatment are not the same for all patients. Adjustments for weight are often necessary: the WHO-recommended dosage forms for FDCs allows for easy adjustment of dosage by weight. Adverse effects may also necessitate changes in the dosage. Hence, any tuberculosis control program using FDCs must also supply single drugs to be used by tuberculosis specialists in particular circumstances.

There are a number of different formulations of FDCs, involving different combinations and different dosages; confusion and incorrect dosing may arise if a country uses more than one FDC formulation, The formulations recommended by WHO and International Union Against Tuberculosis and Lung Disease (IUATLD) should be the only ones used in a country. The National Tuberculosis Program should attempt to have the registration of other formulations withdrawn by the National Drug Regulatory Authority.

There is a theoretical risk that the availability of three- and four-drug FDCs over the counter, as may happen in many countries, would result in more widespread inappropriate use of tuberculosis drugs. In some areas, FDCs have been promoted as an alternative to effective tuberculosis control, potentially with adverse effects for the program. Taking fewer than the recommended number of FDC tablets may expose bacilli to subinhibitory concentration of multiple drugs. In a study that compared patients treated with self-administered FDC with patients given single-drug preparations under direct observation, relapse rates were higher in the group using self-administered FDC.[50]

When three- or four-drug FDCs are used in the intensive phase of treatment, a different two-drug FDC is used in the continuation phase. Patient and physician confusion and error may occur.

Small local manufacturers may not be able to produce FDCs, particularly four-drug FDCs, which may reduce competition and raise prices unless there is international procurement of drugs. A country that uses FDCs will need to provide additional training in drug procurement, treatment recommendations, and patient and provider education.

Although, there are potential advantages to using FDCs, the benefits may be difficult to demonstrate given existing operational, programmatic and regulatory constraints. FDCs are likely to become more widely used, particularly in countries that import antituberculosis drugs, which suggests that measuring their impact is imperative. Each country must carefully weigh the advantages, disadvantages, and appropriate role of FDCs within its program.

DAILY VERSUS INTERMITTENT THERAPY

Intermittent regimens are those in which the individual drugs are given at intervals of more than one day. In vitro experiments have demonstrated that, after a culture of *M. tuberculosis* is exposed to most of the antitubercular drugs, except for thiacetazone for some time it takes several days ("the lag period") before new growth occurs. This formed the basis for intermittent regimens which make treatment observation more convenient and feasible for health workers and patients and achieve a high levels of treatment success with low relapse rates.[51] Intermittent regimens facilitate observation, reduce costs and inconvenience for the patient because of fewer visits, and liberates staff for patient retrieval on alternate days. However, intermittent regimens should be given under direct supervision. Toxicity with intermittent regimens is similar to daily regimens except for rifampicin where adverse effects increased with once weekly or twice weekly regimens. WHO currently recommends that the optimal dosing frequency for new patients with pulmonary TB is daily throughout the course of therapy wherever feasible.[52] These patients may receive a daily intensive phase followed by a three times weekly continuation phase, provided that each dose is directly observed. Three times weekly dosing throughout therapy may be used as another alternative, provided that every dose is directly observed and the patient is not living with HIV or living in an HIV-prevalent setting. However, TB patients with known positive HIV status or living in HIV-prevalent settings should receive daily TB treatment at least during the intensive phase. The optimal dosing frequency is also daily for such patients even for the continuation phase.

MONITORING OF PROGRESS OF CHEMOTHERAPY

There are three approaches for monitoring progress of patients during course of chemotherapy—bacteriological, clinical and radiological assessment.

Bacteriological Assessment

Bacteriological assessment can be done by smear and culture. Although culture is more specific, it is time consuming and costly and there is delay in getting the results. Moreover appropriate facilities are not universally available. Hence, the management of patients is generally based on smear microscopy. Culture can be used to confirm or reject treatment failure and to determine the drug susceptibility pattern in failure cases. It is not necessary to examine the sputum every month. World Health Organization (WHO) and International Union Against Tuberculosis and Lung Disease (IUATLD) recommends that in new sputum smear-positive pulmonary tuberculosis patients, sputum smears should be performed at the end of the second month, during the fifth month and in the last months of 6 months and 8 months treatment regimens. In previously treated sputum positive pulmonary tuberculosis patients, sputum smear should be done at the end of the third month, during the continuation phase (second month after starting continuation) and at the end of treatment. In new sputum smear-negative pulmonary tuberculosis patients, sputum smear should be checked at the end of second month. Sputum smear-negative patients should be monitored clinically; body weight is a useful progress indicator. In extrapulmonary tuberculosis—response to treatment can be monitored only through clinical observation. As in smear negative pulmonary disease, weight of the patient is a useful indicator.

Radiological Assessment

Serial chest X-rays are still preferred by many doctors but assessment by radiographic changes alone can be very misleading. Radiological improvement is evidenced by halting of disease progression, acute lesions (exudative, pneumonia) should clear, cavity either disappears or becomes thin walled, chronic type of lesion heal by fibrosis and by shrinkage of atelectasis but one has to remember that the level of disagreement between readers when chest radiograph was used for follow-up was 27–30% between the readers and in 19–24% of cases individual readers were likely to disagree with their own earlier reading.[53,54]

Clinical Assessment

Clinical assessment is largely subjective. Disappearance of clinical symptoms, general well-being, ability to resume normal activities and weight gain are all pointers to clinical progress. Persistence or re-appearance of symptoms plus weight loss, i.e. objective clinical deterioration indicates the need for further investigations.

ESR and other hematological tests are unreliable and unnecessary in monitoring progress.

CAUSES OF FAILURE OF CHEMOTHERAPY

Standard treatment for 18 months has a potential cure rate of 96% and a relapse rate of less than 5%. Short course chemotherapy of 6–8 months duration including rifampicin at least in the intensive phase can achieve cure rates of 97–99% and a relapse rate of less than 5%. On the whole, the efficacy of current treatment regimens is high: a patient who adheres to treatment has a greater than 98% chance of cure, generally with only one course of treatment. In practice, however, this rate of success is rarely achieved. The main reasons for failure are—inadequate regimen prescribed, irregular drug intake by patient, premature discontinuation of treatment, drug toxicity, initial drug resistance, tuberculosis complicated by diabetes mellitus or empyema, bronchiectasis and wrong diagnosis.

Failure of chemotherapy is indicated most reliably by bacteriological parameters. A patient who is sputum positive even after five months or later of treatment or a sputum smear negative patient who becomes sputum smear positive at 2 months. Failure can also be indicated by the fall and rise phenomena. In this phenomena, sputum containing enormous number of bacilli was smear positive at the beginning. After the start of treatment, the bacillary content of the sputum decreased markedly, the sputum became negative by smear microscopy and positive only by culture—"the fall". After a certain time, the bacillary content increases again and the sputum became positive by smear again-"the rise". Thus, there occurs a fall of the susceptible bacilli and the rise of the resistant mutants of the strain.[55,56] Radiological deterioration is less reliable as radiological changes may be due to secondary infection or other co-existing illness like carcinoma and clinical deterioration is least reliable as symptoms like hemoptysis and cough may persist in spite of absence of disease activity.

Failure cases have a increased chance of having drug resistance and in some cases being a multi-drug resistance. There are many complex problems in the management of resistant/multi-drug resistant cases and such cases should be treated by good specialists in specialized center backed by standard laboratory facilities for drug susceptibility testing, as this opportunity of treatment is the last thing that stands between patient and death.

ROLE OF SURGERY IN PULMONARY TUBERCULOSIS

With modern chemotherapy indication for surgical intervention (thoracoplasty, resection) have narrowed considerably. Indications of surgery are a destroyed lung or lobe, failed chemotherapy, emergencies like recurrent massive hemoptysis and associated complications like empyema, pyopneumothorax and pneumothorax. With the emergence of MDR and XDR-TB, the role of surgery has surfaced due to an inability to ensure complete cure with the available chemotherapy. In MDR-TB patients with localized disease, surgery, as an adjunct to chemotherapy, can improve outcomes provided skilled thoracic surgeons and excellent postoperative care are available.

REFERENCES

1. Fox W. The John Barnwell lecture. Changing concepts in the chemotherapy of pulmonary tuberculosis. American Review of Respiratory Disease. 1968;97:767-90.
2. Tyrrell WF. Bed rest in the treatment of pulmonary tuberculosis. Lancet. 1956;1:821-3.
3. Ramakrishnan CV, et al. The role of diet in the treatment of pulmonary tuberculosis. An evaluation in a controlled chemotherapy study in home and sanatorium patients in south India. Bulletin of the World Health Organization. 1961;25:339-59.
4. A concurrent comparision of home & sanatorium treatment of pulmonary tuberculosis in south India. Bulletin of World health Organization.1959;21:51-145.
5. Dawson JJY, et al. A 5-year-study of patients with pulmonary tuberculosis in a concurrent comparison of home and sanatorium treatment for one year with isoniazid plus PAS. Bulletin of the World Health Organization. 1966;34:533-55.
6. Andrews RH, et al. Prevalence of TB among close family contacts of TB patients in south India, and influence of segregation of the patient on the early attack rate. Bulletin of the World Health Organization. 1960;23:463-510.
7. Kamat SR, et al. A controlled study of the influence of segregation of tuberculous patients for 1 year on the attack rate of TB in a 5 year period in close family controls in south India. Bulletin of the World Health Organization. 1966;34: 517-32.
8. Mitchison DA. Chemotherapy of tuberculosis: a bacteriologist view point. BMJ. 1965;1: 1331-8.
9. Canetti G. Host factors and chemotherapy of tuberculosis. In: Barry VC (Ed). Chemotherapy of tuberculosis. London, Butterworths. 1964;20-38.
10. Controlled trial of 6 months and 8 months regimens in the treatment of pulmonary tuberculosis. First report. American Review of Respiratory Disease. 1978;118:219-28.
11. Controlled clinical trials of four short course (6 months) regimen of chemotherapy for treatment of pulmonary tuberculosis. IIIrd report. East African - British Medical Research Council. Lancet. 1974;2:237-40.

12. Controlled clinical trial of four 6-month regimen of chemotherapy for pulmonary tuberculosis IInd report. IInd East African - British Medical Research Council Study. American Review of Respiratory Disease. 1976;114:471-5.
13. Controlled clinical trial of four short course regimens of chemotherapy for Pulmonary tuberculosis final report. Tubercle, 1983;64:153-6.
14. Controlled clinical trial of four short course regimens of chemotherapy for pulmonary tuberculosis final report. East and central Ailicanl British Medical Research Council 5th collaborative study. Tubercle. 1986;67:5-15.
15. Controlled clinical trial of four short course regimens of chemotherapy for pulmonary tuberculosis 1st Report. American review of Respiratory Disease. 1978;118: 219-28.
16. Controlled clinical trial of 6-8 months regimens of chemotherapy for pulmonary tuberculosis—the result of up to 24 months. Tubercle. 1979;60:201-10.
17. Controlled clinical trial of 6-4 months regimens of chemotherapy for pulmonary tuberculosis. American review of Respiratory Disease. 1979;119: 579-85
18. Long-term follow-up of a clinical trial of 6 months and 4 months regimens of chemotherapy in treatment of pulmonary tuberculosis. Singapore Tuberculosis ServicelBritish Medical Research Council American review of Respiratory Disease 1986;133: 779-83.
19. Controlled clinical trial of 6–8 months regimens of chemotherapy for pulmonary tuberculosis the result of up to 30 months. Tubercle 1981;62: 95-102.
20. Five year follow up a clinical trial of a three–six months regimens of chemotherapy given intermittently in the continuation phase in the treatment of pulmonary tuberculosis. Singapore Tuberculosis Service/British Medical Research Council. American Review of Respiratory Diseases. 1988;137:1147-50.
21. Clinical trial of a three six-months regimens of chemotherapy given intermittently in the continuation phase in the treatment of pulmonary tuberculosis. Singapore Tuberculosis Service/British Medical Research Council. American Review of Respiratory Diseases. 1988;137:1147-50.
22. A controlled clinical trial of oral short course regimens in the treatment of sputum positive pulmonary tuberculosis. Tuberculosis Research Center. International Journal of Tuberculosis and Lung Disease. 1997;1:509-17.
23. Controlled clinical trial of a four short course regimens of chemotherapy for two duration in the treatment of pulmonary tuberculosis. IIIrd report. IIIrd East Ailicanl British Medical Research Council. American review Respiratory Disease. 1978;118:39-48.
24. Controlled clinical trial of a four short course regimens of chemotherapy for two duration in the treatment of pulmonary tuberculosis. IInd report. IIIrd East Ailicanl British Medical Research Council. Tubercle. 1980;61:59-69.
25. Balasubramanian R. Fully intermittent six-months regimen for pulmonary tuberculosis in south India. Indian Journal of Tuberculosis. 1991;38:51-3.
26. Tuberculosis Research Center. Low rate of emergence of drug resistance in sputum positive patients treated with short course therapy. International Journal of Tuberculosis and Lung Disease. 2001;5:40-5.
27. Sputum smears negative pulmonary tuberculosis. Controlled trials of 3 months and 2 months regimens of chemotherapy. Lancet. 1979;1: 1361-4.
28. Controlled clinical trial of 2 months, 3 months and 12 months regimens of chemotherapy for sputum smear negative for pulmonary tuberculosis the result of up to 30 months. Hongkong Chest Service! Tuberculosis Research Center Madras! British Medical Research Council. American Review of Respiratory Diseases. 1981;124:138-42.
29. Controlled clinical trial of 2 months, 3 months and 12 months regimens of chemotherapy for sputum smear negative for pulmonary tuberculosis the result of up to 60 months. American Review of Respiratory Diseases. 1984;130:23-8.

30. Controlled clinical trial of 3 months, 4 months and 6 months regimens of chemotherapy for sputum smear negative for pulmonary tuberculosis the result at five year. Hongkong Chest Service/Tuberculosis Research Center Madras/British Medical Research Council. American Review of Respiratory Diseases. 1989;139:871-6.
31. Controlled clinical trial of 4 short course 6 months regimens of chemotherapy for treatment of pulmonary tuberculosis. IIIrd report East Ailican British Medica Research Council. Lancet. 1974;2:237-40.
32. American Review results at five year of a controlled comparison of a six months and a standard 18 months regimens of chemotherapy for pulmonary tuberculosis. American Review of Respiratory Diseases. 1977;116:3-8.
33. Isoniazid with thiacetazone in the treatment of pulmonary tuberculosis in East Ailican 5th investigation. A co-operative study in East Ailican Hospital, Clinic and laboratories with the collaboration of East Ailican and British Medical Research Council. Tubercle. 1970;51: 123-51.
34. Mitchison DA. How drug resistance emerges as a result of poor compliance during shortcourse chemotherapy for tuberculosis. III International Journal of Tuberculosis and Lung Disease. 1998;2:10-5.
35. Moulding T, Putt A, Reichman L. Fixed-dose combinations of tuberculosis medications to prevent drug resistance. Annals of Internal Medicine. 1995;122:951-4.
36. The promise and reality of fixed-dose combinations with rifampicin. A joint statement of the International Union against Tuberculosis and Lung Disease and the Tuberculosis Programme of the World Health Organization. Tubercle and Lung Disease. 1994;75:180-1.
37. Acceptability, compliance, and adverse reactions when isoniazid, rifampin, and pyrazinamide are given as a combined formulation or separately during three-times-weekly tuberculosis chemotherapy. Hong Kong Chest Service/British Medical Research. American Review of Respiratory Disease. 1989;140:1618-22.
38. Wolde K, et al. Fixed-dose combination short course chemotherapy in the treatment of pulmonary tuberculosis. Ethiopian Medical Journal. 1992;30:63-8.
39. Treatment of tuberculosis: guidelines for national programmes, 3rd edn. Geneva, World Health Organization, 2003 (WHO/CD5/TB/2002.313).
40. Fixed-dose combination tablets for the treatment of tuberculosis: report of an informal meeting held in Geneva, Tuesday 27 Apri/1999. Geneva, World Health Organization, 1999 (document WHO/CDC/CPC/TB/99.267).
41. Blomberg B, et al. The rationale for recommending fixed-dose combination tablets for treatment of tuberculosis. Bulletin of the World Health Organization. 2001;79:61-8.
42. Long MW, Snider DE, Farer LS. US Public Health Service cooperative trial rifampicin-isoniazid regimens in treatment of pulmonary tuberculosis. American Review of Respiratory Disease. 1979;119:879-94.
43. Acocella G, et al. Comparative bioavailability of isoniazid, rifampin, and pyrazinamide administered in free combination and in a fixed triple formulation designed for daily use in tuberculosis chemotherapy. I. Single-dose study. American Review of Respiratory Disease. 1988;138:882-5.
44. Acocella G, et al. Comparative bioavailability of isoniazid, rifampin, and pyrazinamide administered in free combination and in a fixed triple formulation designed for daily use in antituberculosis chemotherapy. 11. Two-month, daily administration study. American Review of Respiratory Disease. 1988;138:886-90.
45. Panchagnula R, et al. Evaluation of rifampicin bioequivalence in fixed-dose combination using the WHO/IUATLD recommended protocol. International Journal of Tuberculosis and Lung Disease. 2000;4:1169-72.
46. Assuring bioavailability of fixed-dose combinations of antituberculosis medications. A joint statement of the International Union Against Tuberculosis and Lung Disease. World Health Organization. International Journal of Tuberculosis and Lung Disease. 1999;3:S282-S3.

47. Fourie PB. Proposed minimum registration requirements for fixed-dose combination anti-tuberculosis drugs. International Journal of Tuberculosis and Lung Disease. 1999;3:S362-S7.
48. Trebucq A, Caudron JM, Pinel J. Requirements for antituberculosis drug tender –requests. International Journal of Tuberculosis and Lung Disease. 1999;3:S358-S61.
49. Ellard GA. The evaluation of rifampicin bioavailabilities of fixed-dose combinations of anti-tuberculosis drugs: procedures for ensuring laboratory proficiency. International Journal of Tuberculosis and Lung Disease. 1999;3:S322-S4.
50. Assessment of a daily combined preparation of isoniazid, rifampicin and pyrazinamide a controlled trial of three 6-month regimens for smear-positive pulmonary tuberculosis. Singapore Tnberculosis Service/British Medical Research Council. American Review of Respiratory Disease. 1991;143:707-12.
51. Chaisson RT, et al. Six month supervised intermittent tuberculosis therapy in Haitian patients with and without HIV infection. American Journal of Respiratory and Critical Care Medicine. 1996;154:1034-5.
52. World Health Organization. Treatment of TB Guidelines - 4th Edition. WHO/HTM/TB/2009.420
53. Fox W. The chemotherapy of Tuberculosis in Developing Countries. In: Head F, Rugbeg NL (eds). Recent Advances in Respiratory Tuberculosis. London, Churchill, 1968: 127-59.
54. Garland LH. Studies on the accuracy of diagnostic procedures. American Journal of Roentgenology and Radium Therapeutic Nuclear Medicine. 1959;82:25-38.
55. Crofton J, Mitchison Da. Streptomycin resistance in pulmonary tuberculosis. BMJ. 1948;2: 1009-15.
56. Mitchison DA. Sensitivity testing. In: Heaf F, Rusby NL (Eds). Recent Advances in Tuberculosis. London Churchill, 1968.

Chapter 17

Anti-tubercular Drug Doses and Regimens for Adults and Children

This chapter deals with drugs, dosage and regimens to treat tuberculosis for adults and children.

Antitubercular drugs with their doses used in new and previously treated patients of tuberculosis are tabulated in Tables 17.1 and 17.2.

Table 17.1: Dose of antitubercular drugs used in new patients of tuberculosis[1,2]

Drugs	Daily		Intermittent	
	Adult	Children*	3-weekly	2-weekly
H	5 (4–6)	10 (10–15)	10 (8–12)	15 (13–17)
R	10 (8–12)	15 (10–20)	10 (8–12)	10 (8–12)
Z	25 (20–30)	35 (30–40)	35 (30–40)	50 (40–60)
E	15 (15–20)	20 (15–25)	30 (25–35)	45 (40–50)
S	15 (12–18)	15 (12–18)	15 (12–18)	15 (12–18)

*Doses modified in 2008.

Abbreviations used: H-Isoniazid, R-Rifampicin, Z-Pyrazinamide, E-Ethambutol, S-Streptomycin

Table 17.2: Doses of antitubercular drugs used in previously treated tuberculosis patients[3]

Drugs	Average daily dosage	Daily dosage (mg)		Type of anti-mycobacterial activity
		Minimum	Maximum	
Group 1 **First line oral agents**				
Pyrazinamide (Z)	25 mg/kg	1200	1500	Bactericidal
Ethambutol (E)	15 mg/kg	800	1200	Bacteriostatic
Rifabutin (Rfb)	5–10 mg/kg	150	600	Bactericidal
Group 2 **Injectable agents**				Bactericidal against actively multiplying organisms
Kanamycin (Km)	15 mg/kg	750	1000	
Amikacin (Am)	15 mg/kg	750	1000	
Streptomycin (S)	15 mg/kg	750	1000	
Capreomycin (Cm)	15 mg/kg	750	1000	
Group 3 **Oral Bacteriostatic second line drugs**				Bacteriostatic
Ethionamide (Eto)	15–20 mg/kg	500–750	1000	
Prothionamide (Pto)	15–20 mg/kg	500–750	1000	
Para-aminosalicyclic acid (PAS)	200–300 mg/kg	10 g	12 g	
Cycloserine (Cs)	10–20 mg/kg	500–750	1000	
Terizidone (Trd)	10–20 mg/kg	500–750	1000	
Group 4 **Fluoroquinolone**				Weakly bactericidal
Moxifloxacin (Mfx)	7.5–10 mg/kg	400	400	
Ofloxacin (Ofx)	15–20 mg/kg	800	1000	
Levofloxacin (Lfx)	7.5–10 mg/kg	500	1000	
Group 5 **Agents with unclear role in treatment of drug resistant TB**				
Clofazimine (Cfz)	4–5 mg/kg	100	300	Bacteriostatic
Linezolid (Lzd)	-	600	1200	
Amoxicillin/clavulanate (Amx/Clv)	2 g/day	500/125 Twice a day	1000/250 Twice a day	Weakly bactericidal
Thioacetazone (Thz)	150 mg/day	-	-	
Imipenem/Cilastatin (Ipm/Cln)	500–1000 mg/ IV every 6 hourly	500	1000	
High dose Isoniazid (high-dose H)	16–20 mg/kg	600	900	
Clarithromycin (Clr)	10–15 mg/kg	500 Twice a day	500 Twice a day	Bactericidal (pH dependent)

WHO recommended treatment regimens for each diagnostic category for adults and children are tabulated in Tables 17.3 and 17.4. Various standard chemotherapy regimens for newly diagnosed patents of tuberculosis by international union against tuberculosis and lung disease are tabulated in Table 17.5. New WHO guideline (2009) for treatment of tuberculosis is tabulated in Table 17.6.

Table 17.3: Recommended treatment regimens for each diagnostic category[1]

TB diagnostic category	TB patients	TB treatment regimens	
		Initial phase (daily or 3 times weekly)[a]	Continuation phase (daily or 3 times weekly)[a]
I	New smear-positive patients; New smear-negative PTB with extensive parencymal involvement; Severe concomitant HIV disease Severe forms of EPTB (Tuberculous meningitis, miliary, pericarditis, peritonitis,B/L or extensive pleural effusion, spinal disease with neurological complications, intestinal, genitourinary)	2 HRZE[b]	4HR or 6 HE dailyc
II	Previously treated sputum smear-positive PTB: Relapse, treatment after interpretation treatment failure[d]	2HRZES/1HRZE	5 HRE
III*	New smear-negative PTB (Other than in category I); Less severe forms of EPTB (lymph node,U/L pleural effusion, bone excluding spine, peripheral joint, skin)	2HRZE[e]	4 HR or 6 HE daily[c]
IV	Chronic and MDR-TB cases[f] (still sputum positive after supervised retreatment)	(6–9) Km Z E Eto Cs Levo	18 E Eto Cs Levo

[a]Direct observation off drug intake is required during the initial phase of treatment in smear-positive cases and always in treatment that includes rifampicin.

[b]Streptomycin may be used instead of ethambutol. In meningeal TB, ethambutol should be replaced by streptomycin. In tubercular meningitis (TBM), spinal TB with neurological complications and other hematogenous tuberculosis continuation phase is prolonged for 3 more months.

[c]This regimen may be associated with a higher rate of treatment failure and relapse compared with the 6 months regimen with rifampicin in the continuation phase.

[d]Whenever possible, drug sensitivity testing is recommended before prescribing category II treatment in failure cases. It is recommended that patients with proven MDR-TB use category IV regimens.

[e]Ethambutol may be omitted during the initial phase of treatment for patients with noncavitary, smear-negative PTB who are known to be HIV negative, patients known to be infected with fully drug-susceptible bacilli, and young children with primary TB.

[f]Contacts of patients with culture proven MDR-TB should be considered for early culture and sensitivity testing

*Recently category III and category I has been merged together and all the new patients of tuberculosis will be treated with category I regimen.

Table 17.4: WHO treatment categories and regiments for children 2010, modified in 2011.[4,5]

TB cases and diagnostic category	Anti-TB drug regimens	
	Intensive phase	Continuation phase
New patient regimen New smear-positive PTB Smear-negative PTB with extensive parenchymal involvement Severe forms of EPTB other than TB meningitis	2HRZE	4HR
New patient regimen Smear-negative PTB without extensive parenchymal involvement Less severe forms of EPTB (e.g TB cervical adenitis)	2HRZ	4HR
New patient regimen TB meningitis	2HRZS[a]	4HR
Retreatment regimen Previously treated smear-positive PTB (relapse, treatment after interruption or treatment failure) *If low risk for MDR TB or risk unknown: continue with retreatment regimen* *If high risk for MDR TB: use MDR TB regimen below*	2HRZES/1HRZE	5HRE
MDR regimen MDR-TB	Individualized regimens	

E, ethambutol; H, isoniazid; R, rifampicin; S, streptomycin; Z, pyrazinamide.

[a:] Other regimens are recommended for treatment of TB meningitits that include replacing streptomycin with ethionamide and treating for 9–12 months.

Recently, guidelines have been changed. The main changes are that all TB types (except TBM and OA TB) in HIV endemic setting should receive a fourth drug in intensive phase 2RHZE/4RH: TBM and osteo-articular TB should receive 2 RHZE/10RH and that streptomycin is no longer recommended as first-line in children.

Table 17.5: Various standard chemotherapy for newly diagnosed patient[7,8]

Recommended standard 6-month regimen	
• 2EHRZ/4HR • 2HRZ/4HR	• 2SHRZ/4HR
Variants of standard 6-month regimen (supervised chemotherapy)	
• $2HRZ/4H_3R_3$ • $2E_3H_3Z_3/4H_3R_3$ • $2E_3H_3R_3Z_3/4H_3R_3$	• $2HRZ/4H_2R_2$ • $2S_3H_3R_3Z_3/4H_3R_3$
Alternative less potent regimens of longer duration	
1. With a potent initial 4-drug phase • 2SHRZ/6HT or 6HE	• $2SHRZ/6S_2H_2Z_2$
2. With a less potent or no initial phase • 2SHR/7HR • 9HR • 2SHE/10 • 12 HT or 12HE	• 2HER/7HR • 2SHT/10HT • 2SHP/10HP • $12S_2H_2$

S = Streptomycin; H = Isoniazid; R = Rifampicin; Z = Pyrazinamide; E = Ethambutol; T = Thiocetazone; P = PAS

Table 17.6: Treatment of TB (WHO 2009 guidelines)[6]

New patient regimen	Retreatment regimen with first line drugs	MDR regimen
1. Should receive a regimen containing 6 months of rifampicin: 2HRZE/4HR 2. Should receive a regimen containing 6 months of rifampicin along with ethambutol: 2HRZE/4HRE where high levels of isoniazid resistance in new TB patients is suspected (presence of resistance to low concentrations of isoniazid (> 1% of bacilli resistant to 0.2 μg/mL but susceptible to 1 μg/mL of isoniazid) 3. Should receive daily TB treatment at least during the intensive phase or for the continuation phase, the optimal dosing frequency is also daily for these TB patients with known positive HIV status and also living in HIV-prevalent settings (defined as countries, subnational administrative units, or selected facilities where the HIV prevalence among adult pregnant women is ≥1% or among TB patients is ≥ 5%)	1. TB patients returning after *defaulting* or *relapsing* from their first treatment course may receive the retreatment regimen containing first-line drugs 2HRZES/1HRZE/5HRE if country-specific data show low or medium levels of MDR in these patients or if such data are not available 2. Should receive daily TB treatment rather than intermittent treatment	1. Use at least 4 drugs certain to be effective 2. Do not use drugs for which there is the possibility of cross-resistance 3. Eliminate drugs that are not safe 4. Include drugs from Groups 1–5 in a hierarchical order based on potency. For further details see chapter on MDR-TB

REFERENCES

1. Treatment of tuberculosis: guidelines for national programmes, 3rd edn. Geneva, World Health Organization, 2003 (WHO/CDS/TB/2003.313).
2. World Health Organization. Report of the meeting on TB medicines for children-July 2008. World Health Organization, Geneva. 2008.
3. Guidelines for the programmatic management of drug-resistant tuberculosis: emergency update 2008. Geneva, World Health Organization, 2008 and 2011 (WHO/HTM/TB/ 2008.402).
4. World Health Organization/FCH/CAH. Guidance for national tuberculosis programmes on the management of tuberculosis in children.WHO/HTM/TB/2006.371.
5. World Health Organization. Guidance for National Tuberculosis and HIV Programmes on the management of tuberculosis in HIV-infected children: recommendations for a public health approach. Geneva: World Health Organization; 2010.
6. World Health Organization. Treatment of TB Guidelines - 4th edn. WHO/HTM/TB/2009.420
7. Jindani A, Nunn AJ, Enarson DA. Two 8-month regimens of chemotherapy for treatment of newly diagnosed pulmonary tuberculosis: international multicentre randomised trial. Lancet. 2004;364:1244-1251.
8. International Union Against Tuberculosis and Lung Disease. Management of tuberculosis: a guide for low income countries. 5th edn. Paris: IUATLD;2000.

Chapter 18

Duration of Treatment in Tuberculosis

INTRODUCTION

This chapter describes the duration of various antitubercular regimens. In general, optimal duration of treatment for various short course regimes is 6–9 months and for standard conventional long-term regimes (without rifampicin) is 1–2 years (Table 18.1).

SPUTUM POSITIVE PULMONARY TUBERCULOSIS

Treatment of newly diagnosed smear-positive patients containing rifampicin throughout and pyrazinamide in the intensive phase (Initial 2–3 months) daily[1-11] or intermittent[5, 6, 15, 16] should be for 6 months. Treatment should be for 8 months if rifampicin is not used in continuation phase (2RHEZ/6HT or HE).[1,2,12,13,14] If pyrazinamide is not used in initial intensive phase then the treatment duration is for 9 months.

SPUTUM SMEAR-NEGATIVE PULMONARY TUBERCULOSIS

Various studies have shown that duration of regimens containing streptomycin, rifampicin, and isoniazid pyrazinamide given daily or intermittently.[17-20] In smear negative patients is at least for 4 months, however, WHO recommended at least 6-month regimen for smear-negative pulmonary tuberculosis.

STANDARD CONVENTIONAL LONG-TERM NON-RIFAMPICIN CONTAINING REGIMEN

Before rifampicin and pyrazinamide become available, patients were treated for prolonged period. Standard conventional long-term regimen containing streptomycin for initial 8 weeks with isoniazid and thioacetazone (STH) practically achieve bacteriological quiescence within 6 months but about of quarter of patients relapsed in next five year.[21] While there is evidence that more than 18 months of good standard conventional treatment produces no additional benefits in terms of treatment success or prevention of relapse.[22] The optimum duration of streptomycin in conventional long-term regimens in 8 weeks.[23]

Table 18.1: Duration of treatment in different regimens

If Z is used during intensive phase—6 months
2RHEZ/4RH
2RHZ/4RH
2SHRZ/4RH
If continuation phase is without R—8 months
2 RHEZ/6 EH/TH
2 RHZ/6 EH/TH
2 SHRZ/6 EH/TH
If Z is not used in intensive phase—9 months
2 RHE/7RH
9 RHE
If R & Z is not used—1–2 years
2STH/10TH
2SHE/10HE
12TH
Such duration is enough for pulmonary tuberculosis as well as extrapulmonary tuberculosis

H-Isoniazid, R-Rifampicin, Z-Pyrazinamide, E-Ethambutol, S-Streptomycin, T-Thioacetazone

Note: In meningeal TB, ethambutol should be replaced by streptomycin. In tubercular meningitis (TBM), spinal TB with neurological complications and other hematogenous tuberculosis continuation phase is prolonged for 3 more months.

REFERENCES

1. Controlled clinical trials of four short course (6 months) regimen of chemotherapy for treatment of pulmonary tuberculosis. IIIrd report. East African – British Medical Research Council. Lancet. 1974; 2:237-40.
2. Controlled clinical trial of four 6-month-regimen of chemotherapy for pulmonary tuberculosis IInd report. IInd East African/British Medical Research Council Study. American review of Respiratory Disease. 1976;114:471-5.
3. Controlled clinical trial of four short course regimens of chemotherapy for pulmonary tuberculosis final report. Tubercle. 1983;64:153-6.
4. Controlled clinical trial of four short course regimens of chemotherapy for pulmonary tuberculosis final report. East and central African/British Medical research Council 5th collaborative study. Tubercle. 1986;67:5-15.
5. Controlled clinical trial of four short course regimens of chemotherapy for pulmonary tuberculosis Ist Report. American Review of Respiratory Disease. 1978;118:219-28.
6. Controlled clinical trial of 6–8-months-regimens of chemotherapy for pulmonary tuberculosis the result of up to 24 months. Tubercle. 1979;60:201-10.

7. Controlled clinical trial of 6 and 4-month-regimens of chemotherapy for pulmonary tuberculosis. American Review of Respiratory Disease. 1979;119:579-85.
8. Long-term follow-up of a clinical trial of 6 months and 4 months regimens of chemotherapy in treatment of pulmonary tuberculosis. Singapore Tuberculosis Service/British Medical Research Council. American Review of Respiratory Disease. 1986;133:779-83.
9. Controlled clinical trial of 6-8-month-regimens of chemotherapy for pulmonary tuberculosis the result of up to 30 months. Tubercle. 1981;62:95-102.
10. Five year follow-up a clinical trial of a three six-month-regimens of chemotherapy given intermittently in the continuation phase in the treatment of pulmonary tuberculosis. Singapore Tuberculosis Service/British Medical Research Council. American Review of Respiratory Diseases. 1988;137:1147-50.
11. Clinical trial of a three six months regimens of chemotherapy given intermittently in the continuation phase in the treatment of pulmonary tuberculosis. Singapore Tuberculosis Service/British Medical Research Council. American Review of Respiratory Diseases. 1988;137:1147-50.
12. A controlled clinical trial of oral short course regimens in the treatment of sputum positive pulmonary tuberculosis. Tuberculosis Research Center. International Journal of Tuberculosis and Lung Disease. 1997;1:509-17.
13. Controlled clinical trial of a four short course regimens of chemotherapy for two duration in the treatment of pulmonary tuberculosis. IIIrd report IIIrd East African/British Medical research Council. American review Respiratory disease. 1978;118:39-48.
14. Controlled clinical trial of a four short course regimens of chemotherapy for two duration in the treatment of pulmonary tuberculosis. IInd report IIIrd East African/British Medical research Council. Tubercle. 1980;61:59-69.
15. Balasubramanian R. Fully intermittent six-month-regimen for pulmonary tuberculosis in south India. Indian Journal of Tuberculosis. 1991;38:51-3.
16. Tuberculosis Research Center. Low rate of emergence of drug resistance in sputum positive patients treated with short course therapy. International Journal of Tuberculosis and Lung Disease. 2001;5:40-5.
17. Sputum smears negative pulmonary tuberculosis. Controlled trials of 3 months and 2 months regimens of chemotherapy. Lancet. 1979;1:1361-4.
18. Controlled clinical trial of 2 months, 3 months and 12 months regimens of chemotherapy for sputum smear-negative for pulmonary tuberculosis the result of up to 30 months. Hongkong Chest Service/Tuberculosis Research Center Madras/British Medical Research Council. American Review of Respiratory Diseases. 1981;124:138-42.
19. Controlled clinical trial of 2 months, 3 months and 12 months regimens of chemotherapy for sputum smear-negative for pulmonary tuberculosis the result of up to 60 months. American Review of Respiratory Diseases. 1984;130:23-8.
20. Controlled clinical trial of 3 months, 4 months and 6 months regimens of chemotherapy for sputum smear-negative for pulmonary tuberculosis the result at five year. Hongkong Chest Service/Tuberculosis Research Center Madras/British Medical Research Council. American Review of Respiratory Diseases. 1989;139:871-6.
21. Controlled clinical trial of 4 short course 6 months regimens of chemotherapy for treatment of pulmonary tuberculosis. IIIrd report East African British Medical Research Council. Lancet. 1974;2:237-40.
22. American Review results at five year of a controlled comparison of a six months and a standard 18 months regimens of chemotherapy for pulmonary tuberculosis. American Review of Respiratory Diseases. 1977;116:3-8.
23. Isoniazid with thiacetazone in the treatment of pulmonary tuberculosis in East African 5th investigation. A cooperative study in East African Hospital, Clinic and laboratories with the collaboration of East African and British Medical Research Council. Tubercle. 1970;51:123-51.

Chapter 19

Treatment of Tuberculosis in Special Conditions—Pregnancy, Liver and Renal Disease

INTRODUCTION

Treatment of tuberculosis poses a difficult clinical problem in special situations like pregnancy, renal insufficiency and liver diseases. There are various concerns regarding dosage, toxicity and way of administration. Present write-up highlights the issue and addresses the clinical queries and problems. Prior to discussing these problems, it is important to know about pharmacokinetic characteristics of individual antitubercular drugs.

PHARMACOKINETICS OF ANTITUBERCULAR DRUGS

Some antitubercular drugs are metabolized in liver; while others are excreted either unchanged or in metabolized form, by renal route. Their secretion in milk, and ability to cross placenta is important in situations of lactation and pregnancy, where there is concern of safety and morbidity of baby.

Isoniazid is rapidly absorbed from gut, metabolized in liver by acetylation and excreted in urine within 24 hours as inactive metabolites. Its half-life varies from one group of population to other, depending upon hepatic acetylation. Half-life is less than 1 hour in rapid acetylators, and more than 3 hours in slow acetylators. It is secreted in milk, but amount is not sufficient to provide antitubercular chemoprophylaxis to infant. It is safe in pregnancy, but risk of hepatitis may be increased in postpartum period.[1] Rifampicin is rapidly absorbed and widely distributed to tissues and bound to plasma protein. Its absorption is reduced if given with food (not of clinical significance), or if given with para-aminosalicylic acid (PAS). It is extensively recycled by enterohepatic circulation, and metabolites formed by deacetylation are excreted in feces. It is found safe in pregnancy, with some risk of postnatal hemorrhage. Ethambutol is rapidly absorbed from gut. It is predominantly excreted in urine as unchanged form or inactive hepatic metabolite (80%).[2] Only 20% is excreted in feces as unchanged drug.[3] Ethambutol is found to be safe in pregnancy, and liver disease. Pyrazinamide is also rapidly absorbed from gut, metabolized in liver to metabolites; pyrazinoic acid and 5-hydroxy-pyrazinoic acid, which are excreted largely by renal route.[4] Its safety in pregnancy is under controversy.[4] Streptomycin is largely concentrated in extracellular fluid. In pregnant lady, it may interfere with development of fetal ear.[5] Plasma half-life is prolonged in newborn, elderly patients and in patients with renal failure. It is excreted unchanged in urine. Pharmacokinetics of amikacin, kanamycin or capreomycin is similar to streptomycin, and found unsafe in pregnancy, where they may cause fetal nephrotoxicity or congenital deafness.[5] They are considered safe in liver disease.

Ethionamide and prothionamide are toxic to liver and teratogenic in pregnant animals. Thus their safety in liver disease and pregnancy is doubtful, and it should not be used in pregnant ladies. They are considered relatively safe in mild renal disease. Cycloserine is about one-third metabolized, and rest excreted in urine. It is not safe in patients with renal failure and alcoholism. In alcoholics, it may lead to seizures. It crosses the placenta in pregnancy, and its safety in this situation is not yet established. PAS is not safe in renal failure. About 80% of drug is excreted in urine, and it should be avoided in severe renal insufficiency, where it may aggravate the problem of metabolic acidosis.[6] Old preparation of tablets interacted with rifampicin absorption, but new preparation of granules has no interaction with it.[7] No studies for its safety, has been done in pregnant ladies, but it has been used safely in pregnancy in past. Thus, adequate data is not available to either recommend or prohibit its use in pregnancy. Fluoroquinolones are also not found safe in animal studies, as they are found to inhibit the growing cartilages of bones. Thus, it is not safe to administer them in pregnancy and childhood. About 80% of levofloxacin is cleared by kidney, and its dose adjustment is recommended in cases of renal insufficiency.[8] This group of drugs are generally safe in cases of liver disease, except ciprofloxacin, which is metabolized in liver. Clofazimine is absorbed from the gastrointestinal tract in amounts varying from 45–70%. It is distributed to most organs, tissues and breast milk, crosses the placenta but not the blood-brain barrier. It is largely excreted unchanged in the feces, both as unabsorbed drug and via biliary excretion. Linezolid is rapidly and extensively absorbed after oral doses with maximum plasma concentration achieved after 1–2 hours. This drug has renal route of excretion mainly. Clarithromycin is rapidly absorbed from intestinal tract and undergoes extensive first-pass metabolism. It has biliary route of excretion predominantly whereas half-life is prolonged in renal impairment.

TREATMENT OF TUBERCULOSIS IN PREGNANCY AND LACTATION

Isoniazid is considered safe in pregnancy, except for some chance of postpartum hepatitis.[1] American Thoracic Society (ATS) recommends supplementation of pyridoxine during pregnancy (25 mg/day).[4] Use of rifampicin and ethambutol is safe in pregnancy. Data regarding other rifamycins (rifabutin and rifapentine) is insufficient, and thus they should be cautiously used. Safety regarding pyrazinamide could not be assured, but WHO and IUATLD recommend its use in pregnancy,[3] because when used for 6 month regimen benefits may outweigh possible risk. Streptomycin may cause congenital deafness, as this drug interferes with development of ear.[5] Other injectables, like amikacin, kanamycin and capreomycin having pharmacokinetics similar to streptomycin, may also cause fetal nephrotoxicity and ototoxicity.[5] One study reported that 17% of babies born to ladies who received streptomycin during pregnancy, develop hearing loss,[9] and thus they are contraindicated. Ethionamide and prothionamide are contraindicated in pregnancy, as they are found teratogenic in animal studies. Cycloserine crosses placenta, and since its safety in pregnancy is not established, it should be avoided, and used only if no other suitable alternatives are available.[5] PAS has been used safely in pregnancy in past, but since no well designed study has been done to ascertain its safety in pregnancy, it should be used in absence of any other alternative. Fluoroquinolones being toxic and inhibitor of growing cartilage in animals, is to be avoided in pregnancy.[9] Animal studies demonstrated teratogenicity (retardation of fetal skull ossification) for clofazimine and crossing of placenta and excretion in milk. However, WHO has approved this drug safe in pregnancy. Similarly, clarithromycin is not safe in pregnancy as higher dose has been associated with embryotoxicity. There are no adequate and well-controlled studies regarding teratogenecity of linezolid in pregnant women. It should be used during pregnancy only if the potential benefit justifies the potential risk to the fetus.

Regarding treatment of tuberculosis in a pregnant lady it is said that, treatment of tuberculosis is far less hazardous than leaving the disease untreated, both with regard to baby and mother. Tuberculosis in pregnant lady may lead to underweight infant or congenital tuberculosis.[10] Risk of miscarriage is much higher in active tuberculosis than risk from the drug treatment, so standard treatment should be given. Treatment regimen for drug sensitive tuberculosis should include rifampicin, isoniazid and ethambutol. Streptomycin should not be used. Opinion regarding use of pyrazinamide is divided, but WHO[3] and IUATLD recommend its use. ATS[4] does not confidently advocate it. According to WHO, 6-month regimen based upon isoniazid, rifampicin and pyrazinamide should be used whenever possible, and ethambutol should be used if a fourth drug is needed during initial phase.[3] Contrary to this, ATS recommends that pyrazinamide should better be avoided in pregnancy, because of lack of sufficient data for its safety.[4] If pyrazinamide is not used, duration of treatment should be 9 months. Although isoniazid, rifampicin and ethambutol cross the placenta, are not found to be teratogenic.[9]

Women taking first-line antitubercular drugs should not be asked for termination of pregnancy, while those on reserve line drugs should be counseled for possible adverse effects. Breastfeeding should not be discouraged, as amount secreted in milk is insufficient to cause any toxic or therapeutic effect. Supplemental pyridoxine is recommended for both nursing mother and her infant, even if no isoniazid is being given to the infant. All antitubercular drugs could be used during lactation, except fluoroquinolones because of possible risk.[9] Baby of woman who has taken rifampicin during pregnancy should receive vitamin K at birth, to avoid the risk of postnatal hemorrhage,[3] as rifampicin may induce metabolism of vitamin K and hamper hepatic synthesis of vitamin K dependent coagulation factors.

Women taking oral hormonal contraceptives, should be counseled for possible contraceptive failure and occurrence of pregnancy, especially in rifampicin containing antitubercular treatment regimen, because of induction of metabolism of contraceptive drug by rifampicin.[11,12] Such ladies should be advised to use nonhormonal contraceptive during, and for one month after treatment with rifampicin containing regimen.[12,13]

TREATMENT OF TUBERCULOSIS IN RENAL INSUFFICIENCY

Treatment of tuberculosis in renal insufficiency poses a difficult clinical problem, because various antituberculosis medications are cleared by kidney. On one side it raises concern of drug induced toxicity, due to impaired excretion by diseased kidney, while on the other side, it raises concern of under treatment of tuberculosis. In later situation, adequate peak serum concentration is usually low, and not of therapeutic use.[4] Another issue of concern is the therapeutic level of antitubercular drugs in patients with end stage renal disease, undergoing hemodialysis, which clears some drugs easily than others.

British Thoracic Society, advocates[11] dose reduction for drugs which are excreted by renal route, while American Thoracic Society[4] prefers increasing the dosing interval instead of decreasing the dose. Administration of drugs which are excreted by kidney should be changed by increasing the dosing interval, if creatinine clearance falls below 30 mL/min (Table 19.1). There is paucity of data to guide the dosing recommendation if creatinine clearance is above 30 mL/min, when standard doses should be prescribed.[4] Rifampicin and isoniazid are eliminated by liver, and they could be given in usual dose.[14] Population with slow hepatic acetylation of isoniazid could be given supplemental pyridoxine to prevent peripheral neuropathy. Alteration in dose of ethambutol which is 80% excreted by kidney,[2] should be made if creatinine clearance falls below 70 mL/min,[4] to lowest possible dose, but if it falls below 30 mL/min, it should be given intermittently as three times a week in dose of 15 to 20 mg/kg body weight.[4] Pyrazinamide is metabolized in liver, but its metabolites, pyrazinoic acid and 5-hydroxy-pyrazinoic acid are excreted by kidney[15,16] and thus drug should be given three times a week, in dose of 25 to 35 mg/kg body weight, to avoid toxicity, if creatinine clearance falls below 30 mL/min[4] (Table 19.1). Apart from this, risk of developing hyperuricemia with pyrazinamide is increased in cases of renal insufficiency. Since streptomycin is predominantly excreted by renal route, and removed by hemodialysis to a significant extent (about 40%),[17] it should be administered three times a week in dose of 12 to 15 mg/kg body weight[4] (Table 19.1) in patients of renal insufficiency with creatinine clearance below 30 mL/min and those on hemodialysis. Since pharmacokinetics of other aminoglycosides is similar to streptomycin, they need similar modification of dose.[4] Renal clearance of fluoroquinolones varies from drug-to-drug. It is greater for levofloxacin than moxifloxacin.[18] Dose adjustment for fluoroquinolones is recommended if

Table 19.1: Dosing recommendation for adult patients with renal insufficiency or undergoing hemodialysis[4]

Drug	Change in frequency	Dose and frequency in patients with creatinine clearance < 30 mL/min or those on hemodialysis
Isoniazid	No change needed	300 mg daily or 900 mg thrice a week
Rifampicin	No change needed	600 mg daily or 600 mg thrice a week
Pyrazinamide	Yes	25–35 mg/kg per dose three times a week
Ethambutol	Yes	15–25 mg/kg per dose three times a week
Levofloxacin	Yes	750–1000 mg per dose three times a week
Cycloserine	Yes	250 mg daily or 500 mg three times a week
Ethionamide	No change needed	250–500 mg daily
PAS	No change needed	4 g/dose twice daily
Streptomycin	Yes	12–15 mg/kg/dose twice or three times a week
Capreomycin	Yes	12–15 mg/kg/dose twice or three times a week
Kanamycin	Yes	12–15 mg/kg/dose twice or three times a week
Amikacin	Yes	12–15 mg/kg/dose twice or three times a week
Clarithromycin	Yes	Usual dose 500 mg twice daily but can be reduced to 250 mg twice daily
Linezolid	No change needed	Usual dose is 600 mg twice daily but can be reduced to 600 mg once daily after 4–6 weeks
Clofazimine	Yes	Begin with 300 mg daily and decreased to 100 mg daily after 4–6 weeks
Amoxicillin and Clavulanic acid	Yes	Dose used is 625 mg twice daily, 1000 mg should not be used.

creatinine clearance is less than 30 mL/min (750 to 1000 mg three times a week).[4] Ethionamide need no or little alteration of administration as it is not excreted by kidney[19] but, if creatinine clearance is less than 30 mL/min dose of ethionamide should be reduced to 250 to 500 mg/day[4] (Table 19.1). Dose of cycloserine should be modified if creatinine clearance falls below 30 ml/min or patient is on hemodialysis. It should be changed to 500 mg thrice a week or 250 mg daily[4] (Table 19.1); Evidence for safety of 250 mg daily dose of cycloserine is not yet established with regard to neuropathy, and 500 mg three times a week, is preferred in this regard. Serum concentrations of drug should be monitored. PAS is not safe in renal disease and should only be given if no other alternative are available, as it may aggravate metabolic acidosis.[6] If it is to be given, it should be given at dose of 4 g/dose, twice daily. Thioacetazone being excreted in urine, it should not be given to patients with renal disease.[20] The pharmacokinetics of the parent drug, linezolid, are not altered in patients with any degree of renal insufficiency but metabolites of linezolid may accumulate in patients with renal insufficiency, with the amount of accumulation increasing with the severity of renal dysfunction. Therefore, no dose adjustment is recommended for patients with renal insufficiency. However, given the absence of information on the clinical significance of accumulation of the primary metabolites, use of linezolid in patients with renal insufficiency should be weighed against the potential risks of accumulation of these metabolites. Clofazimine is safe in patients having renal disease as excretion is mainly through biliary route. In patients with severe renal impairment dose of clarithromycin must be reduced. Imipenem is highly nephrotoxic but addition of cilastatin lessens its toxicity.

Hemodialysis removes the drug before its therapeutic effect, but if the drug is given sufficient time before hemodialysis, so that it gets time to be distributed throughout the body, far less drug is likely to be removed. Administration of drug after hemodialysis, will avoid premature removal of drug on one hand, and facilitate Directly Observed Treatment Short Course (DOTS) on the other hand.[4] Premature removal of second-line drugs, by hemodialysis, may further aggravate the problem of drug resistance by exposing the tubercle bacillus to subtherapeutic drug concentration. Rifampicin, isoniazid and ethambutol are removed to insignificant extent by hemodialysis, but pyrazinamide is removed to a significant extent.[15] Thus supplemental dosing is not needed with isoniazid, rifampicin and ethambutol, in patients of end stage renal disease, undergoing hemodialysis. Similar to streptomycin, about 40% of drugs like kanamycin, amikacin and capreomycin are removed from blood, if they are given just before hemodialysis.[17] Fluoroquinolone[21] and ethionamide[19] are not cleared by hemodialysis and thus their dose need not be altered in this situation. Usually, hemodialysis does not pose significant problem, if drugs are given after the procedure.

Ideally, it is important to monitor serum concentrations of drugs in persons with renal failure who are taking aminoglycosides, cycloserine or ethambutol to provide effective therapeutic drug concentration and also to minimize dose related toxicity. Patients with renal failure may have other comorbid conditions, like diabetes mellitus and gastroparesis, which may further complicate the pharmacokinetics of drugs.[22] Presently there is no data to guide administration of antitubercular drug use in patients undergoing peritoneal dialysis, and for this subset of patients, recommendations of hemodialysis are applicable. The safest regimen that is being advised in patients diagnosed as new cases of tuberculosis with renal insufficiency, is rifampicin, isoniazid and pyrazinamide for two months followed by rifampicin and isoniazid for next four months.[20]

TREATMENT OF TUBERCULOSIS IN LIVER DISEASES

Treatment of tuberculosis, with deranged liver functions presents with two major clinical scenarios. First is use of antitubercular drugs in persons with pre-existing liver disease, and second is antitubercular drug induced hepatotoxicity. Various antitubercular drugs are potentially hepatotoxic, and administration of these drugs may aggravate liver disease, in a patient with compromised liver function. Drugs like ethambutol, streptomycin, kanamycin, amikacin and capreomycin are safe in liver disease as they are neither significantly metabolized, nor toxic to liver.[4]

It is found that, period of latency between start of drug regimen and occurrence of drug induced hepatitis is usually four to nine days.[23] It must be known that, about 10 to 30% of patients receiving antitubercular therapy may normally have transient rise of bilirubin and liver enzymes (Serum glutaryl pyruvate transaminase-SGPT and serum glutaryl oxalate transaminase-SGOT), to about 1 to 3 times the normal, during first two months of therapy, which comes down on continuation of treatment. It is of interest to note that about 10% of patients, who develop mild transaminase elevation (i.e. 1–2% of all adults treated) may have severe hepatitis and liver failure until the drug is discontinued. This clinical condition has case fatality of approximately 10%. Drug induced hepatitis is considered, when serum level of SGPT or SGOT rises more than 150 IU/L on more than three occasions, or greater than 250 IU/L on one occasion, along with values of serum bilirubin more than 34.2 micromol/L (2 mg%).[23] Data indicate that incidence of isoniazid induced clinical hepatitis is lesser than was previously thought. Hepatitis occurs in 0.6% patients, if isoniazid is given alone,[24] but incidence is 1.6% if it is given with drugs, other than rifampicin. With rifampicin, incidence of hepatitis is 2.7%. Risk of drug induced hepatitis, increases with age, and it is 2% in persons aged 50 to 64 years. Rate of fatal hepatitis is 0.023%. If it is given to patient with pre-existing liver disease, it may accumulate in body and further increases risk of drug induced hepatitis.[4] Frequent monitoring of serum level of hepatic transaminases is indicated in this clinical setting.[3] Patients with alcoholic liver disease, are at increased risk of peripheral neuropathy, and should be given pyridoxine prophylactically at dose of 10 mg daily.[3] Rifampicin may cause normal transient hyperbilirubinemia in 0.6% patients. Incidence of hepatitis is 2.7% if it is given with isoniazid, and it is 1.1%, if given with drug other than isoniazid.[24] Clearance of rifampicin, may be impaired, causing serum levels to rise, if it is given to patient with pre-existing liver disease. Careful monitoring of liver functions is indicated in these patients.[3] The first-line drugs isoniazid, rifampicin and pyrazinamide are all associated with hepatotoxicity. Of the three, rifampicin is least likely to cause hepatocellular damage, although it is associated with cholestatic jaundice. Pyrazinamide is the most hepatotoxic of the three first-line drugs. Among the second-line drugs, ethionamide, prothionamide and PAS can also be hepatotoxic, although less so than any of the first-line drugs. Hepatitis occurs rarely with the fluoroquinolones.[25] Chemical structure of ethionamide is similar to isoniazid, and it can cause liver toxicity in about 2% patients, and should be cautiously used in pre-existing liver disease. Para-aminosalicylic acid (PAS) may cause clinical hepatitis in 0.3% cases. Since pharmacokinetics of PAS is not significantly altered in liver disease, it could be used in usual doses and usual regimen.[6] Cycloserine could be safely used in liver disease, except in case of alcohol related hepatitis, where it increases risk of seizures.[5] Thioacetazone is hepatotoxic, and it should be avoided. Fluoroquinolones except ciprofloxacin are safe for use in liver disease.[13] Advanced age, female sex, poor nutritional status, pre-existing liver disease, chronic alcoholism, hepatitis B carrier state and slow acetylator status, are considered risk factors for antitubercular drug induced hepatitis.[23,24,26,27] Several studies have observed relation between serum markers for viral hepatitis and antitubercular drug induced hepatitis. It has been observed, that viral hepatitis complicates treatment more frequently with regimen containing both rifampicin and isoniazid, than in regimen having only one of them or none of them.[23,27] It is often difficult to find the culprit drug, in a multidrug regimen, causing drug induced hepatitis. Regarding this practical problem, it is said that, rise in serum transaminase activity within 15 days of starting regimen, is usually attributed to rifampicin, but if it occurs after one month, it is usually attributed to pyrazinamide.[28] Whether toxicity is due to their additive effect, synergistic effect, hypersensitivity phenomenon or direct effect is still not known. Joint Tuberculosis Committee of British Thoracic Society[29] recommends that liver functions should be monitored weekly in first two weeks, and then at two weekly interval, in patients who have pre-existing liver disease. Recommendation for frequency of monitoring liver functions, in patients with no known risk factors is not clear. If a patient on antitubercular therapy, develops mild transient elevation of serum bilirubin or liver enzymes, treatment need not to be stopped as they usually come down on continuation of treatment. If patient develops hepatitis related symptoms with significant elevation of bilirubin and liver enzymes, treatment should be stopped and viral hepatitis should be ruled out by serology.[29] Drugs should be gradually reintroduced one by one starting from less hepatotoxic drug first, after liver functions come down to normal, with close monitoring for deterioration. In case of stable liver disease, all antitubercular drug could be used, but under close observation for liver functions. In patients with unstable or advanced liver disease, liver function tests should be done at the start of treatment, if possible. If the serum SGPT level is more than 3 times normal before the initiation of treatment, lesser hepatotoxic regimens should be considered. The alternate regimens are devised on the premise that more unstable or severe the liver disease is, fewer the hepatotoxic drugs employed. Possible regimens include those that employ two hepatotoxic drugs (rather than the three in the standard regimen): (a) where 9 months of isoniazid and rifampicin, plus ethambutol (until or unless isoniazid susceptibility is documented) is advocated; or (b) where 2 months of isoniazid, rifampicin, streptomycin and ethambutol is followed by 6–7 months of isoniazid and rifampicin; or (c) where 6–9 months of rifampicin, pyrazinamide and ethambutol is administered.[30] When the liver disease is too serious to permit use of more than one hepatotoxic drug, then a regimen comprising two months of isoniazid, ethambutol and streptomycin, followed by ten months of isoniazid and ethambutol is preferred.[30] In the extreme case of fulminant hepatic failure where antitubercular treatment is indispensable, a regimen devoid of any hepatotoxic drug is prescribed; which is 18–24 months of streptomycin, ethambutol and a fluoroquinolone.[30]

In conclusion, surveying the treatment of tuberculosis with deranged liver functions, one can come across various scenarios. They may reveal themselves as mild derangements in liver enzymes requiring merely a close watch on the liver function without modifying the regimen. At the other side of the spectrum, declining hepatic reserves prohibit the use of any potential hepatotoxic drug—thus considering a substantial revision of the antitubercular regimen. Expert consultation is hence desirable in treating patients with advanced liver disease.

REFERENCES

1. Franks AL, Binkin NJ, Sinder DE Jr, Rokaw WM, Becker S. Isoniazid hepatitis among pregnant and postpartum Hispanic patients. Public Health Rep. 1989;104:151-5.
2. Strauss I, Erhardt F. Ethambutol absorption, excretion and dosage in patients with renal tuberculosis. Chemotherapy. 1970;15:148-57.
3. Treatment of Tuberculosis. Guidelines for National Programmes. World Health Organization document. 2003;annex 2:15-6.

4. American Thoracic Society/Centers for Disease Control and Prevention/Infectious Diseases Society of America: Treatment of Tuberculosis. Am J Respir Crit Care Med. 2003;167:603-62.
5. United States Pharmacopeial Dispensing Information. Drug Information for the Health Care Professional. Vol. I. Englewood, CO: Micromedex; 1999. p. 69-1419.
6. Held H, Fried F. Elimination of para-aminosalicylic acid in patients with renal insufficiency. Chemotherapy. 1977;23:405-15.
7. Horne NW, ed. Modern Drug Treatment of Tuberculosis, 7th edn. London, Chest, Heart and Stroke Association. 1990;7:24-9.
8. Lipsky BA, Baker CA. Fluoroquinolone toxicity profiles: a review focusing on newer agents. Clin Infect Dis. 1999;28:352-64.
9. Briggs GG, Freeman RK, Yaffe SJ, eds. Drugs in Pregnancy and Lactation, 5th edn. Baltimore, MD: Williams & Wilkins; 1998;11:112-7.
10. Jana N, Vasishta K, Jindal SK, Khunnu B, Ghosh K. Perinatal outcome in pregnancies complicated by pulmonary tuberculosis. Int J Gynaecol Obstet. 1994;44:119-24.
11. Chemotherapy and management of tuberculosis in the United Kingdom: recommendations 1998. Thorax. 1998; 53: 536-648.
12. Skolnick JL, et al. Rifampicin, oral contraceptive, and pregnancy. JAMA. 1976;236:1382-6.
13. Frieden T, Espinal M. What is the therapeutic effect and what is the toxicity of antituberculosis drugs ? Toman's Tuberculosis. Case Detection, Treatment and Monitoring. 2nd edn. World Health Organization, Geneva. 2004;110-21.
14. Ellard GA. Chemotherapy of tuberculosis for patients with renal impairment. Nephron. 1993;64:169-81.
15. Malone RS, Fish DN, Spiegel DM, Childs JM, Peloquin CA. The effect of hemodialysis on isoniazid, rifampicin, pyrazinamide and ethambutol. Am J Respir Crit Care Med. 1999;159:1580-4.
16. Ellard GA. Absorption, metabolism and excretion of pyrazinamide in man. Tubercle. 1969;50:144-58.
17. Matzke GR, Halstenson CE, Keane WF. Hemodialysis elimination rates and clearance of gentamycin and tobramycin. Antimicrob Agents Chemother. 1984;25:128-130.
18. Fish DN, Chow AT. The clinical pharmacokinetics of levofloxacin. Clin Pharmacokinet. 1997;32:101-19.
19. Malone RS, Fish DN, Spiegel DM, Childs JM, Peloquin CA. The effect of hemodialysis on cycloserine, ethionamide, para-aminosalicylic acid and clofazimine. Chest. 1999;116: 984-90.
20. Harries A. How does treatment of tuberculosis differ in patients with pregnancy, liver disease, or renal disease? Toman's Tuberculosis. Case Detection, Treatment and Monitoring. 2nd edn. World Health Organization, Geneva. 2004;166-8.
21. Fish DN, Chow AT. Tha clinical pharmacokinetics of levofloxacin. Clin Pharmacokinet. 1997;32:101-19.
22. Peloquin CA. Using therapeutic drug monitoring to dose the antimycobacterial drugs. Clin Chest Med. 1997;18:79-87.
23. Pande JN, Singh SPN, Khilnani GC, Khilnani S, Tandon R. Risk factors for hepatoxicity from antituberculosis drugs: a case control study. Thorax. 1996;51:132-6.
24. Steele MA, Burk RF, DesPrez RM. Toxic hepatitis with isoniazid and rifampcin. Chest. 1991;99:465-71.
25. Guidelines for the programmatic management of drug resistant tuberculosis. Emergency update. 2008;9:82-3.
26. Prasad R, Verma SK, Chaudhary SR, Chandra M. Predisposing factors in Hepatitis induced by antitubercular regimen containing isoniazid, rifampicin and pyrazinamide: A case control study. Journal of Internal Medicine of India. 2006;9:73-8.

27. Kumar A, Misra PK, Mehrotra R, Govil YC, Rana GS. Hepatotoxicity of rifampicin and isoniazid. Is it all drug induced hepatitis ? Am Rev Respir Dis. 1991;143:1350-2.
28. Devoto FM, Gonzalez C, Iannantuono R, Serra HA, Gonzalez CD, Saenz C. Risk factors for hepatotoxicity induced by antitubercular drugs. Acta Physiol Pharma Ther Latin Am. 1997;47:197-202.
29. Ormerord LP, Skinner C, Wales J. (on behalf of the Joint Tuberculosis Committee of the British Thoracic Society). Hepatotoxicity of antituberculosis drugs (editorial). Thorax. 1996;51:111-3.
30. WHO Treatment of Tuberculosis Guidelines. 4th edn. 2009;8:97-8.

Chapter 20

Treatment of Tuberculosis in Special Conditions—Pregnancy, Liver and Renal Diseases—Case-Based Approach

TREATMENT OF TUBERCULOSIS IN PREGNANCY AND LACTATION

Case 1

A 24-year-old, lady having pregnancy of three months, presented with newly diagnosed sputum positive pulmonary tuberculosis. Her liver and renal function were within normal limits. Rifampicin, isoniazid and ethambutol are safe for use in pregnancy. Pyrazinamide is not confidently recommended, because of lack of evidence for safety. Since she was sputum positive, and rapid sputum conversion was needed, she could be given 4 drug regimen of rifampicin, isoniazid, ethambutol and pyrazinamide for 2 months followed by rifampicin and isoniazid for next 4 months, as per World Health Organization (WHO) and International Union Against Tuberculosis and Lung Disease (IUATLD) recommendation, along with prophylactic pyridoxine. The neonate should receive vitamin K injection, to avoid postnatal hemorrhage.

Case 2

A 24-year-old woman having pregnancy of four months, presented with tubercular cervical lymphadenopathy, proved by fine needle aspiration cytology (FNAC). She also underwent chest skiagram, for any pulmonary lesions, with due precautions for radiation exposure to her fetus. Her liver and renal functions were within normal limits. Since this lady was suffering from paucibacillary tubercular condition, pyrazinamide may be avoided. This lady may be kept on regimen of rifampicin, isoniazid and ethambutol for 9 months, along with prophylactic pyridoxine.

Case 3

A 26-year-old lady was suffering from sputum positive pulmonary tuberculosis. She was receiving four drug antitubercular regimen consisting of rifampicin, isoniazid, ethambutol and pyrazinamide, for last one month. While she was on this regimen, she conceived. Since this lady was already on effective antitubercular drug regimen, there was very little risk of disease to fetus. Drugs being used are considered safe in pregnancy, with some doubt about safety of pyrazinamide. Since she has already taken one month of intensive phase of therapy, she may continue to take same drugs for next one month, following which ethambutol and pyrazinamide may be stopped, and rest of drugs to be continued for next four months.

TREATMENT OF TUBERCULOSIS IN RENAL INSUFFICIENCY

Case 1

A 33-year-old male weighing 50 kg, presented with sputum positive new case of pulmonary tuberculosis. His liver functions were within normal limits. His renal functions were deranged with value of blood urea as 98 mg/dL and serum. creatinine as 4 mg/dL. His creatinine clearance was 18.6 mL/min as calculated by formula as:

Creatinine Clearance = {(140 – Age) × Weight in kg}/ 72 × Serum Creatinine [For females above calculated value is multiplied by 0.85]

He may safely be kept on rifampicin and isoniazid without any modification in dose, or interval of administration. Creatinine clearance level below 30 mL/min raises risk of accumulation of pyrazinoic acid and 5-hydroxyl pyrazinoic acid, which are metabolites of pyrazinamide. Thus, it should be given in dose of 1250 mg (25–35 mg/kg body weight) as three times a week. Streptomycin and ethambutol should preferably be avoided.

Case 2

A 50-year-old female weighing 45 kg, presented with sputum positive pulmonary tuberculosis. She has previously taken antitubercular drugs irregularly for 4 months. Her liver functions were within normal limits. Her renal function was deranged, with blood urea as 84 mg/dL and serum. creatinine as 2.25 mg/dL with creatinine clearance of 25 mL/min. This lady should be kept on 5 drug retreatment regimen. Rifampicin and isoniazid are safe in usual doses. Pyrazinamide dose should be altered to 1250 mg three times a week (25-35 mg/kg body weight). Ethambutol and streptomycin, which should preferably be avoided in cases of renal insufficiency, need to be given in this case, but their dose should be modified. Ethambutol could be given in dose of 800 mg three times a week (15 to 20 mg/kg body weight). Streptomycin dose should also be changed to 500 mg three times a week (12 to

15 mg/kg body weight). If this lady undergoes hemodialysis for management of renal insufficiency, drugs should be given after hemodialysis. Ideally serum concentration of drugs should be regularly monitored, to prevent toxicity, and to ensure therapeutic drug concentration.

Case 3

A 50-year-old man weighing 50 kg, presented with sputum positive pulmonary tuberculosis. He has previously taken irregular treatment, for last three years. His sputum culture on BACTEC was positive for *M. tuberculosis*, and bacilli were found resistant to rifampicin and isoniazid. His liver functions were within normal limits. His renal functions were deranged with value of blood urea as 74 mg/dL and S. creatinine as 1.05 mg/dL. His creatinine clearance was 60 mL/min. He could have been kept on reserve line drugs. Since renal functions are not very much compromised, he may be given ethionamide, cycloserine and fluoroquinolone. Injectable drugs (e.g. kanamycin) may be given in dose of 500 mg thrice a week (12 to 15 mg/kg body weight). PAS could be used at dose of 4 g twice a day with hemodialysis. Duration of treatment should be 18 to 24 months. Whatever drugs are given, patient should be regularly monitored for serum drug concentration, and renal function, so as to plan and change the medication as and when needed. If this man undergoes hemodialysis, the drugs should be given after it.

Case 4

A 36-year-old man weighing 58 kg, presented with sputum positive pulmonary tuberculosis. He has previously taken irregular antitubercular treatment. His sputum culture by BACTEC method was positive for *M. tuberculosis*, resistant to rifampicin and isoniazid. His liver functions were within normal limits, but his renal function was impaired with blood urea as 88 mg/dL and serum creatinine as 3.8 mg/dL. His creatinine clearance was 22 mL/min. He should be kept on reserve second-line drugs. Severity of renal insufficiency has left us with very little options, which too are risky. Cycloserine should only be used if this patient undergoes hemodialysis, in dose of 500 mg three times a week. Dose of ethionamide should be changed to 250 mg daily (250 to 500 mg/day). Fluoroquinolone dose should also be changed to 750 mg three times a week. Dose of injectable drugs should also be changed to 500 mg three times a week (12 to 15 mg/kg body weight). PAS is to be avoided. Thioacetazone should not be used.

TREATMENT OF TUBERCULOSIS IN LIVER DISEASE

Case 1

A 42-year-old man presented with fever, anorexia, cough and expectoration for one month. He was diagnosed as a new case of sputum positive pulmonary tuberculosis, and was kept on four drug regimen of rifampicin, isoniazid, ethambutol and pyrazinamide. After 3 weeks he started having vomiting, abdominal pain and yellowish discoloration of eyes and urine. His serum bilirubin was 4.4 mg% and SGPT was 272 IU/L. All of his antitubercular drugs should be stopped, and he should be investigated for viral hepatitis. He should be kept on interim regimen considered safe in liver disease, which should include streptomycin, ethambutol and fluoroquinolone (other than ciprofloxacin). Isoniazid is usually tolerated and can be added in author's opinion. Liver function should be closely monitored. Hepatotoxic drugs like rifampicin and pyrazinamide may be tried one by one after liver function comes down to normal, during frequent monitoring. Many of such patients subsequently tolerate them.

Case 2

A 34-year-old woman, with viral hepatitis having HBsAg positive, presented with sputum positive new case of pulmonary tuberculosis. Her renal functions were within normal limits. Her serum bilirubin was 7.2 mg% and SGPT was 370 IU/L. Since this lady is suffering from chronic active liver disease, all hepatotoxic drugs should be avoided. She may be kept on regimen of streptomycin, ethambutol, and fluoroquinolone along with an oral second-line drug, preferably cycloserine for 18 to 24 months. In case her liver function improves on repeat test, in author's experience isoniazid can also be added.

Case 3

A 38-year-old man, alcoholic, and a known case of cirrhosis of liver, weighing 48 kg, presented as a case of sputum positive pulmonary tuberculosis. He has taken irregular antitubercular treatment for 3 years, but without response. Current liver function profile showed serum bilirubin as 2.2 mg/dL, SGPT as 312 IU/L and SGOT as 280 IU/L. His sputum culture on BACTEC was positive for *M. tuberculosis*, resistant to isoniazid and rifampicin. He should be given reserve antitubercular drugs. Kanamycin, PAS and fluoroquinolones except ciprofloxacin are safe. Ethionamide could be cautiously used, because of risk of drug induced hepatotoxicity. Isoniazid may be given in author's opinion, along with supplemental pyridoxine. Cycloserine should not be used, because it can lead to seizures, especially in this case of alcohol related hepatitis. Thioacetazone being hepatotoxic should be avoided. Thus regimen consists of kanamycin, isoniazid, PAS, ethionamide and ofloxacin (K H PAS Ethio Oflo). Duration of treatment should be 18 to 24 months. Liver function profile should be monitored frequently. Frequency should be weekly for 2 weeks, and then at 2 weekly interval.

Chapter 21

Treatment of Extrapulmonary Tuberculosis

INTRODUCTION

Extrapulmonary tuberculosis (EPTB) has existed as a disease entity for centuries along with the pulmonary tuberculosis though the former has rare occurence. It is a milder form of disease in terms of infectivity as compared to pulmonary tuberculosis. EPTB includes TB of organs other than the lungs. Patients who have both pulmonary and extrapulmonary TB are classified as having pulmonary tuberculosis. The various forms of EPTB are superficial lymphadenitis, pleural disease, bone and joint disease including spine, central nervous system disease, genitourinary disease, gastrointestinal disease, cutaneous disease, cold abscesses of the soft tissues and pericardial disease. Of these, lymphatic (35%), pleural (20%), and bone or joint disease (10%) are the most common in HIV negative as well as HIV positive patients. HIV positive patients are more likely to have disseminated TB than HIV negatives. Extrapulmonary tuberculosis is usually paucibacillary and any treatment regimen that is effective in pulmonary TB is likely to be effective as well in this form of TB. For the purpose of treatment, extrapulmonary tuberculosis can be classified into severe and nonsevere forms as per RNTCP guidelines. Severe forms include meningeal tuberculosis, disseminated TB, spinal tuberculosis with neurological complications, neurotuberculosis, abdominal tuberculosis, bilateral plural effusion/pleurisy, co-infection with HIV, pericardial effusion, genitourinary disease and bone and joint tuberculosis involving more than one site. Nonsevere extrapulmonary tuberculosis includes lymph node tuberculosis, unilateral pleural effusion, bone (excluding spine), peripheral joint and cutaneous tuberculosis. Worldwide, extrapulmonary tuberculosis (EPTB) accounts for approximately 15–20% of tuberculosis (TB) presentations in HIV negative patients[1,2] and more than

50% in HIV infected patients.[2-4] Unlike the much-researched treatment for pulmonary tuberculosis (PTB), treatment of most forms of EPTB is based on only a limited number of controlled clinical trials. Further, the treatment of extrapulmonary tuberculosis differs from that of pulmonary tuberculosis in several ways.[5] This is largely because of difficulty of diagnosis which often lead to empirical treatment without pathological or bacteriological confirmation. However, diagnosis made only on clinical grounds can lead to over diagnosis and unnecessary treatment of large number of patients. Determining a favorable response to anti-TB treatment is more difficult in EPTB than with PTB. For these reasons, clinicians often employ more than adequate anti-TB drug regimens for more than recommended duration rather than following the established guidelines for the treatment of EPTB. This chapter aims to review the various trials and current recommendations for treatment of common extrapulmonary tuberculosis patients.

TUBERCULOUS LYMPHADENITIS

This is the most common form of EPTB in both HIV infected and non-infected patients.[2,3] HIV infected patients usually have evidence of pulmonary disease but only 25–30% of HIV negative patients have evidence of pulmonary involvement.[6,7] Most patients with tuberculous lymphadenitis infected with drug sensitive tubercle bacilli can be effectively managed with the use of modern antimycobacterial drugs like isoniazid (H), rifampicin (R), pyrazinamide (Z), ethambutol (E) and streptomycin (S) employed in various combination chemotherapy regimens. However, the number of drugs required and the ideal duration of treatment for lymph node TB have been an area of intense research. Initially, chemotherapy with two drugs was recommended for up to 18 months.[8] The British Thoracic Society's (BTS) first controlled trial[9] for lymph node TB compared two 18 months regimens: 2SHR/16RH versus 2SHE/16HE. Both the regimens were found to be equally effective. The preliminary results of the second study by the BTS[10] compared an 18 months regimen with 9 months regimen: 2RHE/16RH versus 2RHE/7RH, and found no difference in the response rates. This study clearly established that nine months treatment was as effective as one administered for 18 months. McCarthy and Rudd reported success in 40 out of 41 patients using 2RHZ/4RH regimen.[11] The Tuberculosis Research Center, Chennai in 1990 reported results of their prospective trial evaluating a supervised short-course (6 months) intermittent chemotherapy regimen: 2 $S_3H_3R_3Z_3/4S_2H_2$ in children with lymph node TB.[12] Out of 168 patients finally analyzed, favorable clinical response was noted in most patients at the end of the treatment. Thereafter, the final results of the second study of the BTS[13] compared the regimens: 2RHE/7RH versus 2RHZ/4RH, and observed that the six months regimen was found to be equally effective. In 68 children with tubercular lymphadenitis treated with $2H_3R_3Z_3S_3/4H_2S_2$ and followed up for 36 months over all response rate was found to be 97%.[14] Two other prospective controlled studies have documented that short-course combination chemotherapy given either daily or intermittently for 6 months period is an effective as 9 months of therapy given daily or intermittently.[15,16] The World Health Organization (WHO) recommends that TB-lymphadenitis should be treated for 6 months with 2RHZ/4RH either daily or thrice weekly.[17] However, WHO guidelines 2009 currently recommends that new patients with extrapulmonary TB should receive a regimen containing 6 months of rifampicin (2HRZE/4HR).[18]

Recently, in a multicenter operational study in six Indian states, it was shown that six month thrice weekly DOT for peripheral tubercular lymphadenopathy was satisfactory and there was no evidence of additional benefit of prolonging treatment to 9 months.[19]

During chemotherapy, upto 25% of patients may experience the appearance of new nodes or enlargement, fluctuation or drainage of existing nodes in patients infected with drug sensitive *M. tuberculosis.*[10] In most patients, this phenomenon represents an immunological reaction and not resistance. Drug resistant form of tuberculous lymphadenitis is rarely reported and therefore, most such lymph nodes regress with time and hence the treatment need not be modified. Data are too few to establish guidelines for treatment of drug resistant organisms. The role of surgery in the management of TB lymphadenitis is limited either for diagnostic purposes or in cases who fail to show improvement after an adequate course of chemotherapy or who have discomfort from enlarged or tense, fluctuant nodes.[19] Even nodes with sinus tracts and chronic drainage should undergo trial of chemotherapy prior to surgical removal because initial surgery does not seem to affect the outcome.[10]

PLEURAL EFFUSION

Pleural effusion may occur as a part of primary or post-primary TB. As part of primary TB, the effusion usually resolves even without treatment in 3–4 months time. However, two-thirds of these patients develop active PTB within the ensuing five years[20] and many develop serious restrictive impairment of lung function due to progressive pleural fibrosis. Therefore, to avoid these complications, early diagnosis and treatment of tubercular pleural effusion is important. A six-month anti-TB treatment schedule comprising of 2RHZE/4RH or 2RHZ/4RH daily or thrice weekly supervised regimen with 40 mg of prednisolone per day for first 4 weeks has currently been recommended by WHO for treatment of tuberculous pleural effusion in adults and children.[17] Based on these recommendations in Revised National Control Program (RNTCP), bilateral and moderate pleural effusion are categorized under CAT I where 2RHEZ/4RH thrice weekly is given. Small unilateral pleural effusion are categorized under CAT III where 2RHZ/4 RH thrice weekly is given. Multicentric study has shown that intermittent thrice-weekly treatment for 6 months with three drugs (CAT III) in the intensive phase is effective and safe for unilateral small pleural (less than 1500 mL) effusion in immunocompetent patients.[21] Although CAT III no longer exists in the program. WHO currently recommends to use the regimen 2RHZE/4RH only as there is no longer need of omitting ethambutol during the intensive phase of treatment for patients with extrapulmonary disease who are known to be HIV-negative.[18] Adjunctive treatment with corticosteroids has been shown to accelerate both the resolution of symptoms and reabsorption of fluid.[22]

TUBERCULOUS MENINGITIS (TBM)

The sequelae of TBM are so severe that prompt initiation of anti-TB chemotherapy is mandatory. In tubercular meningitis even with short course treatment, the outcome is related to the stage of the disease at the start of treatment, only a minority of patients with severe disease recover completely. Predictors of poor out come are younger age, advanced stage, neurological sequelae and duration of symptoms. While selecting the drugs, a sound knowledge about the pharmacokinetic properties of the drugs which penetrate blood-brain barrier is desirable. Isoniazid and pyrazinamide are the drugs of choice for central nervous system TB as they penetrate the meninges well.[23] In the absence of inflammation, rifampicin,[24] ethambutol[25] and aminoglycosides[26] can cross the blood brain-barrier negligibly but in its presence, rifampicin and aminoglycosides can penetrate significantly except ethambutol. Ethambutol hardly penetrates the meninges, even in the presence of inflammation and has no demonstrated efficacy in the treatment of tuberculous meningitis. Among the second-line agents, ethionamide[27] and ofloxacin[28] has excellent penetration with or without meningeal inflammation. Cycloserine also penetrates the meninges excellently.

Randomized clinical trials of anti-TB regimens for treatment of TBM have never been validated because of the catastrophic nature of the disease and difficulty in diagnosis. However, anti-TB chemotherapy of TBM is, in most circumstances straightforward. Because the number of tubercle bacillus involved in TBM is small, drug therapy is highly effective. But the optimum duration of treatment is still debatable. The current recommendation of WHO is that TBM may be treated for 9 months with 2SHRZ/7RH regimen given either daily or thrice weekly given the serious risk of disability and mortality.[18]

Despite optimum anti-TB treatment, the mortality in TBM is approximately 20–50% and about 53% may suffer from permanent sequelae, 41% of whom had moderate to severe disability.[29,30] With this background much attention has been focused on the use of adjuvant corticosteroids in stage II and III disease.[30] Corticosteroids improve morbidity and mortality by reducing cerebral edema, cerebral vasculitis and formation of exudate there by preventing the development of hydrocephalus.[29] The development of cerebral tuberculomas with neurological deterioration during anti-TB chemotherapy has been reported in patients with TBM as well as in those with extrameningeal disease,[31] and corticosteroids are probably beneficial in this situation. Recent WHO recommendation for use of corticosteroids in TBM in adults is 60 mg of prednisolone per day for first 4 weeks which is then tapered gradually over several weeks time.[17] Treatment of tuberculous meningitis in patients with AIDS is the same as for HIV negative patients. Prolonged adjunctive therapy with interferon gamma (IFN-γ) and granulocyte colony stimulating factor (G-CSF) may cure an immunocompromised patient with refractory multidrug resistant TBM.[32] The underlying mechanism of action of these new agents is that they activate the monocytes and macrophages against TB in immunocompromised patients. Studies in brain tuberculoma have clearly established the efficacy of short course treatment of 6–9 months in both children and adult.[33]

BONE AND JOINT TUBERCULOSIS

In developing countries, bone and joint TB accounts for upto 20% of all patients with diagnosed active TB.[34] Approximately 14–23% spinal TB patients present with clinically detectable abscess or sinus formation.[35] Neurological signs are present in 6–12% of patients.[35] In about 43% cases, there is radiological evidence of past or present PTB.[35] There is difference of opinion regarding the duration of drug therapy in spinal TB. Most previous studies favor 18–24 months of anti-TB treatment.[36, 37] However, the majority of patients with spinal TB respond to short-course chemotherapy alone, including those with sinuses and abscesses on admission.[38] In a study, comparison was made for 78 patients with 6HR with modified Hong Kong surgery, 78 patients with 6HR, and 79 patients with 9HR with follow-up of 120 months for each group revealed that overall response was 90% in 1st group 94% in 2nd group while 99% in 3rd group.[39] The efficacy of short-course chemotherapy had been tested by the British Medical Research Council (BMRC) Working Party in Hong Kong, Korea and south India. In Hong Kong, all the patients underwent the 'Hong Kong Operation' (which involves resection of lesions and anterior spinal fusion with autologous bone graft) with either 6 months or 9 months of chemotherapy with isoniazid and rifampicin supplemented by streptomycin for 6 months.[35] In Korea, only ambulatory chemotherapy with a regimen of 6 months or 9 months of isoniazid and rifampicin was compared with a regimen of 9 months or 18 months of isoniazid and para-aminosalicylic acid or ethambutol.[38] In a study done at

Chennai, South India, ambulatory chemotherapy with a regimen of 6 months or 9 months of isoniazid and rifampicin was compared with a regimen of 6 months or 9 months of isoniazid plus rifampicin and Hong Kong Operation.[40] After 3 years, all studies showed over 95% of favorable results for regimens containing isoniazid and rifampicin. These results confirmed the efficacy of a short-course regimen of isoniazid and rifampicin for 6 or 9 months for spinal TB and are of particular relevance for countries in which specialized set-up for successful performance of Hong Kong Radical Operation is not feasible. Further, there was no clear evidence that 9 months of chemotherapy with isoniazid and rifampicin had any advantage over 6 months of treatment. In a large series of paraplegic patients treated with chemotherapy alone, 72% were functionally and neurologically normal between one and six years of follow-up and 84% were sufficiently recovered to walk unaided, only 6% were left paralyzed and unable to walk.[41] On the basis of results of these trials, TB of thoracolumbar spine is best treated by a combination of appropriate chemotherapy, including isoniazid plus rifampicin for a period of 6–9 months. The WHO recommends that spinal TB without neurological signs should be treated for 6 months with 2RHEZ/4RH regimen either daily or thrice weekly, while the spinal TB with neurological deficit may be treated for 9 months with 2RHEZ/7RH administered daily or thrice weekly.[17,18] Neurologic signs may sometime develop or worsen during chemotherapy but in the majority of patients these neurological deficits improve.[41]

The role of surgery is yet to be clearly defined but is probably applicable to only a small percentage of patients with severe deforming disease. The role of surgery and drug treatment in the management of patients with tuberculosis of spine were investigated in trial by British Medical Research Council. It was concluded that operative procedure were generally unnecessary, ambulatory short-course treatment regimens were highly effective, and surgery was indicated only in patients aged less than 15 years and having an initial angle of kyphosis more than 30°. When surgery is indicated, anterior and posterior fusions are recommended to reduce kyphosis and improve function of spine. Surgical intervention is not usually necessary in skeletal TB except in spinal TB where spinal cord compression is present or threatened.[42-45]

MILIARY TUBERCULOSIS

The optimal duration of anti-TB therapy in miliary TB has never been tested in large controlled trials. The multitude of infected foci throughout the body and the likelihood of seeding the central nervous system and meninges even in the absence of signs have prompted many investigators to recommend anti-TB treatment for 9–12 months. The 1994 official statement of the American Thoracic Society recommends a 12-month course of chemotherapy for miliary TB in infants and children, and that adults be treated for 6–9 months.[46] It has been recommended by some investigators that patients with proved or suspected HIV infection with miliary TB should receive a minimum of 12 months therapy. This form of TB responds satisfactorily to chemotherapy in most cases despite HIV related immune suppression.[47] The WHO recommends that patients with miliary TB should be treated either with 6 months chemotherapy with 2RHEZ/4RH or 9 months therapy with 2RHEZ/7RH regimen, alternatively supervised thrice weekly variants of these regimens for 6–9 months may be administered successfully.[17,18] Role of corticosteroids in miliary TB remains somewhat controversial, in part because controlled clinical trials have not been conducted so far. Most patients respond promptly and satisfactorily to conventional anti-TB treatment and corticosteroids offer no added benefit. Nonetheless, it is widespread practice to add corticosteroids to the chemotherapeutic regimens in severely ill patients with extreme toxicity due to miliary TB, in an effort to accelerate the clinical response and improved food intake, strength and sense of well-being, thereby reducing the immediate risk. However, actual proof of improved survival with steroids has not been provided via suitable clinical trials.

TUBERCULOUS PERICARDITIS

Tuberculosis is the most common cause of pericardial disease and an important cause of heart failure in developing countries.[48] HIV infection is known to be strongly associated with pericardial tuberculosis[49] and in HIV infected population, TB is the most common cause of a large pericardial effusion.[50] Patients with tuberculous pericarditis may develop constrictive pericarditis[48] or a fistula between a bronchus and pericardium, resulting in pneumopericardium due to rupture of a tuberculous mediastinal lymph node.[51] The WHO recommends 6 months treatment with 2RHEZ/4RH regimen either daily or thrice weekly.[17,18] The response to chemotherapy in pericardial TB is variable and most authorities advocate adjuvant corticosteroid treatment[52] with or without pericardiocentesis and/or pericardiectomy. Adjuvant prednisolone during the initial weeks of chemotherapy significantly reduce the risk of death due to pericarditis and also reduces the need for repeated pericardiocentesis,[53] defervescence is rapid and arrhythmias are controlled within 2–3 days. Whether or not corticosteroids will diminish the likelihood of late constrictive pericarditis is not known. Currently WHO recommends use of prednisolone 60 mg/day for first 4 weeks followed by 30 mg/day for next 4 weeks and then gradual tapering over several weeks in adult patients with tuberculous pericarditis.[17,18]

ABDOMINAL TUBERCULOSIS

Intestinal TB usually responds well to standard anti-TB treatment. Although no controlled trials have determined the optimal type of therapy or duration, conventionally, patients with abdominal TB have been treated with antituberculosis drug regimens of 9-12 months duration.[54,55] Recently, a six-month short-course chemotherapy regimen has been found to be as effective as the standard twelve months regimen in the treatment of patients with all forms of abdominal TB.[56] The current WHO recommendation is that abdominal TB should be treated for 6 months with 2RHEZ/4RH regimen either daily or supervised thrice weekly.[17,18] Surgery is indicated for massive bleeding, obstruction, free perforation and confined perforation with abscess or sinus formation. Although widely used, there is no evidence that corticosteroids have a role in any form of abdominal TB.

GENITOURINARY TUBERCULOSIS

For the treatment of genitourinary TB randomized control trial specific to genitourinary disease, comparing different treatment regimens have not been performed. Although success has been reported with 4-months of chemotherapy for genitourinary TB,[57] most chest physicians would prefer to adhere to proven standard short-course chemotherapy.[58] Some investigators suggest that the possibility of covert prostatic infection which is more difficult to eradicate might be appropriately dealt with by treating all the patients with renal TB for upto 2 years.[59] No data exist to support this point of view and this seems to be an unnecessary precaution. Further, in urinary TB there are fewer organisms sometimes 100 times less than in PTB and the organisms in kidney are invariably excreted intermittently, there are high concentrations of isoniazid, rifampicin and pyrazinamide in urine, isoniazid and rifampicin pass readily into renal cortices in concentration high enough to kill tubercle bacilli, all standard drugs penetrate the kidney, ureters, bladder and prostate in concentration that are lethal to tubercle bacilli. With this background, there seems no rationale to prolong the duration of treatment. The WHO recommends 6 months treatment with 2RHEZ/4RH either daily or thrice weekly.[17,18] There is no convincing evidence of the utility of steroids to prevent stricture formation during the course of therapy.[60] A few patients eventually require either ablative or reconstructive surgery. The surgical management of genitourinary TB is largely reserved for severe or life-threatening complications such as hemorrhage, severe hypertension or suspicion of malignancy.[61]

OCULAR TUBERCULOSIS

Ocular manifestations of TB are rare, occurring in only 1.4% of patients.[62] Once the diagnosis of ocular tuberculosis is made, systemic TB therapy should be initiated at once. Systemic treatment is successful in the vast majority of cases. Any patient with disease highly suspicious for ocular TB should be treated with a multidrug regimen of proven efficacy because pulmonary infection and other foci of infection may coexist. It is the author's experience that almost all the patients with ocular TB can be treated successfully with either 6 months therapy with 2RHZ/4RH regimen given daily or thrice weekly. Recent WHO guidelines 2009 recommends 6 months treatment with 2RHEZ/4RH given daily or thrice weekly.[18]

UPPER RESPIRATORY TRACT TUBERCULOSIS

Tuberculosis of the upper respiratory tract occurs in about 1.8% of TB admissions[63] and is usually a complication of PTB—the result of surface contact by sputum heavily laden with tubercle bacilli. Hematogenous spread is seldom the cause and primary TB of the tonsil is rare.[64] Patients with tuberculous laryngitis are very infectious. This is relatively uncommon condition and occurs in about 1% of those with extensive pulmonary disease. The principles of anti-TB chemotherapy that apply to patients with extensive PTB apply to those with upper airway disease. The time required to achieve negative sputum bacteriology, however is substantially longer than that reported for patients with comparable pulmonary disease who receive equally effective drug regimens.[63] Delayed sputum conversion may occur because there usually is more extensive PTB in patients with tuberculous laryngitis, or it may relate to a general defect in host defense, which also predispose to upper airway disease. Gastrointestinal TB is frequent in patients with tuberculous laryngitis, hence a prompt and careful attention should be given to abdominal complaints and physical findings. Corticosteroids may be beneficial in selected, seriously ill patients who have difficulty eating or swallowing anti-TB drugs because of painful laryngeal ulcers, pharyngitis or disease of the oral cavity. A short course of prednisolone 40–60 mg/day with a rapid tapering after 2–3 weeks may be administered when laryngitis threatens the airway.

CUTANEOUS TUBERCULOSIS

The mainstay of treatment for all forms of cutaneous TB is the anti-TB therapy. Current WHO guidelines 2009 recommends 6-month treatment with 2RHEZ/4RH given daily or supervised thrice weekly.[18] Combination chemotherapy is recommended for patients with extracutaneous disease and multiple skin lesions and for those with profound immunosuppression. With the exception of TB cutis miliaris disseminata, most forms of cutaneous TB respond to chemotherapy and carry a good prognosis. A paradoxical skin reaction sometimes occurs in patients undergoing anti-TB therapy, particularly in anergic patients treated for cutaneous TB. During chemotherapy, fluctuant swellings appear that on aspiration yield pus. Smear and culture for

M. tuberculosis are often positive and the isolates usually retain its susceptibility to the patient's treatment regimen. This paradoxical response is thought to represent an immunologic phenomenon, not resistance, and typically responds to continued chemotherapy.

CONCLUSION

Although the anti-TB drug regimens for treatment of most forms of EPTB have not been studied extensively in controlled clinical trials, the available information suggests that all forms of EPTB can be managed effectively with short-course chemotherapy regimens administered daily or thrice weekly for duration of 6–9 months. The difficulty of defining a clear-cut end point for assessing the efficacy of treatment of extrapulmonary tuberculosis has led to varying duration of treatment. Since all anti-TB drugs diffuse well into all tissues and the burden of tubercle bacilli involved in all form of EPTB is small, it is unreasonable to consider that EPTB requires a different or more prolonged course of chemotherapy than does PTB. Patients with HIV positive and negative EPTB respond equally well to short-course chemotherapy. As the mycobacterial load in all forms of EPTB is low, emergence of required drug resistance in EPTB is seldom a problem. This fact is of utmost importance because clinicians might misdiagnose drug resistance in an otherwise drug sensitive EPTB patient who sometimes presents with paradoxical worsening of the lesion during anti-TB chemotherapy. It is to be noted that such paradoxical response is well reported phenomenon. Such lesions subside in due course of time with continued chemotherapy or after completion of treatment.

REFERENCES

1. US Department of Health and Human Services, Public Health Service, Centre for Disease Control. Tuberculosis in the United States. Publication No. [CDC] 808322, June 1980.
2. Hart CA, Beeching NJ, Duerden BI. Tuberculosis into the next century. J Med Microbiol. 1996;44:1-34.
3. Shafer RW, Edlin BR. Tuberculosis in patients infected with human immunodeficiency virus: perspective on the last decade. Clin Infect Dis. 1996;22:683-704.
4. Nunn P, Gicheha C, Hayes R, et al. Cross-sectional survey of HIV infection among patients with tuberculosis in Nairobi, Kenya. Tubercle Lung Dis. 1992;73:45-9.
5. Ramanatahn M, et al. Abdominal tuberculosis a presumptive diagnosis. Singapur Medical Journal. 1997;38:364-8.
6. Shrinker KA, Mathison GE, Goetz MB. Comparison of mycobacterial lymphadenitis among persons infected with human immunodeficiency virus and seronegatives controls. Clin Infect Dis. 1992;15:601-5.
7. Priel I, Dolev E. Tuberculous lymphadenitis: A survey of 94 cases. J Infect Dis. 1982;146: 710-4.
8. Kilpatrick GS, Douglas AC. Superficial glandular tuberculosis treatment with chemotherapy. BMJ. 1957;2:612-4.

9. Campbell IA, Dyson AJ. Lymph node tuberculosis: a comparison of treatments 18 months after completion of chemotherapy. Tubercle. 1979;60:95-8.
10. British Thoracic Society Research Committee. Short-course chemotherapy for tuberculosis of lymph nodes: a controlled trial. BMJ. 1985;290:1106-8.
11. Mc Carthy OR, Rudd RM. Six months chemotherapy for lymph node tuberculosis. Respir Med. 1989;83:425-7.
12. Balasubramanian R, Ramachandran R. Management of nonpulmonary forms of tuberculosis: review of TRC studies over two decades. Indian Journal of Pediatrics. 2000;67:S34-S40.
13. British Thoracic Society Research Committee. Six months versus nine months chemotherapy for tuberculosis of lymph nodes: final results. Respir Med. 1993;87:621-3.
14. Jawahar MS, et al. Short-course chemotherapy for tuberculous lymphadenitis in children. British Medical Journal. 1990;301:359-62.
15. Campbell IA, Ormerod LP, Friend JAR. et al. Six months versus nine months chemotherapy for tuberculosis of lymph node: final results. Respir Med. 1993;87:621-3.
16. Yurn APW, Wong SHW, Tam CM, et al. Prospective randomized study of twice weekly six-month and nine-month chemotherapy for cervical tuberculous lymphadenopaty. Otolaryngol Head Neck Surg. 1997;116:189-2.
17. WHO/CDS/TB/03.313. Treatment of Tuberculosis: Guidelines for National Tuberculosis Programme. World Health organization, 2003.
18. World Health Organization. Treatment of TB Guidelines - 4th edn. WHO/HTM/TB/2009.420
19. Jindal SK, Aggarwal AN, Gupta D, Ahmed Z, Gupta KB, Janmeja AK, et al. Tuberculous lymphadenopathy: a multicentre operational study of 6-month thrice weekly directly observed treatment. Int J Tuberc Lung Dis 2013;17:234-9.
20. Patiala J. Initial tuberculous pleuritis in the Finnish armed forces in 1939-45 with special reference to eventual post pleuritic tuberculosis. Acta Tuberc Scand. 1954;36(Suppl):1-16.
21. Sharma SK, Solanki R, Mohan A, Jain NK, Chauhan LS. Outcomes of Category III Dots treatment in immuno Competent patients with tuberculous pleural effusion. Int J Tuberc Lung Dis. 2012;16:1505-9.
22. Lee CH, Wang WJ, Lan RS, et al. Corticosteroids in the treatment of tuberculous pleurisy: a double blind placebo controlled, randomized study. Chest. 1988;94:1256-9.
23. Forgan Smith R, Ellard GA, Newton D, Mitchison DA. Pyrazinamide and other drugs in tuberculous meningitis. Lancet. 1973;2:374-8.
24. Sippel JE, Mikhail IA, Girgis NI. Rifampicin concentration in cerebrospinal fluid of patients with tuberculous meningitis. Am Rev Respir Dis. 1974;109:559-60.
25. Pilheu JA, Maglio F, Cetranglo R, Pleus AD. Concentration of ethambutol in the cerebrospinal fluid after oral administration. Tubercle. 1971;52:117-22.
26. Buggs CW, Pilling MA, Bronstein B, Hirshfeld JW. The absorption, distribution and excretion of streptomycin in man. J Clin Invest. 1946;25:94-102.
27. Donald PR, Seifart HI. Cerebrospinal fluid concentrations of ethionamide in children with tuberculous meningitis. J Pediatr. 1989;115:483-6.
28. Pioget JC, Wolff M, Singlas E, et al. Diffusion of ofloxacin into cerebrospinal fluid of patients with purulent meningitis or ventriculitis. Antimicrob Agents Chemother. 1989;33:933-6.
29. Alzeer AH, Fitz Gerald JM. Corticosteroids and tuberculosis: risks and use as an adjunct therapy. Tubercle Lung Dis. 1993;74:6-11.
30. Ramachandran P, Duraipandian M, Reetha AM, et al. Long-term status of children treated for tuberculous meningitis in south India. Tubercle. 1989;70:235-9.
31. Teoh R, Humphries MJ, O' Mahony G. Symptomatic intracranial tuberculoma developing during treatment of tuberculosis: a report of 10 patients and review of the literature. Q J Med. 1987;63:449-60.

32. Raad I, Hachem R, Leeds N, et al. Use of adjunctive treatment with interferon gamma in an immunocompromised patient who had refractory multidrug resistant tuberculosis of the brain. Clin Infect Dis. 1996;22:572-4.
33. Rajeshwari R, et al. A controlled clinical trial of short-course chemotherapy for tuberculoma of the brain. Tubercle and Lung Disease. 1995;76:111-7.
34. Curie MA. Profile of spine and joint tuberculosis in Pakistan's Afghan frontier. Ann R Coll Surg. 1984;66:105-7.
35. Medical Research Council Working Party on Tuberculosis of the Spine. A controlled trial of 6 months and 9 months regimens of chemotherapy in patients undergoing radical surgery for tuberculosis of the spine in Hong Kong. Tubercle. 1986;67:243-59.
36. Hodgson AR, Stock FE. Anterior spinal fusion. A preliminary communication on the radical treatment of Pott's disease and Pott's paraplegia. Br J Surg. 1956;44:266-75.
37. Hodgson AR, Stock FE. Anterior spinal fusion for treatment of tuberculosis of the spine. J Bone Joint Surg. 1960;42-A:295-310.
38. Medical Research Council Working Party on Tuberculosis of the Spine. Controlled trial of short course regimens of chemotherapy in the ambulatory treatment of spinal tuberculosis. Results at 3 years of a study in Korea. J Bone Joint Surg. 1993;75 B:240-8.
39. Short course chemotherapy for tuberculosis of the spine. A compassion between ambulant treatment and radical surgery – A 10 year report. Journal of Bone and Joint Surgery. British Volume. 1999;81:464-71.
40. Indian Medical Research Council–British Medical Research Council. A controlled trial of short course regimens of chemotherapy in patients receiving ambulatory treatment or undergoing radical surgery for tuberculosis of the spine. Indian J Tuberc. 1989;36(suppl):1-21.
41. Pattison PRM. Pott's paraplegia: an account of the treatment of 89 consecutive patients. Paraplegia. 1986;24:77-91.
42. Fancourt GJ, Edben P, Garner P, et al. Bone tuberculosis results and experience in Leicestershire. Br J Dis Chest. 1986;80:265-72.
43. Thirteenth report of MRC working party on TB of spine. Journal of Bone and Joint surgery. British volume. 1998;80:456.
44. Parthasarathy R, et al. Short course chemotherapy for tuberculosis of spine. A comparison between ambulant and radical surgery. Journal of Bone nad Joint Surgery. British volume. 1998;81:464.
45. Upadhyay SS, et al. Longitudinal changes in spinal deformity after anterior spinal surgery for tuberculosis of spine in adults. A comparative analysis between radical and debridement surgery. Spine. 1994;90:542-9.
46. American Thoracic Society. Treatment of tuberculosis and tuberculosis infection in adults and children. Am J Respir Crit Care Med. 1994;149:1359-74.
47. Small PM, Schester GF, Goodman PC, et al. Treatment of tuberculosis in patients with advanced human immunodeficiency virus infection. N Engl J Med. 1991;324:289-94.
48. Desai HN. Tuberculous pericarditis. A review of 100 cases. S Afr Med. 1979;55:877-80.
49. Elliott AM, Luo N, Tembo G, et al. Impact of HIV on tuberculosis in Zambia: a cross-sectional survey. BMJ. 1990;301:412-5.
50. Cegieleski JP, Lwakatare J, Dukes CS, et al. Tuberculous pericarditis in Tanzanian patients with and without HIV infection. Tubercle Lung Dis. 1994;75:429-34.
51. Paredes C, Del Campo F, Zamarron C. Cardiac tamponade due to tuberculous mediastinal lymphadenitis. Tubercle. 1990;71:219-20.
52. Allen MB, Cooke NJ. Corticosteroids and tuberculosis. BMJ. 1991;303:871-2.
53. Strang JIG, Kakaza HHS, Gibson DG, et al. Controlled trial of prednisolone as an adjunct in the treatment of tuberculous constrictive percarditis in Transkei. Lancet. 1987;2:1418-22.
54. Anand BS, Nanda R, Sachdev GK. Response of tuberculous stricture to antituberculous treatment. Gut. 1988;29:62-9.

55. Chuttani HK, Sarin SK. Intestinal tuberculosis. Indian J Tuberc. 1985;32:117-9.
56. Balasubramanian R, Narayana M, Balambal R, Tripathy SP, Sundaraman R, Venkatesan P. Randomized controlled trial of short-course chemotherapy in abdominal tuberculosis: a five year report. Int J Tuberc Lung Dis. 1997;1:44-51.
57. Gow JG, Barbosa S. Genito-urinary tuberculosis. A study of 1117 cases over a period of 34 years. Br J Urol. 1984;56:449-55.
58. Wong SH, Lan WY, Ho KK, et al. The management of urinary tuberculosis: a logical approach. Br J Urol. 1984;56:349-53.
59. O'Dea MJ, Moore SB, Greene LF. Tuberculous prostatitis. Urology. 1987;11:483-5.
60. Gow JG. Results of treatment in a large series of cases of genitourinary tuberculosis and the changing pattern of the disease. Br J Urol. 1970;42:647-55.
61. Garcia–Radriguez JA, Gracia Sanchez JE, Munoz Bellido JL, et al. Genitourinary tuberculosis in Spain: review of 81 cases. Clin Infect Dis. 1994;18:557-61.
62. Rosen PH, Spalton DJ, Graham EM. Intraocular tuberculosis. Eye. 1990;4:486-92.
63. Rohwedder JJ. Tuberculosis of the upper respiratory tract. Sixteen cases in a general hospital. Ann Intern Med. 1974;80:708-13.
64. McDowell C. Destructive primary tuberculosis of the faucial tonsil. Am Rev Tuberc. 1954;69: 612-7.

Chapter 22

Corticosteroids in Tuberculosis

INTRODUCTION

Intact cellular immunity is crucial in the prevention of tuberculosis (TB). Drugs like corticosteroids depress the cellular immunity and may predispose patients to tuberculosis infection and progression of disease. It was therefore suggested in the past that adjuvant corticosteroids therapy should not be administered in the presence of TB.[1] The advent of HIV has further complicated the issue because physicians may be hesitant to administer corticosteroids in a HIV positive tuberculosis patient who is already immunosuppressed and at increased risk for opportunistic infections. The actual risk of tuberculosis in steroid treated patients is unknown, various reports have confirmed the development of tuberculosis in steroid-treated patients.[2-4] However, several other studies[5-7] have revealed a very low incidence of tuberculosis in corticosteroid treated patients. Adjunctive treatment with corticosteroids in certain forms of tuberculosis has been found to decrease the morbidity and mortality associated with tuberculosis, provided the patient receives adequate antituberculosis drug therapy simultaneously.[8,9] This chapter aims to review the indications and rationale of use of corticosteroids in tuberculosis.

INDICATIONS OF CORTICOSTEROIDS IN TUBERCULOSIS

Purpose of corticosteroid therapy in tuberculosis is to diminish the host inflammatory response that may be producing additional tissue damage. There are specific clinical conditions in which the benefit of corticosteroid treatment has been clearly documented.[10,11] Corticosteroid adjuvant therapy may need to be administered in following clinical settings: 1) In seriously ill preterminal stage of tuberculosis to buy sometime for chemotherapy to become effective,[12] 2) to control drug hypersensitivity reactions,[13] 3) in tuberculosis of serous sacs, i.e. pericarditis,[14] peritonitis, and pleural effusion to prevent fibrosis and adhesion and to hasten absorption of fluid, 4) in tuberculous meningitis to prevent morbidity and mortality due to adhesion, particularly in stage II and III disease,[15] 5) occasionally for suppression of lymph node enlargement during chemotherapy, e.g. where mediastinal lymph nodes are causing bronchial obstruction or occasionally for the management of tuberculous endobronchitis.[16]

Seriously ill Preterminal Stage of Tuberculosis

Corticosteroid seems to play a beneficial role in making antitubercular therapy effective in treating seriously ill preterminal stage patients of tuberculosis. A controlled trial was conducted by Tuberculosis Society of Scotland between 1956–1957 in order to establish role of steroids in management of TB. Prednisolone group with 44 patients (ATT and Prednisolone) as well as control group with 46 patients (ATT only) were observed for a duration of 6 months.[12] The anti-inflammatory action of the corticosteroids might be expected to reduce the toxic effects of TB in severely ill patients as significant weight gain, fall in erythrocyte sedimentation rate and radiological improvement was observed. Rate of sputum conversion was also higher at the end of 5 months though not significantly as compared to control group.[12]

Control of Severe Drug Hypersensitivity Reactions

It may be noted that steroids may be used to lessen anti-tubercular therapy induced hypersensitivity reactions. It was proven by the above-mentioned trial as development of rashes in 25% of patients within two weeks of withdrawal of prednisolone suggesting that concurrent administration with ATT from beginning of treatment results in desensitization and withdrawal may lead to mild hypersensitivity.[13] It has been observed that using prednisolone in the dose of 40 mg/day or less during the continuation phase of antitubercular treatment in few cases complicated by allergy or toxic reaction to such drugs is beneficial. It can be inferred that steroids are important in controlling reaction in order to provide effective chemotherapy.

Tuberculous Meningitis (TBM)

Corticosteroids have documented benefits in reducing inflammation and increased intracranial tension. They reduce cerebral edema and inflammation, and prevent CSF block. They suppress both immunity and inflammation, an action that could be desirable in patients with TBM. A recent randomized placebo-controlled study documented the benefits of steroid use in patients with stage II and stage III disease.[10] Some authorities now routinely include steroids at stage II and III treatment regimens, as well as for spinal cord disease and significant cerebral edema.[17] In 1992, a subcommittee of the Infectious Disease Society of America concluded that moderate evidence favored the routine use of corticosteroids in cases of TBM.[18] Steroids often mute some of the signs and symptoms of TBM, including fever, headache, malaise and delirium. With use of steroids, CSF protein content and leukocyte count may normalize more rapidly than otherwise. A frequent interpretation of the conflicting data on steroid use in TBM concludes that in some subsets of patients they are quite helpful, but in others they may be unnecessary or even harmful, particularly when the specific diagnosis may not have been established. But in general, it seems best to use steroids and accept the risk if patient's condition is critical. The utility of steroid therapy in cases of impending or established spinal block is now virtually unchallenged.[19,20] Recent WHO recommendation for use of corticosteroids in TBM is 60 mg of prednisolone per day for first 4 weeks which is then tapered gradually over several weeks time.[21,22]

Pleural Effusion

Pleural disease in tuberculosis is thought to result from rupture of a subpleural caseous focus into the pleural space.[23] Hypersensitivity to tubercle bacillus also plays role in the occurrence of pleural effusion. Adjunctive treatment with corticosteroids has been shown to accelerate both the resolution of symptomatology and reabsorption of pleural fluid.[24] However, usage must be employed judiciously and probably should be withheld in patients with HIV infection or HIV risk. One of the common sequelae of pleural tuberculosis is residual pleural thickening which may occur in as many as 50% patients with tuberculous pleurisy.[25] Neither clinical characteristics nor pleural fluid biochemistry and cytology are predictive of the ultimate development of pleural thickening,[25] and neither corticosteroid therapy nor repeated therapeutic thoracentesis prevents this complication.[25,26] The WHO recommended dosage of prednisolone for pleural effusion is 40 mg daily for 4 weeks.[21,22] In tuberculous empyema, corticosteroids have no role in treating the problem of extensive residual pleural scarring and calcification.[27]

Pulmonary Tuberculosis

Endobronchial tuberculosis in children may represent a special situation in which anti-TB chemotherapy alone may not result in prompt or satisfactory reduction of illness.[28] It is speculated that caseation in peribronchial lymph nodes makes it difficult for drugs to reach all of the infected tissue.[29] This condition may therefore merit the use of corticosteroids to help control the inflammatory response and resulting bronchial compression.[30] The only study demonstrated that administering corticosteroids within the first 4 months of illness of children with endobronchial tuberculosis resulted in significantly more rapid resolution of the disease.[11] The recommended corticosteroid regimen in such a case is a 37 days therapy, with prednisolone 3 mg/kg/day for initial 3 days, 2 mg/kg/day for next 3 days, 1 mg/kg/day for next 24 days, 0.5 mg/kg/day for next 4 days, and 0.25 mg/kg/day for last three days. Whether steroid therapy is beneficial in reversing bronchostenosis in endobronchial TB is unclear. Many studies[11,16,31,32] have shown that the effect of corticosteroids is difficult to predict when the mechanism of airway narrowing includes fibrosis and inflammation. Only the inflammation may respond to steroid therapy. Stenotic lesions may need to be treated with repeated dilatations.[33] Unfortunately, no data are available to determine whether there is a beneficial effect on the long-term outcome in terms of bronchiectasis and bronchial stenosis. Thus, routine corticosteroid adjunctive therapy is not recommended in endobronchial tuberculosis. In pulmonary TB, it seems reasonable not to routinely use corticosteroids except in life-threatening disease because of more rapid clinical and radiological improvement observed during the initial period of corticosteroid therapy.[34]

Miliary Tuberculosis

The role of corticosteroids in miliary TB remains somewhat controversial, in part because controlled clinical trials have not been conducted in this type of tuberculosis. Most patients respond promptly and satisfactorily to conventional chemotherapy and corticosteroids are of benefit in selected patients with meningeal,[10] pericardial[14] involvement or when rare and clearly aberrant immunologic phenomenon appear (e.g. immune complex nephritis[35] and histiocytic hemophagocytosis),[36] and deterioration of organ function (particularly gas exchange) continues despite adequate anti-TB therapy. Replacement doses of corticosteroids should be used if adrenal insufficiency is suspected, with the knowledge that rifampicin increases exogenous corticosteroid metabolism.[37] Decision to administer corticosteroids in miliary tuberculosis is not free from risks especially with increasing trend of MDR-TB. Further in a severely immunocompromised patient, other inapparent opportunistic infections may co-exist and if not addressed properly, may progress during corticosteroid therapy. Opportunistic infections and gastric hemorrhage due to use of corticosteroids have been reported.[38] As yet, no suitable clinical trials have provided actual proof of improved survival with steroids in miliary TB.

Pericardial Tuberculosis

In tuberculous pericarditis, corticosteroids nonspecifically suppress inflammation, thereby lessening the hemodynamic sequelae as the anti-TB drugs eliminate the organism. The exudation of fluid abates and reabsorption of fluid commences. A noticeable decrease in heart size often occurs within 2–3 days and it may return to normal within 2 weeks. Defervescence is rapid and arrhythmias are controlled within 2–3 days. The corticosteroids may be withdrawn over next 6–8 weeks without recrudescence of symptoms. Whether or not corticosteroids will diminish the likelihood of late constrictive pericarditis is not known. Corticosteroids may lessen (but do not eliminate) the risk of pericardial related mortality in acute disease but they do not affect long-term constrictive complications. It has to be recognized that corticosteroid treatment is not a panacea in the management of tuberculous pericarditis and it does not eliminate the necessity for pericardiocentesis and ancillary agents to control heart failure or even pericardiectomy. Earlier, an initial regimen of 60–80 mg of prednisolone/day had been used with tapering over 8–11 weeks.[14,39] Recently, WHO has recommended prednisolone 60 mg/day for first 4 weeks followed by 30 mg/day for next 4 weeks and then gradual tapering over several weeks.[21,22] Steroid metabolism is increased when rifampicin is co-administered and the steroid dosage may need to be increased.[37]

Genitourinary Tuberculosis

In general, routine use of corticosteroids has not been recommended in conservative management of genitourinary tuberculosis.[39] There is no convincing evidence of the utility of steroids to prevent stricture formation during the course of the therapy.[40]

Tuberculosis of Upper Airway

Corticosteroids may be helpful in selected seriously ill patients who have difficulty in eating or swallowing anti-TB medication because of painful laryngeal ulcers, pharyngitis or disease of the oral cavity. A short course of prednisolone 40–60 mg/day with a rapid tapering after 2–3 weeks may be administered when laryngitis threatens the airway.

Management of Antituberculosis Drug Induced Fever

Fever due to tuberculosis *per se* usually responds to ATT within first two weeks of treatment with an effective treatment regimen. The persistence of fever after two weeks in drug sensitive tuberculosis should raise the suspicion of other foci of infection. In the absence of a focus being found, the possibility of a drug fever should be considered. In many instances, withdrawal of the offending drug can be achieved but this requires significant trial and error. An alternative approach is to use corticosteroids in cases where withdrawl of offending drug is not possible because of problem of drug resistance. Prednisolone 40 mg/day will in most instances resolve the fever and allow continuation of therapy.[41]

Treatment of BCG Scar

One of the long-term problem with BCG immunization is development of hypertrophic or keloid scars. To avoid this, lower portion of deltoid should be used for BCG vaccination. Once the scar/keloid develops, 3–4 injections of triamcinolone at monthly interval will cause the scar to atrophy.

Steroid Treatment in HIV Positive TB Patients

As steroids are immunosuppressants, the apprehension is that steroids may further depress cellular immunity and increase risk of opportunistic infection in HIV positive patients. However, WHO recommends that HIV positive TB patients are still likely to benefit from use of steroids and indications for steroid treatment in HIV positive tuberculosis patient are the same as for HIV negative TB patients.[21,22]

DOSE AND DURATION OF CORTICOSTEROIDS[42]

The dosage and duration of corticosteroid therapy in various conditions has not been clearly defined. However, it depends on the severity of the disease. In severely ill preterminal stage of tuberculosis, prednisolone should be initiated at higher dose (50–60 mg/day) in preferably oral (equivalent dosage intravenously in case of comatose state) maintaining at same dose till emergency and then tapered off 5 mg/week till the last dose should be 2.5 mg/day for one week and stopped finally. In case of pericardial tuberculosis, it has been recommended to prescribe prednisolone 60 mg/day for first 4 weeks followed by 30 mg/day for next 4 weeks and then gradual tapering over several weeks. However, in case of less severe conditions like pleural effusion prednisolone should be started at lower dose (30–40 mg/day), maintained for next four to six weeks and then tapered off thereafter in a similar fashion.

CONCLUSION

Corticosteroids are potent immunosuppressant drugs which may increase the risk of tuberculosis infection and progression to disease. Injudicious use of corticosteroid in patients with tuberculosis may lead to risk of MDR-TB particularly in the era of HIV pandemic. So, corticosteroids should never be given to patients with tuberculosis unless they are receiving adequate anti-TB therapy. Further, in a severely ill patient, inapparent opportunistic infections may coexist and if not addressed properly, may progress during corticosteroid therapy. When the treatment regimen contains rifampicin, dosage of prednisolone needs to be increased.

REFERENCES

1. American Thoracic Society. The effect of cortisone and/or corticotrophin on tuberculosis infection in man. Am Rev Tuberc. 1952;66:245-56.
2. Sahn SA, Lakshminarayan S. Tuberculosis after corticosteroid therapy. Br J Dis Chest. 1976;70:195-205.

3. Abbott MR, Smith DD. Mycobacterial infections in immunosuppressed patients. Med J Aust. 1981;1:351-3.
4. Skogberg K, Ruutu P, Tukiainen P, Valtonen V. Effect of immunosuppressive therapy on the clinical presentation and outcome of tuberculosis. Clin Infect Dis. 1993;17:1012-7.
5. Smyllie HC, Connolly CK. Incidence of serious complications of corticosteroid therapy in respiratory disease. Thorax. 1968;23:571-81.
6. Schatz M, Patterson R, Kloner R, Falk J. The prevalence of tuberculosis and positive tuberculin skin tests in a steroid-treated asthmatic population. Ann Intern Med. 1976;84:261-5.
7. Cowie RL, King LM. Pulmonary tuberculosis in corticosteroid treated asthmatics. S Afr Med J. 1987;72:849-50.
8. Alzeer AH, FitzGerald JM. Corticosteroids and tuberculosis: risks and use as adjunct therapy. Tubercle Lung Dis. 1993;74:6-11.
9. Senderovitz T, Viskum K. Corticosteroids and tuberculosis. Respir Med. 1994;88:561-5.
10. Girgis NI, Farid Z, Kilpatrick ME, Sultan Y, Mikhail A. Dexamethasone adjunctive treatment for tuberculous meningitis. Pediatr Infect Dis J. 1991;10:179-83.
11. Nemir RL, Cardona J, Vaziri F, Toledo R. Prednisone as an adjunct in chemotherapy of lymph node-bronchial tuberculosis in childhood: a double blind study. Am Rev Respir Dis. 1966;95:402-10.
12. Tuberculosis Society of Scotland. Prednisolone in the treatment of pulmonary tuberculosis: a controlled trial. BMJ. 1957;ii:1131-4.
13. Barnes PF, Chan LS, Wong SF. The course of fever during treatment of pulmonary tuberculosis. Tubercle. 1987;68:255-60.
14. Strang JG, Kakasa HHS, Gibson DG, et al. Controlled clinical trial of complete open surgical drainage and prednisolone in the treatment of tuberculous pericardial effusion in Transkei. Lancet. 1988;(2):759-64.
15. Humphries MK, Teoh R, Lau J, Gabrial M. Factors of prognostic significance in Chinese children with tuberculous meningitis. Tubercle. 1990;71:161-8.
16. Chan HS, Pang JA. Effect of corticosteroids on deterioration of endobronchial tuberculosis during chemotherapy. Chest. 1989;96:1195-6.
17. Humphries M. The management of tuberculous meningitis. Thorax. 1992;47:577-81.
18. McGowan, JE Jr, Chesney PJ, Crossley KB, La Force FM. Guidelines for the use of systemic glucocorticosteroids in the management of selected infections. J Infect Dis. 1992;165:1-13.
19. Parsons M. The treatment of tuberculous meningitis. Tubercle. 1989;70:79-82.
20. Molais A, Le Frock JL. Tuberculous meningitis. Med Clin North Am. 1985;69:315-31.
21. WHO/CDS/TB/03.313. Treatment of Tuberculosis: Guidelines for National Tuberculosis Programme. World Health organization, 2003.
22. World Health Organization. Treatment of TB Guidelines - 4th edn. WHO/HTM/TB/2009.420
23. Falk A, Stead WW. Antimicrobial therapy of primary tuberculous pleurisy with effusion; its effects upon the incidence of subsequent tuberculous relapse. Am Rev Tuberc. 1956;74: 897-902.
24. Lee CH, Wang WJ, Lan RS, et al. Corticoisterids in the treatment of tuberculous pleurisy: a double blind placebo controlled, randomized study. Chest. 1988;94:1256-9.
25. Barbas CS, Cukier A, De Varvalho CR, et al. The relationship between pleural fluid findings and the development of pleural thickening in patients with pleural tuberculosis. Chest. 1991;100:1264-7.
26. Large SK, Levick RK. Aspiration in the treatment of primary tuberculous pleural effusion. BMJ. 1958;1:1512-4.
27. Berger HW, Mejia E. Tuberculous pleurisy. Chest. 1973;63:88-92.
28. Nakvi AJ, Nohl-Oser HC. Surgical treatment of bronchial obstruction in primary tuberculosis in children: report of seven cases. Thorax. 1979;34:464-9.

29. Rana SR, Saena SB, Gumbs RV. Tuberculous mediastinal lymphadenitis with a chestwall mass. Pediatr Radiol. 1985;15:127-8.
30. Durfee ML, Nemir RL, Sewell EM, et al. The treatment of tuberculosis in children. Am Rev Respir Dis. 1969;99:304-7.
31. Lee JH, Park SS, Lee DH, Shin DH, Yang SC, Yoo BM. Endobronchial tuberculosis. Clinical and bronchoscopic features in 121 cases. Chest. 1992;102:990-4.
32. Ip MSM, So SY, Lam WK, Mok CK. Endobronchial tuberculosis revisited. Chest. 1986;89: 727-30.
33. Vanden Brande PM, Van de Mierop T, Verben K, Demedts M. Clinical spectrum of endobronchial tuberculosis in elderly patients. Arch Intern Med. 1990;150:2105-8.
34. Malik SK, Martin CS. Tuberculosis, corticosteroid therapy, and pulmonary function. Am Rev Respir Dis. 1969;100:13-8.
35. Shribman JH, Eastwood JB, Uff J. Immune complex nephritis complicating miliary tuberculosis. BMJ. 1983;287:1593-4.
36. Monier BM, Fauroux B, Chevalier JY, et al. Miliary tuberculosis with acute respiratory failure and histiocytic haemophagocytosis. Successful treatment with extracorporeal lung support and epipodophyllotoxin VP (16-213). Acta Paediatr. 1992;81:725-7.
37. Mc Allister WAC, Thompson PJ, Al-Habet SM, et al. Rifampicin reduces effectiveness and bioavailability of prednisolone. BMJ. 1983;286:923-5.
38. Munt PW. Miliary tuberculosis in the chemotherapy era: a clinical review in 69 American adults. Medicine. 1972;51:139-55.
39. Horne NW, Tulloch WS. Conservative management of renal tuberculosis. Br J Urol. 1975;47: 481-7.
40. Gow JG. Results of treatment in a large series of cases of genitourinary tuberculosis and the changing pattern of the disease. Br J Urol. 1970;42:647-55.
41. Chung KF, Snashoull PD. Suppression of prolonged fever during treatment of pulmonary tuberculosis: importance of using twice versus single daily dose of prednisolone. Postgrad Med J. 1983;59:373-5.
42. Prasad R, Nautiyal RG. Use of corticosteroids in tuberculosis. Journal of Internal Medicine of India. 2001;4:194-7.

Chapter 23

Management of Retreatment Cases in Tuberculosis

INTRODUCTION

Tuberculosis retreatment refers to treatment in a patient of tuberculosis who has been previously treated for more than four weeks with antituberculosis drugs and who are now smear or culture positive for *Mycobacterium tuberculosis.*[1] The management of retreatment cases in tuberculosis (TB) involves management of entities like relapse, failure and treatment after default and poor adherence to previous treatment. All of these entities may imply different approaches and physician handling these problems requires adequate knowledge of appropriate retreatment regimens. Retreatment patients correspond to the greater part of the problem and the major source of complications. In the two largest high-tuberculosis burden countries (China and India), retreatment cases accounted for upto 20% of sputum smear-positive cases.[2] Retreatment forms the most complex part of the problem because these patients have already had the opportunity to receive a curative treatment; therefore, excluding relapse cases, most retreatment cases arise due to errors during the implementation or administration of the previous treatment regimen.[3] This chapter aims at management of retreatment cases in tuberculosis.

The retreatment of TB involves entities such as relapse, failure, treatment after default, and poor patient adherence to the previous treatment.

RELAPSE

Relapse is defined as a patient previously treated for TB who has been declared cured or treatment completed, and is diagnosed with bacteriologically positive (smear or culture) tuberculosis.[1,4] However, there can be certainty that a patient has completed all their medication only when treatment administration is directly observed. If the treatment was not supervised, the authenticity of a relapse can be questioned. The rapidly dividing population of bacilli is eliminated early in effective therapy as shown by early clinical responses and clearing of live bacilli from sputum within 2 months in 80% of patients. The remaining subpopulations, i.e. mainly the persisters of *M. tuberculosis* account for relapse cases. For this reason, it is theoretically accepted that relapses exhibit the same pattern of resistance as that of the patient's initial TB; hence the same initial treatment could be administered. If the relapse occurs several years after the initial treatment, re-infection is more likely than relapse.[5, 6] Though this is not simple to demonstrate, the indication for the same initial treatment scheme still applies. Although relapses are usually due to susceptible bacilli, it is still advisable to carry out drug susceptibility test (DST) to first-line anti-TB drugs before the commencement of treatment for relapse cases. However, when DST is conducted in the field, the incidence of resistance among relapse patients increases significantly compared to that seen in initial cases. This might be explained by irregularities in drug intake but also by selection of initial single or multiple resistances. This situation has led to the recommendation that, in low- and middle-income countries like india and under Revised National Tuberculosis Control Program (RNTCP) conditions, relapses be treated with a reinforced first-line drug regimen,[3] administered for a longer period of time which is in the form of Category II regimen of WHO (2SRHEZ/RHEZ/5RHE either daily or thrice weekly).

DEFAULTERS OR TREATMENT AFTER DEFAULT

A person who returns to treatment, positive bacteriologically, following interruption of treatment for 2 months or more of anti-TB treatment.[1] There are two different kinds of defaulters: one who abandons all of their drugs, and others who omit one of them. Those who abandon all of their drugs usually do not incur an elevated risk of selection of resistance, since the drugs were effective when the patient took the treatment, and there were no favorable conditions for selection of the naturally resistance mutants. When the effect of the treatment was interrupted due to default, the entire bacillary population resumes growth, as before the initial treatment. Thus, in these cases, it is adequate to reintroduce the initial treatment regimen or better with a reinforced first-line drug regimen or a Cat II regimen. The situation is entirely different when the patient abandons one of the drugs while undergoing treatment. It generates the conditions for the selection of microorganisms spontaneously resistant to the drugs the patient continues taking.[4] This is the reason why fixed dose combinations (multiple drugs incorporated into one) are superior to individual drugs, and are strongly recommended in international recommendations of WHO and International Union Against Tuberculosis and Lung Disease (IUALTD) when DOTS (Directly observed treatment, short-course) is not possible since drug resistance may be less likely to develop and further, because when treatment is interrupted,[7] simultaneously all drugs will be stopped together and this would prevent resistant organisms being selected.

FAILURE

Failure is defined on the basis of two aspects bacteriologically, i.e. on sputum smear and culture status. In low- and middle-income countries like India where cultures are less frequently used, sputum smears are used to define failures. Failure for initially smear-positive patients (Category I and Category II) is defined as sputum smear-positive at the end of the fifth month of treatment or later.[1] Failure for initially smear-negative patients (Category III) regimen is defined as who became smear-positive during treatment.[1]

Based on culture, failure is defined as the reappearance, while the patient is receiving treatment and after the negative conversion of cultures, of bacteriological activity.[1,4] It is also considered treatment failure when cultures do not become negative during the course of treatment. For the initial 6-month treatment scheme with rifampicin (R) in both phases, i.e. Category I, failure is considered when sputum cultures are still positive at the end of the fourth month. For the 8-month treatment scheme, without R in the continuation phase, i.e. 2RHEZ/6HE, failure is not diagnosed before the end of the fifth month.[1,8] The failure is due to a population of bacilli that is metabolically active and proliferates during the treatment, which creates favorable conditions for selection of naturally resistant mutant bacilli present in the original population. Therefore, the failure situation should imply resistance to all of the drugs being administered at the time when failure was diagnosed; hence the importance of carrying out DST to first-line drugs. However, some studies show that upto 50% of failures exhibit drug susceptibility in drug susceptibility testing,[9,10] and can be cured with an initial or reinforced first-line drug-based scheme, i.e Category II regimen.[11] The contributing factors for this could be the imperfect correlation between DST results and the behavior of bacilli *in vivo*, and the extremely small fraction of patients in whom negative conversion of cultures take > 4 months despite well-documented susceptibility to drugs.

POOR ADHERENCE TO TREATMENT

This may be much more common than thought especially in the latter months of treatment when most of the patient are already relieved of symptoms. When this situation is continued over a period of time, it results in creating a favorable environment for naturally resistant mutant bacilli to develop.[3]

DRUG RESISTANT TUBERCULOSIS

Drug Resistance in New Cases

The management of new patients suspected of having contracted drug-resistant strains of *M. tuberculosis*, i.e. primary resistance or now known as "resistance in new cases" should be essentially similar to the lines of treatment of other new patients. They should be given the same initial standardized treatment recommended by the National Tuberculosis Program (NTP), i.e. Category I regimen; however, as resistance is highly suspected, drug susceptibility testing (DST) to first-line drugs should be carried out. If these tests confirm MDR, but if the patient shows a favorable clinical progression, the initial regimen should perhaps remain unchanged, since some reports have demonstrated that 20–50% of these new patients with MDR-TB are cured by standard regimens.[10] If the clinical response is not favorable, the initial treatment must be interrupted in favor of a new regimen following the basic principles of drug resistance treatment detailed later. Nonetheless, some authors advocate the administration of empirical treatments with upto seven drugs until DST results are available, with further adaptation of the regimen subsequent to these results.

Drug Resistance in Retreatment Cases

First and foremost, requirement before starting a retreatment regimen is to assess the possibility whether the person carries resistance strain or not. The two basic approaches for this is by establishment of prior TB treatments and DST reports.[3] In the case of failure, partial default on medication, sustained poor compliance of the patient, or chronicity with multiple previous treatments, the presence of resistance to one or more drugs is very likely whereas in the case of relapse or total treatment default, it can be assumed that there is no resistance. A comprehensive history of previous TB treatments requires complete chronology of the previous introduction and cessation of drugs, including administered doses and pharmacological associations of prior regimens. This allows the evaluation of real or masked monotherapies previously received by the patient. The main predictor of resistance to a particular drug is the demonstration of its prior use in monotherapy for more than one month.[3, 12] Sometimes resistance develops if the patient was on the functional equivalent of two drugs, depending on the drugs concerned. For example, pyrazinamide is not considered a good companion drug to prevent resistance. If a patient was receiving functionally only rifampicin and pyrazinamide in the initial phase (because of resistance to isoniazid and ethambutol), resistance to rifampicin may develop. Thus, it is crucial to consider which functional drugs the patient received between the time of DST specimen collection and the time of the new regimen design (i.e. consider whether resistance has developed to any of the functional drugs).

In practice, the quality of information collected through this medical history is better than that from DST, which can take > 3 months (when carried out by conventional methods on solid media) and may also fail due to insufficient growth of cultures. Susceptibility testing for isoniazid, rifampicin, the fluoroquinolones, and the injectable agents is fairly reliable. For other agents it is less reliable, and basing individualized treatments on DST for these agents should be avoided. The clinical effectiveness or ineffectiveness of a drug cannot be predicted by DST with 100% certainty.[16,17] DST to pyrazinamide (Z) requires Bactec, a radiometric method not available in most low-income countries.[13-17] It should be pointed out that drug resistance, as detected in the DST, reflects the inefficacy of this drug in culture media, but drug susceptibility does not necessarily correspond to the efficacy of the drug within a new regimen; the latter can be estimated in view of the history of previous treatments. Laboratories too vary in reliability and errors may occur in laboratory also and it is often seen that different sensitivity pattern reports are obtained from different laboratories at different times. Therefore, the DST results should not be relied uncritically especially without the background of previous drug history. At present, it appears that DST results concerning second-line drugs such as kanamycin (Km) and ofloxacin/ciprofloxacin could be of great help, but not DST to other drugs.[16]

Category II Regimen for Retreatment TB Patients

In the case of failure, partial default on medication, or chronicity with multiple previous treatments, the presence of resistance to one or more drugs is very likely. The reinforced first-line drug 8–9 month regimen (Category II regimen employed in India) can cure most relapses and treatment defaults (the most common sources of patients for retreatment) and a variable proportion of initial failures. The difficulty with the 8–9 month regimen is the group representing failure of the initial treatment and patients carrying multidrug resistant strains of *M. tuberculosis*. Short-course chemotherapy (SCC) for patients infected with drug-resistant strains may create even more resistance to the drugs in use. This has been termed the "amplifier effect" of SCC[18] which implies that resistant strains in bacterial population are selected repeatedly when a regimen is used continuously over a long period in a given community and these become dominant strains. The argument against Category II regimen for retreatment cases by many physicians is the fear of adding a single drug to a failing regimen, causing emergence of further drug resistance, particularly MDR. Therefore, in the case of failure of an initial 6-month regimen, i.e. Category I regimen, there is a high risk of resistance to H and R and so, if an 8-month regimen or Category II regimen is prescribed, it would amount to masked monotherapy with ethambutol during the last 5 months of treatment.[3] This entails a high risk of amplifying resistance to ethambutol and will not cure the patient. Likewise, if the patient has been initially infected with an MDR strain of *M. tuberculosis* (primary MDR) and fails to respond to the initial 6-month regimen, selection of resistance to ethambutol and pyrazinamide during the initial 2 months of treatment is very likely, because the combination of these two drugs is weak, in the context of inefficiency of H and R. In this case, administration of the 8-month treatment regimen would be equivalent to masked monotherapy with streptomycin in the initial phase, with a high risk of amplifying resistance to streptomycin.[3] No sufficient data are available on the response of patients with TB who have multidrug resistance to SCC with first-line drugs under routine countrywide control program conditions. Currently, the only few available data are from patients treated in limited or special settings[19, 20] or in few clinical trials.[21-23] A retrospective study to assess the results of treatment with first-line drugs for patients enrolled in the WHO and the International Union Against Tuberculosis and Lung Disease's global project on drug-resistance surveillance was carried out in 6 countries. These data suggest that standard short-course chemotherapy, based on first-line drugs, was an inadequate treatment for some patients with drug-resistant TB.[10] A study from Vietnam[22] had reported 80% of Category I failure cases to have MDR-TB. A recent study done from a rural area of Tamil Nadu showed that out of Category I regimen using DOTS treatment; only 17% (10 of 60) had organisms resistant to isoniazid and rifampicin (MDR-TB) from sputum collected of 60 patients out of 74 cases declared as failures (smear positive at 5/6 months of treatment) to Category I regimen.[23]

These findings suggest that the current WHO policy of administration of the 5 first-line drugs as standard retreatment regimens needs to be revisited according to the availability of resources and DST, the prevalence of multidrug resistant TB, and the prevailing quality of TB control. Although the proportion of failures is small, in a high burden country such as India, the absolute number of failures is high. A change in the present policy to use 'stronger regimens' for these patients will have other implications. Providing culture and drug susceptibility testing for such a large number of patients across the country is logistically and economically non-feasible in low-income countries like India. Under the new guidelines of RNTCP (Revised National Tuberculosis Control Program in India), any patient who fails a Category I or III treatment regimen or any Category II patient who remains smear positive at the end of the fourth month of treatment or later will be identified as "*MDR-TB suspect*" and will be subjected to sputum culture and DST.[24] Timely identification of DR-TB and adequate second-line treatment regimens (Category IV regimens see below) administered early in the course of the disease are essential to stop primary transmission. Experience has shown that implementing a DR-TB control program substantially strengthens overall TB control for both drug-susceptible and drug-resistant cases.[25]

Non-MDR

These include patients with mono-resistant TB and patients with poly-resistant TB other than MDR-TB. *Mono-resistance* refers to resistance to a single first-line drug, and *poly-resistance* refers to resistance to two or more first-line drugs but not to both isoniazid and rifampicin. Cases with mono- or poly-resistance will be identified during the course of case-finding for MDR-TB. Treatment of patients infected with mono-or poly-resistant strains using standardized SCC has been associated with increased risk of treatment failure and further acquired resistance, including the development of MDR-TB.[22, 26]

Treatment of such patients include using regimens which are considered "modifications" of Category I or Category II treatment and the adjusted treatment continued for the indicated length of time.[18] When a decision has been made to modify standardized SCC, the most effective regimen should be chosen from the start to maximize the likelihood of cure; effective drugs should not be withheld for later use. They are not classified as Category IV (see below) treatments, which are regimens designed to treat MDR-TB. Definitive randomized or controlled studies have not been performed to determine the best treatment for various patterns of drug resistance, except for streptomycin resistance.[18]

Chronic TB Case

A chronic case of TB is defined as a TB patient who remains smear-positive after completing a retreatment regimen.[1] Chronic cases form the most complex part of problem encompassing patients undergoing retreatment because they have been received multiple treatments, are thought to carry higher degree of resistance strains to primary line drugs and second-line drugs (SLDs) depending on their usage. The management of this high-risk group entails DST for at least the primary line drugs and DST for SLD if there is previous history of treatment with SLD and commencement of standardized or individualized regimen based on resource setting as detailed below.

MDR-TB

Among the few drugs available for the treatment of tuberculosis (TB), only isoniazid (H) and rifampicin (R) are highly effective. Curing TB patients with resistance to at least both of these drugs, multidrug-resistant tuberculosis (MDR-TB), is therefore very difficult and presents huge challenges worldwide. As per RNTCP report, the number of patients who were registered under Category II during the year 2006 was 185, 718 (RNTCP Central TB Division, India: Personal communication). Out of these, the total number of patients declared cured was 113845, i.e. 61.3% and the number of patients who were classified as failure, treatment default and died during Category II treatment were 10400 (5.6%), 30643 (16.5%), and 3157 (1.7%) respectively. Based on studies done, assuming that approximate 50% of Category II failures have MDR pattern of resistance then according to this report the probable number of MDR patients would then be approximately 5200 (i.e. 50% of 10400). Also taking into account the possibility that MDR strains would have been present in patients who died and defaulted during the course of treatment, so then assuming that 50% of these two categories were also MDR, the total number of MDR patients in the year 2006 in India under RNTCP would be around 27,671 (50% of total of Category II Failure + Died + Default). According to the WHO/IUATLD 4th global survey, the estimated prevalence of primary and acquired MDR-TB in India is 2.8% (95% CI, 2.3–3.4%) and 17.2% (95% CI, 15.0–19.7), respectively[27] and the number of estimated cases of MDR-TB in India during 2006 was 110,132 (95% CI, 79,975–142,386).[27] This huge deficit between the two figures speaks volumes of huge number of patients being treated outside the tuberculosis control program of our country and also throws light on the grim situation our country faces when it comes to discrepancies in management of DR-TB between the private and government sector.

The diagnosis of MDR-TB should be based on the patient's treatment history (failure of standard regimens, exposure to patients with MDR-TB, etc.) and on the results of DST[28] against H and R, for which reliability approaches 100%.[29] Even then, it takes three months or more to confirm the diagnosis. During this period, they can spread the multidrug-resistant disease to others. WHO with the Stop TB Partnership, UNITAID and the Foundation for Innovative New Diagnostics (FIND) together unveiled a new policy endorsing use of Line Probe Assays[30] and GeneXpert MTB/RIF[31] in low resource countries like India. The advantages include rapid screening of patients with MDR-TB risk within 2 hours to 2 days as compared to 2–3 months for conventional cultures.

The number of drugs needed to constitute a good retreatment regimen in the patients with MDR-TB is one of the most controversial topics debated and the conclusion is that clinical trials, comparing different number and type of drugs, are necessary to develop the evidence base for the most appropriate treatment of MDR-TB. The statement from the American Thoracic Society/Centers for Disease Control and Prevention/Infectious Diseases Society of America (ATS/CDC/IDSA) states that regimens employing four to six medications appear to be associated with better results.[32] They concluded that acceptable results have been obtained using more than four drugs, with favorable responses varying between 65%[33] and 85.5%.[34] However, the problem with administration of four, six, or more drugs is a high probability of intolerance by the patient who will default from treatment or will refuse to take it when faced with the appearance of severe side effects. It is not insignificant that in the 30–54.4% of patients experienced side effects that compelled them to discontinue one or two drugs.[33,35] A study from India showed that 16 out of 39 patients, i.e. 41% developed side effects and out of which 8 patients (21.1%) developed significant side effects that required the stoppage/change of drugs.[36] Given the significant global increase in MDR-TB in recent years, more solid evidence validating the various recommendations will certainly come to light in the near future.

Now for the treatment of MDR-TB patients whether to use individualized or standardized regimen the main principles of individualized regimen being the selection of treatment based on the individual DST results and elaboration of aggressive therapeutic regimens in settings that allow close follow-up of patients by skilled professionals. Several published studies have reported the efficacy of this strategy.[37–43] This is, however, a highly expensive approach that is difficult to implement in the majority of middle- and low-income countries like India which bear the high burden of MDR-TB. As many countries have employed very few second-line drugs in recent years, the microorganisms would be expected to be more susceptible to these than would be assumed from the often unreliable DST results.[3] For this reason, the WHO recommendations for the treatment of MDR-TB favored the use of standardized treatment regimens in such circumstances.[44,45] Standard treatment regimens for these MDR-TB patients facilitate their management, reduce the number of specialist physicians needed and reduce the overall cost of treatment by five to ten times. The efficacy of this strategy has been confirmed by reports in the literature.[46]

DOTS-Plus is an integral component of RNTCP to manage MDR-TB to be implemented through program infrastructure.[24] The strategy is designed to manage MDR-TB using second-line anti-TB drugs within the DOTS strategy in low- and middle-income countries like India. Therefore in every DOTS implementing unit of the country, DOTS would be prioritized above DOTS-Plus with the view that DOTS reduces the emergence of MDR-TB, and therefore the need for DOTS-Plus over time. The RNTCP under DOTS-PLUS will be using a standardized treatment regimen (STR) Category IV regimen, comprising of 6 drugs (kanamycin, levofloxcin, ethionamide, cycloserine, pyrazinamide and ethambutol) during 6–9 months of the intensive phase and 4 drugs (levofloxcin, ethionamide, cycloserine and ethambutol) during the 18 months of the continuation phase. *Para*-aminosalicylic acid (PAS) is included in the regimen as a substitute drug if any bactericidal drug (kanamycin, ofloxacin/levofloxcin, ethionamide and pyrazinamide) or any 2 bacteriostatic (ethambutol and cycloserine) drugs are not tolerated. This Category IV regimen is highly suitable for high TB prevalence as well low to middle income countries like India. Injectable agent should be given at least 6 months and the whole treatment duration is minimum of 18 months beyond sputum conversion. Fully standardized second-line treatment have shown to be feasible and cost-effective in MDR-TB treatment.[47]

PREVENTION OF RETREATMENT CASES

Tuberculosis is still a curable disease and the main crux is the initial treatment which is said to be most important and safest bet in curing the disease without any relapse and preventing drug resistant strains from developing. However, the irony of the fact is the irrational and improper use of ATT, be it in dosage, duration, quality of drugs or even in the number of drugs which is still rampant in our country. Even though by March 2006 nationwide DOTS coverage had been achieved, however the ground reality is that private sector in India[48] still continues to play a big role in management of TB patients. A recent study in India to analyze the prescription patterns of private doctors for TB patients found that 33 different regimens were prescribed by 449 doctors and 45% doctors did not practice current NTP/ WHO recommended regimens and 75% doctors made prescription errors.[49] This is probably an area which our country can be benefitted by proper education of both practioners and public alike. Sensing this need, WHO came up with the Stop TB Strategy (which aims to reduce dramatically the burden of TB by 2015) and one of the main components of this strategy is by scaling up public-private mix (PPM) to bridge down the gap between the private and government sector by engaging all care providers, including public, nongovernmental and private providers, and other approaches to ensure adherence to international standards of TB care.

CONCLUSION

Presently in our country which is still lacking in resources, all retreatment cases should be given Category II regimen under DOTS (2SRHEZ/RHEZ/5RHE either daily or thrice weekly) and ideally if possible their sputum cultures should be sent for DST even before the start of the retreatment regimen to identify the drug resistant strains at the earliest. Efforts to ensure that good, reliable and adequate number of laboratory services for the timely diagnosis of drug resistant strains be made available throughout the country. Now that DOTS has been implemented throughout our country and the foremost aim at present is the fast implementation of DOTS-Plus program throughout the country at the earliest. Along with this, proper education on the management aspects of retreatment cases including drug resistant and multidrug resistant TB should be imparted to all the practioners of the country. The proper use of second-line drugs must be ensured to cure existing multidrug resistant tuberculosis, to reduce transmission of MDR-TB and to prevent the emergence of XDR-TB.

REFERENCES

1. World Health Organization. Treatment of TB Guidelines - 4th edition. WHO/HTM/TB/2009.420
2. Global tuberculosis control: surveillance, planning, financing. WHO report 2008. Geneva, World Health Organization, 2008 (WHO/HTM/TB/2008.393).
3. Caminero JA. Management of multidrug-resistant tuberculosis and patients in retreatment. Eur Respir J. 2005;25:928-36.
4. Caminero JA. Guía de la tuberculosis para médicos especialistas. [Tuberculosis Guide for Specialist Physicians]. Paris, International Union Against Tuberculosis and Lung Disease, 2003.
5. Caminero JA, Pena MJ, Campos-Herrero MI, et al. Exogenous reinfection with tuberculosis on a European island with a moderate incidence of disease. Am J Respir Crit Care Med. 2001;163:717-20.
6. Van Rie A, Warren R, Richardson M, et al. Exogenous reinfection as a cause of recurrent tuberculosis after curative treatment. N Engl J Med. 1999;341:1174-9.
7. Moulding T, putt A, reichman L. Fixed dose combinations of tuberculosis medications to prevent drug resistance. Annals of Internal Medicine. 1995;122:951-4.
8. Enarson Da, Rieder HL, Arnadottir T, Trébucq A. Management of tuberculosis: a guide for low income countries. 5th edn. Paris, International Union Against Tuberculosis and Lung Disease, 2000.
9. Tuberculosis Research Center, Indian Council of Medical Research. Low rate of emergence of drug resistance in sputum positive patients treated with short course chemotherapy. Int J Tuberc Lung Dis. 2001;5:40-5.
10. Prasad R, Verma SK, Garg R, Jain A, Anand SC, Hosmane GB, et al. Drug susceptibility pattern of Mycobacterium tuberculosis isolates from patients of category-II failure of pulmonary tuberculosis under directly observed treatment short-course from north India, Biosci Trends. 2012;6:110-4.
11. Espinal ma, kim sj, suarez pg, et al. Standard short-course chemotherapy for drug-resistant tuberculosis: treatment outcomes in 6 countries. JAMA. 2000;283:2537-45.
12. Mitchison DA. The segregation of streptomycin-resistant variants of *Mycobacterium tuberculosis* into groups with characteristic levels of resistance. J Gen Microbiol. 1951;5:596-604.
13. Caminero JA. Guía de la tuberculosis para médicos especialistas. [Tuberculosis Guide for Specialist Physicians]. Paris, International Union Against Tuberculosis and Lung Disease, 2003.
14. Iseman MD. Treatment of multidrug-resistant tuberculosis. N Engl J Med. 1993;329:784-91.
15. Ortega A. Retratamientos en tuberculosis. [Retreatment in tuberculosis]. Rev Clin Esp. 1987;180:269-74.
16. Kim SJ. Drug-susceptibility testing in tuberculosis: methods and reliability of the results. Eur Respir J. 2005;25:564-9.
17. Canetti G. Present aspects of bacterial resistance in tuberculosis. Am Rev Respir Dis. 1965;92:687-703.
18. Guidelines for the programmatic management of drug resistant tuberculosis—WHO 2008.
19. Garcia-Garcia M, Ponce-de-Leon A, Jiménez-Corona M, et al. Clinical consequences and transmissibility of drug-resistant tuberculosis in Southern Mexico. Arch Intern Med. 2000;160:630-6.
20. Coninx R, Mathieu C, Debacker M, et al. First-line tuberculosis therapy and drug-resistant *Mycobacterium tuberculosis* in prisons. Lancet. 1999;353:969-73.
21. Mitchinson D, Nunn AJ. Influence of initial drug resistance on the response to short-course chemotherapy of pulmonary tuberculosis. Am Rev Respir Dis. 1986;133:423-30.
22. Quy HWT, Lan NTN, Borgdoff MW, et al. Drug susceptibility among failures and relapse cases of tuberculosis: Is standard re-treatment regimen adequate? Int J Tub Lung Dis. 2003;7:631-6.

23. Santha T, Gopi PG, Rajeswari R, Selvakumar N, Subramani R, Chandrasekaran V, et al. Is it worth treating category I failure patients with Category II regimen? Indian J Tuberc. 2005;52:203-6.
24. DOTS PLUS guidelines, Revised National Tuberculosis Control Programme, Central TB Division Directorate General Health Services, Ministry of Health & Family Welfare, Nirman Bhawan, New Delhi. Sep 2008.
25. Kim JY, et al. From multidrug-resistant tuberculosis to DOTS expansion and beyond: making the most of a paradigm shift. *Tuberculosis (Edinb).* 2003;83:59-65.
26. Tuberculosis Research Centre, Chennai, India. Low rate of emergence of drug resistance in sputum positive patients treated with short-course chemotherapy. Int J of Tub and Lung Dis. 2001;5:40-5.
27. WHO IUALTD Global Project on Anti-Tuberculosis Drug Resistance Surveillance (2002-2007), Fourth Global Report (2008).
28. American Thoracic Society. Treatment of drug-resistant tuberculosis. Am Rev Respir Dis. 1966;94:125-7.
29. Kim SJ. Drug-susceptibility testing in tuberculosis: methods and reliability of results. Eur Respir J. 2005;25:564-9.
30. WHO Press Release New Rapid Test for DR-TB for developing Countries Geneva, June 30 2008.
31. Towards universal access to diagnosis and treatment of multidrug-resistant and extensively drug resistant tuberculosis by 2015. WHO progress report 2011. WHO/HTM/TB/2011.3.
32. American Thoracic Society Documents. American Thoracic Society/Centers for Disease Control and Prevention/Infectious Diseases Society of America: treatment of tuberculosis. Am J Respir Crit Care Med. 2003;167:603-62.
33. Goble M, Iseman MD, Madsen LA, Waite D, Ackerson L, Horsburgh R. Treatment of 171 patients with pulmonary tuberculosis resistant to isoniazid and rifampin. N Engl J Med. 1993;328:527-32.
34. Park SK, Kim CT, Song SD. Outcome of chemotherapy in 107 patients with pulmonary tuberculosis resistant to isoniazid and rifampin. Int J Tuberc Lung Dis. 1998;2:877-84.
35. Geerligs WA, Altena R, de Lange WCM, van Soolingen D, van der Werf TS. Multidrug-resistant tuberculosis: long-term treatment outcome in the Netherlands. Int J Tuberc Lung Dis. 2000;4:758-64.
36. Prasad R, Verma SK, Sahai S, Kumar S, Jain A. Efficacy and safety of kanamycin, ethionamide, PAS, and cycloserine in multiresistant resistant pulmonary tuberculosis patients. Ind J Chest Dis Allied Sci. 2006;48:183-6.
37. Mukherjee J, Socci A, Acha J, et al. The PIH guide to management of multidrug-resistant tuberculosis. International edition. Boston, MA, USA: Partners in Health, 2003.
38. Mukherjee JS, Rich ML, Socci AR, et al. Programmes and principles in treatment for multidrug-resistant tuberculosis. Lancet. 2004;363:474-81.
39. Tahaoglu K, Törün T, Sevim T, et al. The treatment of multidrug-resistant tuberculosis in Turkey. N Engl J Med. 2001;345:170-4.
40. Narita M, Alonso P, Lauzardo M, Hollender ES, Pitchenik AE, Ashkin D. Treatment experience of multidrug-resistant tuberculosis in Florida, 1994–1997. Chest. 2001;120:343-8.
41. Chan ED, Laurel V, Strand MJ, et al. Treatment and outcome analysis of 205 patients with multidrug-resistant tuberculosis. Am J Respir Crit Care Med. 2004;169:1103-9.
42. Park SK, Lee CM, Heu JP, Song SD. A retrospective study for the outcome of pulmonary resection in 49 patients with multidrug-resistant tuberculosis. Int J Tuberc Lung Dis. 2002;6:143-9.
43. Evan W Orenstein BS, Sanjay Basu, N Sarita Shah, et al. Treatment outcomes among patients with multidrug-resistant tuberculosis: systematic review and meta-analysis. Lancet Infect Dis. 2009;9:153-61.

44. Crofton J, Chaulet P, Maher D, et al. Guidelines for the management of drug-resistant tuberculosis. WHO/TB/96.210.Geneva, Switzerland: WHO, 1997.
45. Prasad R. Management of multidrug resistance tuberculosis practitioner's view point. Indian J Tub. 2007;54:3-11.
46. Van Deun A, Hamid Salim MA, Kumar Das AP, Bastian I, Portaels F. Results of a standardised regimen for multidrug resistant tuberculosis in Bangladesh. Int J Tuberc Lung Dis. 2004;8:560-7.
47. Suarez PG, et al. Feasibility and cost-effectiveness of standardised second-line drug treatment for chronic tuberculosis patients; a national cohort study in Peru. Lancet. 2002;359:1980-9.
48. Uplekar MW, Shepard DS. Treatment of tuberculosis by private general practitioners in India. Tubercle. 1991;72:284-90.
49. Prasad R, Nautiyal RG, Mukherji PK, Jain A, et al Treatment of new pulmonary tuberculosis patients: what do allopathic doctors do in India? Int J Tuberc Lung Dis. 2002;6:895-902.

Chapter 24

Drug Resistant and Multidrug Resistant Tuberculosis: Current Status

INTRODUCTION

Drug resistant tuberculosis has been reported since the early days of introduction of antitubercular chemotherapy, but multidrug resistant tuberculosis (MDR-TB) has been an area of growing concern, and is posing threat to global efforts of tuberculosis control. The exact magnitude of the problem of MDR-TB worldwide was not known till the 1994–97 global project on antituberculosis drug resistance surveillance initiated by WHO and International Union Against Tuberculosis and Lung Disease (IUATLD). Prevalence of MDR-TB mirrors the functional state and efficacy of tuberculosis control programs and realistic attitude of the community towards implementation of such programs.[1] With potent antitubercular drugs and effective treatment strategies like DOTS presently available worldwide, we hope to prevent the further development of MDR-TB. More than 400,000 cases of MDR-TB emerge every year as a result of poor management of drug sensitive as well as drug resistant TB. This chapter aims to review the present scenario of multidrug-resistant tuberculosis.

DEFINITION

Drug resistant tuberculosis is defined as a case of tuberculosis excreting bacilli resistant to one or more antitubercular drugs. Multidrug resistant tuberculosis (MDR-TB) is defined as disease due to *M. tuberculosis* that is resistant to isoniazid and rifampicin with or without resistance to other drugs (the culture and drug susceptibility test result being from an RNTCP accredited laboratory). Mono-resistance is defined as resistance to one antituberculosis drug where as poly-resistance is defined as resistance to more than one antituberculosis drug, other than both isoniazid and rifampicin.

TYPES OF DRUG RESISTANCE

Drug resistance may be of two types—Primary and Acquired. Primary drug resistance may be defined as drug resistance in a patient who has not received any antitubercular treatment in the past. The resistance that develops in a patient who has received prior chemotherapy is defined as acquired drug resistance. Recently the terms "resistance in new cases" and "resistance in previously treated cases" have been proposed for use because of the difficulty to confirm the validity of the patients past history of treatment. When one is not sure whether the resistance is primary or acquired due to concealed history of previous treatment or unawareness of treatment taken before, it is known as initial drug resistance. Thus, initial resistance is primary resistance plus some undisclosed acquired resistance. Combined resistance is defined as the sum of primary and acquired resistance.

PREVALENCE OF MDR-TB: GLOBAL

A review by WHO of a series of 63 surveys of drug resistant TB carried out between 1985–1994 led to the conclusion that the problem of drug resistance was global.[2] The overall percentages of resistance to different antituberculosis drugs obtained from different surveys done throughout the world are shown in Tables 24.1 and 24.2. The rate of MDR-TB was very low in most of the surveys ranging from 0–10.8% in the case of primary resistance and from 0–48% for acquired resistance. Multidrug resistance was reported to range from 0.5–14.3% in surveys where there was no distinction between primary and acquired resistance. In most regions of the world, the rates of MDR-TB were very low,[2] except in New York and Nepal where high rates of acquired type MDR-TB were reported. It is evident that prevalence of drug resistant tuberculosis varied considerably throughout the world. The reasons for this variation in different surveys were the degree of selection of patient studied, the degree of misuse of drugs, the quality of enquiry regarding previous treatment and the inadequate culture and drug susceptibility facilities in many parts of the world.

Considering the limitation of the previous studies, a WHO/IUATLD global project of drug resistance surveillance spread over 35 countries in 5 continents was carried out between 1994–1997.[3] Median prevalence of primary and acquired multidrug resistance was reported to be 1.4% (0–14.4%) and 13% (0–54.4%), respectively (Tables 24.1 and 24.2). Particularly high prevalence of multi-drug resistance was found in the former Soviet Union, Asia, Argentina and the Dominican Republic. The WHO for the first time introduced the term MDR 'hotspot' where high prevalence of MDR has been observed. The 'hotspots' referred to the countries or regions where the combined prevalence of MDR TB exceeded 5%. The report concluded that resistance to anti-TB drugs was found in all 35 countries and regions surveyed, suggesting again that the problem was global.

Table 24.1: Global primary/initial drug resistance

Study	Any Drug	Any H %	Any S %	Any R %	Any E %	H+R %
Cohn, et al. review of 63 surveys (1985–1994)[2]	-	0 – 16.9	0.1–23.5	0 – 3.0	0 – 4.2	0 – 10.8
WHO-IUATLD 1994–1997 surveillance[3]	9.9 (2.0–40.6)	7.3 (1.5–31.7)	6.5 (0.3–8.0)	1.8 (0–16.8)	1.0 (0–9.9)	1.4 (0–14.4)
WHO-IUATLD 1996–1999 surveillance[6]	10.7 (1.7–36 .9)	6.2 (0–28.1)	5.2 (0.3–32.4)	1.2 (0–15.8)	0.6 (0–11.1)	1.0 (0–14.1)
WHO-IUATLD 1999–2002 surveillance[12]	10.2 (0–57.1)	5.7 (0–42.6)	6.3 (0–51.5)	1.4 (0–15.6)	0.8 (0–24.8)	1.1 (0–4.2)
WHO-IUATLD 2002–2007 surveillance[14]	17 (0–56.3)	10.3 (0–42.4)	10.9 (0–51.5)	3.7 (0–22.7)	2.5 (0–24.8)	2.9 (0–22.3)
M/XDR-TB Global report on surveillance and response 2010[14]						1.5 (0–28.3)
Global TB report 2012[15]						3.7 (0–32.3)

Table 24.2: Global acquired drug resistance

Study	Any Drug	Any H %	Any S %	Any R %	Any E%	H+R%
Cohn–et al. review of 63 surveys (1985–1994)[2]	-	4–53.7	0–19.4	0–14.5	0–13.7	0–48.0
WHO-IUATLD 1994–1997 surveillance[3]	36.0 (5.3–100)	-	-	-	-	13.0 (0–54.4)
WHO-IUATLD 1996–1999 surveillance[6]	23.3 (0–93.8)	19.6	12.4 (0–53.4)	12.0 (0–50.0)	5.9 (0–32.1)	9.3 (0–48.2)
WHO-IUATLD 1999–2002 surveillance[12]	18.4 (0–82.1)	14.4 (0–71)	11.4 (0–77.1)	8.7 (0–61.4)	3.5 (0–54.2)	7.0 (0–58.3)
WHO-IUATLD 2002–2007 surveillance[14]	35 (0–85.9)	27.7 (0–81.2)	20.1 (0–83.5)	17.5 (0–62.5)	10.3 (0–54.3)	15.3 (0–62.5)
M/XDR-TB Global report on surveillance and response 2010[14]						7.9 (0–61.6)
Global TB report 2012[15]						20 (0–65)

A second WHO/IUATLD global project on drug resistance surveillance in 58 countries/geographical sites was carried out in 1996–1999.[4] Trends of drug resistance were also observed from 28 sites. Median prevalence of primary and acquired multidrug resistance was reported in 1% (0–14%) and 9% (0–48%), respectively. Of the 58 sites surveyed drug resistance among new and previously treated cases were reported in 54 and 48 sites, respectively. Most of the previous 'hotspots' of MDR-TB were confirmed again; however new areas in Russia and China were added. This global survey tested a total of 61,415 patients with tuberculosis (Median per site 661; range 41–12675). These sites accounted for 610,000 (18%) of 3.3 million cases of tuberculosis reported to WHO in 1997 and 1.5 billion (26%) of the world's 5.8 billion inhabitants. Several countries including 11 of the 22 world tuberculosis high burdened countries had not yet been surveyed. A mathematical model had estimated the magnitude of MDR-TB worldwide and suggested that in year 2000, 3% (273,000; 95% CI, 185,000–414,000) of all new and previously treated TB cases were MDR-TB.[5] The trend analysis confirmed that MDR-TB was not a major problem in countries implementing TB control according to international guidelines for several years. Botswana, Chile, Cuba and Czech Republic and Uruguay have all showed very low prevalence of MDR-TB confirming that efficient TB control prevents the outset and spread of MDR TB.[4,6-11]

A third WHO/IUATLD global project on drug resistance surveillance in 77 countries/geographical sites was carried out in 1999–2002[12] representing 20% of the global total of new smear-positive TB cases. It included 39 settings not previously included in global project and reported trends for 46 settings. Median prevalence of primary and acquired multidrug resistance was reported in 1.1% (0–14.2%) and 7% (0–58.3%), respectively (Tables 24.1 and 24.2). This report analyzed the distribution of MDR prevalence (among new cases) from 74 settings. After analysis the cut-off value for hotspots was reset to MDR prevalence of more than 6.5% among new cases. There were 10 countries regarded as hotspots with MDR-TB prevalence, viz. Ecuador (6.6%), Henan (7.8%), Latvia (9.3%), Lithuania (9.4%), Liaoning (10.4%), Estonia (12.2%), Uzbekistan (13.2%), Tomsk Oblast (13.7%), Israel (14.2%) and Kazakhstan (14.2%). Despite the expansion in coverage of drug-resistance surveillance for both new and previously treated cases in recent years, data on drug resistance are still not available for more than 100 countries. To estimate the levels of drug resistance in places where direct data are not available, Matteo Zignol, et al.[13] had developed statistical models for settings where data were available and applied them to places where they are not. After their analysis they have revealed the total number of MDR-TB cases estimated to have occurred worldwide in 2004 is 424,203 (95% CI, 376,019–620,061), or 4.3% (95% CI, 3.8%–6.1%) of all new and previously treated TB cases. Three countries—China, India, and the Russian Federation—accounted for 261,362 (95% CI, 180,779–414,749) MDR-TB cases, or 62% of the estimated global burden. In the same year, the total number of MDR-TB cases was 2.7% (95% CI, 2.4–3.8%) of 8,987,743 new cases (242,794,95% CI, 209,363–350,291) and 18.4% (95%CI, 14.2–31.7%) of previously treated cases (181,408; 95% CI, 135,276–319,017). This study provides a new comprehensive set of estimates of the incidence of MDR-TB in 184 countries and globally. They have found lower rates of MDR-TB in countries of Central Europe such as Hungary, Macedonia and Turkey in comparison to previous studies. Their study showed a positive correlation between proportion of patients who had previously received treatment and proportion of MDR-TB cases among new cases.

A fourth WHO/IUATLD global project on drug resistance surveillance included drug susceptibility test results (DST) from 91,577 patients from 93 settings in 81 countries and 2 special administrative regions (SARs) of China collected between 2002 and 2007, and representing 35% of the global total of notified new smear-positive TB cases.[14] It included data from 33 countries that have never been previously reported. New data were included from the high TB burden countries like India, China, Russian Federation, Indonesia, Ethiopia, Philippines, Vietnam, Thailand and Myanmar. Between 1994 and 2007 a total of 138 settings in 114 countries and 2 SARs of China had reported data to the global project. The median prevalence of primary and acquired MDR-TB globally was 2.9% (95%CI, 2.2–3.6%) and 15.3% (95% CI, 9.6–21.1%), respectively. The global population weighted proportion of multidrug resistance among all TB cases was 5.3%(95% CI, 3.9–6.6%). It is estimated that 489,139 MDR-TB cases emerged in 2006 globally and the global proportion of multidrug resistance among all new and previously treated cases is 4.8%. According to the new data, China and India carry approximately 50% of the global burden and Russia a further 7% in 2008. Multidrug and extensively drug-resistant TB (M/XDR-TB) 2010 global report on surveillance and response, estimated that 440,000 (95% CI, 390,000–510,000) cases of MDR-TB emerged globally in 2008. Among all incident TB cases globally, 3.6% (95% CI, 3.0–4.4%) are estimated to have MDR-TB. These estimates, which lie in the same range as the previous ones, are based on more data and a revised methodology. Almost 50% of MDR-TB cases worldwide are estimated to occur in China and India. In 2008, MDR-TB caused an estimated 150,000 deaths.[14]

The Global Tuberculosis Report 2012 summarizes the latest status of progress in global surveillance of anti-TB drug resistance, using the most recent data on multidrug resistance TB (MDR-TB), extensively drug-resistant TB (XDR-TB). Data on drug resistance has been systematically collected and analyzed from 135 countries worldwide (70% of WHO's 194 Member States). This includes 63 countries that have continuous surveillance systems based on routine diagnostic drug susceptibility testing (DST) of all TB patients and 72 countries that rely on special surveys of representative samples of patients. During the past 4 years, most of the 27 high MDR-TB and 22 high TB burden countries have expanded coverage of surveillance of drug resistance to obtain more accurate estimates of the burden of MDR-TB. Globally, 3.7% (95% CI, 2.1–5.2%) of new cases and 20% (95% CI, 13–26%) of previously treated cases estimated to have MDR-TB. Proportions of MDR TB in new TB cases ranged from 0% to 32.3% and were highest in Belarus (32.3%), Estonia (22.9%), Kazakhstan (30.3%), Kyrgyzstan (26.4%), the Republic of Moldova (19.4%) and Uzbekistan (23.2%). The proportion of MDR-TB in previously treated TB cases with at country level ranged from 0 to 65.1%. Countries or subnational areas with the highest reported proportions were Azerbaijan (Baku city, 55.8% in 2007), Belarus (75.6% in 2011), Estonia (57.7% in 2011), Kazakhstan (51.3% in 2011), Kyrgyzstan (51.6% in 2011) the Republic of Moldova (63.5% in 2011), Tajikistan (53.6% in 2011) and Uzbekistan (62.0% in 2011). There is an estimated number of 310,000 cases of MDR-TB among the notified cases of TB across the globe in 2011. India, China and Russian Federation contribute to almost 60% of the estimated global burden of MDR-TB.[15]

TRENDS IN MDR-TB: GLOBAL

The global project has collected data from 114 countries and 2 SARs of China and trend analysis includes data from all global reports between 1994 and 2007, as well as data provided between the publication of reports. Analysis were limited to countries reporting three data points or more. Proportions of MDR-TB, isoniazid resistance, and any resistance were examined. Declining trends in MDR-TB were noted in USA, Hong Kong, SAR, China among all TB cases. Hong Kong, SAR, China also showed significant decreases in any resistance among all cases and isoniazid resistance and MDR-TB among new cases. Both countries reported declining TB notifications. Denmark showed significant declines in any drug resistance in both new and combined TB cases. Puerto Rico showed declining trends in any resistance and MDR-TB among combined cases. Singapore showed a significant decrease in prevalence of MDR-TB among all TB cases; however numbers were very small. Countries of the Baltic region (Estonia, Latvia, and Lithuania) showed relatively stable trends in MDR-TB among new cases, with a slow but significant increase in MDR-TB among new cases in Lithuania. The proportion of resistance remained high in these countries, ranging from 9.8% (95% CI, 8.2–11.7) in Lithuania to 13.2% (95% CI, 9.7–17.5) in Estonia. These trends in MDR-TB were coupled with declining TB notification rates in all three countries. Estonia has shown the most rapid decline at about 8% per year. Increasing trends in resistance were reported to the global project from Orel and Tomsk Oblasts of the Russian Federation. These countries showed a statistically significant increase in the proportion of MDR-TB among new TB cases as well as increases in absolute numbers of cases. Both regions showed increase in isoniazid resistance though neither were statistically significant. Both regions showed a slowly declining TB notification rate. During this same time period, TB notification rates for the whole of the Russian Federation have remained stable. The Republic of Korea and Peru have shown increasing trends in MDR-TB, any resistance and isoniazid resistance among new cases. In Peru and the Republic of Korea increase in isoniazid and any resistance were found to be statistically significant. The increase in MDR-TB was statistically significant in the Republic of Korea. The Republic of Korea has shown a steadily declining TB notification rate from 1994 until 2003. From 2004, the TB notification rate has increased slowly; however, this is likely due to expansion of the national surveillance system into the private sector.

The Russian Federation, which was able to provide high-quality continuous surveillance data from 12 of its oblasts and republics, reported proportions of 23.8–28.3% MDR-TB among new TB cases in three of its oblasts in the northwest part of the country. Other Russian oblasts were found to have proportions of MDR-TB as low as 5.4% among new TB cases. Tajikistan, in its first ever survey, found proportions of 16.5% MDR-TB among new TB cases and 61.6% MDR-TB among previously treated TB patients in Dushanbe city and Rudaki district, the highest proportion ever reported among previously treated TB patients. To date, 12 countries have reported nationwide or subnational proportions of MDR-TB of 6% or more among new TB cases. Five of these countries also report MDR-TB proportions of 50% or more among previously treated cases. All of these settings are located in the Eastern Part of Europe or in Central Asia.[14]

PREVALENCE OF MDR-TB: INDIA

Though the development of drug resistance in India was noted since the beginning of the chemotherapeutic era, it was based on clinical perception and several isolated reports, which failed to give an idea of the national situation as a whole. The first definite step was taken in this direction in 1965–67, when the ICMR conducted two surveys to estimate the prevalence of drug resistance.[16,17] Since then several studies have been conducted by various authors in different parts of the country. The total prevalence of primary/initial drug resistance (Table 24.3) was observed to be about 20.49% (5.3–34.9%)[6,12-14,16-30] and multidrug resistance among new cases varied between 0–5%.[20-30] A study conducted by Tuberculosis Research Center, Chennai in collaboration with the National Tuberculosis Institute, Bengaluru using WHO/IUATLD guidelines between 1999-2002 including 6 districts in India showed that incidence of primary MDR-TB ranged from 0.7–2.8%.[28-30] The overall impression as seen in Table 24.3 is that the primary and initial drug resistance has remained more or less constant over the years, including initial multidrug resistance. According to the third Global Report of WHO, total prevalence of drug resistance among new cases in India (Wardha) is 19.8% and MDR is 0.5%.[12]

Table 24.3: Primary/initial drug resistance (India)

Study	Total Prevalence	H %	S %	R %	H+R %
ICMR (1968)[16]	20.4	14.7	12.5	-	-
ICMR (1969)[17]	22	15.5	13.8	-	-
Krishnan Swamy KV, et al. 1976[19]	-	10.6	9.5	-	-
Trivedi, et al. (1988)[18]	20	13.9	7.4	0	0
Chandrasekharan, et al. (1990)[20]	21.2	17.4	5.7	3	1.3
Chandrasekharan, et al. (1992)[21] Rural	34.9	32.8	5.1	4.4	3.4
Urban	20.5	17.3	4.1	2.9	1.4
Parmasivan, et al. (1993)[22] North Arcet of (1985–89)	25.0	13.0	4.0	2.0	1.6
Pondicherry (1985–1991)	13.9	6.0	4.0	0.9	0.7
Gupta, et al. (1993)[23]	19.5	10.1	7.6	3	0.7
Jain, et al. (1993)[24]	-	18.5	-	0.6	0.4
Jena, et al. (1996)[25]	7.9	2.9	4.9	1	0.4
Parmasivan, et al. (2000)[26] (Tamil Nadu)	18.8	15.4	6.8	4.4	3.4
R Prasad, et al. (2001)[27]	27.4	15.6	11.7	3.9	5.0
WHO-IUATLD (1996–1999)[6]	18.8	15.4	6.8	4.4	3.4
Paramasivan, et al. (2002)[28] North Arcot (South)1999	27.7	23.4	12.4	2.8	2.8
Raichur (South) 1999–2000	21.9	18.7	7.2	2.5	2.5
WHO–IUATLD (1999–2002)[12] Wardha	19.8	15.2	7.6	0.5	0.5
Sofia et al (2004)[29] Bangalore City	27.7	13.7	22.5	2.6	2.2
Mahadeo, et al. (2005)[30] Mayurbhanj 2000–2002	5.3	2.5	3.9	0.7	0.7
Hoogli 2000–2001	16.7	10.3	13.7	3.0	3.0
Zignol M, et al. (2006)[13]	-	-	-	-	2.4
WHO/IUATLD (2002–2007)[14]	-	11.7	9.9	2.2	2.8
M/XDR-TB Global report on surveillance and response 2010[14]					2.3
WHO-TB report 2012[15]					2.1

The prevalence of acquired drug resistance (Table 24.4) ranged from 25–100%[3,6,12-14,17,18,24,28,31-35] in several studies. The acquired multidrug resistance rates also varied from 6–100%[24,28,32-35] in the same time period. In a study conducted in Gujarat, it was found that 95% of the R resistant strains were also resistant to H or S or both. The WHO-IUATLD surveillance[3] in India noted the combined prevalence of drug resistance to be 13.3% (95% CI, 10.9–14.9%) in 1998; however, this was done on a small sample of 2240 people around Delhi city and therefore was not representative of the

Table 24.4: Acquired drug resistance (India)

Study	Total Prevalence %	H %	S %	R %	H+R %
ICMR (1969)[16]	32 (22–74)	15–69	12–63	-	-
Trivedi, et al. (1988)[18]					
1980	50.1	34.5	26	2.8	95% of R resistant were resistant to H or S or both
1986	65.3	55.8	-	37.3	-
Dutta M, et al. 1993[31]	-	67.0	26.0	12.0	6.0
Jain, et al. (1992)[24] Delhi	50.7	50.7	-	33.3	33.3
outside Delhi	78.8	78.8	-	61.5	61.5
Chowgule, et al. (1998)[32]	25.6	15	53.6	66.8	10.7
WHO-IUATLD Surveillance (1994–1997)[3]	32.4	28.8	18.1	14	13.3
WHO-IUATLD Surveillance (1999–2002)[6]	50.0	50.0	12.5	25.0	25.0
Shah AR, et al. (2002)[33]	58.67	57.18	35.58	37.47	35.1
Deivanayagam (2002)[34]	71.0	66.3	35.6	55.5	54. 8
Paramasivan, et al. (2002)[28]	81.0	81.0	56.2	69.0	69.0
North Arcot (South) Raichur (South)	100.0	100.0	36.4	100.0	100.0
R Prasad, et al. (2003)[35]	79.2	48.6	36.6	34.4	29.5
Zignol M, et al. (2006)[13]	-	-	-	-	14.7
WHO-IUATLD (2002–2007) surveillance[14]	-	36.8	26.2	18.1	17.2
M/XDR-TB Global report on surveillance and response 2010[14]					17.2
WHO-TB report 2012[15]					15.0

country.[3] The WHO-IUATLD global drug resistance surveillance carried out between 1996-1999 reported that the median prevalence of primary and acquired MDR-TB to be 3.4% (95% CI, 1.8-5.7%) and 25% (95% CI, 7.3-52.3%), respectively.[4] Study conducted in two districts of South India showed that acquired drug resistance ranged from 69-100%.[22] Zignol, et al. estimated the incidence of primary and acquired MDR-TB cases to be 44,653 cases (95% CI, 13,547-85,068) among 1,824,395 new cases or 2.4% (95% CI, 1-5%) and 42,760 cases (95% CI, 6068-171,774) among 290,019 previously treated cases or 14.7% (95% CI, 2.1-56.9%), respectively. The estimated incidence of MDR-TB among new and previously treated cases was 87,413 (4.1%) of all the TB cases in India.[13] The fourth global surveillance of WHO-IUATLD, carried out in 2002–2007 also reported new data from Gujarat giving the first reliable source of data with regard to MDR-TB among previously treated cases in India. Data from nine sites in India show that drug resistance among new cases is relatively low; however, new data from Gujarat indicate that 17.2% MDR among retreatment cases is higher than previously anticipated and it is estimated that 110,132 (95% CI, 79, 975–142, 386) MDR-TB cases emerged in India in 2006, representing over 20% of the global burden. The estimated prevalence of primary and acquired MDR-TB in India is 2.8% (95% CI, 2.3–3.4%) and 17.2% (95% CI, 15.0–19.7), respectively. The estimated prevalence among all TB cases is 4.9% (95% CI, 3.9-6.2%).[14] In India, estimates based on subnational drug resistance data showed that percentage of MDR among new TB cases is 2.3 (1.8–2.8), and in previously treated patients is 17.2 (14.9–19.5). Estimated number of MDR-TB patients in India is 99,000 (95% CI, 79 000–120 000).[14] The estimated prevalence of MDR-TB among notified pulmonary TB patients in India is 5.3% (95% CI, 3.6–6.2%). The estimated prevalence among notified new pulmonary TB patients in 2.1% (95% CI, 1.5–2.7%) and in retreatment pulmonary TB patients is 15% (95% CI, 13–17%). India accounted far an estimated 64,000 cases of MDR-TB among the notified TB cases in 2011.[15] These studies were conducted in different states mostly in institutions and tertiary care centers and they do not reflect the overall status of drug resistance problem in India. It is therefore necessary to conduct a country wide multi-center drug resistance surveillance comprising both rural and urban areas in order to have a picture of the total situation in the country.

HIV INFECTION AND MULTIDRUG RESISTANT TUBERCULOSIS

There is a well-documented association between TB and human immunodeficiency virus (HIV). Outbreaks of drug resistant forms of tuberculosis among HIV infected patients have been widely documented in nosocomial and other congregate settings[36,37] but little information is available about the association of HIV and drug resistant TB on a population level.[38,39] The primary reason for the lack of information is that HIV and anti-TB drug susceptibility testing have not been sufficiently accessible for joint surveys under routine conditions. The accelerating and amplifying influence of HIV infection and the delay in recognition and diagnosis of tuberculosis were found to contribute to outbreaks of MDR-TB among HIV infected patients in USA.[36,40-42] Shafer, et al.[43] studied temporal trends and transmission patterns in New York city using restriction fragment length polymorphism (RFLP) and found clustering of MDR-TB cases, particularly among HIV infected persons who suffered disproportionately from drug-resistant disease, findings consistent with the above scenario. A subsequent survey of 167 consecutive cases of tuberculosis seen at five New York hospitals during 1992 and 1993 demonstrated that HIV-infected persons were significantly more likely to have been recently infected with MDR-TB; indeed, 79% of the drug-resistant cases were shown by RFLP to be clustered with the clear implication of recent transmission.[43] In the Fourth WHO/IUATLD global drug surveillance report,[14] Eight settings in seven countries reported data on drug resistance stratified by HIV status: Cuba, Honduras, Latvia, the Russian Federation (Tomsk Oblast), Spain (Barcelona and Galicia), Ukraine (Donetsk Oblast) and Uruguay. Four countries were not able to discriminate between negative and unknown HIV status. The data reported from the majority of countries were not strong enough to examine an association between HIV and drug resistance. However, the data available from Donetsk Oblast, Ukraine, and Latvia indicated a significant association between HIV and MDR-TB. Additional information on risk factors including history of hospitalization or imprisonment were not available for this analysis, so the specific reasons for the association are not known. Both countries have a high underlying prevalence of MDR-TB, as well as an emerging HIV epidemic, that initially was concentrated among risk groups, but has now become more generalized. However, several studies in India and other South East Asian countries, having high prevalence of HIV seropositivity, have reported very low prevalence of MDR-TB in HIV seropositive patients contrary to Western literature. Main reasons for an association between HIV/AIDS and multidrug-resistant tuberculosis may be because of the acquired rifamycin resistance associated with HIV infection among TB patients under treatment and anti-TB drug malabsorption which has been documented in patient cohorts in settings of high HIV prevalence. In addition HIV infected patients and drug resistant TB patients may have similar risk factors such as history of hospitalization. It is also possible that HIV infected TB cases may be more susceptible to infection once exposed. HIV infected TB cases are more likely to be smear negative, and delayed diagnosis of drug resistance as well as unavailability of treatment have led to high death rates in people living with HIV. Both of these factors may suggest a lower rate of transmission. However, HIV infected cases progress rapidly to disease, and in settings where MDR-TB is prevalent, this may lead to rapid development of a pool of drug resistant TB patients, or an outbreak. Despite some of the weakness in these data and subsequent analysis, the association between HIV and MDR-TB is concerning particularly given the implications for the clinical management of these patients. Rapid progression to death in HIV-infected MDR-TB patients in both outbreaks and treatment cohorts has been widely documented.[36,44] Antiretroviral treatment for HIV does appear to benefit coinfected MDR-TB patients; however, co-management of treatment for both diseases is very complicated.

Currently, most TB Control Programs in high burden countries do not have the diagnostic infrastructure to either detect an outbreak nor the programmatic capacity to manage an outbreak. Given the impact on mortality, outbreaks should be avoided at all costs. The development of infection control measures in congregate settings as well as diagnostic screening tools to rapidly identify drug resistant TB are a priority, for all countries, but particularly for those with high prevalence of HIV or MDR-TB. From a global perspective, routine diagnosis of both HIV and drug resistant TB should be scaled up for patient benefit. Better surveillance data may help in developing an understanding of the relationship between HIV and MDR-TB.

RISK FACTORS OF MDR-TB

Several risk factors have been identified in the causation of multidrug resistant tuberculosis of which the three most important are—previous treatment with antitubercular drugs which may be inappropriate, incomplete or erratic, high prevalence of drug resistant tuberculosis in the community and contact with a patient known to have drug resistant tuberculosis. In patients with previous treatment or disease, the odds of resistant tuberculosis were 4–7 times higher than for persons with no history of past treatment. Other factors that may be responsible for increased risk of MDR-TB are—coinfection with HIV, socioeconomically deprived groups in slums, prisons, correctional facilities, day care centers, intravenous drug abusers and other immunocompromised states as in transplant recipients, anticancer therapy patients, and patients with diabetes mellitus. Radiologically far advanced pulmonary tuberculosis with cavitary lesions were four times as likely to harbor drug resistant organisms.

SOURCES AND CAUSES OF MDR-TB

Though unfortunate, yet a reality is that multidrug resistance is a man-made problem. Drug resistant tuberculosis results largely from poorly managed care of TB.[45] The sources are many and the causes multifactorial. To blame for this are the government, the pharmaceutical industry, doctors, patients and their families each of whom contribute in their own way to add up to the problem. The government plays its share by providing poor infrastructure in the National Tuberculosis Control Program, unnecessary administrative control on purchase and distribution of drugs with no proper mechanism on quality control and bioavailability tests. The pharmaceutical industry in its turn contributes by manufacturing drugs of uncertain bioavailability in fixed dose or inappropriate drug combinations, poor storage condition of drugs and substitution by inferior quality drugs by pharmacies. The doctor, by his lack of knowledge regarding doses, duration of treatment, side effects and standard regimens, frequent change of brand names and poor patient motivation, contributes the lion's share to the problem. In one of the studies where prescriptions of 449 doctors were analyzed, 75% of the doctors were found to have made some prescription error.[46] Added to this is the poor teaching and training facilities for them. Noncompliant patients due to monetary lack, lack of information, side effects of drugs and social myths and misconceptions often do not adhere to treatment. Comorbid conditions like diabetes, HIV, psychiatric conditions, the habits of smoking and alcoholism make the patient more vulnerable. To sum up, multidrug resistant tuberculosis usually result from inadequate drug therapy in multibacillary cases of tuberculosis, addition of single drug in cases of failure, difficulty in obtaining drugs by the poor due to lack of financial resources or social insurances, frequent shortage of second-line antituberculous drugs by poor management and/or financial constrains, use of drugs or combination of drugs (FDC) with unproven bioavailability, lack of motivation at the beginning of treatment and inadequate self administration of drugs without direct observation in the intensive phase of therapy.

CONTROL OF MDR-TB

The primary aim in the control of multi-drug resistant tuberculosis is to prevent its development in the first place. This can be done by Directly Observed Treatment Short-Course (DOTS), which is the most cost-effective way of treatment and prevention of MDR tuberculosis. At the same time since MDR-TB cases respond poorly to short-course chemotherapy, careful introduction of second-line drugs to treat MDR-TB to reduce further transmission of such strains will be required.[47] To control the emergence of drug resistant and multidrug resistant tuberculosis, WHO in 1998 had proposed the work plan known as 'DOTS-Plus' for which WHO had established Green light committee.[48] The primary aims of committee were to approve, conduct and oversee pilot projects based on guidelines for establishing 'DOTS-Plus' pilot projects. 'DOTS-Plus' is a comprehensive management strategy to control tuberculosis and multi-drug resistant tuberculosis. Following the roll out and successful implementation of "DOTS-Plus" pilot projects for the management of drug resistant TB between 2000 and 2005, a new Stop TB Strategy was launched in 2006. The new Stop TB Strategy includes the diagnosis and the management of drug resistant TB.[49] The launch of the Stop TB Strategy was followed by the Global Plan to Stop TB, 2006–2015 that provided targets for scale-up and budgets required for the implementation of the strategy Stop TB partnership.[50] To combat the threat of XDR-TB, WHO convened a Global Task Force on XDR-TB in October 2006 and recommended to strengthen basic activities to control TB and HIV/AIDS, to avoid additional emergence of M/XDR-TB as well as acceleration of treatment of MDR and XDR-TB cases with universal access to sound management of M/XDR-TB by 2015 in all countries and near to universal access in the high burden countries by 2010.[51] The revised plan recommended the treatment of 1.6 million M/XDR-TB cases by 2015 instead of 800,000 MDR-TB cases. It will require integration of M/XDR-TB activities into general

TB control activities. It will include the strengthening of laboratory services for adequate and timely diagnosis of M/XDR-TB, surveillance of M/XDR-TB, development and implementation of sound TB infection control policies, Advocacy Communication and Social Mobilization to sustain political commitment and resource mobilization and the promotion of research and development into new diagnostics, drugs, vaccines and operational research on MDR-TB management. It is expected that full implementation of this response plan will save the lives of thousands of people infected by M/XDR-TB and will be able to prevent and control M/XDR-TB.

CONCLUSION

MDR-TB has been an area of growing concern and posing threat to control of TB. It is estimated that more than 400,000 cases of MDR-TB emerge every year globally as a result of poor management of sensitive as well as drug resistant TB cases. MDR-TB is a man-made problem and its emergence can be prevented by prompt diagnosis and effective treatment of all TB cases. The DOTS-Plus proposed by WHO highlights the comprehensive management strategy to control MDR-TB. Laboratory services for adequate and timely diagnosis of MDR-TB must be strengthened and programmatic management of MDR-TB must be scaled up as per target set by global plan. It must be emphasized that optimal treatment of MDR-TB alone will not curb the epidemic. Efforts must be focused on the effective use of first-line drugs in every new patient, so as to prevent the ultimate emergence of multidrug resistance. The proper use of second-line drugs must be ensured to cure existing multidrug resistant tuberculosis, to reduce transmission of MDR-TB and to prevent XDR-TB. Sound infection control measures to avoid further transmission of MDR-TB and research towards development of new diagnostics, drugs and vaccines should be promoted to control MDR-TB.

REFERENCES

1. Multidrug resistant tuberculosis. ICMR. 1999;29:105-14.
2. Cohn DL, Bustreo F, Raviglione MC. Drug resistant tuberculosis. Review of the worldwide situation and the WHO/IUATLD Global Surveillance Project. International Union Against Tuberculosis and Lung Disease. Clin Infect Dis. 1997;24:S121-30.
3. Pablos-Mendez A, Biokin N, Rieder HL, Bustreo F, Cohn DL, Lambregts van Weezenbeek, et al. Global surveillance for antituberculosis drug resistance, 1994-1997. World Health Organization–International Union Against Tuberculosis and Lung Disease Working Group on Antituberculosis Drug Resistance Surveillance. N Engl J Med. 1998;338:1641-9.
4. Espinal MA, Laszlo A, Simonsen L, et al. Global trends in resistance to antituberculosis drugs. N Engl J Med. 2001;344:1294-303.
5. Dye C, Espinal MA, Watt CJ, Mbiaga C, Williams BG. Worldwide incidence of multidrug resistant tuberculosis. J Infect Dis. 2002;185:1197-202.
6. World Health Organization. Antituberculosis drug resistance in the world: prevalence and trends. Report No. 2. WHO/CDS/TB/2000. 278. Geneva: WHO, 2000.

7. Dye C, William BG, Espinal MA, Raviglione MC. Erasing the world's slow strain: Strategies to beat multidrug-resistant tuberculosis. Science. 2002;295:2042-6.
8. National Tuberculosis Programme. Tuberculosis in Latvia 1991-2000. Riga. 2001;21-3.
9. Robert J, Trystram D, Pernot-Truffot C, Jarlier V. Surveillance de la tuberculose a bacilles multiresistants en France en 1998. Bull Epidemiol Hebdo. 2002;16:71-2.
10. Robert J, Trystram D, Pernot-Truffot C, Carbonelle B. Surveillance of *Mycobacterium tuberculosis* drug resistance in France, 1995-1997. Int J Tuberc Lung Dis. 2000;4:665-72.
11. Centers for Disease Control. Reported tuberculosis in the United States 2000. Atlanta, GA: US Department of Health and Human Services, CDC, August 2001.
12. WHO-IUALTD Global Project on Antituberculosis Drug Resistance Surveillance (1999-2002), Third Global Report (2003).
13. Zignol M, Hosseini MS, Wright A, Weezenbeek CL, Nunn P, Watt CJ, et al. Global incidence of multidrug-resistant tuberculosis. J Infect Dis. 2006;194:479-85.
14. WHO-IUALTD Global Project on Antituberculosis Drug Resistance Surveillance (2002-2007), Fourth Global Report (2008), updated 2010.
15. Global tuberculosis report 2012. WHO/HTM/TB/2012.6.
16. ICMR, Prevalence of drug resistance in patients with pulmonary tuberculosis presenting for the first time with symptoms at chest clinics in India - I. Findings in urban clinics among patients giving no history of previous chemotherapy. Indian J Med Res. 1968;56:1617-30.
17. ICMR, Prevalence of drug resistance in patients with pulmonary tuberculosis presenting for the first time with symptoms at chest clinics in India - II. Findings in urban clinics among all patients, with or without history of previous chemotherapy. Indian J Med Res. 1969;57:823-35.
18. Trivedi SS, Desai SC. Primary antituberculosis drug resistance and acquired rifampicin resistance in Gujarat, India Tubercle. 1988;69:37-42.
19. Krishnaswamy KV, Rahim MA. Primary drug resistance in pulmonary tuberculosis. Indian J Chest Dis. 1976;28:233-7.
20. Chandrasekaran S, Chauhan MM, Rajalaksmi R, Chaudhuri K, Mahadev B. Initial drug resistance to antituberculosis drugs in patients attending an urban district tuberculosis centre. Ind J Tub. 1990;37:215-6.
21. Chandrasekaran S, Jagota P, Chaudhuri K. Initial drug resistance to antituberculosis drugs in urban and rural district tuberculosis programme. Ind J Tub. 1992;39:171-5.
22. Paramasivan CN, Chandrasekaran V, Santha T, Sudarsanam NM, Prabhakar R. Bacteriological investigations for short course chemotherapy under the tuberculosis programme in two districts in India. Tuber Lung Dis. 1993;74:23-7.
23. Gupta PR, Singhal B, Sharma TN, Gupta RB. Prevalence of initial drug resistance in tuberculosis patients attending a chest hospital. Ind J Med Res. 1993;97:102-3.
24. Jain NK, Chopra KK, Prasad G. Initial and acquired isoniazid and rifampicin resistance to *M. tuberculosis* and its implications for treatment. Ind J Tub. 1992;39:121-4.
25. Jena J, Panda BN, Nema SK, Ohri VC, Pahwa RS. Drug resistance pattern of *Mycobacterium tuberculosis* in a chest disease hospital of armed forces. Lung India. 1995;13:56-9.
26. Parmasivan CN, Bhaskaran K, Venkataraman, Chandrasekhran V, Narayanan PR. Survilence of drug resistance in tuberculosis in the state of Tamil Nadu. Ind J Tub. 2000;47:27-33.
27. Prasad R, Suryakant, Mukerji PK, Gupta AK, Garg R, Rizvi DM, et al. Initial drug resistance in patients of pulmonary tuberculosis attending a tertiary care center. Ind J Tub. 2001;48:159.
28. Paramasivan CN, Venkata raman P, Chandrashekhran V, Bhatt S, Narayanan PR. Surveillance of drug resistant in tuberculosis in two districts of south India. Int J Tuberc Lung Dis. 2002;6:479-84.
29. Sofia V, Balasangameshwara VH, Jagannatha PS, Kumar P. Initial drug resistant among tuberculosis patients under DOTS programme in Banglore city. Ind J Tuberc. 2004;52:17-21.

30. Mahadeo B, Kumar P, Agrawal SP, Chauhan LS, Sriknataramu N. Surveillance of drug resistant to antituberculosis drugs in districts of Hoogli in West Bengal and Myurbhanj in Orissa. Indian J Tuberc. 2005;52:5-10.
31. Datta M, Radhamani MP, Selvaraj R, Paramasivan CN, Gopalan BN, Sudeendra CR, et al. Critical assessment of smear-positive pulmonary tuberculosis patients after chemotherapy under the district tuberculosis programme. Tub Lung Dis. 1993;74:180-6.
32. Chowgule RV, Deodhar L. Pattern of secondary acquired drug resistance to antituberculosis drug in Mumbai, India—1991–1995. Indian J Chest Dis Allied and Sci. 1998;40:23-31.
33. Shah AR, Agarawal SK, Shah KV. Study of drug resistance in previously treated tuberculosis patients in Gujarat, India. Int J Tuberc Lung Dis. 2002;6:1098-101.
34. Deivanayagam CN, Rajasekaran S, Venkatesan R. et al. Prevalence of acquired MDR-TB and HIV coinfection. Indian J Chest Dis Allied Sci. 2002;44:237-42.
35. Prasad R, Suryakant, Mukerji PK, Gupta AK, Garg R, Rizvi DM, et al. Acquire drug resistance in patients of pulmonary tuberculosis attending a tertiary care center. Int J Tuberc Lung Dis. 2003;11 (Suppl): S3O3 (Abstract).
36. Edlin BR, Tokars, JI, Grieco MH, et al. An outbreak of multidrug-resistant tuberculosis among hospitalized patients with the acquired immunodeficiency syndrome. N Engl J Med. 1992;326:1514-21.
37. Moro ML, et al. An outbreak of multidrug-resistant tuberculosis involving HIV infected patients of two hospitals in Milan, Italy. AIDS. 1998;12:1095-102.
38. Kenyon TA, et al. Low levels of drug resistance amidst rapidly increasing tuberculosis and human immunodeficiency virus co-epidemics in Botswana. Int J Tuberc Lung Dis. 1999;3:4-11.
39. Chum HJ, et al. An epidemiological study of tuberculosis and HIV infection in Tanzania, 1991-1993. AIDS. 1996;10:299-309.
40. Frieden TR, Sterling T, Pablos-Mendez A, Kilburn JO, Cauthen GM, Dooley SW. The mergence of drug-resistant tuberculosis in New York City. N Engl J Med. 1993;328:521-6.
41. Coronado VG, Beck-Sague CM, Hutton MD, et al. Transmission of multidrug-resistant *Mycobacterium tuberculosis* among persons with human immunodeficiency virus infection in an urban hospital: epidemiologic and restriction fragment length polymorphism analysis. J Infect Dis. 1993;168:1052-5.
42. Busillo C, Lessnau K-D, Sanjana V, et al. Multidrug-resistant *Mycobacterium tuberculosis* in patients with human immunodeficiency virus infection. Chest. 1992;102:797-801.
43. Shafer RW, Small PM, Larkin C, et al. Temporal trends and transmission patterns during the emergence of multidrug-resistant tuberculosis in New York City: a molecular epidemiologic assessment. J Infect Dis. 1995;152:171-6.
44. Mac-Arthur A Jr, et al. Characteristics of drug resistance and HIV among tuberculosis patients in Mozambique. Int J Tuberc Lung Dis. 2001;5:894-902.
45. Philip C Hopewell, Madhukar Pai, Dermot Maher, Mukund Uplekar, Mario C Raviglione. International standards for tuberculosis care. Lancet Infect Dis. 2006;6:710-25.
46. Prasad R, Nautiyal RG, Ahuja RC, et al. Treatment of new pulmonary tuberculosis patients: what do allopathic doctors do in India? Int J Tuberc Lung Dis. 2002;6:895-902.
47. Espinal MA, Kim SJ, Surarez PG, et al. Standard short course chemotherapy for drug resistant tuberculosis: treatment outcome in six countries. JAMA. 2000;283:2537-45.
48. DOTS-Plus and Green Light Committee, www.who.int/gtb/policyrd /dotsplus.htm.
49. *The Global MDR-TB & XDR-TB response Plan 2007-2008.* World Health Organization Document, 2007 WHO/HTM/TB/2007.387.
50. Stop TB Partnership and World Heath Organization, *The global plan to Stop TB 2006–2015*, Geneva, Switzerland: World Health Organization 2006.
51. WHO Global XDR-TB task force meeting, Oct 2006. Available at:http://www.who.int/tb/xdr/taskforcereport_oct06.pdf.

Chapter 25

Drug Resistant and Multidrug Resistant Tuberculosis: Management

INTRODUCTION

Drug resistant tuberculosis (DR-TB) has been reported since the early days of introduction of antitubercular chemotherapy, but recently multidrug resistant tuberculosis (MDR-TB) has been an area of growing concern, and is posing threat to global efforts of tuberculosis control. Prevalence of MDR-TB, in a community, mirrors the functional state and efficacy of tuberculosis control program and realistic attitude of the community towards implementation of such programs.[1] Management of DR-TB and MDR-TB is difficult, much expensive, challenging and quite often leads to treatment failure. This chapter aims to illustrate the diagnosis and treatment of drug resistant and multidrug resistant tuberculosis.

DEFINITION

Drug resistant tuberculosis is defined as a case of tuberculosis excreting bacilli resistant to one or more antitubercular drugs. Multidrug resistant tuberculosis (MDR-TB) is defined as disease due to *M. tuberculosis* that is resistant to isoniazid and rifampicin with or without resistance to other drugs (the culture and drug susceptibility test result being from an RNTCP accredited laboratory). Mono-resistance is defined as resistance to one antituberculosis drug where as poly-resistance is defined as resistance to more than one antituberculosis drug, other than both isoniazid and rifampicin.

MECHANISM OF DRUG RESISTANCE

Drug resistance in tuberculosis occurs by random single step spontaneous mutation at a low but predictable frequency in large bacterial populations.

There is no convincing evidence for the role of plasmids or transposons as in other bacterial pathogens. The probability of drug resistant mutants in the case of rifampicin is 10^8, for INH, streptomycin and ethambutol is 10^6 and for ethionamide, cycloserine, capreomycin and thiacetazone 10^3. The probability of resistance developing in a 2.5 cm cavity which harbors 10^8–10^9 bacilli is 10^6 for INH and 10^8 for rifampicin and 10^{14} for INH and rifampicin together. In reality therefore, only one of the bacilli in 10^{14} organisms will be resistant to both isoniazid and rifampicin. This illustrates a very fundamental principle that multidrug resistant tuberculosis is a man-made problem.[3]

GENETIC BASIS OF DRUG RESISTANCE

Dramatic discoveries in the field of molecular biology in the last few years have greatly increased our understanding of the mechanism of drug resistance. The findings of such discoveries led to the conclusion that the primary mechanism of multiple drug resistance in tuberculosis is due to alterations in individual drug target genes.[1] Isoniazid resistance has been found to be due to a defect in the Kat G gene which codes for the catalase peroxidase enzyme. Mutation in Kat G, Inh A and ahp C (alkyl hydroperoxide reductase) genes are found in upto 90% of isoniazid resistance. Rifampicin resistance (> 96%) has been associated with mutations in the rpo B gene,[2] pyrazinamide resistance (72–97%) to pncA mutations, ethambutol (47–65%) to mutations in emb AB gene, streptomycin resistance with rrs or rpsL mutations and fluoroquinolone resistance (75–94%) with substitutions in gyr A gene. Apart from these 11 genes, additional genes and mechanisms may play a role particularly in association with lower levels of resistance.[3]

VIRULENCE AND DRUG-RESISTANT STRAINS

The traditionally received wisdom about drug resistant strains of tuberculosis that they are less virulent was based substantially on the observation by Cohn, et al.[4] that virulent strains of *M. tuberculosis*, when selectively bred in the laboratory for high-level resistance to INH, became significantly less capable of producing progressive infection in animal models. This was associated with loss of catalase activity by bacilli. Snider, et al. observed that there is no or a lesser risk of infection when contacts are exposed to tubercular bacilli resistant to high concentration of INH and SM.[5] Ordway, et al.[6] have observed that some MDR-TB strains that exhibit in vitro growth rates and animal virulence characteristics comparable to the most virulent, wild type drug susceptible strains. Frieden, et al.[7] in their report of multi-institutional spread of notorious 'Strain W' in New York City reported despite mutation in the Kat G locus; strain was catalase positive and grows rapidly in culture media and animals. Overall, evidences indicate that current drug-resistant strains have demonstrated the capacity to produce progressive disease in both normal and immunosuppressed contacts.

IMPACT OF DRUG RESISTANCE ON THE OUTCOME OF CHEMOTHERAPY

In early treatment era, it was recognized that the resistance with isoniazid (H) and streptomycin (S) was associated with increased risk of treatment failure[8] but in current situation, the loss of single drug to resistance is potentially less significant because of availability and use of potent agents such as rifampicin, pyrazinamide, ethambutol (E). The most reliable data on treatment outcome were derived from British Medical Research Council (BMRC) short course chemotherapy trials performed in East Africa, Hong Kong, Singapore.[9] Failure rate of isoniazid (H), rifampicin (R), pyrazinamide (Z) and streptomycin (S) containing regimen among such cases, was less than 5% in contrast to approximately 20% failure rate among cases assigned to less potent regimens. Thus it is possible to obtain good result with use of six months short-course chemotherapy with isoniazid, rifampin, pyrazinzmide and streptomycin or ethambutol when initial susceptibility test indicates resistance to isoniazid and/or streptomycin. It was also confirmed in Indian study that strains resistant to isonizid, streptomycin, or both neither pose a major problem nor affect the result of treatment in a big way provided proper regimens are used. On the contrary, patients infected with organisms resistant to rifampicin, isoniazid or both have a high rate of treatment failure[10-12] and this forms a major threat to tuberculosis control programs particularly for countries like India with poor resources.[13] Four separate studies from New York city between 1995-1996 on response to therapy for patient with MDR-TB[14-17] reported better outcome can be demonstrated with early recognization of resistance and administration of effective drugs.

DIAGNOSIS OF DRUG RESISTANT AND MULTIDRUG RESISTANT TUBERCULOSIS

It is needless to emphasize that early diagnosis and treatment of drug resistant and multidrug resistant tuberculosis is of paramount importance not only from the patient's perspective but also for the community at large; failing this, there will be propagation of the deadly drug resistant bacilli, decreased chances of cure for the patient, increasing cost of therapy and unnecessary drug toxicity. The diagnosis of drug resistant and multidrug resistant tuberculosis is based on—clinical, radiological and bacteriological evidences.

Clinical Evidence

This comprises of the signs and symptoms and past history of antitubercular therapy. History of prior treatment with antitubercular drugs is most important. The other important aspects of the history include contact with a known case of resistant tuberculosis and patient's place of residence which may have a high prevalence of drug resistance. The salient points in the past treatment history should include the drugs and regimens followed, dosage of drugs and duration of each course of treatment, regularity in taking the drugs, response to treatment in terms of relief of symptoms and bacteriological indices if available, and any adverse drug reactions suffered. The ICMR in its study has shown that longer duration of chemotherapy and single drug therapy in the past was associated with greater degrees of resistance.[10] In the context of our country where illiteracy is the main culprit, several difficulties may be encountered in eliciting reliable information. Some of the common problems faced by the physician include unawareness or forgetfulness of the patient so that he is unable to give a proper history, poor record keeping of prescriptions, sputum examination reports and X-rays, drugs dispensed by private practitioners without a proper prescription and the practice of prescribing combipacks making it impossible for the patient to remember the names. MDR-TB Suspect is defined as a TB patient who fails an RNTCP Category I or III treatment regimen and any RNTCP Category II patient who is sputum smear positive at the end of the fourth month of treatment or later.[18] It must be remembered that clinical evidences are the least reliable for the diagnosis of drug resistant and multidrug resistant tuberculosis. However, clinical deterioration in the presence of sputum smear positivity and/or radiological worsening can be considered due to resistance.

Radiological Evidence

Though radiology is not a very reliable indicator for predicting drug resistance, yet it serves to complement the clinical and bacteriological evidence of the patient. The presence of multiple or giant cavities and destroyed lung increases the probability of drug resistance. Change in size of cavities, increase in size of existing lesions and appearance of new lesions are signs of disease progression and activity. Serial X-rays showing worsening in the forms as described above at the end of three months of regular and adequate chemotherapy can make one suspicious of drug resistance. These radiological findings at the end of three months in addition to positive sputum and/or clinical worsening can be diagnosed as resistant tuberculosis.[19] However, one should also realize that radiological worsening may be due to pneumonia, pulmonary embolism and supervening carcinoma.

Bacteriological Evidence

The bacteriological criteria serve as the gold standard in the detection of drug resistant tuberculosis. This is based on sputum smear microscopy and culture of *M. tuberculosis* and drug susceptibility testing (DST) to the various primary and second-line antitubercular drugs. Sputum smear microscopy, after starting standard chemotherapy can show a positive, negative or suboptimal response. While positive response is characterized by sputum conversion at 2/3 months of chemotherapy, a negative response could mean persistent smear positivity at the end of 3 months of adequate chemotherapy and a suboptimal response by an initial fall in the sputum grade followed by a gradual rise—the so-called 'fall and rise' phenomenon[20] while the patient is on antitubercular therapy. The last two patterns increase the probability of drug resistant tuberculosis. The confirmation of the presence of drug resistance is obtained by culture of *M. tuberculosis* and drug susceptibility testing. Even the definition of drug resistance is one that is based on susceptibility test results, i.e confirmed MDR-TB case is a MDR-TB suspect who is sputum culture positive and whose TB is due to *M. tuberculosis* that are resistant in-vitro to at least isoniazid and rifampicin[18] (the culture and DST result being from an accredited laboratory). Ideally DST should be done in all patients undergoing retreatment, but since this is not feasible in an Indian set-up, it is better to do DST for MDR-TB suspects. It is, however, noteworthy that culture and sensitivity in spite of continuing to be the gold standard for diagnosis of tuberculosis and drug resistance, is not foolproof and one has to keep in mind the limitations of this highly specific test. This is because the technique is complex and it is difficult to perform sensitivity tests accurately even when skilled personnel are available and laboratory facilities are of a high standard. This is true even in highly industrialized nations such as the United Kingdom and the United States. In the United Kingdom, retesting of 234 strains of drug resistant bacilli by a reference laboratory showed discordant reports in 50–70% of the results reported by local laboratories.[19] Additional limitations are the difficulty and unreliability of testing susceptibility to second-line drugs. In the United States, 43 laboratories which were having above average laboratory standards tested the results of a reference laboratory. The results obtained were as follows—consistently good in 23, adequate in 9 and poor in 11. The WHO thus concluded that the wide scale on which unreliable sensitivity tests are reported, even in technically advanced countries, gives a cause for concern.[21-23] However recently due to setting up of supranational reference laboratory network, there is improvement in quality susceptibility testing of national reference laboratories and surveys carried out within the WHO/IUATLD global project on drug resistance surveillance. These initiatives apply to surveillance and not to clinical practice.[24] Susceptibility testing for isoniazid, rifampicin, the fluoroquinolones, and the injectable agents is fairly reliable. For other agents, it is less reliable, and basing individualized treatments on DST for these agents should be avoided. The clinical effectiveness or ineffectiveness of a drug cannot be predicted by DST with 100% certainty.[25]

Laboratories performing culture/susceptibility testing are situated in only a few major cities in India. The WHO definition of resistance based on drug susceptibility reports therefore becomes only a theoretical exercise in our country in most occasions.[20] The laboratories vary in reliability; errors occur in laboratories, different sensitivity reports are obtained of the same patient from different laboratories due to sampling of different populations of bacilli and different techniques employed. Standardization, coordination and cross checking facilities with reference laboratories do not exist in our country by and large, thus magnifying the problem. On this background, it is pertinent to reaffirm that drug susceptibility testing should not be accepted uncritically, they should be correlated with prior treatment history, smear result and X-ray and should be used as a guide for future therapies and not dictate treatment options. If sensitivity report does not fit with other available evidences, it should be discussed with a microbiologist and the test repeated.

Rapid Culture Technique

In this technique, culture time is reduced from an average 38.5 days to 18 days. Technique usually applied is Bactec system and Mycobacterial Growth Indicator Tube (MGIT). In Bactec, 7H12, and in MGIT, 7H9 middle Brooke media are used. In Bactec method, the released radiolabeled carbon dioxide is detected that indicates growth of *M. tuberculosis* whereas in MGIT the oxygen sensitive fluorescent compound is used to detect growth of *M. tuberculosis*. The rapid culture technology take much shorter time as compared to LJ media.[26,27] A higher degree of concordance has been documented between susceptibility data from the Bactec system and those obtained by conventional solid media method.[28] In fact the rapid radiometric system offers a substantially more quantitative approach to the determination of susceptibility than other method,[29] another major advantage of Bactec system that it can also perform susceptibility test for pyrazinamide.

Molecular Biological Technique

For identification of resistance associated mutation molecular techniques like—DNA sequencing, line probe assay (LiPA), DNA microarrays, molecular beacons, single strand conformation polymorphism, fluorescent resonance energy transfer probes, other PCR based techniques or mycobacteriophages-based assays like—FAST Plaque TB and Luciferase receptors phages (LRPs) have been used. WHO with the Stop TB Partnership, UNITAID and the Foundation for Innovative New Diagnostics (FIND) together unveiled a new Policy endorsing use of Line Probe Assays in low resource countries. There are two types, the geno type MTB-DR assay and INNO-LiPA Rif.TB assay. Advantages include rapid screening of patients with MDR-TB risk and results within 2 days as compared to 2–3 months for conventional cultures. At present their use is limited to culture isolates and direct testing of sputum specimens. They are not recommended as a complete replacement to the conventional culture and DST.[30] Currently, LiPA is not useful for detecting mutations responsible for drug resistance in second-line drugs. The Xpert MTB/RIF assay enables simultaneous detection of *Mycobacterium tuberculosis* (MTB) and rifampicin resistance and it was endorsed by WHO in 2010. The Xpert

MTB/RIF was found to be highly sensitive (98%) and specific (98%) in detecting tuberculosis and rifampicin resistance (a reliable proxy for MDR) directly from sputum, in less than two hours. The assay is robust enough to be performed outside of conventional laboratories, at district and subdistrict level of health system but requires uninterrupted power supply. Widespread implementation of Xpert MTB/RIF would greatly enhance the diagnostic capacity for TB and MDR TB; its accuracy and ease of use represents a major milestone for TB and MDR TB care and control.[31] Molecular techniques involves detection of resistant genes or DNA sequencing of *M. tuberculosis* by amplification of nucleic acid and its identification. The polymerase chain reaction single strand conformational polymorphism (PCR SSCP)[32] and restriction fragment length polymorphism (RFLP)[33,34] analysis are usually applied. The PCR when compared with culture results, the sensitivity, specificity, and positive predictive value were found 83.5%, 99% and 94.2%, respectively. RFLP gives fingerprint of strains which is specific for each strain of *M. tuberculosis,* so has more valuable place for molecular epidemiology in differentiating the strains. Overall, RFLP analysis has immense potential as a tool to study transmission patterns and the natural histories of primary and reinfection tuberculosis specifically in HIV infected patients[34] while luciferase reporter assay rapid system based on enzyme luciferase, involves the introduction of this enzyme into *M. tuberculosis* via a reporter phage system. Exposure of luminous *Mycobacterium* to antimicrobial agents would block luminous activity in the sensitive bacilli but with no effect on resistant bacilli. This method requires substantial growth of *Mycobacterium* population (about 10^6) yet, the potential of such methodology is intriguing, perhaps playing a role in industrial screening of large numbers of compounds for antimycobacterial activity.[35] The expectation that molecular techniques would surpass conventional methods has yet not been realized because most of techniques still require detailed and systemic evaluation using standard techniques as references before their application in clinical setting. These techniques might be used as complement to the standard methods.[36]

TREATMENT OF DRUG RESISTANT AND MULTIDRUG RESISTANT TUBERCULOSIS

The WHO recommends that treatment of drug resistant and multidrug resistant tuberculosis should be ideally carried out in a hospital that has a specialized unit for dealing with such cases with trained doctors and laboratory personnel. There should be standard laboratory facilities for carrying out reliable drug susceptibility testing and uninterrupted supply of drugs. The management of multidrug resistant tuberculosis is an area that has been shrouded in a lot of myths and misconceptions, and therefore utterly chaotic. Though guidelines in general have been laid down by the WHO, which have been found cost effective and feasible in resource limited countries, but they may not be applicable to every patients where individualized treatment regimens depending on reliable sensitivity report may be used. Use of standardized or individualized treatment regimens is currently subject of operational studies to assess the feasibility and cost-effectiveness. In some countries, a standardized regimen for certain groups of patients may be more appropriate than an individualized regimen, while in others the converse may be best. Most of the guidelines for the management of drug resistant TB are primarily for high income nations, where expert diagnostics and optimal care are available. Low income nations will inevitably require different approaches than those of the more affluent, industrialized nations. Individualized regimens are based on individual DST and prior treatment history, require close follow-up by skilled professionals and incur high cost. Management issues in second-line drugs are complex, especially when individualized treatment regimens are used. Drugs are frequently changed as a result of adverse effects, delayed DST results and poor response to treatment. Standardized regimens for middle to low income nations are based on DRS data from representative patient populations. Such regimens reduce the number of specialist physicians needed and cost of tretment by 5–10 times. WHO has designed the DOTS-Plus regimen for managing MDR-TB in resource poor nations like India. Even in countries where reliable DST is available, standardized regimens may be chosen as a strategy over individualized regimens for the following reasons: Interpretation of DST to some of the first- and second-line drugs is difficult and could mislead regimen design. Standardized regimens can give guidance to clinicians and prevent basing decisions on DST that is not reliable, turn around time for many culture-based DST methods is long, the laboratory may not perform DST of certain drugs, or may perform them at different times. Results from rapid methods (molecular) may be available within days, but only for certain first-line drugs such as isoniazid and rifampicin. Many laboratories perform second-line DST only after resistance to first-line drugs is confirmed. Accounting for the effectiveness of the 5 drug groups, it is a known fact that the first-line drugs are more powerful, cheaper and effective. Given the circumstances, it would be ideal to add one or more first-line drugs to any regimen-based on the appropriate DST.

Second-Line Drugs and Their Dosage

The second-line drugs used for treatment of drug resistant and multidrug resistant tuberculosis are given in Table 25.1 with their dosages in decreasing potency from top-to-bottom against *M. tuberculosis*. It is generally thought that, second-line drugs are frequently associated with very high rates of unacceptable adverse drug reactions, needing frequent interruption and change of regimen, but in clinical practice, it is observed that these drugs are fairly tolerated. Author himself in one of study reported that 41% patients, experience some side effects but only 21.1% patients required stoppage or change of drug in their study of 39 patients of MDR-TB.[37] Thus, it is practically possible to treat the patients of MDR-TB with these drugs.

Table 25.1: Doses of antitubercular drugs used in previously treated patients of TB

Drugs	Average daily dosage	Daily dosage (mg)		Type of anti-mycobacterial activity
		Minimum	Maximum	
Group 1 First-line oral agents Pyrazinamide (Z) Ethambutol (E) Rifabutin (Rfb)	 25 mg/kg 15 mg/kg 5–10 mg/kg	 1200 800 150	 1500 1200 600	 Bactericidal Bacteriostatic
Group 2 Injectable agents Kanamycin (Km) Amikacin (Am) Streptomycin (S) Capreomycin (Cm)	 15 mg/kg 15 mg/kg 15 mg/kg 15 mg/kg	 750 750 750 750	 1000 1000 1000 1000	Bactericidal against actively multiplying organisms
Group 3 Fluoroquinolones Moxifloxacin (Mfx) Levofloxacin (Lfx) Ofloxacin (Ofx)	 7.5–10 mg/kg 7.5–10 mg/kg 15–20 mg/kg	 400 500 400	 400 1000 1000	 Weakly bactericidal
Group 4 Oral bacteriostatic second-line drugs Ethionamide (Eto) Prothionamide (Pto) Para-aminosalicyclic acid (PAS) Cycloserine (Cs) Terizidone (Trd)	 15–20 mg/kg 15–20 mg/kg 200–300 mg/kg 10–20 mg/kg 10–20 mg/kg	 500–750 500–750 10 g 500–750 500–750	 1000 1000 12 g 1000 1000	 Bacteriostatic
Group 5 Agents with unclear role in treatment of drug resistant TB Clofazimine (Cfz) Linezolid (Lzd) Amoxicillin/clavulanate Thioacetazone (Thz) Imipenem/Cilastatin (Ipm/Cln) High dose isoniazid (high-dose H) Clarithromycin (Clr)	 4–5 mg/kg 1200 mg/day 2 g/day 150 mg/day 500–1000 mg/IV every 6 hourly 16–20 mg/kg 10–15 mg/kg	 100-200 600 500/125 Twice a day - 500 every 6 hourly 600 500 twice a day	 300 1200 1000/250 Twice a day - 1000 every 6 hourly 900 500 twice a day	 Bacteriostatic Weakly bactericidal Bactericidal (pH dependent)

Cross-Resistance

Cross-resistance has been reported between thioamides and thioacetazone (one way resistance—strains resistance to thioacetazone are susceptible to thioamides, the reverse is seldom the case), kanamycin/amikacin with streptomycin,[38] rifampicin with rifapentine, and rifabutin (> 70% strains)[39] and among various derivatives of fluoroquinolones.[40] Cross-resistance between the fluoroquinolones is almost complete. Limited evidence suggests that the third-generation fluoroquinolones (notably moxifloxacin) do not have complete cross-resistance with the older generations and may have enhanced clinical benefit due to their low MICs, enhanced antimycobacterial activity, and improved biochemical structure providing metabolic stability and long half-life, theoretically reducing the selection of resistant mutants. While the clinical benefit of newer-generation fluoroquinolones has been validated in one small retrospective study,[41] more clinical and laboratory research is needed to understand the extent of fluoroquinolone cross-resistance and its clinical relevance. Cross-resistance has also been reported between ethionamide and INH,[42] amikacin and kanamycin,[38] amikacin and capreomycin.[38] Strains resistant to streptomycin/kanamycin/amikacin are still sensitive to capreomycin. It is ineffective to use two drugs of the same group or to use a drug potentially ineffective because of cross-resistance.

General Principles for Designing Treatment Regimen for Mono and Poly Drug Resistant-TB

Definitive randomized or control study have not been performed to determine the best treatment for various patterns of drug resistance except for streptomycin resistance. The recommendation in these guidelines are based on evidences from the pre-rifampicin era, observational studies, general principles of microbiology and therapeutics in TB, extrapolations from established evidence and expert opinion. When a decision has been made to modify standard short-course chemotherapy, the most effective regimen should be chosen from the start to maximize the likelihood of cure. Effective drugs should not be withheld for later use. The regimen should be based on previous treatment history, DST pattern and the possibility of strain of *M. tuberculosis*, having acquired new resistance while awaiting DST result. WHO has suggested regimen (Table 25.2) for mono and poly drug resistance when DST results are highly reliable and further acquired resistance while awaiting DST results is not a factor.[43]

General Principles for Designing Treatment Regimens for Multidrug Resistant Tuberculosis[44-50]

Early suspicion, diagnosis and appropriate treatment of MDR-TB is essential to prevent morbidity, mortality and transmission of MDR-TB. Treatment should be initiated in a specialized center with standard laboratory facilities.

Table 25.2: Suggested regimen for mono and poly drug resistance

Pattern of drug resistance	Suggested regimen	Minimum duration of treatment (months)	Comments
H (± S)	R, Z and E	6–9	A fluoroquinolone may strengthen the regimen for patients with extensive disease
H and Z	R, E and fluoroquinolones	9–12	A longer duration of treatment should be used for patients with extensive disease
H and E	R, Z and fluoroquinolones	9–12	A longer duration of treatment should be used for patients with extensive disease
R	H, E, fluoroquinolones, plus at least 2 months of Z	12–18	An injectable agent may strengthen the regimen for patients with extensive disease
R and E (± S)	H, Z, fluoroquinolones, plus an injectable agent for at least the first 2–3 months	18	A longer course (6 months) of the injectable agent may strengthen the regimen for patients with extensive disease
R and Z (± S)	H, E, fluoroquinolones, plus an injectable agent for at least the first 2–3 months	18	A longer course (6 months) of the injectable agent may strengthen the regimen for patients with extensive disease
H, E, Z (± S)	R, fluoroquinolones, plus an oral second-line agent, plus an injectable agent for the first 2–3 months	18	A longer course (6 months) of the injectable agent may strengthen the regimen for patients with extensive disease

H = isoniazid; R = rifampicin; E = ethambutol; Z = pyrazinamide; S = streptomycin

Single drug should not be added to failing regimen. Intermittent therapy is not effective in multidrug resistant tuberculosis and should be avoided. Past history of drugs taken by the patient and drugs commonly used in the country and prevalence of resistance to first- and second-line drugs should be taken into consideration when designing a standardized regimen. Regimens should consist of at least four drugs with either certain, or almost certain, effectiveness. If the evidence about the effectiveness of a certain drug is unclear, the drug can be part of the regimen, but it should not be depended upon for success. Often, more than four drugs may be started if the susceptibility pattern is unknown, effectiveness is questionable for

Table 25.3: Grouping of antituberculosis drugs

Group	Drugs
Group 1 First-line oral agents	Ethambutol (E); Pyrazinamide (Z); Rifabutin (Rfb)
Group 2 Injectable agents	Kanamycin (Km); Amikacin (Amk); Capreomycin (Cm) Streptomycin (S)
Group 3 Fluoroquinolones	Moxifloxacin (Mfx); Levofloxacin (Lfx); Ofloxacin (Ofx)
Group 4 Oral bacteriostatic 2nd line agents	Ethionamide (Eto); Prothionamide (Pto); Cycloserine (Cs); Terizidone (Trd); p-aminosalicylic acid (PAS)
Group 5 (drugs with unclear efficacy or unclear role in MDR-TB treatment, not recommended by WHO for routine use in MDR-TB patients)	Clofazimine (Cfz); Linezolid (Lzd); Amoxicillin/Clavulanate (Amx/Clv); Thioacetazone (Thz); Imipenem/Cilastatin (Ipm/Cln); High-dose isoniazid (high-dose H); Clarithromycin (Clr)

an agent(s) or if extensive, bilateral pulmonary disease is present. Design treatment regimens with a consistent approach based on the hierarchy of the five groups of antituberculosis drugs (Table 25.3).

Use any first-line oral agent (Group-1) to which isolate is sensitive, use one injectable (Group-2), one fluoroquinolone (Group-3) and add as many second-line bacteriostatic agents (Group-4) to make up at least 4 effective drugs. Group-5 drugs are not recommended for routine use except where an adequate regimen is impossible with Group 1–4. Do not use ciprofloxacin as an antituberculosis drug. When possible, pyrazinamide, ethambutol and fluoroquinolones should be given once per day as the high peaks attained in once-a-day dosing may be more efficacious. Once-a-day dosing is permitted for other second-line drugs depending on patient tolerance; however ethionamide/prothionamide, cycloserine and PAS have traditionally been given in split doses during the day to reduce adverse effects. The drug dosage should be determined by body weight. Most drugs should be started at full dose, except cycloserine, ethionamide and PAS, in which case the dose of the drug can be increased over a two-week period (drug ramping).[42,44] The injectable agent should be continued for a minimum of 6 months, and for at least 4 months after the patient first becomes and remains smear- or culture-negative. Review of the patient's cultures, smears, X-rays and clinical status may also aid in deciding whether or not to continue an injectable agent longer than the above recommendation, particularly in the case of patients for whom the susceptibility pattern is unknown, effectiveness of one or more agents is questionable, or extensive or bilateral pulmonary disease is present.[25] Treatment of adverse drug effects should be immediate and adequate in order to minimize the risk of treatment interruptions and prevent increased morbidity and mortality due to serious adverse effects.

The minimum duration of treatment is 18 months after culture conversion preferably each dose is given as directly observed therapy (DOT) throughout the treatment. At least therapy should be under direct observation preferably for 3–4 months or till the sputum conversion. If directly observed treatment is not possible, adherence to treatment must be ensured by intense health education to patient and family member at start of treatment and during each follow-up visits and other adherence measures like checking empty blister packs. No drug should be kept in reserve and the most powerful drugs (bactericidal) should be used initially and in maximum combination so as to ensure that the first battle is won and won permanently. DST of drugs with high reproducibility and reliability (and from a dependable laboratory) should be used to guide therapy. Do not depend on DST in regimen design for ethambutol, pyrazinamide, and Group 4 and 5 drugs. Pyrazinamide can be used for the entire treatment if it is judged to be effective. Many DR-TB patients have chronically inflamed lungs, which theoretically produce the acidic environment in which pyrazinamide is active. Alternatively, in patients doing well, pyrazinamide can be stopped with the injectable phase if the patient can continue with at least three certain, or almost certain, effective drugs. Use adjunctive measures appropriately, including surgery and nutritional and social support. All measures should be taken to persuade and encourage patients not to stop treatment despite all its discomforts as it is the last that stands between patient and death.[44-50]

DOTS-Plus

DOTS-Plus now programatic management of drug resistant tuberculosis (PMDT) is an integral component of RNTCP to manage MDR-TB to be implemented through program infrastructure. The strategy is designed to manage MDR-TB using second-line anti-TB drugs within the DOTS strategy in low- and middle-income countries like India. Therefore in every DOTS implementing unit of the country, DOTS would be prioritized above DOTS-Plus with the view that DOTS reduces the emergence of MDR-TB, and therefore the need for DOTS-Plus overtime. The RNTCP under DOTS-Plus will be using a standardized treatment regimen (STR) Category IV regimen, comprising of 6 drugs (kanamycin, levofloxacin, ethionamide, cycloserine, pyrazinamide, and ethambutol) during 6–9 months of the intensive phase and 4 drugs (levofloxacin, ethionamide, cycloserine and ethambutol) during the 18 months of the continuation phase. *p*-aminosalicylic acid (PAS) is included in the regimen as a substitute drug if any bactericidal drug (kanamycin, levofloxacin, pyrazinamide and ethionamide) or any 2 bacteriostatic (ethambutol and cycloserine) drugs are not tolerated. This Category IV regimen is highly suitable for high TB prevalent nations as well as low to middle income countries like India. Injectable agent should be given at least for 6 months and the whole treatment duration is minimum of 18 months

Table 25.4: Suggested regimen for drug resistant/multidrug resistant tuberculosis before or without or unreliable DST reports

		Drug regimen	Duration in months	Drugs given (Responders)	Duration in months	Drugs given (Non-responders)
I	Misused drugs like SHE and THZ	Rifampicin Isoniazid Ethambutol Pyrazinamide ± Streptomycin	2–3*	Rifampicin Isoniazid Ethambutol ± Pyrazinamide	9	Treat as Group II or Take help of DST result
II	Misused drugs like SHREZ THZ	Streptomycin Isoniazid Rifampicin Ethambutol Pyrazinamide	2–3*	Rifampicin Isoniazid Ethambutol ± Pyrazinamide	9	Treat as Group III or Take help of DST result
III	Failed after adequate 5 drugs (SHREZ)	Kanamycin Fluoroquinolone (Levofloxacin/ Ofloxacin) Ethionamide Cycloserine Pyrazinamide Ethambutol	6–9	Ethionamide Fluoroquinolone (Levofloxacin/ Ofloxacin) Cycloserine Ethambutol	18	Treat as Group IV or Take help of DST result and consider surgery
IV	Failed on group III treatment	Capreomycin PAS Moxifloxacin High-dose INH Clofazimine Linezolid Amoxycillin/ Clavulanate	6–12	PAS Moxifloxacin High-dose INH Clofazimine Linezolid Amoxycillin/Clavulanate	18	Consider surgery

* depending on sputum conversion can be used for 3–6 months if toxicity does not intervene
R-rifampicin. H-isoniazid. E-ethambutol. Z-pyrazinamide. S-streptomycin. THZ-thiacetazone.

beyond sputum conversion. Fully standardized second-line treatment have shown to be feasible and cost-effective in DR-TB treatment.[18,49]

In our Indian set-up, most of the time either DST results are not available or if available they are usually highly unreliable. Keeping this fact in mind, depending upon past history of antituberculosis treatment author himself has used four groups of regimen in treating resistant/multidrug resistant tuberculosis and found to be effective.[37] The suggested regimen by author is given in Table 25.4.

Duration of Treatment

The optimal duration of therapy for MDR-TB has not been clearly established and duration remains questionable. WHO guidelines recommend continuing therapy for a minimum of 18 months after culture conversion until there is conclusive evidence to support a shorter duration of treatment. Extension of therapy to 24 months may be indicated in chronic cases with extensive pulmonary damage. This is, however, a highly expensive approach that is difficult to implement in the majority of middle- and low-income countries like India which bear the high burden of MDR-TB. The duration of injectables is also controversial. The 2006 and 2008 WHO guidelines advise at least 6 months or at least 4 months after smear or culture conversion. WHO guideline 2011 advise atlest 8 months of injectable. In addition duration has to be decided in correlation with other factors also like other drugs in the regimen, bacteriological status and drug toxicity.[44]

Monitoring of Treatment

Monitoring of treatment should be done with bacteriological, radiological and clinical methods. Sputum specimens should be obtained for semi-quantitative smear and culture every month from third month onwards during the intensive phase of therapy. Sputum conversion is defined as two sets of consecutive negative smears and cultures, from samples collected at least 30 days apart. Both bacteriological techniques (smear and culture) should be used to monitor patients throughout therapy. After sputum conversion smear examination and culture are done once in three months till the end of therapy.[44] If such large number of smears and cultures for follow-up is not possible, then at least five smears and cultures must be done for follow-up (4, 6, 12, 18 and 24 months), X-ray should be done every 6 months whereas clinical monitoring preferably should be done every month.[37]

Adjuvant Therapies

In addition to the administration of antimicrobial drug therapy, various other treatment modalities may play a significant role in management of patients. These include surgery, collapse therapy, laser therapy, immunomodulation therapy and gene therapy.

Surgery

The most common operative procedure is resection surgery. It is adjunct to chemotherapy and should not be considered as last resort. Chemotherapy should be given at least for two months prior to surgery and continued for 12–24 months after resection. It is indicated in patients who remain sputum positive, with resistance to large number of drugs; and localized pulmonary disease.[44]

Collapse Therapy

It is a reversible surgical therapy which involves collapse of lung by artificial pneumoperitonium or pneumothorax used for cavity containing diseased lung with concept that compression of the cavity will change the local environment in a manner which will inhibit the mycobacteria. This therapy does not appear to be of general utility, although artificial pneumoperitonium and pneumothorax may be helpful in highly selected cases.[51] However, controlled studies are lacking.

Laser Therapy

This has also been tried as an adjunct to chemotherapy in some countries such as Russia for the treatment of drug resistant TB. This is effective in multicavitary disease with heavy bacterial loads particularly when there is an increased chance of failure of medical treatment. It is thought to have a role in the rapid killing of bacteria, increases and improves penetration of antitubercular drugs in walled off lesions and helps in early closure of cavities and is of proven benefit in tracheal and bronchial stenosis due to endobronchial growth. It also reduces the trauma of surgery and postoperative complications.

Immunotherapy or Immunomodulation

Therapeutic modulation of the immune system to enhance the host's immunity to control tuberculosis and to shorten the durations of chemotherapy required to 'cure' patients with drug susceptible disease has been tried with some success. *Mycobacterium vaccae* have shown transiently favorable results when given to drug resistant tuberculosis who had failed chemotherapy.[52] Immune modulation can be affected by enhancing proinflammatory cytokines like IL-2, IL-12, IFN-γ, TNF-γ, inhibiting the anti-inflammatory cytokines like IL-4, IL-5, IL-10, addition of serum to enhance humoral factors or diverting the harmful Th_2 immune pathway to the beneficial Th_1 response by vaccination utilizing *M. vaccae*. However, these therapies are adjuncts and have proved useful in selected cases of drug resistant tuberculosis and randomized control trials, have failed to confirm the utility of this therapy.[53] Beneficial effect of parenterally used interferon gamma (IFN-α) have been reported in disseminated disease attributable to mycobacteria other than tuberculosis that was refractory to chemotherapy.[54] Favorable results were reported following one month use of inhaled IFN-γ, 500 microgram thrice weekly. Cytokine therapy has been shown to have clinical utility in modifying the inflammatory manifestation of the lepromatous type of disease.[55] Interleukin-2 (IL-2) was used to restore antigen responsiveness, presumably via enhancing IFN-γ production. Thalidomide has been shown to inhibit the in-vitro release of TNF-α from peripheral blood monocytes. In patients with active tuberculosis, it induces a significant gain in weight.[56] However, the possibility that thalidomide agents may ameliorate tissue injury in tuberculosis needs further study.[57,58] The potential role of diverse agents such as transfer factor, indomethacin, and levamisole is yet to be established.[59] Levamisole as adjunct to drug treatment has been reported to cause more rapid radiological clearing in the treated group. However, it did not significantly affect the clinical outcome.[60] *Mycobacterium w* (commercially available as Immuvac) has been extensively studied as an effective immunomodulator for treatment of leprosy. It enhances bacterial killing and lesion clearance when used as an adjuvant to multidrug therapy for leprosy. *Mycobacterium w* shares antigens with *M leprae* as well as *M. tuberculosis* suggesting its application in treatment of drug resistant tuberculosis. A randomized control study has demonstrated that this drug may be responsible for overall reduction of duration of therapy, with no change in sputum conversion rate compared with the traditional short- course chemotherapy in new as well as retreatment cases of tuberculosis.[61,62] Another advantage though not proven, may be that Immuvac effect would be longer lasting and could take care of defaulters more meaningfully than chemotherapy alone, leading to a reduction in relapse rate and the emergence of MDR TB. Recently, a randomized control trial has been initiated in 2007 and is under progress in order to establish its efficacy and safety as an adjunct therapy in new pulmonary tuberculosis (Category I) patients.

Gene Therapy

The decoding of the human genome provides another fascinating aspect in the future therapeutic intervention of tuberculosis. By identifying resistance genes, it will be possible to detect drug resistance before start of therapy and also to develop drugs that target these specific genes, enabling us to considerably reduce the duration of therapy.[63]

Role of Steroids

The adjuvant use of corticosteroids in DR-TB patients has been shown not to increase mortality and can be beneficial in conditions such as severe respiratory insufficiency, severe drug induced rashes and central nervous system or pericardial involvement. Prednisone is commonly used, starting at approximately 1 mg/kg and gradually decreasing the dose to 10 mg per week when a long course is indicated. Corticosteroids may also alleviate symptoms in patients with an exacerbation of obstructive pulmonary disease or when patient is in a very low general condition. In these cases, prednisone may be given in a short course, tapering over 1–2 weeks, starting at approximately 1 mg/kg and decreasing the dose by 5–10 mg per day. Injectable corticosteroids are often used initially when a more immediate response is needed.[44]

OUTCOME OF TREATMENT

The outcome of treatment of multidrug resistant tuberculosis is not very favorable and varied from 50–80% in different studies. In a retrospective analysis of 171 immunocompetent patients treated over a ten-year period (1973–1983) at the National Jewish Hospital in Denver, the overall favorable outcome was only a little over 50%.[64] All patients were treated with individually tailored regimens in which they received at least 3 or 4 drugs which they had not received previously, or to which they were known to be susceptible. Of the 134 patients evaluated for efficacy, 65% became culture negative and 35% failed to respond. Of those who became culture negative, 14% eventually relapsed giving an overall favorable outcome in 56% of patients. Of the patients who failed, 46% died of tuberculosis. In the Cape Province South Africa, the 5 year outcome of 240 MDR-TB patients was death in 48%, cure in 33%, 15% were respiratory disabled and 13% were still bacteriologically positive.[65] However, not all the reports are so grim. In a retrospective analysis reported from South Korea, of 107 patients with MDR-TB treated with at least four drugs to which they had not been exposed to before, or to which they were known to be susceptible, in 63 patients with sufficient follow-up data, 52 (82.5%) responded to chemotherapy. There was no subsequent relapse among the patients who responded, and there were no tuberculosis related deaths. The author concluded that, MDR-TB responds relatively well to carefully selected regimens. However, the mean period of follow-up was only 17 months.[66] Experience of scientists of TRC, Chennai with MDR-TB has been equally discouraging. In about 170 patients with MDR-TB over a 12-year-period (1986–1997) all but two of whom were HIV negative, only one-third had a favorable outcome, and one-third died. These patients were treated with regimens which included at least three or four of the following drugs: ethionamide, ethambutol, pyrazinamide, cycloserine, streptomycin or kanamycin, PAS, thioacetazone and high dose isoniazid (600 mg) with 10 mg of pyridoxine. Goble, et al. in a study on 171 patients showed poor outcome after a mean follow-up period of 5 years, in which only 56% patients responded, and 20% of the mortality was attributed to TB.[64] Khanna, et al.[67] used kanamycin (6 months), cycloserine, ethionamide and sodium PAS for 18 months in hospitalized patients and observed bacteriological conversion in 10 out of 14 patients (71%). Purohit, et al.[68] used kanamycin (6 months), ethionamide, sodium PAS and isoniazid for 18 months on domiciliary basis and bacteriological conversion was achieved in 73% of the patients. In another study by Rupak Singla, et al.[69] bacteriological quescence was achieved in 78% of the patients who completed the full therapy. Prasad, et al.[37] observed 75.5% sputum and culture conversion rate at the end of two years in 45 patients of MDR pulmonary tuberculosis patients by using kanamycin, ethionamide, PAS and cycloserine regimen. Out of 45 patients 34 (75.5%) patients were decleared cured, these patients followed for average 17.4 months (3–60 months) two patients relapsed (5.7%) so long-term outcome was around 70%. This cohort had greater long-term success rates 75% vs 56% and lower TB death rates, 12% vs 22% than the earlier one. Markers of response in order of reliability are bacteriology of sputum, radiology followed by the clinical picture. A systematic review and meta-analysis of the available therapeutic studies on the treatment of multidrug resistant tuberculosis showed that the overall treatment success estimate was 62% (95% CI, 58–67%); however, the heterogeneity in study characteristics led to significant variation in reported treatment outcomes. Individualized treatment regimens had higher treatment success (64%, 95% CI 59–68%) than standardized regimens (54%, 95% CI 43–68%), although the difference was not significant. The proportion of patients treated successfully improved when treatment duration was at least 18 months, and if patients received directly observed therapy throughout treatment. Studies that combined both factors had significantly higher pooled success proportions (69%, 95% CI 64–73%) than other studies of treatment outcomes (58%, 95% CI 52–64%).[70] The outcome for patients with MDR-TB is not very favorable in immunocompetent patients, the response in HIV positive patients is even bleaker. In the outbreaks of MDR-TB in and around New York city, between 1988 and 1992, predominantly in HIV infected individuals, mortality was in the order of 80% and the mean duration from diagnosis to death was 4–16 weeks. In a study of 173 patients hospitalized from 1983 to 1993 with MDR-TB, of whom 52% were known to be HIV infected, 55% of the patients in the cohort died; mortality was significantly greater for HIV positive than HIV negative (72% versus 20%) patients. The median duration of survival of MDR-TB patients was 22 days to 1 month. In HIV positive patients, only appropriate therapy was associated with prolonged survival.[64]

CONCLUSION

The subject of drug resistant and multidrug resistant tuberculosis is a vast one and an area of growing concern among clinicians, epidemiologists, public health workers worldwide. New researches in the areas involving molecular biology and application of these in the field of epidemiology could help in better understanding of the mechanisms of drug resistance and development of newer diagnostic tools and effective drugs to control multidrug resistant tuberculosis. Till such time multidrug resistant tuberculosis must be managed very effectively to reduce morbidity and mortality and transmission of multi-drug resistance tuberculosis. It must also be emphasized that even optimal treatment of multidrug resistance tuberculosis will not alone curb the epidemic. Efforts must be focused on the effective use of first-line drugs in every new case so as to prevent the ultimate emergence of multidrug resistant tuberculosis.

REFERENCES

1. Multidrug resistant tuberculosis. ICMR. 1999;29(10 and 11):105-14.
2. Jin DT, Gross CA. Mapping and sequencing of mutations in the *E. coli* rpoB gene that lead to rifampicin resistance. J Mol Biol. 1988;202:45-58.

3. Multidrug Resistant Tuberculosis. Chest. 1993;104(4):1194-8.
4. Cohn ML, Kovitz C, Oda U, Middlebrook G. Studies on isoniazid and tubercle bacilli, II : the growth requirements, catalase activities, and pathogenic properties of isoniazid-resistant mutants. Am Rev Tuberc. 1954;54:641-64.
5. Spider DE, Kelly GD, Cauthen GM, Thompson NJ, Kilburn JO. Infection and disease among contacts of tuberculosis cases with drug-resistant and drug-susceptible bacilli. Am Rev Respir Dis. 1985;132:125-32.
6. Ordway DJ, Sonnenberg MG, Donahue SA, Belisle JT, Orme IM. Drug-resistant strains of *Mycobacterium tuberculosis* exhibit a range of virulence for mice. Infect Immun. 1995;63:741-3.
7. Frieden TR, Sherman LF, Maw KL, et al. A multi-institutional outbreak of highly drug-resistant tuberculosis: epidemiology and clinical outcome. JAMA. 1996;276:1229-35.
8. Stewart SM, Crofton JW. The clinical significance of low degrees of drug resistance in pulmonary tuberculosis. Am Rev Respir Dis. 1964;89:811-29.
9. Mitchison DA, Nunn AJ. Influence of initial drug-resistance on the response to short-course chemotherapy of pulmonary tuberculosis. Am Rev Respir Dis. 1986;133:423-30.
10. Chandrasekaran S, Jagota P, Chaudhuri K. Initial drug resistance to antituberculosis drugs in urban and rural district tuberculosis programme. Ind J Tub. 1992;39:171-5.
11. Paramasivan CN, Chandrasekaran V, Santha T, Sudarsanam NM, Prabhakar R. Bacteriological investigations for short course chemotherapy under the tuberculosis programme in two districts in India. Tuber Lung Dis. 1993;74:23-7.
12. Jain NK, Chopra KK, Prasad G. Initial and acquired isoniazid and rifampicin resistance to *M. tuberculosis* and its implications for treatment. Ind J Tub. 1992;39:121-4.
13. Mathew R. Santha T, Parthasarathy R, Rajaram K, Paramasivan CN, Janardhanam B, et al. Response of patients with initially drug-resistant organisms to treatment with short-course chemotherapy. Indian J Tuberc. 1993;40:119-23.
14. Salomon N, Perlman DC, Friedmann P, Buchstein S, Kreiswirth BN, Mildvan D. Predictors and outcome of multidrug-resistant tuberculosis. Clin Infect Dis. 1995;21:1245-52.
15. Turett GS, Telzak EE, Torian LV. Improved outcomes for patients with multidrug-resistant tuberculosis. Clin Infect Dis. 1995;21:1238-44.
16. Telzak EE, Sepkowitz K, Alpert P, et al. Multidrug-resistant tuberculosis in patients without HIV infection. N Engl J Med. 1995;333:907-11.
17. Park MM, Davis AL, Schluger NW, Cohen H, Rom WN. Outcome of MDR-TB patients, 1983-1993 prolonged survival with appropriate therapy. Am J Respir Crit Care Med. 1996;153: 317-24.
18. DOTS-PLUS guidelines, Revised National Tuberculosis Control Program, Central TB Division Directorate General Health Services, Ministry of Health and Family Welfare, Nirman Bhawan, New Delhi. Publishers (P) Ltd. 2008.
19. National Consensus on MDR Tuberculosis Research Forum India. 1999.
20. Toman K. Tuberculosis Case Detection, Treatment and Monitoring. Jaypee Brothers Medical Publishers (P). Ltd. 2nd Ind. Ed. New Delhi, 2004.
21. Marks J. Cited in Fox, W. Bulletin of the international union against tuberculosis. 1972;47:49.
22. Wichelhausen RH and Robinson LB. American review of respiratory diseases. 1969;99:1.
23. Guidelines for the management of Drug Resistant Tuberculosis, Global Tuberculosis Program. WHO/TB/96.210.
24. Laszlo A, et al. Quality assurance program for drugs susceptibility testing of *Mycobacterium tuberculosis* in the WHO/IUATLD supranational laboratory network: first round of proficiency testing. International journal of tuberculosis and Lung Disease. 1997;1:231-8.
25. Treatment of tuberculosis: guidelines—4th edn. WHO/HTM/TB/2009.420.
26. Casal M, Gutierrez J, Vaquero M. Comparative evaluation of the mycobacteria growth indicator tube with the BACTEC 460 TB system and Löwenstein-Jensen medium for isolation of mycobacteria from clinical specimens. Int J Tuberc Lung Dis. 1997;1:81-4.

27. Rivera AB, Tupasi TE, Grimaldo ER, Cardano RC, Co VM. Rapid and improved recovery rate of *Mycobacterium tuberculosis* in mycobacteria growth indicator. Int J Tuebrc Lung Dis. 1997;1:454-9.
28. Heifets LB. Clinical Mycobacteriology. Philadelphia : WB Saunders, 1996.
29. Kiehn TE. The diagnostic mycobacteriology laboratory of the 1990s. Clin Infect Dis. 1993;17:S447-54.
30. WHO Press Release New Rapid Test for DR-TB for developing Countries Geneva, 2008.
31. Towards universal access to diagnosis and treatment of multidrug-resistant and extensively drug resistant tuberculosis by 2015. WHO progress report 2011. WHO/HTM/TB/2011.3.
32. Telenti A, Imboden P, Marchesi F, Schmidheini T, Bodmer T, et al. Direct automated detection of rifampin resistant *Mycobacterium tuberculosis* by polymerase chain reaction and single-strand conformation polymorphism. Antimicrob Agents Chemother. 1993a;37:2054-8.
33. Shoemaker SA, Fisher JH, Jones WE Jr, Scoggin CH. Restriction fragment analysis of chromosomal DNA defines different strains of *Mycobacterium tuberculosis* complex: analysis of restriction fragment heterogenicity using cloned DNA probes. Am Rev Respir Dis. 1986;133:1065-8.
34. Cohn DL, O'Brien RJ. The use of restriction fragment length polymorphism (RFLP) analysis for epidemiological studies of tuberculosis in developing countries. Int J Tuberc Lung Dis. 1998;2:16-26.
35. Dubow MS. Antituberculosis drug screening [commentary]. Lancet. 1993;342:448-9.
36. Hazbon MH. Recent advances in molecular methods for early diagnosis of tuberculosis and drug resistant tuberculisis. Biomedica. 2004;24(Suppl):149-62.
37. Prasad R, Verma SK, Sahai S, Kumar, Jain A. Efficacy and safety of kanamycin, ethionamide, PAS, and cycloserine in multidrug resistant pulmonary tuberculosis patients. Ind J Chest Dis Allied Sci. 2006;48:183-6.
38. Tsukamura M, Mzumo. Cross resistant relationships among the aminoglycoside antibiotics in *Mycobacterium tuberculosis*. J Gen Microbiol. 1995;98:611.
39. Venkataraman P, Paramsivan CN, Prabhakar R. In vitro activity of rifampicin, rifapentine and rifabutin against south Indian isolates *Mycobacteirum tuberculosis*. Ind J Tub. 1993;40:17.
40. Jain NK, Surpal BB, Khanna SP, Fatma T. In vitro activity of ofloxacin against clinical isolates of *Mycobacterium tuberculosis*. Ind J Tub. 1996;43:183-6.
41. Yew WW, Chan CK, Leung CC, et al. Comparative roles of levofloxacin and ofloxacin in the treatment of multidrug-resistant tuberculosis: Preliminary results of a retrospective study from Hong-Kong. Chest. 2003;124:1476-81.
42. Canetti G, Kreis B, Thibur R, Gay P, Oe-Lirzin M. Donnees actualles su la resistance primare deus la tuberculose pulmonaire de "L" adulte in France, deuxieme enquiete In Centre d'Etudes sur la resistance Primaire (1) aunees 1865-66. Rev Tuberc Pneumol. 1967;31:433-74.
43. Drug-resistant tuberculosis: A survival guide for clinicians. San Francisco, Franis J. Curry National Tuberculosis Center and California Department of Health Services, 2004.
44. Guidelines for the programmatic management of drug-resistant tuberculosis—WHO 2008, 2011.
45. Prasad R. Management of multidrug resistance tuberculosis practitioner's view point. Indian J Tub. 2007;54:3-11.
46. Treatment of tuberculosis: Guidelines for national programmes. Geneva, WHO 2003 (WHO CDS/TB/2003.313)
47. Crofton J Chaulet P, Maher D. Guidelines for the management of drug resistant tuberculosis, Geneva,WHO, 1997 (Document WHO/TB/96: 210).
48. Mukerjee JS, Rich ML, Socci AR, et al. Programmes and principles in treatment of multidrug resistant tuberculosis. Lancet. 2004;363:474-81.
49. Suarez PG, et al. Feasibility and cost-effectiveness of standardized second-line drug treatment for chronic tuberculosis patients; a national cohort study in Peru. Lancet. 2002;359:1980-9.

50. Mukherjee J, Socci A, Acha J, et al. The PIH guide to management of multidrug-resistant tuberculosis. International edition. Boston, MA, USA: Partners in Health, 2003.
51. Nitta AT, Iseman MD, Newell JD, Madsen LA, Goble M. Ten-year experience with artificial pneumoperitoneum for end-stage, drug-resistant pulmonary tuberculosis. Clin Infect Dis. 1993;16:219-22.
52. Etemadi A, Farid R, Stanford JL. Immunotherapy for drug-resistant tuberculosis [Letter]. Lancet. 1992;340:1360-1.
53. Stanfort JL. Frontiers in mycobacteriology. Symposium sponsored by National Jewish Center for Immunology and Respiratory Medicine, Vail, Colorado, 1997.
54. Holland SN, Eisenstein EM, Kuhns DB, et al. Treatment of refractory disseminated nontuberculous mycobacterial infection with interferon gamma. N Engl J Med. 1994;330: 1348-55.
55. Kaplan G. Recent advances in cytokine therapy in leprosy. J Infect Dis. 1993;167:S18-S22.
56. Moller DR, Wysocka M, Greenlee BM. Inhibition of IL-12 production by thalidomide. J Immunol. 1997;159:5157-17.
57. Tremontana JM, Utaipat U, Molloy A, Akarasewi P, Burroughs M, Makonkawkeykoon S, et al. Thalidomide treatment reduces tumor necrosis factor-alpha production and enhances weight gain in patients with pulmonary tuberculosis. Mol Med. 1995;1:384-97.
58. Klausner JD, Makonkawkeyoon S, Akarasewi P, Nataka K, Kasinerk W, Cooral L, et al. The effect of thalidomide on the pathogenesis of human immunodeficiency virus type 1 and *Mycobacterium tuberculosis* infection. J Acquir Immune Defic Syndr Hum Retroviral. 1996;11:247-57.
59. Edwards D, Kirkpatrick CH. The immunology of mycobacterial diseases. Am Rev Respir Dis. 1986;134:1062-71.
60. Singh MM, Kumar P, Malaviya AN, Kumar R. Levamisole as an adjunct in the treatment of pulmonary tuberculosis. Am Rev Respir Dis. 1981;123:277-9.
61. Patel N, Deshpande MM, Shah M. Effect of an immunomodulator containing *Mycobacterium w* on sputum conversion in pulmonary tuberculosis. J Indian Med Assoc. 2002;100:191-3.
62. Patel N, Trapathi SB. Improved cure rates in pulmonary tuberculosis category II (retreatment) with *Mycobacterium w.* J Indian Med Assoc. 2003;101:680-2.
63. Ian Smith. Stop TB : Is DOTS the Answer ? Ind J Tub. 1999;46:81-9.
64. Goble M, Iseman MD, Madson LA, Waite, D, Ackerson L, Horsburg CR Jr. Treatment of 171 patients with pulmonary tuberculosis resistant to isoniazid and streptomycin. N Engl J Med. 1993;328:527.
65. Schaaf HS, Botha P, Beyers N, Gie RP, Vermeulen HA, Groenewald P, et al. The 5-year outcome of multidrug resistant tuberculosis patients in the Cape Province of South Africa. Trop Med Int Health. 1996;1:718.
66. Park SK, Kim CT, Song SD. Outcome of chemotherapy in 107 patients with pulmonary tuberculosis resistant to isoniazid and rifampicin. Int J Tuber Lung Dis. 1998;2:877.
67. Khanna BK. Treatment of long-term tuberculosis treatment failures. Ind J Tub. 1985;32:171.
68. Purohit SD, Gupta M, Agnihotri SP, Madan A, Gupta PR. Management of chemotherapy failures. Ind J Tub. 1991;38:3.
69. Singla R, Myneedu VP, Jaiswal A, Puri MM, Jain RC. Ethionamide, cycloserine, isoniazid, sodium PAS and kanamycin in retreatment of drug failure pulmonary tuberculosis patients. Ind J Tub. 1995;42:23.
70. Evan W Orenstein BS, Sanjay Basu, Sarita Shah, N et al. Treatment outcomes among patients with multidrug-resistant tuberculosis: systematic review and meta-analysis. Lancet Infect Dis. 2009;9,153-61.

Chapter 26

Multidrug Resistant Tuberculosis: Case-Based Management

CASE I

TS, a 18-year-old female diagnosed as pulmonary tuberculosis in 1995 and was prescribed rifampicin, isoniazid and ethambutol which she stopped herself after four months due to improvement. After five months of asymptomatic period, she again developed symptoms and prescribed rifampicin, isoniazid and ethambutol which she stopped after one month due to drug intolerance. Next time she received rifampicin, isoniazid, ethambutol and pyrazinamide in fix dose combination of controversial quality for next three months without any improvement. Thereafter, treatment was changed to streptomycin, rifampicin, isoniazid, ethambutol and pyrazinamide for next two months, without any response. Then she received Category II treatment under Revised National TB Control Program (RNTCP) for nine months and still her sputum remained positive for acid-fast bacilli (AFB). In June 1997, she was hospitalized and her sputum was sent for culture and sensitivity for *Mycobacterium tuberculosis* and was treated with daily streptomycin, rifampicin, isoniazid, ethambutol and pyrazinamide in adequate doses under supervision. After four months of regular treatment her sputum remained positive for AFB. Her sputum culture and sensitivity report revealed resistance to rifampicin, isoniazid and streptomycin. Considering the past history of treatment, radiological, symptomatic deterioration and sensitivity report, she was diagnosed as MDR-TB. She was treated with injection kanamycin 0.75 g, PAS 10 g (in two divided doses), ethionamide 500 mg and cycloserine 500 mg daily. 300 mg of isoniazid was also given (Fig. 26.1A). Her sputum smear was examined every month for AFB. Kanamycin was stopped after 4 months

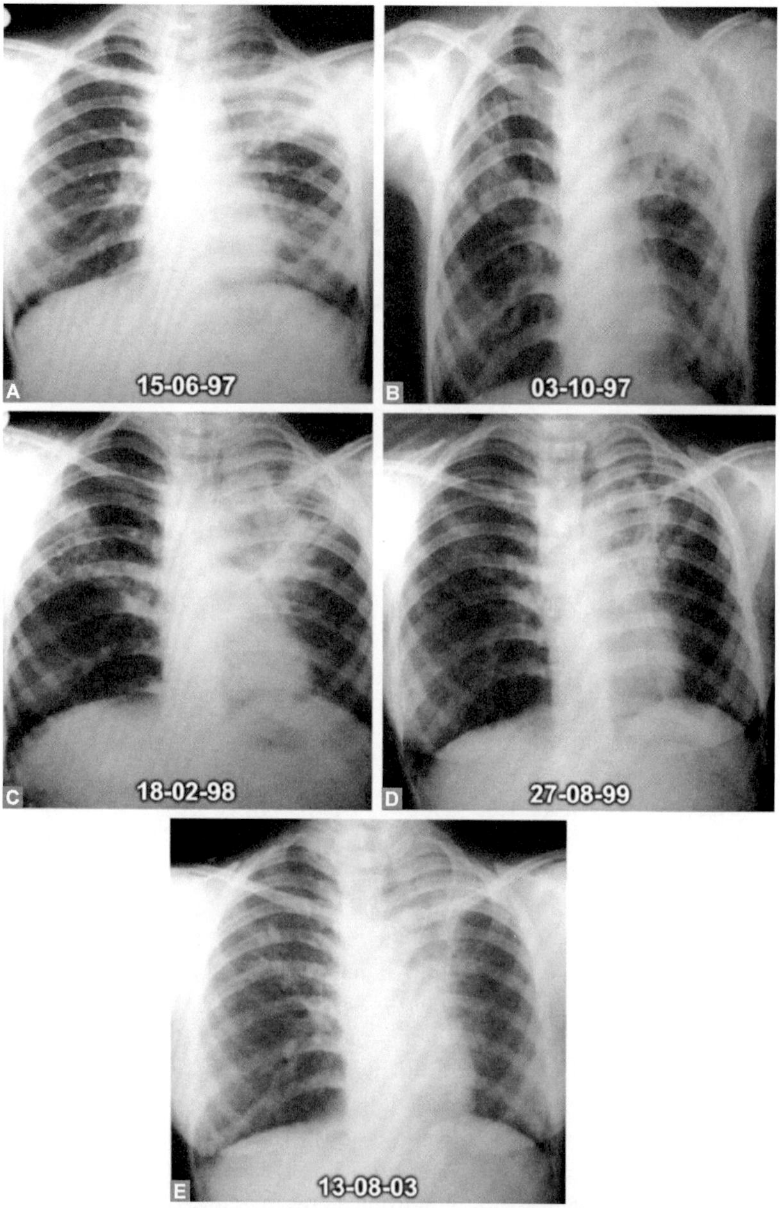

Figs 26.1 A to E : Chest X-rays of patients undergoing treatment

when her sputum smear became negative for AFB (Fig. 26.1B). Rest of the treatment was continued for a period of 18 months (Figs 26.1C and D). At the end of the treatment, sputum smear and culture were negative for MTB. On subsequent follow-up for next five years, there was no relapse (Fig. 26.1E).

CASE II

SS, a 15-year-old female, weighing 35 kg was diagnosed as a sputum positive new case of pulmonary tuberculosis in February 1998, with bad family history of her brother, who died of pulmonary tuberculosis after prolonged treatment for 4 years. She was prescribed 4 drug regimen comprising rifampicin, isoniazid, ethambutol and pyrazinamide in adequate doses, which she took regularly for 2 month, without any significant improvement clinically, radiologically as well as bacteriologically. Then she sought advice from other physician who added streptomycin and sparfloxacin to her previous regimen of 4 drugs. She took 6 drug regimen regularly for 6 months with negligible response clinically and radiologically. Subsequently she consulted us, when her sputum was positive for AFB and was also sent for culture and sensitivity for *Mycobacterium tuberculosis*. In light of her previous treatment experiences and outcomes, she was suspected as a case of primary MDR-TB. Pending sensitivity report, she was started on kanamycin 0.75 g, isoniazid 300 mg, PAS 8 g (in two divided doses), ethionamide 500 mg and cycloserine 500 mg daily in single dose, in September 1998 (Figs 26.2A to C). With the passage of time, she showed improvement clinically and radiologically, when her sputum became negative after 4 months. At the same time her sputum culture and sensitivity report from 4 different laboratories (sent at beginning of treatment) showed lots of discrepancies, with 2 of them labeling her as a case of MDR-TB while other labeling her as polydrug resistance other than MDR. Regardless of conflicting sensitivity reports we adhered to our regimen. Kanamycin was stopped after she became sputum negative, and rest of the treatment was continued for another 20 months. At the end of 2 years of treatment, she was smear and culture negative with dramatic clearing of chest radiograph and weight gain of about 7 kg (Figs 26.2D and E). She was followed for 5 years (till 2002), without any relapse (Fig. 26.2F).

CASE III

MR, 32-year-old male, weighing 43 kg was diagnosed as a case of pulmonary tuberculosis in 1992 and was treated with 2RHEZ/4RHE and declared cured. He has relapsed in 1994 and was again treated by different doctors for two years with different inadequate regimens with drug including streptomycin, rifampicin, isoniazid, ethambutol and pyrazinamide without any response. He consulted another physician and took kanamycin (2 months), ethionamide, (2 months), isoniazid and thiacetazone for one year without any response. He came to us in September 1997 with complaints of cough, fever, loss of appetite and weight. His serial chest X-rays showed progressive deterioration and his sputum was positive for AFB (Fig. 26.3A). Sputum was sent for culture and sensitivity for MTB. Pending the culture and sensitivity report, he was prescribed streptomycin, rifampicin, isoniazid, ethambutol

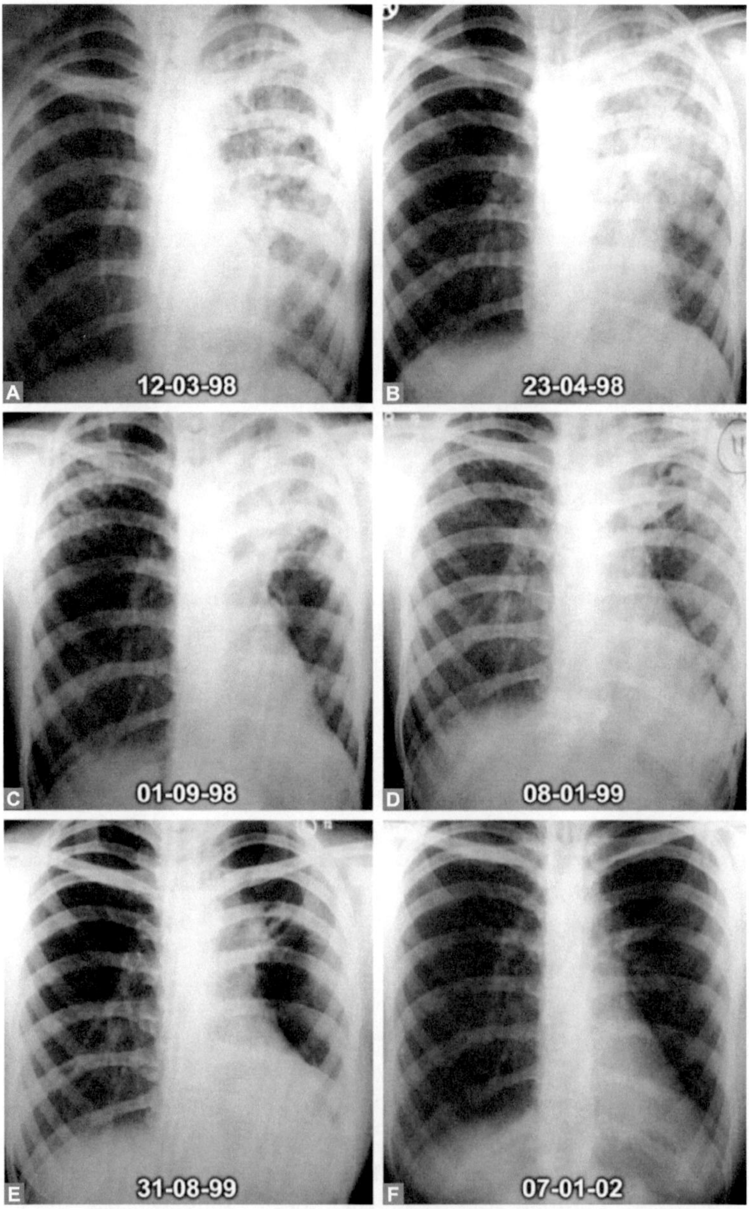

Figs 26.2 A to F: Chest X-rays of patients undergoing treatment

and pyrazinamide in adequate doses with intensive health education. At the end of three months of regular treatment, he did not respond clinically and his sputum remained positive for AFB. Sputum culture (sent at the time of starting five drug) and sensitivity showed resistance to streptomycin, pyrazinamide, PAS and ethionamide with susceptibility to rifampicin, isoniazid, ethambutol, thiacetazone and cycloserine. However in view of past

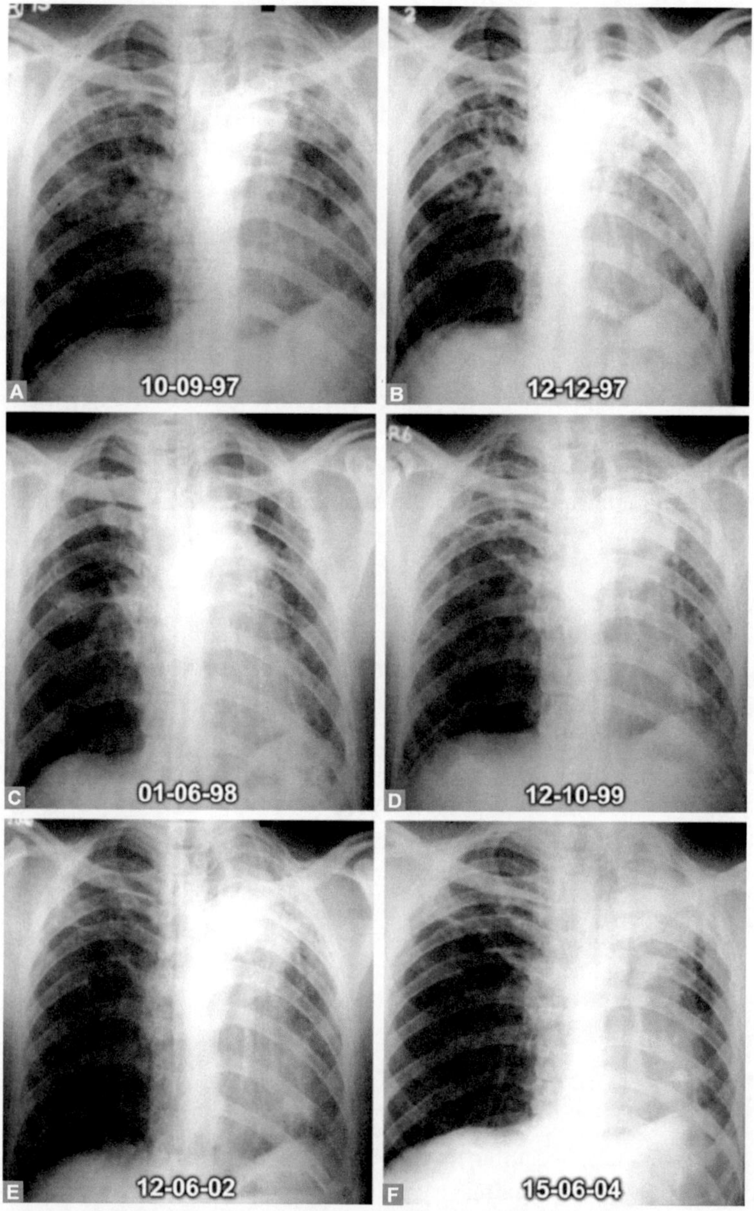

Figs 26.3 A to F: Chest X-rays of patients undergoing treatment

history of ATT, his sensitivity report was ignored and was assumed as a case of MDR-TB and treatment was changed to injection kanamycin 0.75 g, PAS 10 g (in two divided doses), ethionamide 500 mg, pyrazinamide 1500 mg and ofloxacin 600 mg daily in December 1997 (Fig. 26.3B). 300 mg of isonizid was also given. His sputum smear was examined for AFB every month. Patient developed gastric intolerance in the beginning of treatment, however, all the drugs were continued. Injection kanamycin was stopped after 6 months in June 1998 (Fig. 26.3C), when his sputum became negative for AFB and rest of the drugs were continued for another 18 months. Patient responded clinically, radiologically and bacteriologically. Sputum smears for AFB and cultures were negative for MTB at the end of the treatment (Fig. 26.3D). Till now, after five years of regular follow-up, he has not relapsed (Fig. 26.3E and F).

CASE IV

NK, a 27-year-male, weighing 40 kg presented with bilateral pulmonary tuberculosis with previous antitubercular treatment. Different doctors treated him for 4 years for pulmonary tuberculosis with different regimens in various combinations with drugs including streptomycin, isoniazid, rifampicin, ethambutol and pyrazinamide. His sputum was positive for AFB, which was sent for culture and sensitivity for *M. tuberculosis*. Pending culture report, treatment was started with five drug regimen of streptomycin 0.75 g, isoniazid 300 mg, rifampicin 450 mg, ethambutol 800 mg and pyrazinamide 1000 mg, daily in single dose, which he took regularly for 2 months without any clinical, radiological or bacteriological response. Sputum culture and sensitivity sent earlier, revealed drug resistance to streptomycin, isoniazid and rifampicin. On basis of this report, and previous history of treatment, he was kept on kanamycin 0.75 g, ethionamide 500 mg, ofloxacin 600 mg, ethambutol 800 mg and pyrazinamide 1000 mg daily in single dose. Isoniazid in single dose of 300 mg daily was also added. He responded clinically and bacteriologically, but his chest radiograph revealed no change on left side (which was destroyed), with some clearing of shadows in right lung. Sputum conversion occurred after 6 months of treatment, when kanamycin was stopped, and rest of drugs were continued for next 18 months. At the end of treatment, his sputum was negative for AFB and he has gained weight of 6 kg, but radiographical shadows persisted without much change, which in all likelihood will persist throughout his life and may be source of infection and hemoptysis in future (Fig. 26.4A to D).

CASE V

NR, 35-year-male, weighing 40 kg, presented with bilateral pulmonary tuberculosis, with previous history of antitubercular treatment, from different doctors in various inadequate regimens, using streptomycin, isoniazid, rifampicin, ethambutol and pyrazinamide. At the time of presentation to us in January 2001 (Fig. 26.5A), his sputum was positive for AFB, which was also sent for culture and sensitivity for *M. tuberculosis*. Pending sensitivity report, he was kept on regimen containing streptomycin 0.75 g, isoniazid 300 mg, rifampicin 450 mg, ethambutol 800 mg and pyrazinamide 1000 mg. Despite 4 months of regular treatment, there was no response on clinical,

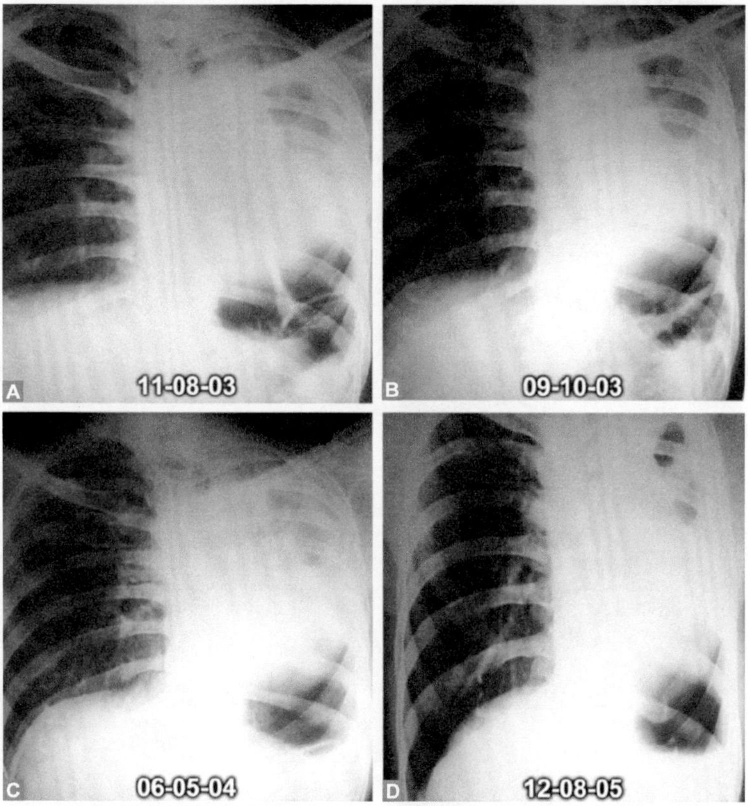

Figs 26.4 A to D: Chest X-rays of patients undergoing treatment

radiological and bacteriological parameters (Fig. 26.5B). Sputum sensitivity sent at the beginning of treatment reported resistance to streptomycin, isoniazid, ethambutol and rifampicin. In light of this sensitivity report, previous inadequate treatment and lack of response to 4 months treatment of 5 drugs, he was diagnosed as a case of MDR-TB, and kept on kanamycin 0.75 g, isoniazid 300 mg, PAS 8 g (in two divided doses), ethionamide 500 mg and cycloserine 500 mg daily in single dose (Fig. 26.5C). After one month of this therapy, he developed psychosis with suicidal tendency, which was managed by antipsychotic drugs, and cycloserine was replaced by ofloxacin 600 mg daily in single dose. His sputum became negative for AFB after 6 months of treatment, when kanamycin was stopped, and rest of drugs continued for next 18 months till April 2003 (Figs 26.5D to F), when he became smear and culture negative, and declared cured. While he was on this regimen, chest radiographic picture deteriorated, but sputum smear always remained negative. Considering this radiological deterioration as intercurrent pyogenic infection, we adhered to our antitubercular regimen with some appropriate antibiotics. He was followed up for 2 years, without any relapse, although he experienced occasional bouts of streaking of sputum during follow-up period, which used to improve with conservative treatment (Fig. 26.5G).

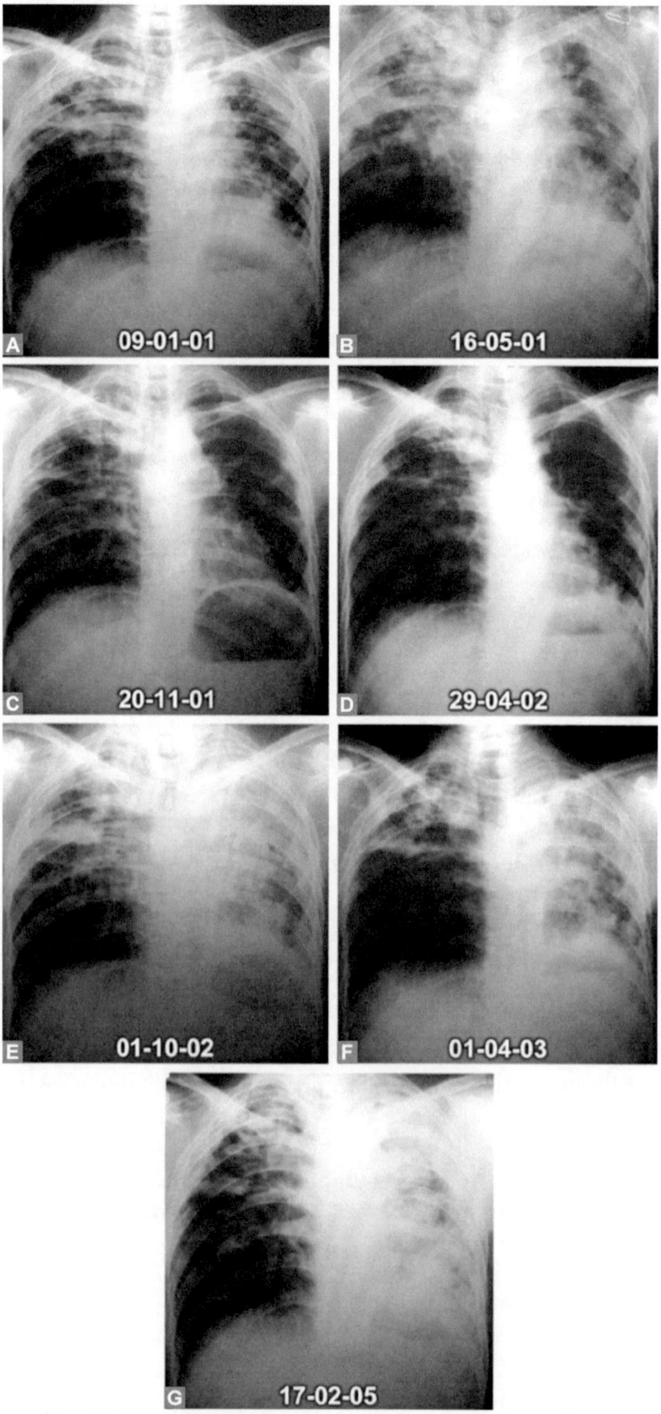

Figs 26.5 A to G: Chest X-rays of patients undergoing treatment

CASE VI

AV, a 22-year-old female diagnosed as a new case of sputum positive pulmonary tuberculosis in 2006 (Fig. 26.6A). She was started on a regimen based on rifampicin, isoniazid, ethambutol, pyrazinamide from private practitioner. She developed vomiting and gastritis after which she stopped her antituberculosis drugs. She then consulted multiple private practitioners taking the prescribed treatment consisting of primary line of anti-TB drugs for 1–2 months then stopping at her own with partial relief of symptoms each time. In May 2008, (Fig. 26.6B) she presented to us, her sputum was found to be positive for AFB, sputum was sent for culture and

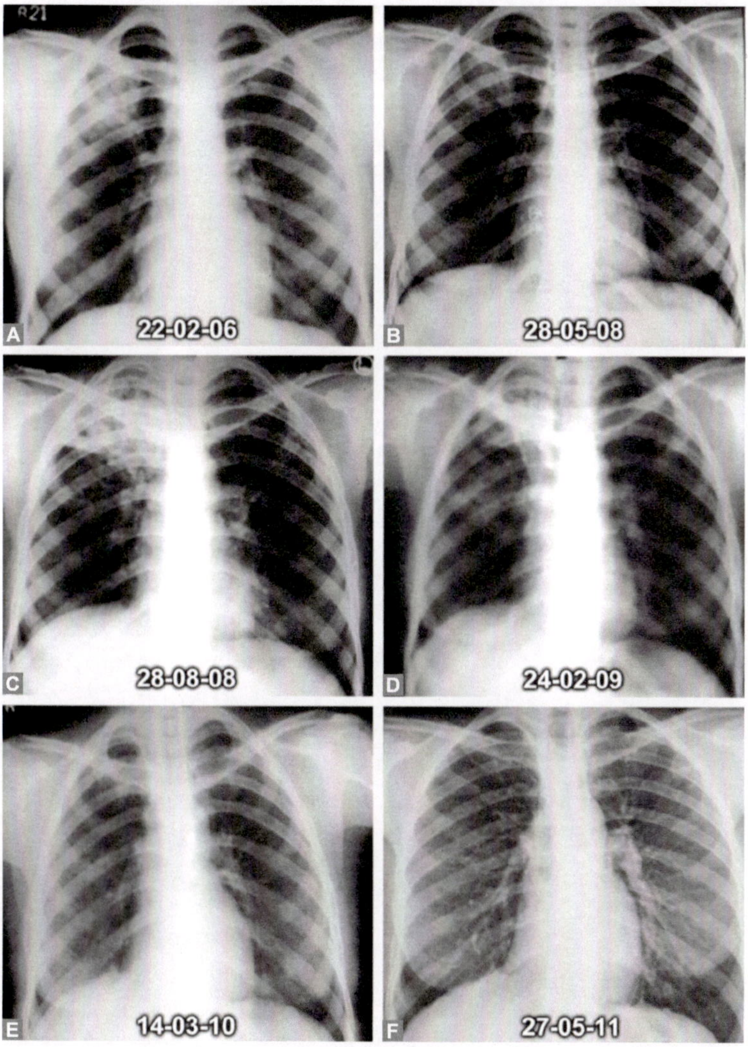

Figs 26.6 A to F: Chest X-rays of patients undergoing treatment

sensitivity for mycobacterial tuberculosis and she was started on a five drug regimen consisting of rifampicin, isoniazid, ethambutol, pyrazinamide and streptomycin. Her sputum culture sensitivity received in August 2008 (Fig. 26.6C) showed growth of *Mycobacterium tuberculosis*, which was resistant to rifampicin and isoniazid. She was started on regimen for MDR TB consisting of injection kanamycin, pyrizinamide, ethambutol, ethionamide, cycloserine and ofloxacin. Her clinical condition improved, sputum for AFB and culture for *Mycobacterium* became negative 4th month onwards. Kanamycin and pyrizinamide were stopped after 6 months (Fig. 26.6D). Rest of the treatment was continued for 18 months (Fig. 26.6E). Patient responded clinically, radiologically and bacteriologically. Sputum and culture were negative for *Mycobacterium tuberculosis* at the end of treatment in 2010. On subsequent follow up for one year she was asymptomatic (Fig. 26.6F).

Chapter 27

Multidrug Resistant Tuberculosis—Monitoring of Treatment and Adverse Drug Reaction

INTRODUCTION

The initial evaluation serves to establish a baseline and may identify patients who are at increased risk for adverse effects or poor outcomes. The monitoring of treatment and the management of adverse effects may have to be more intensive in patients with pre-existing conditions or conditions identified at the initial evaluation (diabetes mellitus, renal insufficiency, acute or chronic liver disease, thyroid disease, mental illness, drug or alcohol dependence, HIV infection, pregnancy, lactation and others). This chapter aims to addresses the monitoring requirements for the treatment of drug resistant tuberculosis (DR-TB), adverse effects associated with different second-line drugs, strategies for the early detection and treatment of adverse effects and also adverse effects in human immunodeficiency virus (HIV) coinfected patients with DR-TB.

PRETREATMENT SCREENING AND EVALUATION

The required initial pretreatment clinical investigation includes a thorough medical history and physical examination. The recommended initial evaluation and monitoring during treatment of DR-TB are shown in Table 27.1.

MONITORING PROGRESS OF TREATMENT

Clinically, the most important way to monitor response to treatment is through regular history taking and physical examination. The classic symptoms of TB like cough, sputum production, fever and weight loss generally improve within the first few months of treatment and should be monitored frequently by health-care providers. Patients should be monitored closely for signs of

Table 27.1: Pretreatment evaluation and monitoring during MDR-TB treatment

Monitoring evaluation	Recommended frequency
Evaluation by clinician	At baseline, and at least monthly until conversion, then every 2–3 months
Screening by DOT worker	At every DOT encounter
Sputum smears and cultures	For follow-up examination four sputum specimens will be collected and examined by smear and culture at least 30 days apart from the 3rd to 7th month of treatment (i.e. at the end of the months 3, 4, 5, 6 and 7) and at 3-monthly intervals from the 9th month onwards till the completion of treatment (i.e. at the end of the months 9, 12, 15, 18, 21 and 24)
Weight	At baseline and then monthly
Drug susceptibility	At baseline in programs doing individualized treatment or in programs doing standardized treatments that need to confirm MDR-TB. For patients who remain culture-positive, it is not necessary to repeat DST within less than 3 months of treatment
Chest radiograph	At baseline, and then every 6 months
Serum creatinine	At baseline, then monthly if possible while receiving an injectable drug. Every 1–3 weeks in HIV-infected patients, diabetes and other high-risk patients
Serum potassium	Monthly while receiving an injectable agent. Every 1–3 weeks in HIV-infected patients, diabetics and other high-risk patients
Thyroid stimulating hormone (TSH)	Every 6 months if receiving ethionamide/prothionamide and/or PAS; and monitor monthly for signs/symptoms of hypothyroidism. TSH is sufficient fo screening for hypothyroidism; it is not necessary to measure hormone thyroid levels
Liver serum enzymes	Periodic monitoring (every 1–3 months) in patients receiving pyrazinamide for extended periods or for patients at risk for or with symptoms of hepatitis. For HIV-infected patients, do monthly monitoring
HIV screening	At baseline, and repeat if clinically indicated
Pregnancy tests	At baseline for women of childbearing age, and repeat if indicated
Hemoglobin and white blood count	If on linezolid, monitor weekly at first, then monthly or as needed based on symptoms; there is little clinical experience with prolonged use. For HIV-positive patients on an ART regime that includes AZT, monitor monthly initially and then as needed, based on symptoms
Lipase	Indicated for work up of abdominal pain to rule out pancreatitis in patients on linezolid, stavudine, didanosine and zalcitabine
Lactic acidosis	Indicated for work up of lactic acidosis in patients on linezolid or antiretroviral treatment
Serum glucose	If receiving gatifloxacin, monitor glucose frequently (weekly) and educate patient on signs and symptoms of hypoglycemia and hyperglycemia

treatment failure. The recurrence of TB symptoms after sputum conversion, for example, may be the first sign of treatment failure. For children, height and weight should be measured regularly to ensure that they are growing normally. A normal growth rate should resume after a few months of successful treatment. Objective laboratory evidence of improvement often lags behind clinical improvement. The chest radiograph may be unchanged or show only slight improvement, especially in retreatment patients with chronic pulmonary lesions. Chest radiographs should be taken at least every six months, when a surgical intervention is being considered, or whenever the patient's clinical situation has worsened. The most important objective evidence of improvement is conversion of the sputum smear and culture to negative. While sputum smear is still useful clinically because of its much shorter turnaround time. Sputum culture is much more sensitive and is necessary to monitor the progress of treatment. Sputum examinations are also dependent on the quality of the sputum produced, so care should be taken to obtain adequate specimens. Persistently positive sputum and cultures for *Mycobacterium tuberculosis* bacilli should be assessed for nontuberculous mycobacteria (NTM), as overgrowth with NTM in lung damage secondary to TB is not uncommon. In such cases, although DR-TB may be adequately treated, treatment may need to be directed towards the NTM as well sputum conversion is slower in DR-TB than in drug-susceptible TB. Paucibacillary culture results should not be automatically regarded as negative when treating DR-TB. Acquired drug resistance and treatment failure often begin with the growth of one or two colonies on a sputum culture. Culture conversion should not be considered to be equivalent to cure. A certain proportion of patients may initially convert and later revert to positive sputum culture. Sputum smears and cultures should be monitored closely throughout treatment. These guidelines recommend that the tests should be performed monthly before smear and culture conversion, with conversion defined as two consecutive negative smears and cultures taken 30 days apart. After conversion, the minimum period recommended for bacteriological monitoring is monthly for smears and quarterly for cultures. Programs with adequate culture capacity may choose to do cultures more frequently, every 1–2 months, after conversion. Specimens for monitoring do not need to be examined in duplicate, but doing so can increase the sensitivity of the monitoring. For patients who remain smear- and culture-positive during treatment or who are suspects for treatment failure, DST can be repeated. It is usually not necessary to repeat drug susceptibility testing (DST) within less than three months of completion of treatment.

MONITORING FOR ADVERSE EFFECTS DURING TREATMENT

Close monitoring of patients is necessary to ensure that the adverse effects of second-line drugs are recognized quickly by health-care personnel.

The ability to monitor patients for adverse effects daily is one of the major advantages of Directly Observed Therapy (DOT) over self-administration of DR-TB treatment. The majority of adverse effects are easy to recognize. Commonly, patients will volunteer that they are experiencing adverse effects. However, it is important to have a systematic method of patient interviewing since some patients may not reveal even severe adverse effects. Other patients may be distracted by one adverse effect and forget to tell the health-care provider about others. Laboratory screening is invaluable for detecting certain adverse effects that are more occult. The recommendations based on the experience of several DOTS-Plus projects [1] for the minimal frequency of essential laboratory screening is given in Table 27.1. More frequent screening may be advisable, particularly for high-risk patients. Nephrotoxicity is a known complication of the injectable drugs, both of aminoglycosides and of capreomycin. This adverse effect is occult in onset and can be fatal. The optimal timing for checking serum creatinine is unknown, but most current treatment programs for DR-TB check serum creatinine at least monthly. In addition, patients with a history of renal disease (including comorbidities such as HIV and diabetes), advanced age or any renal symptoms should be monitored more closely, particularly at the start of treatment. An estimate of the glomerular filtration rate may help to further stratify the risk of nephrotoxicity in these patients. Electrolyte imbalance is a known complication of the antituberculosis injectable drugs, most frequently with capreomycin. It is generally a late effect occurring after months of treatment, and is reversible once the injectable drug is suspended. Since electrolyte imbalance is often occult in the early stages and can be easily managed with electrolyte replacement, serum potassium should be checked at least monthly in high-risk patients, and in all those taking capreomycin.[2] Hypothyroidism is a late effect provoked by PAS and ethionamide. It is suspected by clinical assessment and confirmed by testing the serum level of thyroid stimulating hormone (TSH). The use of these agents together can produce hypothyroidism in upto 10% of patients.[3] Since the symptoms can be subtle, it is recommended that patients are screened for hypothyroidism with a serum TSH at 6–9 months, and then tested again every 6 months or sooner if symptoms arise. The dosing of thyroid replacement therapy should be guided using serum levels of TSH. Goiters can develop due to the toxic effects of PAS, ethionamide or prothionamide.

MANAGEMENT OF ADVERSE EFFECTS

Second-line drugs have many more adverse effects than the first-line antituberculosis drugs. Proper management of adverse effects begins with patient education. Before starting treatment, the patient should be instructed in detail about the potential adverse effects that could be produced by the prescribed drug regimen. Prompt evaluation, diagnosis and treatment of adverse effects are extremely important, even if the adverse effect is not particularly dangerous. Patients may have significant fear and anxiety about an adverse effect if they do not understand why it is happening. These emotions in turn may augment the severity of the adverse effect, as in the case of nausea and vomiting. If the adverse effect is mild and not dangerous, continuing the treatment regimen, with the help of ancillary drugs if needed, is often the best option. In patients with highly resistant TB, a satisfactory replacement drug may not be available, so that suspending a drug will make the treatment regimen less potent. Some adverse effects may disappear or diminish with time, and patients may be able to continue receiving the drug if sufficiently motivated. The adverse effects of a number of second-line drugs are highly dose dependent. Reducing the dosage of the offending drug is another method of managing adverse effects, but only in cases where the reduced dose is still expected to produce adequate serum levels and not compromise the regimen. With cycloserine and ethionamide, for example, a patient may be completely intolerant at one dose and completely tolerant at a slightly lower dose. Unfortunately, given the narrow therapeutic margins of these drugs, lowering the dose may also affect efficacy, so every effort should be made to maintain an adequate dose of the drug according to body weight.

Pyridoxine (vitamin B_6) should be given to all patients receiving cycloserine or terizidone to help prevent neurological adverse effects. The recommended dose is 50 mg for every 250 mg of cycloserine (or terizidone) prescribed. Psychosocial support is an important component of the management of adverse effects. The common adverse effects, the likely responsible antituberculosis agents and the suggested management strategies are given in Table 27.2.

CONCLUSION

The initial evaluation, timely and intensive monitoring for, and management of, adverse effects caused by second-line drugs are essential components of DR-TB control programs. Poor management of adverse effects increases the risk of default or irregular adherence to treatment, and may result in death or permanent morbidity. The physicians should be familiar with the common adverse effects of MDR-TB therapy. Patients experiencing adverse effects should be referred to specialists who have experience in treating the adverse effects. It is rarely necessary to suspend antituberculosis drugs completely. Ancillary drugs for the management of adverse effects should be available.

Table 27.2: Common adverse effects, suspected agent(s) and management strategies of antituberculous drugs used in drug resistant patients of TB

Adverse effect	Suspected agent	Suggested management strategies
Seizures	Cs H Fq	• Suspend suspected agent pending resolution of seizures • Initiate anticonvulsant therapy (e.g. phenytoin, valproic acid) • Increase pyridoxine to maximum daily dose (200 mg per day) • Restart suspected agent or reinitiate suspected agent at lower dose, if essential to the regimen • Discontinue suspected agent if this can be done without compromising regimen • Anticonvulsant is generally continued until MDR-TB treatment is completed or suspected agent discontinued • History of previous seizure disorder is not a contraindication to the use of agents listed here if a patient's seizures are well controlled and/or the patient is receiving anticonvulsant • Patients with history of previous seizures may be at increased risk for development of seizures during MDR-TB
Peripheral neuropathy	Cs Lzd H S Km Am Cm Eto/Pto Fq	• Increase pyridoxine to maximum daily dose (200 mg per day) • Change injectable to capreomycin if patient has documented susceptibility to capreomycin • Initiate therapy with tricyclic antidepressants such as amitriptyline. Nonsteroidal anti-inflammatory drugs or acetaminophen may help alleviate symptoms • Lower dose of suspected agent, if this can be done without compromising regimen • Discontinue suspected agent if this can be done without compromising regimen
		• Patients with comorbid disease (e.g. diabetes, HIV, alcohol neuropathy (dependence) may be more likely to develop peripheral neuropathy, but these conditions are not contraindications to the use of the agents listed here • Neuropathy may be irreversible; however, some patients may experience improvement when offending agents are suspended
Hearing loss	S Km Am Cm Clr	• Document hearing loss and compare with baseline audiometry if available • Change parenteral treatment to capreomycin if patient has documented susceptibility to capreomycin • Decrease frequency and/or lower dose of suspected agent if this can be done without compromising the regimen (consider administration three times per week) • Discontinue suspected agent if this can be done without compromising the regimen • Patients with previous exposure to aminoglycosides may have baseline hearing loss. In such patients, audiometry may be helpful at the start of MDR-TB therapy • Hearing loss is generally not reversible • The risk of further hearing loss must be weighed against the risks of stopping the injectable in the treatment regimen • While the benefit of hearing aids is minimal to moderate in auditory toxicity, consider a trial use to determine if a patient with hearing loss can benefit from their use

Contd...

Contd...

Adverse effect	Suspected agent	Suggested management strategies
Psychotic symptoms	Cs H Fq Eto/Pto	• Stop suspected agent for a short period of time (1–4 weeks) while psychotic symptoms are brought under control • Initiate antipsychotic therapy • Lower dose of suspected agent if this can be done without compromising regimen • Discontinue suspected agent if this can be done without compromising regimen • Some patients will need to continue antipsychotic treatment throughout MDR-TB therapy • Previous history of psychiatric disease is not a contraindication to the use of agents listed here but may increase the likelihood of psychotic symptoms developing during treatment • Psychotic symptoms are generally reversible upon completion of MDR-TB treatment or cessation of the offending agent
Depression	Cs Fq Eto/Pto H	• Offer group or individual counseling • Initiate antidepressant therapy • Lower dose of suspected agent if this can be done without compromising regimen • Discontinue suspected agent if this can be done without compromising regimen • Socioeconomic conditions and chronic illness should not be underestimated as contributing factors to depression • Depressive symptoms may fluctuate during therapy and may improve as illness is successfully treated • History of previous depression is not a contraindication to the use of the agents listed but may increase the likelihood of depression developing during treatment
Hypothyroidism	PAS Eto/Pto	• Initiate thyroxine therapy • Completely reversible upon discontinuation of PAS or ethionamide/prothionamide. • The combination of ethionamide/prothionamide with PAS is more frequently associated with hypothyroidism than the individual use of each drug
Nausea and vomiting	Eto/Pto PAS H E Z	• Assess for dehydration; initiate rehydration if indicated • Initiate antiemetic therapy • Lower dose of suspected agent if this can be done without compromising regimen • Discontinue suspected agent if this can be done without compromising regimen rarely necessary • Nausea and vomiting universal in early weeks of therapy and usually abate with time on treatment and adjunctive therapy • Electrolytes should be monitored if vomiting is severe • Reversible upon discontinuation of suspected agent • Severe abdominal distress and acute abdomen have been reported with the use of clofazimine. Although these reports are rare, if this effect occurs, clofazimine should be suspended
Gastritis	PAS Eto/Pto	• H2-blockers, proton-pump inhibitors, or antacids • Stop suspected agent(s) for short periods of time (e.g 1–7 days) • Lower dose of suspected agent, if this can be done without compromising regimen • Discontinue suspected agent if this can be done without compromising regimen • Severe gastritis, as manifested by hematemesis, melena or hematechezia, is rare • Dosing of antacids should be carefully timed so as to not interfere with the absorption of antituberculosis drugs (take 2 hours before or 3 hours after antituberculosis medications) • Reversible upon discontinuation of suspected agent(s)

Contd...

Contd...

Adverse effect	Suspected agent	Suggested management strategies
Hepatitis	Z H R Eto/Pto PAS Fq	• Stop all therapy pending resolution of hepatitis • Eliminate other potential causes of hepatitis • Consider suspending most likely agent permanently • Reintroduce remaining drugs, one at a time while monitoring liver function • History of previous hepatitis should be carefully analyzed to determine most likely causative agent(s); these should be avoided in future regimens. • Generally reversible upon discontinuation of suspected agent
Renal toxicity	S Km Am Cm	• Discontinue suspected agent • Consider using capreomycin if an aminoglycoside had been the prior injectable in regimen • Consider dosing 2–3 times a week if drug is essential to the regimen and patient can tolerate (close monitoring of creatinine) • Adjust all antituberculosis medications according to the creatinine clearance • History of diabetes or renal disease is not a contraindication to the use of the agents listed here, although patients with these comorbidities may be at increased risk for developing renal failure • Renal impairment may be permanent
Electrolyte disturbances (hypokalemia and hypomagnesemia)	Cm Km Am S	• Check potassium. • If potassium is low, also check magnesium (and calcium if hypocalcemia is suspected) • Replace electrolytes as needed • If severe hypokalemia is present, consider hospitalization • Amiloride 5–10 mg QD or spironolactone 25 mg QD may decrease potassium and magnesium wasting and is useful in refractory cases • Oral potassium replacements can cause significant nausea and vomiting. Oral magnesium may cause diarrhea
Optic neuritis	E Eto/Pto	• Stop E • Refer patient to an ophthalmologist • Usually reverses with cessation of E • Rare case reports of optic neuritis have been attributed to streptomycin
Arthralgias	Z Fq	• Initiate therapy with nonsteroidal anti-inflammatory drugs • Lower dose of suspected agent if this can be done without compromising regimen • Discontinue suspected agent if this can be done without compromising regimen • Uric acid levels may be elevated in patients on pyrazinamide. Allopurinol appears not to correct the uric acid levels in such cases • Symptoms of arthralgia generally diminish overtime, even without intervention

Isoniazid (H), Rifampicin (R), Ethambutol (E), Pyrazinamide (Z), Streptomycin (S), Kanamycin (Km), Amikacin (Am), Capreomycin (Cm), Fluoroquinolones (Fq) Ethionamide (Eto), Prothionamide (Pto), P-aminosalicylic acid (PAS), Cycloserine (Cs), Clofazimine (Cfz), Linezolid (Lzd), Clarithromycin (Clr).

REFERENCES

1. Nathanson E, Gupta R, Huamani P, Leimane V, Pasechnikov AD, Tupasi TE, et al. Adverse events in the treatment of multidrug-resistant tuberculosis: results from the DOTS-Plus initiative. International Journal of Tuberculosis and Lung Disease. 2004;8:1382-4.
2. Shin S, Furin J, Alcantara F, et al. Hypokalaemia among patients receiving treatment for multidrug-resistant tuberculosis. Chest. 2004;125:974-80.
3. Furin JJ, Mitnick CD, Shin SS, Bayona J, Becerra MC, Singler JM, et al. Occurrence of serious adverse effects in patients receiving community-based therapy for multidrug-resistant tuberculosis. International Journal of Tuberculosis and Lung Disease. 2001;5:648-55.

Chapter 28

Multidrug Resistant Tuberculosis—Management in Special Situation

INTRODUCTION

Compared to drug sensitive tuberculosis, drug resistant tuberculosis (DR-TB) is more demanding in terms of cost of treatment, duration of treatment, higher adverse reactions to second-line drugs, resources required by the treatment providers, and the prolonged adherence required by the patients. To add to these issues certain associated special situations make the treatment of multidrug resistant tuberculosis and extensively drug resistant tuberculosis (M/XDR-TB) more difficult.[1,2] This chapter outlines the management of M/XDR-TB in special conditions and situations like pregnancy, breastfeeding, contraception, children, diabetes mellitus, renal insufficiency, liver disorders, seizure disorders, psychiatric disorders and substance dependence.

M/XDR-TB IN PREGNANCY

There is a lack of experience in treating pregnant women with M/XDR-TB. Although teratogenicity has been demonstrated in only a few of the drugs used to treat M/XDR-TB, all except ethambutol have uncertain safety information available. This all makes treating M/XDR-TB during pregnancy very challenging. It is prudent to solicit the opinion of an experienced gynecologist/obstetrician and chest physician while treating such patients.[3-7] All female patients of childbearing age should be tested for pregnancy upon initial evaluation. Pregnancy is not a contraindication for treatment of M/XDR-TB, which poses great risks to the lives of both mother and fetus.[8,9] However, birth control is strongly recommended for all nonpregnant women receiving therapy for M/XDR-TB because of the potential consequences for both mother and fetus resulting from frequent and severe adverse drug reactions. M/XDR-TB patients found to be pregnant prior to treatment initiation or whilst on treatment are evaluated in consultation with a gynecologist/obstetrician taking into consideration the factors like: risks and benefits of M/XDR-TB treatment, severity of the M/XDR-TB, gestational age and potential risk to the fetus. The risks and benefits of treatment should be carefully considered, with the primary goal of smear conversion to protect the health of the mother and child, both before and afterbirth. Since the majority of teratogenic effects occur in the first trimester, therapy may be delayed until the second trimester. The decision to postpone the start of treatment should be agreed by both patient and doctor after analysis of the risks and benefits. When therapy is started, three or four oral drugs with demonstrated efficacy against the infecting strain should be used and then reinforced with an injectable agent and possibly other drugs immediately postpartum.[10] For the most part, aminoglycosides should not be used in the regimens of pregnant patients and can be particularly toxic to the developing fetal ear. Capreomycin may also carry a risk of ototoxicity but is the injectable drug of choice if an injectable agent cannot be avoided. Ethionamide can increase the risk of nausea and vomiting associated with pregnancy, and teratogenic effects have been observed in animal studies. If possible, ethionamide should be avoided in pregnant patients. Further management of M/XDR-TB patients who are pregnant prior to initiation of M/XDR-TB treatment or whilst on M/XDR-TB treatment are based on the duration of pregnancy. If the duration of pregnancy is < 20 weeks, the patient should be advised to opt for a Medical Termination of Pregnancy (MTP) in view of the potential severe risk to both the mother and fetus. If the patient is willing, she should be referred to a Gynecologist/Obstetrician for MTP following which M/XDR-TB treatment can be initiated if the patient has not started M/XDR-TB treatment or continued if the patient is already on M/XDR-TB treatment. For patients who are unwilling for MTP or have pregnancy of > 20 weeks, the risk to the mother and fetus needs to be explained clearly and a modified M/XDR-TB should be started like: For patients in the first trimester (≤ 12 weeks), kanamycin and ethionamide are omitted from the M/XDR-TB regimen and PAS is added. For patients who have completed the first trimester (> 12 weeks), kanamycin is replaced with PAS. Postpartum, PAS may be replaced with kanamycin and continued until the end of the intensive phase. Pregnant M/XDR-TB patients need to be monitored carefully both in relation to the treatment and the progress of the pregnancy. This approach should lead to good results, since the patient should be smear negative at the time of parturition, and mother and infant do not need to be separated. Breastfeeding should be encouraged as long as the patient is sputum negative.

M/XDR-TB IN BREASTFEEDING

Timely and properly applied chemotherapy is the best way to prevent transmission of tubercle bacilli to the baby. A woman who is breastfeeding and has drug-resistant TB should receive a full course of antituberculosis treatment. In lactating mothers on treatment, most antituberculosis drugs will be found in the breast milk in concentrations that would equal only a small fraction of the therapeutic dose used in an infant. However, any effects on infants of such exposure during the full course of M/XDR-TB treatment have not been established. Therefore, when resources are available, it is recommended to provide infant formula options as an alternative to breastfeeding. The mother and her baby should not be completely separated. However, if the mother is sputum smear-positive, the care of the infant should be left to family members until she becomes sputum smear-negative, if this is feasible. When the mother and infant are together, this common time should be spent in well-ventilated areas or outdoors. In some settings, the mother may be offered the option of using a surgical mask or an N-95 respirator until she becomes sputum smear-negative.

M/XDR-TB IN CONTRACEPTION

All women of childbearing age who are receiving M/XDR-TB therapy should be advised to use birthcontrol measures because of the potential risk to both mother and fetus. There is no contraindication to the use of oral contraceptives with the non-rifamycin containing regimens. It should be remembered that oral contraceptives might have decreased efficacy due to vomiting and drug interactions with second line drugs. These patients should be advised to take their contraceptives apart from times when they may experience vomiting caused by the antituberculosis treatment. Patients who vomit at any time directly after, or within the first two hours after, taking the contraceptive tablet, should use a barrier method of contraception until a full month of the contraceptive tablets can be tolerated. Thus for prevention of pregnancy, the use of barrier methods (condoms/diaphragm), IUDs (CuT) or depotmedrox-progesterone are recommended based on individual preference and eligibility. Similarly all women of child bearing age identified as DR TB suspects should be advised to use a reliable and appropriate contraceptive method till the results of culture and Drug Susceptibility Test (DST) are available. For patients with mono- and poly-resistant TB that is susceptible to rifampicin, the use of rifampicin interacts with the contraceptive drugs resulting in decreased efficacy of protection against pregnancy. A woman on oral contraception while receiving rifampicin treatment may choose between two options: following consultation with a physician, use of an oral contraceptive pill containing a higher dose of estrogen (50 μg); or use of another form of contraception.

M/XDR-TB IN CHILDREN

There is only limited reported experience with the use of second-line drugs for extended periods in children. Frank discussion with family members is critical, especially at the outset of therapy. The risks and benefits of each drug should be carefully considered in designing a regimen. Children with drug-resistant TB generally have primary resistance transmitted from an index case with drug-resistant TB. When DST is available it should be used to guide therapy, although children with paucibacillary TB are often culture-negative. Nevertheless, every effort should be made to confirm drug-resistant TB bacteriologically by the use of DST and to avoid exposing children unnecessarily to toxic drugs. The treatment of culture-negative children with clinical evidence of active TB disease and contact with a documented case of drug-resistant TB should be guided by the results of DST and the history of the contact's exposure to antituberculosis drugs.[11] M/XDR-TB is life-threatening, and no antituberculosis drugs are absolutely contraindicated in children. Children who have received treatment for drug-resistant TB have generally tolerated the second-line drugs well.[11,12] Fluoroquinolones have been shown to retard cartilage development in beagle puppies,[13] experience with the use of fluoroquinolones in humans has not demonstrated similar effects[14,15.] It is considered that the benefit of fluoroquinolones in treating M/XDR-TB in children outweighs any risk. Additionally, ethionamide, PAS and cycloserine have been used effectively in children and are well tolerated. In general, dose of antituberculosis drugs should be according to body weight as given in Table 28.1. Monthly monitoring of body weight is therefore especially important in pediatric cases, with adjustment of doses as children gain weight.[16] Dose of all drugs, including the fluoroquinolones, should be given at the higher end of the recommended ranges whenever possible, except ethambutol.[11,17] Ethambutol should be dosed at 15 mg/kg, and not at 25 mg/kg as sometimes used in adults with M/XDR-TB, as it is more difficult to monitor for optic neuritis in children. In children who are not culture-positive initially, treatment failure is difficult to assess. Persistent abnormalities on chest radiograph do not necessarily signify a lack of improvement. In children, weight loss or, more commonly, failure to gain

Table 28.1: Pediatric dosing of second-line antituberculosis drugs

Drug	Daily dose (mg/kg)	Frequency	Maximum daily dose
Streptomycin	20–40	Once daily	1g
Kanamycin	15–30	Once daily	1g
Amikacin	15–22.5	Once daily	1g
Capreomycin	15–30	Once daily	1g
Ofloxacin	15–20	Once or twice daily	800 mg
Levofloxacin	7.5–10	Once daily	750 mg
Moxifloxacin	7.5–10	Once daily	400 mg
Ethionamide	15–20	Once or twice daily	1g
Prothionamide	15–20	Once or twice daily	1g
Cycloserine	10–20	Once or twice daily	1g
Para-aminosalicylic acid	150	Twice daily	12 g

weight adequately, is of particular concern and often one of the first signs of treatment failure. This is another key reason to monitor weight carefully in children. Anecdotal evidence suggests that adolescents are at high risk for poor treatment outcomes. Early diagnosis, strong social support, individual and family counseling and a close relationship with the medical provider may help to improve outcomes in this group.

M/XDR-TB IN DIABETES MELLITUS

Diabetes must be managed closely throughout the treatment of M/XDR-TB.The health care provider should be in close communication with the physician who manages the patient's diabetes. Diabetic patients with M/XDR-TB are at risk for poor outcomes. In addition, the presence of diabetes mellitus may potentiate the adverse effects of antituberculosis drugs, especially renal dysfunction and peripheral neuropathy. Oral hypoglycemic agents are not contraindicated during the treatment of M/XDR-TB but may require the patient to increase the dosage. Use of ethionamide or protionamide may make it more difficult to control insulin levels. Creatinine and potassium levels should be monitored more frequently, often weekly for the first month and then at least monthly thereafter.

M/XDR-TB IN RENAL INSUFFICIENCY

Renal insufficiency due to longstanding TB disease itself, previous use of aminoglycosides or concurrent renal disease, is not uncommon. Great care should be taken in the administration of second-line drugs in patients with renal impairment. Consideration needs to be taken that M/XDR-TB patients require aminoglycosides for 6 months or more. Other drugs, which also might require dose or interval adjustment in presence of mild to moderate renal impairment, are: ethambutol, quinolones, cycloserine and PAS.[11] In the presence of severe renal impairment many other drugs may also require adjustments as given in Table 28.2. In M/XDR-TB patients, blood urea and serum creatinine should be monitored prior to treatment initiation, monthly for three months after treatment initiation and then every three months whilst injection kanamycin is being administered. In patients with mild renal impairment, the dose of aminoglycosides may be reduced. In the presence of severe renal failure, the aminoglycoside therapy should be discontinued and replaced with other potent non-nephrotoxic antituberculosis drugs.[18]

M/XDR-TB IN LIVER DISORDERS

Pyrazinamide is the most hepatotoxic of the three first-line drugs (rifampicin, isoniazid, pyrazinamide). Among the second-line drugs, ethionamide, protionamide and PAS can also be hepatotoxic, although less so than any

Table 28.2: Adjustment of antituberculosis medication in renal insufficiency

Drug	Change in frequency	Recommended dose and frequency for patients with creatinine clearance < 30 ml/min or for patients receiving hemodialysis
Isoniazid	No change	300 mg once daily, or 900 mg three times per week
Pyrazinamide	Yes	25–35 mg/kg per dose three times per week (not daily)
Ethambutol	Yes	15–25 mg/kg per dose three times per week (not daily)
Ofloxacin	Yes	600–800 mg per dose three times per week (not daily)
Levofloxacin	Yes	750–1000 mg per dose three times per week (not daily)
Moxifloxacin	No change	400 mg once daily
Cycloserine	Yes	250 mg once daily, or 500 mg/dose three times per week
Terizidone	-	Recommendations not available
Prothionamide	No change	250–500 mg per dose daily
ethionamide	No change	250–500 mg per dose daily
Para-aminosalicylic acid	No change	4 g/dose, twice daily
Capreomycin	Yes	12–15 mg/kg per dose two or three times per week (not daily)
Kanamycin	Yes	12–15 mg/kg per dose two or three times per week (not daily)
Amikacin	Yes	12–15 mg/kg per dose two or three times per week (not daily)
Clarithromycin	Yes	Usual dose 500 mg twice daily but can be reduced to 250 mg twice daily
Linezolid	No change needed	Usual adult dose is 600 mg twice daily
Clofazimine	Yes	Begin at 300 mg daily and decrease to 100 mg after 4 to 6 weeks
Amoxycillin and-clavulanic acid	Yes	Dose used is 625 mg twice daily,1000 mg should not be administered

of the first-line drugs. Hepatitis occurs rarely with the flouroquinolones. The potential for hepatotoxicity is increased in elderly, alcoholics and in patients with pre-existing liver disease. In general, most of second line drugs can be safely used in presence of mild hepatic impairment, as they are relatively less hepatotoxic than the first-line drugs. However, pyrazinamide should be avoided in such patients. All other drugs can be used, but close monitoring of liver enzymes is advised. If significant aggravation of liver inflammation occurs, the drugs responsible may have to be stopped. Once a patient on second line drugs develops hepatitis, other etiologies should also be excluded such as viral hepatitis, alcoholic hepatitis, drug induced hepatitis by non-TB drugs.[19]

M/XDR-TB IN SEIZURE DISORDERS

TB might itself involve central nervous system and may cause seizures. However when seizures present for the first time during anti-TB therapy, they are likely to be the result of an adverse effect of one of the anti-TB drugs. Among second line drugs, cycloserine, ethionamide and fluoroquinolones have been associated with seizures. Some patients requiring treatment for M/XDR-TB will have a past or present medical history of a seizure disorder. The first step in evaluating such patients is to determine whether the seizure disorder is under control and whether the patient is taking anti-seizure medication to control the disorder. If the seizures are not under control, initiation or adjustment of anti-seizure medications will be needed prior to the start of M/XDR-TB therapy. In addition, if other underlying conditions or causes for seizures exist, they should be corrected. Pyridoxine should be given with cycloserine to prevent seizures. Cycloserine should however be avoided in patients with active seizure disorders that are not well controlled with medication. In cases where no other drug is appropriate, cycloserine can be given and the anti-seizure medication adjusted as needed to control the seizure disorder. The risk and benefits of using cycloserine should be discussed with the patient and the decision on whether to use cycloserine are made together with the patient. Antiepileptic drugs may have drug interactions with cycloserine and quinolones. Hence, close monitoring of serum levels of anti-epileptic drugs should be done.[19,20]

M/XDR-TB IN SUBSTANCE DEPENDENCE

Patients with substance dependence disorders should be offered treatment for their addiction. Complete abstinence from alcohol or other substances should be strongly encouraged, although active consumption is not a contraindication for antituberculosis treatment. If the treatment is repeatedly interrupted because of the patient's dependence, therapy should be suspended until successful treatment or measures to ensure adherence have been established. Good DOT gives the patient contact with and support from health-care providers, which often allows complete treatment even in patients with substance dependence. Cycloserine will have a higher incidence of adverse effects in patients dependent on alcohol or other substances, including a higher incidence of seizures. However, if cycloserine is considered important to the regimen, it should be used and the patient closely observed for adverse effects, which are then adequately treated.

M/XDR-TB IN PATIENTS WITH PSYCHOSIS

There is a high baseline incidence of depression and anxiety in patients with M/XDR-TB, often connected with the chronicity and socioeconomic stress factors related to the disease. For M/XDR-TB patients with a concurrent psychiatric illness, it is advisable to have an evaluation carried out by a psychiatrist before the start of treatment for M/XDR-TB. The initial evaluation documents any pre-existing psychiatric condition and establishes a baseline for comparison if new psychiatric symptoms develop while the patient is on treatment. Any identified psychiatric illness at the start or during treatment should be fully addressed. If a health care worker with psychiatric training is not available, the treating health care provider should document any psychiatric conditions the patient may have at the initial evaluation. Treatment with psychiatric medication, individual counseling, and/or group therapy may be necessary to manage the patient suffering from a psychiatric condition or adverse psychiatric effect due to medication.[21,22] Fluoroquinolones and ethionomide have been associated with psychosis. Pyridoxine prophylaxis may minimize risk of neurologic and psychiatric adverse reactions. Cycloserine may cause severe psychosis and depression leading to suicidal tendencies. However, the use of cycloserine is not absolutely contraindicated for the psychiatric patient. Adverse effects of cycloserine may be more prevalent in the psychiatric patient, but the benefits of using this drug often outweigh the potential higher risk of adverse effects. Close monitoring is recommended if cycloserine is used in patients with psychiatric disorders. If patient on cycloserine therapy develops psychosis, anti-psychotic treatment should be started and cycloserine therapy should be temporarily suspended. Once symptoms resolve and patient is stabilized cycloserine therapy may be resumed. Such patients may require anti-psychotic treatment till anti-TB treatment is completed. When any patient on M/XDR-TB treatment develops psychosis, other etiologies such as psycho-social stresses, depression, hypothyroidism, illicit drug and alcohol use, should also be looked for. All health-care workers treating drug-resistant TB should work closely with a mental health specialist and have an organized system for psychiatric emergencies.[21,22]

REFERENCES

1. WHO/IUATLD. Global Project on Anti-tuberculosis Drug Resistance Surveillance. Anti-tuberculosis drug resistance in the world. Report No.2. HO/CDS/TB/2000.278.
2. World Health Organization. The WHO/IUATLD. Global Project on Antituberculosis Drug Resistance Surveillance: Antituberculosis drug resistance in the world. Report No.3.Geneva: Switzerland; 2004.WHO/CDS/TB/2004.
3. Drobac PC, del Castillo H, Sweetland A, Anca G, Joseph JK, Furin J, et al. Treatment of multidrug-resistant tuberculosis during pregnancy: long-term follow-up of 6 children with intrauterine exposure to second-line agents. Clin Infect Dis. 2005;40:1689-92.
4. Shin S, Guerra D, Rich M, Seung KJ, Mukherjee J, Joseph K, et al. Treatment of multidrug-resistant tuberculosis during pregnancy: a report of 7 cases. ClinInfect Dis. 2003;36:996-1003.
5. Duff P. Antibiotic selection in obstetric patients. Infect Dis Clin North Am. 1997;11:1-12.
6. Valleho JG, Surke Jr. Tuberculosis and pregnancy Clinic Chest Med. 1992;13:693-707.
7. Hamadeh MA, Glassroth J. Tuberculosis and Pregnancy: Chest 1992;101:1114-20.1.
8. Figueroa-Damián R, Arredondo-García JL. Neonatal outcome of children born to women with tuberculosis. Archives of Medical Research, 2001;32:66-9.

9. Brost BC, Newman RB. The maternal and fetal effects of tuberculosis therapy. Obstetrics and Gynecology Clinics of North America. 1997;24:659-73.
10. Duff P. Antibiotic selection in obstetric patients. Infectious Disease Clinics of North America. 1997;11:1-12.
11. Swanson DS, Starke JR. Drug resistant tuberculosis in pediatrics. Pediatric Clinics of North America. 1995;42:553–81.
12. Mukherjee JS, Joseph JK, Rich ML, Shin SS, Furin JJ, Seung KJ, et al. Clinical and programmatic considerations in the treatment of MDR-TB in children: a series of 16 patients from Lima, Peru. International Journal of Tuberculosis and Lung Disease. 2003;7:637-44.
13. Takizawa T, Hashimoto K, Minami T, Yamashita S, Owen k. The comparative arthropathy of fluoroquinolones in dogs. Human and Experimental Toxicology. 1999;18:392-9.
14. Warren RW. Rheumatologic aspects of pediatric cystic fibrosis patients treated with fluoroquinolones. Pediatric Infectious Disease Journal. 1997;16:118-22.
15. Hampel B, Hullmann R, Schmidt H. Ciprofloxacin in pediatrics: worldwide clinical experience based on compassionate use—safety report. Pediatric Infectious Disease Journal. 1997;16(1):127-9.
16. Loebstein R, Koren G. Clinical pharmacology and therapeutic drug monitoring in neonates and children. Pediatric Review. 1998;19:42-428.
17. Siberry GK, Iannone R, eds. The Harriet Lane handbook, 15th edn. Baltimore, Mosby. 2000.
18. Ruckenstein MI. Vertigo and disequilibrium with associated hearing loss. Otolaryngol Clin North Am. 2000;33:535-62.
19. Braunwald E. Harrison's Principle of Internal Medicine. 15th edn. New York: McGraw- Hill, 2001.
20. WHO. Treatment of tuberculosis: guidelines for national programmes. WHO/CDS/TB 2003.313. Geneva: WHO 2003.
21. Lansdown FS, Beran M, Litwak T. Psychotoxic reaction during ethionamide therapy: Am Rev Resp Dis. 1967;95:1053-5.
22. Patel AM, McKeon J. Avoidance and management of adverse reactions to antituberculosis drugs. Drugs Saf. 1995;12:1-25.

Chapter 29

Multidrug Resistant Tuberculosis Contacts: Management

INTRODUCTION

Opportunities to halt the transmission of resistant mycobacteria in communities and to treat drug resistant tuberculosis (DR-TB) in a timely fashion are often squandered. The main reasons are lack of investigation of contacts of MDR-TB patients, failure to ask patients presenting with active TB disease about any history of exposure to DR-TB, and lack of access by national treatment programs to second line regimens and/or drug susceptibility testing (DST). Close contacts of DR-TB patients are defined as people living in the same household, or spending many hours a day together with the patient in the same indoor living space. The available data indicate that close contacts of DR-TB patients who develop active TB most commonly have drug-resistant disease.[1-5] While all contacts of TB require investigation, DR-TB requires the most vigilance. Because of the severe risk of morbidity and mortality of extensively drug resistant tuberculosis (XDR-TB), contact tracing of cases of XDR-TB should be given the highest level of alertness and priority. This chapter aims to outlines the management of symptomatic adults and children who have or have had a known contact with a DR-TB patient.

MANAGEMENT OF SYMPTOMATIC ADULT CONTACTS OF PATIENTS WITH MDR-TB

All close contacts of DR-TB cases should be identified through contact tracing and evaluated for active TB by a physician. If the contact appears to have active TB disease, culture and DST should be performed. If DST is not available, or while DST results are awaited, an empirical regimen based either on the resistance pattern of the index case or on the most common resistance pattern in the community may be started. Delay in the diagnosis of MDR-TB and start of appropriate treatment can lead to increased morbidity and mortality as well as unchecked amplification and transmission of drug-resistant strains of TB. When investigation of a symptomatic adult contact yields no evidence of TB, a trial of a broad-spectrum antibiotic, particularly one that is not active against TB can be used. If the patient continues to have symptoms, chest computed tomography and bronchoscopy for smear and culture should be considered if available. Where these diagnostic tools are not available or the results are not conclusive, a diagnosis should be based on the clinical information at hand. If the initial investigation is not suggestive of active TB but the contact remains symptomatic, repeat physical examinations, smears and cultures should be performed monthly with repeat chest X-ray as needed.

MANAGEMENT OF SYMPTOMATIC PEDIATRIC CONTACTS OF PATIENTS WITH MDR-TB

DR-TB should be suspected in children with active TB in the following situations: a child who is a close contact of an DR-TB patient, a child who is a contact of a TB patient who died while on treatment when there are reasons to suspect that the disease was DR-TB and children with bacteriologically proven TB who are not responding to first line drugs given with direct observation. The diagnosis of TB is more difficult in children than in adults. Symptoms of TB in young children can be nonspecific, e.g. chronic cough or wheeze, failure to thrive and recurrent fevers. Bacteriological confirmation may be difficult to obtain because of the inability of children to generate a sputum sample, as well as the paucibacillary nature of pediatric TB and the increased likelihood of extrapulmonary TB in children. While every effort should be made to establish a bacteriological diagnosis in a child with suspected DR-TB, in practice pediatric cases are often not confirmed bacteriologically. Use of scoring systems that have been produced to aid screening and diagnosis of active TB is strongly recommended.[6] Symptomatic pediatric household contacts should receive an evaluation by a physician, including history and physical examination, Tuberculin skin testing with purified protein derivative (PPD), radiological examination (chest X-ray examination and computerized tomography (CT), sputum smear, culture and DST. Every effort should be made to establish a bacteriological diagnosis in a child with suspected DR-TB. Bacteriological confirmation may include more aggressive measures such as induced sputum, gastric aspirate, lymph node aspirate or other relevant sample, plus culture and DST[6] and HIV counseling and testing in areas of high HIV prevalence or if parent(s) known, or suspected to be, HIV-infected.When the tuberculin (PPD) skin test result is > 5 mm but the chest radiograph and gastric aspirate or sputum smear are negative, the symptomatic child can be treated with a broad spectrum antibiotic that is not active against TB, such as trimethoprim/sulfamethoxazole. The child should be followed closely, with evaluations including smear test and culture on samples from induced sputum or gastric aspirates, or sputum samples whenever possible, as well as chest X-rays. The optimal frequency of these evaluations has not yet been determined. It is not clear whether the frequency of evaluation recommended for adults can be applied to children. If a child's clinical condition is highly suggestive of TB, or progressively deteriorates, empirical therapy designed according to the DST pattern of the strain from the index case can be started. Children with DR-TB who are incorrectly entered in short course chemotherapy (SCC) may suffer significant and protracted morbidity as a result of ongoing active disease, with the possibility of lifelong disability or even death. Because children with TB may never become sputum smear-positive, it is reasonable to initiate empirical DR-TB therapy based on the DST pattern of the contact. If DST of the contact is not available, therapy can be based on the common DST patterns of resistance in the community.

CHEMOPROPHYLAXIS OF CONTACTS OF DR-TB INDEX CASES

The only chemoprophylaxis regimens to have been studied are based on isoniazid and, to a lesser extent, rifampicin. Since by definition MDR-TB is resistant to both of these drugs, it is unlikely that use of these drugs to treat latent infection caused by an MDR-TB strain will prevent the development of active TB disease. Contacts of MDR-TB patients in whom latent infection is diagnosed may not be infected with the same strain; some may be infected with isoniazid susceptible strains, particularly in high-burden areas where many different strains of TB may circulate in homes, schools, workplaces, etc. Studies from high-burden TB areas have shown that approximately one-half to two-thirds of household members had the same strain of TB, as determined by genetic testing.[7-9] Close contacts of DR-TB patients should receive careful clinical follow-up for a period of at least two years. If active disease develops, prompt initiation of treatment with a regimen designed to treat DR-TB is recommended. On the basis of the currently available evidence, WHO does not recommend the universal use of second-line drugs for chemoprophylaxis in DR-TB contacts.

REFERENCES

1. Kritski AL, Marques MJO, Rabahi MF, Viera MA, Werneck-Barroso E, Carvalho CE, et al. Transmission of tuberculosis to close contacts of patients with multidrug-resistant tuberculosis. American Journal of Respiratory and Critical Care Medicine. 1996;153:331-5.
2. Schaaf HS, Van Rie A, Gie RP, Beyers N, Victor TC, Van Helden PD, et al. Transmission of multidrug-resistant tuberculosis. Pediatric Infectious Disease Journal. 2000;19:695-9.
3. Teixeira L, Perkins MD, Johnson JL, Keller R, Palaci M, do Valle Dettoni V, et al. Infection and disease among household contacts of patients with multidrug-resistant tuberculosis. International Journal of Tuberculosis and Lung Disease. 2001;5:321-8.

4. Schaaf HS, Gie RP, Kennedy M, Beyers N, Hesseling PB, Donald PR. Evaluation of young children in contact with adult multidrug-resistant pulmonary tuberculosis: A 30-month follow-up. Pediatrics. 2002;109:765-71.
5. Bayona J, Chavez-Pachas AM, Palacios E, Llaro K, Sapag R, et al. Contact investigations as a means of detection and timely treatment of persons with infectious multidrug-resistant tuberculosis. Int J Tuberc Lung Dis. 2003;7:501-S509.
6. Guidance for national tuberculosis programmes on the management of tuberculosis in children. Geneva, World Health Organization. 2006(WHO/HTM/TB/2006.371; WHO/FCH/CAH/2006.7).
7. Verver S, Warren RM, Munch Z, Richardson M, van der Spuy GD, Borgdorff MW, et al. Proportion of tuberculosis transmission that takes place in households in a high-incidence area. Lancet. 2004;363:212-4.
8. Schaaf HS, Vermeulen HAS, Gie RP, Beyers N, Donald PR. Evaluation of young children in household contact with adult multidrug-resistant pulmonary tuberculosis cases. Pediatric Infectious Disease Journal. 1999;18:494-500.
9. Steiner P, Rao M. Drug-resistant tuberculosis in children. Seminars in Pediatric Infectious Diseases. 1993;4:275-82.

Chapter 30

Multidrug Resistant and Extensively Drug Resistant Tuberculosis: Prevention

INTRODUCTION

Tuberculosis is a very important aspect of medical diseases throughout the world. It occurs world wide and remains an important cause of morbidity and mortality in many countries. According to WHO, in 2011, there were an estimated 8.7 million new cases of tuberculosis and an estimated 12 million prevalent cases causing death to 1.4 million people. There were an estimated 2.2 million (25% of the total cases) new cases in India and 0.30 million people are dying every year in our country due to tuberculosis. It is a cause for concern as India stands first in terms of absolute number of cases, closely followed by China.[1] It is a real paradox because pathogenesis, transmission, prevention, diagnosis and specific therapy are all well-known for tuberculosis.

Ideally good chemotherapy should achieve 100% sputum conversion if correct regimens are prescribed and taken. There will be hardly any relapse if duration of treatment has been sufficient and there will be no emergence of drug resistance. Every treatment failure should be regarded as a failure by the doctor. He has either prescribed a bad or unreliable regimen or he has failed to ensure that the patient takes the regimen as prescribed.[2-4] Drug resistant tuberculosis has been reported since the early days of introduction of anti-TB chemotherapy, but multidrug resistant tuberculosis (MDR-TB) and more recently extensively drug resistant tuberculosis (XDR-TB) has been an area of growing concern, and is posing threat to global efforts of tuberculosis control. Prevalence of drug resistant TB mirrors the functional state and efficacy of tuberculosis control programs and realistic attitude of the community towards implementation of such programs.[5] Poor TB control generates MDR-TB and the misuse of 2nd line drugs generates XDR-TB. Drug resistance in our country is due to inadequate tuberculosis control services, less well-trained doctors in modern chemotherapy, widespread inadequate treatment by private practitioner of various systems of medicine and quacks and inadequate management of already drug resistant tuberculosis.[6-9] Drug resistant tuberculosis is one of the important reasons of morbidity and mortality in tuberculosis.

The fourth WHO-IUATLD, global drug resistance surveillance carried out in 2002–2007, in 93 settings in 81 countries reported median prevalence of primary and acquired multidrug resistant tuberculosis (MDR-TB) as 2.9% and 15.3% respectively. It is estimated that 440,000 MDR-TB cases emerged in 2008 globally. Data from nine sites in India show that drug resistance among new cases is relatively low. The estimated prevalence of primary and acquired MDR-TB in India is 2.8% and 17.2% respectively. It is estimated that 99,000 MDR-TB cases emerged in India in 2008, representing over 20% of the global burden. In 2006, XDR-TB was reported in all regions of the world and it has become a serious emerging threat to global public health especially in countries with a high prevalence of Human Immunodeficiency Virus (HIV). Combining data from 46 countries, 5.4% of MDR-TB cases were found to have XDR-TB. Eight countries reported XDR-TB in more than 10% of MDR-TB cases; six of these countries were located in Eastern Europe and Central Asia. To date, a cumulative total of 84 countries have confirmed at least one case of XDR-TB.[10,11] Although isolated reports, both published and unpublished, indicate the existence of XDR-TB in India, it is not possible as yet to estimate its magnitude and distribution from the available data. According to the data reported on XDR-TB from India, it varied from 1.5 to 11% of MDR-TB cases.[12-14] XDR-TB has raised the possibility that the current drug susceptible TB will be replaced with a form of TB with severely restricted treatment options. This would halt the progress made in recent years to control TB globally. Thus it is evident that, MDR-TB and XDR-TB is a man made problem and its emergence can be prevented. Management of MDR-TB and XDR-TB is more difficult, complicated, challenging and more costlier and so the saying "Prevention is better than cure" holds strength here. The present write up gives an overview for the prevention of MDR-TB and XDR-TB.

GENERAL GUIDELINES FOR THE PREVENTION OF MDR- AND XDR-TB

1. No single drug therapy. Drug resistance usually follows and is permanent. Never add a single drug to a failing regimen. If he is getting worse, his bacilli may be resistant to all drugs being used. Adding one drug is the same as giving one drug alone. The patient will soon develop resistance to the new drug also.[15]
2. All the drugs should be administered in single dose preferably, as serum peak concentration of drug has greater and more prolonged inhibitory effect on tubercle bacilli compared to minimum inhibitory concentration

(MIC) in the serum following administration of the same dose in two divided doses.[16,17]

3. Use only standard, time tested drug regimens recommended by various national and international agencies.
4. Use drugs in adequate doses and for adequate duration.
5. Never use unreliable chemotherapy even for a short time.
6. Always prescribe good quality medicines if you are prescribing fixed dose combinations, make sure that they are of good quality as supported by frequent bioavailability test.[18-20]
7. Be kind and sympathetic to the patient. He is much more likely to come back and complete his treatment if he has confidence in you and believes that you are his well-wisher.
8. Follow-up the patient regularly, motivate and make sure that patient takes full recommended course of treatment for adequate duration, i.e. 6–9 months for short course chemotherapy and 1–2 years for long-term treatment. If possible make sure that some one sees the patient taking every dose (directly observed therapy).
9. Always assess adverse effects due to medications and address them quickly and adequately.[21]
10. Use rifampicin only in tuberculosis or leprosy. Avoid misuse of rifampicin as it is one of the most potent anti-tuberculosis drugs available at present. Development of resistance to rifampicin will lead to multidrug resistant tuberculosis (MDR-TB).
11. Relapse after good and adequate treatment is rare. If relapse has occurred after good and adequate treatment or after too short duration of regular treatment, such cases can be treated with previously used drug regimens. Five drug (2SHREZ/1HRZE/5HRE) regimen either daily or thrice weekly would be much effective and safe.[15]
12. In the group of previously treated patients with one or several courses of chemotherapy and who remain sputum positive (by smear and/or culture) three subpopulations can be observed. (a) Patients existing bacilli still sensitive to all drugs. (b) Patients existing bacilli resistant to atleast isoniazid but sensitive to rifampicin. (c) Patients bacilli resistant to atleast, isoniazid and rifampicin. The respective proportion of the three subpopulations varies according to chemotherapy applied in the community and number of courses of chemotherapy and type of regimens received by the patients. In the patients who have failed after the first course of chemotherapy, the proportion of patients existing bacilli sensitive to all drugs is usually higher than the proportion of two other subpopulations. For such patients, WHO retreatment regimens or category-II regimens of five drugs (2SHRZE/1HRZE/5HRE) or (2 $S_3H_3R_3E_3Z_3/1H_3R_3E_3Z_3/5H_3R_3E_3$) or even 4 drugs regimen (HRZE/HRE) under direct supervision can cure majority of patients having either

sensitive bacilli or bacilli resistant to isoniazid and/or streptomycin but still sensitive to rifampicin.[15,22]

13. In patients who have failed after several courses of previous treatment perhaps with bad or unreliable drug regimens or after two or more courses of chemotherapy under National Tuberculosis Control Program (last being the fully supervised standard WHO retreatment regimen of five drugs), the proportion of patients with MDR-TB can be as much as 50–70%. Treatment of such patients requires expertise and must be carried out under a specialist/specialized center as planning of treatment is very complex and a mistake at this stage can be fatal.[22-24]
14. Early suspicion, diagnosis and appropriate treatment of MDR-TB is essential to prevent morbidity, mortality and transmission of MDR-TB. Under RNTCP, a MDR suspect refers to any patient who fails a category I or III treatment regimen or any category II patient who remains smear positive at the end of the fourth month of treatment or later.[25] Ideally every such patient should be subjected to culture and drug sensitivity testing (DST) for *Mycobacterium tuberculosis* from a quality accredited laboratory, before starting a retreatment regimen. Subsequently, when the culture and DST report confirms MDR-TB, an appropriate treatment regimen containing atleast 4 new drugs, the patient has not taken previously or to which the bacilli is considered to be sensitive are given. There are 5 groups of anti-tuberculosis drugs. Include drugs from group 1–5 in hierarchical order. Use any first line oral agent such as Pyrazinamide (Z), Ethambutol (E), Rifabutin (Rfb) (Group-1) to which isolate is sensitive, use one injectable-Kanamycin (Km), Capreomycin (Cm), Amikacin (Am) (Group-2), one fluoroquinolone-Levofloxacin (Lfx), Moxifloxacin (Mfx), Ofloxacin (Ofx) (Group-3) and add as many second line bacteriostatic agents-Ethionamide (Eto), Protionamide (Pto), Cycloserine (Cs), Terizidone (Trd) and Para-aminosalicylic acid (PAS) (Group-4) to makeup atleast 4 effective drugs. Group-5 drugs such as Clofazimine (Cfz), Linezolid (Lzd), Amoxicillin/Clavulanate (Amx/Clv), Thiacetazone (Thz), Imipenem/Cilastatin (Ipm/Cln), High-dose isoniazid (High dose-H) and Clarithromycin (Clr) are not recommended for routine use except where an adequate regimen is impossible with Group 1–4. In standardized treatment, drug resistance surveillance (DRS) data from representative patient populations are used to base regimen design in the absence of individual DST. All patients in a defined group or category receive the same regimen. This type of treatment regimen is followed in resource poor, low income nations like India. The Government of India has thereby introduced the DOTS Plus/Category IV as standardized treatment for MDR-TB patients which consists of 6–9 months of intensive phase comprising of kanamycin, levofloxacin, ethionamide, cycloserine, pyrazinamide, ethambutol followed by 18

months of continuation phase comprising of levofloxacin, ethionamide, cycloserine and ethambutol. Para-amino salicylic acid (PAS) is included in the regimen as a substitute drug if any bactericidal drug (kanamycin, levofloxacin, ethionamide and pyrazinamide) or two bacteriostatic drugs (ethambutol and cycloserine) are not tolerated. Till DOTS Plus gets introduced in the whole country, all care providers must use proper and appropriate regimens in MDR-TB.

15. Avoid widespread misuse of second line anti-tuberculosis drugs (SLD's) like ethionamide/prothionamide, cycloserine, PAS, kanamycin/capreomycin, fluoroquinolones (levofloxacin, ofloxacin, moxifloxacin), clofazimine, macrolides, etc. in suspected resistant cases if you are not well-trained to manage such cases as these are the only drugs available at present which have some hope of cure. Inappropriately using these valuable drugs might convert a MDR-TB case into extensively drug resistant tuberculosis (XDR-TB). A preliminary study by the author among sixty MDR suspect patients showed 88.8% of MDR and 72.2% MDR suspect cases had taken SLD's for more than one month. The most commonly used SLD was fluoroquinolones (63.36%), ethionamide (47.72%) and kanamycin (40.9%).[26]
16. Some physicians (especially engaged in management of drug resistant cases) feel keeping certain drugs in reserve but this is a serious error. It is a prescription for losing one battle after another. Physicians treating such patient should note that the most powerful drugs available should be used initially and in maximum combination so as to ensure that the first battle is won and won permanently.
17. Treatment of tuberculosis benefits both the community and the patient. Thus, any public/private healthcare provider undertaking to treat a patient with TB is assuming an important public health responsibility that includes not only prescribing an appropriate regimen but also ensuring adherence to the treatment until treatment is completed. Therefore, the responsibility for successful treatment of TB is placed primarily on the provider or program initiating therapy, rather than on the patient.[27,28] All measures should be taken to ensure adherence by persuading and encouraging such patients and their family members not to stop treatment despite all its discomfort as it is the last that stands between the patient and death.[23,24]
18. Delay in recognition of MDR-TB, prolonged periods of infectiousness, crowded wards, and mixing TB and HIV patients all contribute to nosocomial transmission. However, in view of its seriousness, every program or physician attempting to treat MDR-TB should also undertake a systematic review of current practices and ensure that everything possible is done to prevent transmission among patients and to staff by implementation of adequate infection control precautions.[29]

19. Extrapulmonary drug resistant tuberculosis is treated with the same strategy and duration as pulmonary drug-resistant tuberculosis. If the patient has symptoms suggestive of central nervous system involvement and is infected with drug-resistant tuberculosis, the regimen should use drugs that have adequate penetration into the central nervous system.[30] Rifampicin, isoniazid, pyrazinamide, protionamide/ethionamide and cycloserine have good penetration into the cerebrospinal fluid (CSF); kanamycin, amikacin and capreomycin do so only in the presence of meningeal inflammation; PAS and ethambutol have poor or no penetration. The fluoroquinolones have variable CSF penetration, with better penetration seen in the later generations.

CONCLUSION

In conclusion, the emergence of multidrug resistant tuberculosis and extensively drug resistant tuberculosis is a man-made problem and is always due to medical error. If our tuberculosis control program is effectively implemented, all doctors can prescribe reliable regimens using reliable drugs and if they can ensure (by directly observed treatment and education of the patient and his family) that it is taken as prescribed, virtually all patients should be cured without any relapse and no drug resistance should occur. Laboratory services for adequate and timely diagnosis of MDR-TB and XDR-TB must be strengthened and programmatic management of MDR-TB and XDR-TB must be scaled up as per target set by global plan. It must be emphasized that optimal treatment of MDR-TB alone will not curb the epidemic. Efforts must be focused on the effective use of first line drugs in every new patient so as to prevent the ultimate emergence of multidrug resistance and extensively drug resistant TB. The proper use of second-line drugs in every patient of MDR-TB must be ensured to cure existing multidrug resistant tuberculosis, to reduce transmission of MDR-TB and to prevent XDR-TB.

REFERENCES

1. Global tuberculosis control—surveillance, planning, financing: WHO Report 2012.WHO/HTM/TB/2012.6.
2. Crofton J. The prevention and management of drug resistant tuberculosis. Bull Int Un Tuberc Lung Dis. 1989;62:6.
3. Crofton J, Horne N, Miller F. Clinical tuberculosis. Macmillan Education Limited. 1992.
4. Editorial. Multidrug resistance in Tuberculosis. Ind J Tub. 1994;41:1.
5. Prasad R. MDR TB: Current status (Review article). Indian J Tub. 2005;52:121-31.
6. Mahmoudi A, Iseman MD. Pitfalls in the care of patients with Tuberculosis. JAMA. 1993; 270:65.
7. Uplekar MW, Shepard DS. Treatment of tuberculosis by private general practitioners in India. Tubercle. 1991;72:284.
8. Prasad R, Nautiyal RG, Ahuja RC, et al. Treatment of new pulmonary tuberculosis patients: What do allopathic doctors do in India? Int J Tuberc Lung Dis. 2002;6:895-902.

9. Performance in Private Sector in Several Parts of World, International Standards for TB Care. Lancet Infect Dis. 2006;6:710-25.
10. WHO-IUATLD-Global Project on Anti-Tuberculosis Drug Resistance Surveillance (2002-2007), Fourth Global Report. 2008.
11. World Health Organization. Multidrug and extensively drug-resistant TB (M/XDR-TB): 2010 global report on surveillance and response.WHO/HTM/TB/2010.
12. Udwadia Z, Jain S, Rodrigues C, Mehta A.XDR-TB in India: What's in a name? The Lancet Infectious diseases. 2007;7:441-2
13. Mondal R, Jain A. XDR *Mycobacterium tuberculosis* isolates, India (letter). Emerg Infect Dis 2007. available from http:/www.cdc.gov/EID/content/13/9/ 1429.htm
14. Thomas A, Ramachandran R, Rehman F, et al. Management of multi drug resistant tuberculosis in the field: Tuberculosis Research Centre Experience. Indian J Tuberc. 2007;54: 117-24.
15. Caminero JA. Management of multidrug resistant tuberculosis and patients in retreatment. Eur Respir J. 2005;25:928-36.
16. Tuberculosis Research Centre, Indian Council of Medical Research. Low rate of emergence of drug resistance in sputum positive patients treated with short course chemotherapy. International Journal of Tuberculosis and Lung Diseases. 2001;5:40-5.
17. Tuberculosis Chemotherapy Centre, Madras. A concurrent comparison of INH and PAS with 3 regimens of INH alone in the domiciliary treatment of pulmonary tuberculosis in South India. Bulletin of the World Health Organisation. 1960;23:535-85
18. Acocella G. Studies of bioavailability in man. Bull Int Un Tuberc Lung Dis. 1989;64:40.
19. Editorial. Multidrug formulations. Ind J Tub. 1988;35:161.
20. Good manufacturing practices for pharmaceutical products. WHO Expert Committee on Specifications for Pharmaceutical Preparations. Thirty-second report. Geneva,World Health Organization. 1992. (WHO Technical Report Series, No..823), Annex 1.
21. Guidelines for the programmatic management of drug-resistant tuberculosis—WHO. 2008, 2011.
22. Mitchison DA, Nunn AJ. Influence of initial drug resistance on the response to short course chemotherapy of pulmonary tuberculosis. Am Rev Respir Dis. 1986;133:423.
23. Iseman MD, Madsen LA.Treatment of multidrug resistant tub. N Engl J Med. 1993;329:784.
24. Crofton J, Chaulet P, Maher D. Guidelines for the management of drug resistant tuberculosis. WHO Global Tuberculosis Programme, Geneva 1997. WHO/TB/96, 210.
25. DOTS PLUS guidelines, Revised National Tuberculosis Control Programme, Central TB Division Directorate General Health Services, Ministry of Health & Family welfare, Nirman Bhawan ,New Delhi. Sep 2008, 2012.
26. Anand SC, Prasad R, Garg R, et al. Observational Study to assess the use of second line drugs in patients with Tuberculosis. Poster session presented at National Conference on Pulmonary Diseases. (NAPCON 2008) at Lucknow on 6–9 Nov 2008.
27. Centers for Disease Control and Prevention. Treatment of tuberculosis: American Thoracic Society, CDC, and Infectious Diseases Society of America. MMWR Morb Mortal Wkly Rep. 2003;52(RR-11):44.
28. Treatment of Tuberculosis. Guidelines for National Programmes.World Health Organisation-Geneva. 1993, 1997, 2003, 2009.
29. Basu S, et al. Prevention of nosocomial transmission of extensively drug resistant tuberculosis in rural South African district hospitals: an epidemiological modelling study. Lancet. 2007; 370:1500-7.
30. Holdiness MR. Cerebrospinal fluid pharmokinetics of antituberculosis drugs. Clinical Pharmacokinetics. 1985;10:532-4.

Chapter 31

Extensively Drug Resistant Tuberculosis: Current Status and Management

INTRODUCTION

Drug resistant tuberculosis has been reported since the early days of the introduction of chemotherapy but recently extensively drug resistant tuberculosis (XDR-TB) has been an area of growing concern and is posing a threat to control of tuberculosis. The emergence of XDR-TB across the world raises the possibility that the current epidemic of mostly drug susceptible TB will be replaced with a form of TB with severely restricted treatment options. If this happens it would jeopardize the progress made in recent years to control TB and patients would have to be managed like TB patients before the antibiotic era. XDR-TB is a man made problem and its emergence can be prevented by prompt diagnosis and effective treatment with second line drugs in MDR-TB cases. The concept of XDR-TB as a distinct clinical entity was first developed at the Center for Disease Control and Prevention (CDC) in March 2005 and the term was introduced into public use in October 2005 at the 36th World Conference on Lung Health in Paris where data on second-line drug resistance from a global survey of supranational TB reference laboratories conducted by CDC and the World Health Organization, as well as treatment outcomes of XDR-TB patients in Latvia, were first presented.[1,2] Shortly thereafter, the cluster of TB deaths with resistance to second-line drugs in HIV-infected persons in Kwa Zulu-Natal was presented at a conference in Denver in February 2006.[3] This chapter aims to review the definition, epidemiology, diagnosis, treatment and control of XDR-TB.

DEFINITION

The original definition for XDR-TB published in the Morbidity and Mortality Weekly Report in March 2006 was provisionally defined as those persons with TB whose isolates were resistant to isoniazid and rifampicin and atleast three of the six main classes of Second Line Drugs (SLDs) (aminoglycosides, polypeptides, fluoroquinolones, thioamides, cycloserine, and para-aminosalicylic acid).[4] But in October 2006, at an emergency meeting of the Global XDR-TB task force, the World Health Organization in consideration of the difficulty to test some second line drugs and the fact that some forms of drug resistance are less treatable than others, revised the case definition of XDR-TB as 'TB with resistance to at least isoniazid and rifampicin as well as further resistance to a fluroquinolone and a second line injectable agent (kanamycin, amikacin or capreomycin).[5] The term "extremely" drug resistant XXDR-TB has now been proposed for cases resistant to all available first and second line drugs.[6,7]

EPIDEMIOLOGY

Global

Limited data exist in the literature about extensively drug-resistant tuberculosis (XDR-TB) and second-line drug resistance patterns among MDR-TB patients. Centers for Disease Control and Prevention, USA surveyed the Network of Supranational Reference Laboratories for *M. tuberculosis* isolates that were resistant to second-line anti-TB drugs during 2000–2004.[8] Of 23 eligible laboratories, 14 (61%) contributed data on 17,690 isolates, which reflected drug susceptibility results from 48 countries. Of 3,520 (19.9%) MDR TB isolates, 347 (9.9%) met criteria for XDR TB. Among XDR-TB patients, combination drug-resistance patterns included 90 (3.4%) with resistance to aminoglycosides, capreomycin and fluoroquinolones; 102 (3.4%) with resistance to aminoglycosides, fluoroquinolones, and thioamides; and 94 (3.8%) with resistance to fluoroquinolones, thioamides, and para-aminosalicyclic acid. Nearly half (n = 167, 48.1%) of all XDR-TB isolates were resistant to all 4 first line drugs, bringing the total to > 7 drugs to which the isolate was resistant. Among the group of industrialized nations, 53 (6.5%) MDR-TB patients met criteria for XDR-TB. Among patients from Russia and Eastern Europe, 55 (13.6%) MDR-TB patients met criteria for XDR-TB. Among patients from the Republic of Korea, 200 (15.4%) MDR-TB patients, who accounted for 1.7% of all *M. tuberculosis* isolates tested, met criteria for XDR-TB. Data from patients undergoing retreatment for TB in Hong Kong showed that 30 (17%) MDR-TB isolates were resistant to > 3 second-line drugs, thereby meeting criteria for XDR-TB.[9] A drug-resistance survey of 447 culture-positive new patients and patients undergoing retreatment in Abkhazia, Republic of Georgia, found that of 63 MDR-TB patients, 2 (3%) had additional resistance to 3 second-line drug classes, consistent with XDR-TB.[10] More recently, clusters of XDR-TB have been reported in South Africa and Iran[11,12] and have been associated with HIV infection and rapid and high death rates. In the Fourth WHO/IUATLD anti-TB drug resistance surveillance report, thirty five countries and 2 SARs have reported data on XDR-TB. The quality assurance for laboratory testing was variable among countries reported. Out of total 4012 MDR-TB cases, 301 (7%) were XDR-TB cases.[13] In general, absolute numbers of XDR-TB cases were low in Central and Western Europe, the Americas and in the Asian countries that reported data. The XDR-TB proportion among MDR-TB in these settings varied from 0% in 11 countries to 30% in Japan. These countries have a relatively low MDR-TB burden, so this represents few absolute cases. A more significant problem lies in the countries of the former Soviet Union. Of the 9 countries that reported, approximately 10% of all MDR-TB cases were XDR ranging from 4.0% in Armenia to almost 24.0% in Estonia; however these proportions represent a much larger absolute number of cases. In a study conducted in Lima, Peru on 810 patients referred for individualized antituberculous drug therapy from 1999–2002, 48 (7.4%) patients of total 651 patients tested had XDR-TB, and the remaining 603 were all MDR-TB.[14] Recently released data from South Africa showed that of 996 or 5.6% of 17, 615 MDR isolates collected from 2004 to October 2007 were XDR-TB. Proportions varied across provinces with Kwa Zulu-Natal reporting 656 or 14% of 4701 MDR cases as XDR-TB. Selection and testing practices varied across the country and over time; however all isolates correspond to individual cases. Data for XDR-TB from 46 countries that have reported continuous surveillance or representative surveys of second-line drug resistance among MDR-TB cases. Combining data from these countries, 5.4% of MDR-TB cases were found to have XDR-TB. Eight countries reported XDR-TB in more than 10% of MDR-TB cases; six of these countries were located in Eastern Europe and Central Asia. To date, a cumulative total of 84 countries have confirmed at least one case of XDR-TB.[15]

India

Although isolated reports, both published and unpublished, indicate the existence of XDR-TB in the country, it is not possible as yet to estimate its magnitude and distribution from the available data. Drug susceptibility test results (DST) of second line anti-tuberculous drugs should be interpreted with great caution due to limited capacity of laboratories, absence of quality-assurance and lack of standardized methodology. According to the data reported on XDR-TB from India, it varied from 1.5 to 11% of MDR-TB.[16-19] Subnational survey from India in 2006 in the state of Gujarat reported XDR TB in 3.2% (95% CI, 1.2%–6.6%) of all MDR-TB patients.[15] In a recent study, XDR-TB was found is 8.5% of MDR-TB case. Furthermore, 42.3% of MDR-TB cases were resistant to either ofloxacin or kanamycin (Pre XDR-TB) which in studies have shown to be an independent prognostic factor of poor outcome and survival in patients with MDR-TB.[16]

FACTORS RESPONSIBLE FOR XDR-TB

Drug resistance in *M. tuberculosis* is due to the accumulation of mutations in the genome. Mismanagement of MDR-TB cases primarily results in this form of TB, mainly by the following reasons: Faulty or improper treatment, non-adherence to treatment guidelines, inappropriate, incomplete or erratic use of second line drugs and moreover use of poor quality second line drugs.

A report from South Korea revealed that XDR-TB was significantly associated with the cumulative duration of previous TB treatment received with second-line drugs.[20,21] Little or no access to reliable laboratory for drug susceptibility testing against first and second line drugs, lack of experience, poor training and skills to manage drug resistant TB and factors linked to poor control practices for example, lack of measures to ensure adherence to treatment and treatment of tuberculosis in unmonitored private sectors played a major role in originating XDR-TB. The two strongest risk factors for XDR-TB are: Failure of an anti-TB regimen that contains second-line drugs including an injectable agent and a fluoroquinolone and close contact with an individual with documented XDR-TB or with an individual for whom treatment with a regimen including second-line drugs is failing or has failed.[22]

DIAGNOSIS

A clinical diagnosis of XDR-TB is not possible. In a patient of MDR-TB who is on second-line anti-tubercular treatment who has 6th month follow-up culture is positive, is said to be 'XDR-TB suspect'. And the culture isolate is to be sent for DST for second-line drugs. In addition, any category IV patient who has culture converted but is found to have 2 consecutive positive cultures subsequently, would also be suspected of treatment failure. In such cases, the culture isolate of the second positive culture would be sent for second-line DST (mainly kanamycin and fluoroquinolone).[23] The only way to diagnose XDR-TB currently is by drug susceptibility testing to first and second line drugs which may take upto 16 weeks if done by conventional method which involves growth of the bacteria on solid culture media like LJ media. DST against second-line drugs should not be carried routinely on account of its difficulty, cost and poor reliability. Even in well-developed countries, where multiple methods are available for performing DST for second-line drugs, interpretation of the results requires cautious analysis by experienced staff since the concentrations used for each drug has not been standardized and the definitions of resistance vary widely, even between the best laboratories. DST of drugs such as Group 4 and 5 drugs (Table 31.1) does not have high reproducibility and reliability; guidelines strongly caution against basing individual regimens on DST of these drugs. As a general rule if by drug history, a patient has used a drug for over a month with persistently positive smears or cultures, the strain should be considered as "probably resistant" to that drug, even if DST is reported as susceptible.[22] More rapid tests like radiometric methods have been used, e.g. BACTEC 460, MGIT 960, in which the bacteria are inoculated into a radio-labeled broth with and without the drug to be tested and growth in broth is measured. The time to detection with the MGIT 960 system was 12.7 days compared with 20 days with the solid media. The combination of MGIT and BACTEC detected 171 (95%) of all isolates with a time to detection of *M. tuberculosis* of 9.9 days compared with 9.7 days with BACTEC and 20.2 days with solid medium proving that MGIT was a valuable alternative to the radiometric system.[24,25] No rapid molecular tests for detection of XDR-TB are currently available; as a result, conventional and the newer liquid DST techniques are considered the most reliable methods for determining XDR-TB. Some of the newer liquid and agar techniques can determine the presence of XDR-TB within 14 days. Other, more rapid systems are also being tested for identification of drug resistance, e.g. colorimetric assays, broth-based assays for rapid detection of *Mycobacterium* and for resistance to isoniazid and rifampicin. Genotypic methods for detecting specific genetic mutations and responsible for certain types of drug resistance are available for only MDR-TB, e.g. Genotype MTB-DR assay, INNO LiPA assay.[26,27] Studies for resistance to second line antituberculosis drugs by genotypic methods are in pipeline. In a study, sensitivity and specificity of the Genotype MTB DRsl test was found to be 87% and 96% respectively for fluoroguinolones; 100% for amikacin; 77% and 100% respectively, for kanamycin; 80% and 98% respectively for capreomycin and 57% and 92% respectively for ethambutol.[28]

TREATMENT

Treatment of XDR-TB is more difficult and expensive. Less powerful agents (second line and group V agents) are required for treatment because R and H cannot be used and they have to be used for a longer duration also. The treatment can be an individualized regimen or a standardized one, depending on the previous drugs taken by the patient (by constructing a drug-o-gram), the degree of resistance in the community and the financial status of the patient. A drug may be considered likely to be effective if the baseline DST shows susceptibility to that drug; if no DST results are available, a drug may still be considered likely to be effective if the patient has not received the drug for atleast 1 month.[27]

Management Guidelines for Patients with Documented or Almost Certain, XDR-TB

Hierarchical system of drug groups usage applies in XDR-TB also. Atleast 5 drugs with proven susceptibility or which are most likely to be effective should be used. (Table 31.1) Use any Group 1 agents that may be effective.

Table 31.1: Grouping of anti-tuberculosis drugs

Group 1 First line oral agents	Ethambutol (E); Pyrazinamide (Z); Rifabutin (Rfb)
Group 2 Injectable agents	Kanamycin (Km); Amikacin (Amk); Capreomycin (Cm); Streptomycin (S)
Group 3 Fluoroquinolones	Moxifloxacin (Mfx); Levofloxacin (Lfx); Ofloxacin (Ofx)
Group 4 Oral bacteriostatic second line agents	Ethionamide (Eto); Prothionamide (Pto); Cycloserine (Cs); Terizidone (Trd); Para-aminosalicylic acid (PAS)
Group 5 (drugs with unclear efficacy or unclear role in MDR-TB treatment, not recommended by WHO for routine use in MDR-TB patients)	Clofazimine (Cfz); Linezolid (Lzd); Amoxicillin/clavulanate (Amx/Clv); Thioacetazone (Thz); Imipenem/cilastatin (Ipm/Cln); High-dose isoniazid (high-dose H); Clarithromycin (Clr)

Use an injectable agent to which the strain is susceptible and consider an extended duration of use (12 months or possibly the whole treatment). If resistant to all injectable agents, it is recommended to use one the patient has never used before (strain may be resistant to injectable in vitro, though not necessarily in vivo). Use a later-generation fluoroquinolone such as moxifloxacin. Use all Group 4 agents that have not been used extensively in a previous regimen or any that are likely to be effective. Use two or more agents from Group 5. Consider high-dose isoniazid treatment if low-level resistance is documented. Consider adjuvant surgery if there is localized disease. Ensure strong infection control measures. Treat HIV disease if present. Provide comprehensive monitoring and full adherence support.

Under programmatic management of drug resistant tuberculosis (PMDT), government of India has a standardized treatment for the management of XDR-TB patients. Prospectively named "Category V", the regimen consist of 7 drugs, with 2 reserve/substitute drugs. The dosages of the drugs would vary as per the weight of the patient (≤ 45 kg or > 45 kg). All drugs are to be given on a daily basis under supervision of a DOT provider. Injection of capreomycin is to be given 6 days/week. The details of the drugs and dosages are in Table 31.2.

The reserve/substitute drugs would be used in the following conditions:

- If the patient was on PAS during their category IV treatment, PAS will be replaced with one of the reserve drugs in the category V regimen.
- If the patient is unable to tolerate one or more of the drugs
- If the patient is found to be resistant to capreomycin.

The Category V regimen would be of 24–30 months duration, with 6–12 months intensive phase (IP) and 18 months continuation phase (CP). The intensive phase will consist of capreomycin, PAS, moxifloxacin, high dose-INH (600–900 mg), clofazamine, linezolid, and amoxicillin/clavulanate while the continuation phase will consist of PAS, moxifloxacin, high dose-INH

Table 31.2: Dosages of second line drugs used for XDR-TB

Drugs	Dosage/day	
	≤ 45 kg	> 45 kg
Capreomycin (Cm)	750 mg OD	1000 mg OD
Na PAS	10 g OD	12 g OD
Moxifloxacin (Mfx)	400 mg OD	400 mg OD
High dose INH (High dose-H)	600 mg OD	900 mg OD
Clofazimine (Cfz)	200 mg OD	200 mg OD
Linezolid (Lzd)	600 mg OD	600 mg OD
Amoxyclav (Amx/Clv)	875/125 mg BD	875/125 mg BD
Pyridoxine	100 mg OD	100 mg OD
Reserve/substitute drugs		
Clarithromycin (Clr)	500 mg BD	500 mg BD
Thiacetazone (Thz)	150 mg OD	150 mg OD

(600–900 mg), clofazamine, linezolid, and amoxicillin/clavulanate. Reserve/Substitute drugs would be clarithromycin and thiacetazone. The change from IP to CP will be done only after achievement of culture conversion, i.e. 2 consecutive negative cultures taken at least one month apart. In case of delay in culture conversion, the IP will be extended from 6 months up to a maximum of 12 months.[23] In case of extension, the DOTS-Plus site committee, which will be responsible for initiating and monitoring the category V regimen, can decide on administering capreomycin injection intermittently (3 times/week) for the months 7–12.

MONITORING OF TREATMENT

No randomized controlled trials have been conducted on XDR-TB, regarding the appropriate duration of treatment or regarding the appropriate monitoring techniques. Therefore, it is largely based on consensus.[23] Essentially, the treatment should be given directly observed for a minimum of 6 days/week as treatment success is critical. Ensure strict compliance and prompt identification and management of side effects.

Baseline Evaluation

- Complete blood count with platelets
- Thyroid function test
- Liver function test
- Kidney function test
- Serum electrolytes
- Blood sugar
- Pregnancy test

- All patients would be offered HIV testing after pretest counseling, unless known to be HIV positive
- Chest X-ray
- Surgical evaluation.

Follow-up Schedule

a. Culture monthly during IP starting after 3 months of starting treatment, i.e. 3, 4, 5, and 6, 7 and quarterly during CP i.e. 9, 12, 15, 18, 21 and 24. In case of extension of IP due to delay in culture conversion, the followup schedule will be modified accordingly.
b. Other tests.
    - Complete blood count—weekly in first month, then monthly to rule out bone marrow suppression, anemia as a side effect of linezolid
    - Renal function tests, serum electrolytes—monthly during the period that the capreomycin is being administered
    - Liver function tests—monthly in IP and 3 monthly during CP
    - CXR—6 monthly
    - Thyroid function tests and other tests when clinically indicated.

Assess side effects due to drugs and manage appropriately. Smear status at 6th month may be used as a surrogate marker for response to treatment and those who remain smear positive at 6 months can be considered for change of treatment.[28]

OUTCOMES OF TREATMENT

A study was conducted in Peru between 1999 and 2002, on 810 patients with unsuccessfully treated TB. Of the 651 patients tested, 48 had XDR-TB and 603 had multidrug-resistant TB (MDR-TB). None of the XDR-TB patients were coinfected with HIV. More than 60% of XDR-TB patients were cured after receiving the bulk of their personalized treatment at home or in community-based settings. Frequent contact with healthcare workers afforded many benefits and was an important element of success. Healthcare workers ensured a high level of treatment adherence and promptly detected circumstances requiring additional attention. Psychosocial needs were also assessed continuously and addressed through a range of interventions. This showed that ambulatory form of treatment is successful, and can be widely implemented in resource-poor settings.[27] In a retrospective Cohort study of 608 patients with MDR-TB in Russia between 2000 and 2004, 29 (4.8%) patients had XDR-TB. 48.3% of XDR-TB had treatment cure or completion.[29] The largest outbreak of XDR-TB is certainly the one that occurred in the Kwa Zulu-Natal region in South Africa in an HIV-positive population, characterized by a high mortality rate.[12] Out of 544 patients studied, 221 had MDR-TB; of these, 53 were defined as XDR-TB. Of the 53 patients, 44 had been tested for HIV and all were HIV-positive; 52 of 53 patients died, on average, within 25 days, including those treated with antiretroviral drugs. So XDR-TB outbreaks in HIV-infected patients appear to be common and is extremely difficult to treat.[5,20,30,31]

ROLE OF SURGERY

With the emergence of MDR and XDR-TB, the role of surgery has again surfaced due to an inability to ensure complete cure with the available chemotherapy. In XDR-TB patients with localized disease, surgery, as an adjunct to chemotherapy, can improve outcomes provided skilled thoracic surgeons and excellent postoperative care are available. It is adjunct to chemotherapy and should not be considered as last resort. Chemotherapy should be given atleast for two month prior to surgery and continued for 12–24 months after resection. It is indicated in patients who remain sputum positive, with resistance to large number of drugs; and localized pulmonary disease.[22]

Most common operative procedure in patients with pulmonary DR-TB is resection surgery.[32] Resection surgery should be timed to offer the patient the best possible chances of cure with the least morbidity, for example, when the disease is still localized to one lung or one lung lobe. In other words, surgery should not be considered as a last resort. Specialized surgical facilities should include stringent infection control measures, since infectious substances and aerosols are generated in large quantities during surgery and during mechanical ventilation and postoperative pulmonary hygiene maneuvers. Computerized tomography, pulmonary function testing and quantitative lung perfusion/ventilation are recommended as part of the preoperative work-up. It has been shown that overall cure rate was substantially higher (81% v/s 56%) when surgery was more frequently and aggressively applied in cases of resistant pulmonary tuberculosis.[33,34] The same principle can be applied to surgically feasible XDR-TB patients.

HIV AND XDR-TB

The treatment of DR-TB in patients with HIV is very similar to that in patients without HIV except that ART plays a crucial role, as mortality in XDR-TB/HIV patients without the use of ART is extremely high.[11,22] Adverse effects are more common in patients with HIV. The multiple medicines involved in DR-TB with recognized high toxicity risks, often combined with ART, results in a high incidence of adverse effects. Some toxicities are common to both anti-tuberculosis treatment and ART, which may result in added rates of adverse events. Monitoring needs to be more intense for both response to therapy and adverse effects. The use of thioacetazone is not recommended for patients with HIV or for routine use in populations with high rates of HIV.[35] Immune reconstitution inflammatory syndrome (IRIS) may complicate therapy.

XDR-TB IN PEDIATRIC PATIENTS

Children with DR-TB generally have primary resistance transmitted from an index case with DR-TB. When DST is available, it should be used to guide therapy, although children with paucibacillary TB are often culture negative. Nevertheless, every effort should be made to confirm DR-TB bacteriologically by the use of DST and to avoid exposing children unnecessarily to toxic drugs. The treatment of culture-negative children with clinical evidence of active TB disease and contact with a documented case of DR-TB should be guided by the results of DST and the history of the contact's exposure to anti-tuberculosis drugs.[36] There is only limited reported experience with the use of second-line drugs for extended periods in children. The risks and benefits of each drug should be carefully considered in designing a regimen. Frank discussion with family members is critical, especially at the outset of therapy. DR-TB is life-threatening, and no anti-tuberculosis drugs are absolutely contraindicated in children. Children who have received treatment for DR-TB have generally tolerated the second-line drugs well.[36,37] Experience with the use of fluoroquinolones has not demonstrated side effects in humans, so it is considered that the benefit of fluoroquinolones in treating DR-TB in children outweighs any risk.[38,39] Additionally, ethionamide, PAS and cycloserine have been used effectively in children and are well-tolerated. In general, anti-tuberculosis drugs should be given according to body weight (Table 31.3). Monthly monitoring of body weight is therefore especially important in pediatric cases, with adjustment of doses as children gain weight. All drugs, including the fluoroquinolones, should be dosed at the higher end of the recommended ranges whenever possible, except ethambutol. Ethambutol should be dosed at 15 mg/kg, and not at 25 mg/kg as sometimes used in adults

Table 31.3: Pediatric dosing of second-line antituberculosis drugs

Drug (mg/kg)	Daily dose	Frequency daily dose	Maximum
Streptomycin	20–40	Once daily	1 g
Kanamycin	15–30	Once daily	1 g
Amikacin	15–22.5	Once daily	1 g
Capreomycin	15–30	Once daily	1 g
Ofloxacin	15–20	Twice daily	800 mg
Levofloxacin	7.5–10	Once daily	750 mg
Moxifloxacin	7.5–10	Once daily	400 mg
Ethionamide	15–20	Twice daily	1 g
Prothionamide	15–20	Twice daily	1 g
Cycloserine	10–20	Once or twice daily	1 g
Para-aminosalicylic acid	150	Twice or thrice daily	12 g

with DR-TB, as it is more difficult to monitor for optic neuritis in children. In children who are not culture-positive initially, treatment failure is difficult to assess. Persistent abnormalities on chest radiograph do not necessarily signify a lack of improvement. In children, weight loss or more commonly, failure to gain weight adequately, is of particular concern and often one of the first or only signs of treatment failure. This is another key reason to monitor weight carefully in children.[22]

XDR-TB IN PREGNANCY

All female patients of childbearing age should be tested for pregnancy upon initial evaluation. Pregnancy is not a contraindication for treatment of active DR-TB, which poses great risks to the lives of both mother and fetus.[22,40,41] However, birth control is strongly recommended for all non-pregnant women receiving therapy for DR-TB because of the potential consequences for both mother and fetus resulting from frequent and severe adverse drug reactions. The risks and benefits of treatment should be carefully considered, with the primary goal of smear conversion to protect the health of the mother and child, both before and after birth. The following are some general guidelines:

- Start treatment of drug resistance in second trimester or sooner if condition of patient is severe. Since the majority of teratogenic effects occur in the first trimester, therapy may be delayed until the second trimester. The decision to postpone the start of treatment should be agreed by both patient and doctor after analysis of the risks and benefits. It is based primarily on the clinical judgment resulting from the analysis of life-threatening signs/symptoms and severity of the disease. When therapy is started, three or four oral drugs with demonstrated efficacy against the infecting strain should be used and then reinforced with an injectable agent and possibly other drugs immediately postpartum.[42]
- Avoid injectable agents. For the most part, aminoglycosides should not be used in the regimens of pregnant patients and can be particularly toxic to the developing fetal ear. Capreomycin may also carry a risk of ototoxicity but is the injectable drug of choice if an injectable agent cannot be avoided.
- Avoid ethionamide. Ethionamide can increase the risk of nausea and vomiting associated with pregnancy, and teratogenic effects have been observed in animal studies. If possible, ethionamide should be avoided in pregnant patients.

Breastfeeding

A woman who is breastfeeding and has active DR-TB should receive a full course of anti-tuberculosis treatment. Timely and properly applied chemotherapy is the best way to prevent transmission of tubercle bacilli to her baby. In lactating mothers on treatment, most antituberculosis drugs will be found in the breast milk in concentrations that would equal only a small fraction of the therapeutic dose used in an infant. However, any effects on infants of such exposure during the full course of DR-TB treatment have not been established. Therefore, when resources are available, it is recommended to provide infant formula options as an alternative to breastfeeding. However, if the mother is sputum smear-positive, the care of the infant should be left to family members until she becomes sputum smear-negative, if this is feasible. When the mother and infant are together, this common time should be spent in well-ventilated areas or outdoors. In some settings, the mother may be offered the option of using a surgical mask or an N-95 respirator until she becomes sputum smear-negative.

Contraception

There is no contraindication to the use of oral contraceptives with the non-rifamycin containing regimens. Patients who vomit directly after taking an oral contraceptive can be at risk of decreased absorption of the drug and therefore of decreased efficacy. These patients should be advised to take their contraceptives apart from times when they may experience vomiting caused by the antituberculosis treatment. Patients who vomit at any time directly after, or within the first two hours after, taking the contraceptive tablet, should use a barrier method of contraception until a full month of the contraceptive tablets can be tolerated.

WHO RESPONSE STRATEGIES FOR XDR-TB[43]

To combat the threat of XDR-TB, WHO convened a Global Task Force on XDR-TB on 17 October 2006 and recommended to strengthen basic activities to control TB and HIV/AIDS and to avoid additional emergence of MDR-TB and XDR-TB as well as acceleration of treatment of MDR and XDR-TB cases with universal access to sound management of MDR and XDR-TB by 2015 in all countries and near to universal access in the high burden countries by 2010. The revised plan recommended the treatment of 1.6 million MDR-TB and XDR-TB cases by 2015 instead of 800,000 MDR-TB cases. During this meeting, eight recommendations were put forward to the international TB community, outlining key areas of response, beginning with strengthening of basic TB and HIV/AIDS control and proper management of MDR-TB. The eight recommendations are:

- Strengthening basic activities to control TB and HIV/AIDS, as detailed in the 'Stop TB Strategy and the Global Plan,' to avoid additional emergence of MDR-TB and XDR-TB;
- Scaling-up the programmatic management of MDR-TB and XDR-TB to reach the targets set forth in the global plan;

- Strengthening laboratory services for adequate and timely diagnosis of MDR-TB and XDR-TB;
- Expanding surveillance of MDR-TB and XDR-TB to better understand the magnitude and trends of drug resistance and the links with HIV;
- Fostering sound infection-control measures to avoid MDR-TB and XDR-TB transmission to protect patients, health workers, others working in congregate settings and the broader community, especially in high HIV prevalence settings;
- Strengthening advocacy, communication and social mobilization for sustained political commitment and a patient-centered approach to treatment.

CONTROL OF XDR-TB

The primary aim in the control of extensively drug resistant tuberculosis is to prevent its development in the first place. This can be done by directly observed treatment short course (DOTS), which is the most cost-effective way of treatment and prevention of MDR tuberculosis. At the same time-since MDR-TB and XDR-TB cases respond poorly to short course chemotherapy, careful introduction of second line drugs to treat MDR-TB and proper management of MDR-TB cases to prevent XDR-TB cases, should be ensured to reduce further transmission of such strains.[44] Since new drugs for tuberculosis are unlikely to come up in the near future, the key to success remains in prompt and correct diagnosis and effective treatment of infectious patients. Apart from a strong tuberculosis control program, there is also a need for a continuous and periodic survey of drug resistance which will provide information on the type of chemotherapy to be used for the treatment of patients and also serve as a useful parameter in evaluation of current and past chemotherapy programs. There is a need for revision of guidelines of national programs based on levels of resistance, training of professionals in private sector, strengthening of existing National Tuberculosis Control Program, and by ensuring compliance enhancing measures like providing free/subsidized anti-tubercular drugs, supervised treatment and health education.

CONCLUSION

Overall, the emergence of XDR-TB is a reminder that TB control globally needs a massive commitment by scientific, political and financial authorities. In practice, one of the first priorities is to diagnose rapidly and correctly XDR-TB. This means to increase the laboratory capacity, e.g. to allow the reference laboratories in each country to perform correctly DST for all the SLD necessary to diagnose XDR-TB. Molecular tests to rapidly identify isoniazid and rifampicin resistance are available and together with drug susceptibility testing for SLD, will play a great role in early diagnosis, but large investments in personnel and facilities are necessary to make it feasible in resource poor nations. New researches in the areas involving molecular biology and application of these in the field of epidemiology could help in better understanding of the mechanisms of drug resistance, development of newer diagnostic tools and effective drugs to control drug resistant tuberculosis. Till such time extensively resistant tuberculosis must be managed very effectively with careful use of second line drugs to reduce morbidity and mortality and transmission. It must also be emphasized that even optimal treatment of multi-drug resistant tuberculosis and extensively-drug resistant tuberculosis will not alone curb the epidemic; efforts must be focused on the effective use of first line drugs in every new patients so as to prevent the ultimate emergence of multidrug resistant tuberculosis, extensively drug resistant tuberculosis and extreme drug resistant tuberculosis (XXDR-TB) or total drug resistant tuberculosis (TDR-TB).

REFERENCES

1. Shah NS, Wright A, Drobniewski F, et al. Extreme drug resistance in tuberculosis (XDR-TB): Global survey of supranational reference laboratories for *Mycobacterium tuberculosis* with resistance to second-line drugs. Int J Tuberc Lung Dis. 2005;9:S77.
2. Holtz TH, Riektsina V, Zarovska E, Laserson KF, Wells CD, et al. XDR-TB: Extreme drug-resistance and treatment outcome under DOTS-Plus, Latvia, 2000–2002. Int J Tuberc Lung Dis. 2005;9:S258.
3. Moll A, Gandhi NR, Pawinski R, Andrews J, Zeller K, et al. Identification of a multidrug-resistant tuberculosis cluster as a cause of death among HIV coinfected patients in rural South Africa. 13th Conference on Retroviruses and Opportunistic Infections; 7 February 2006; Denver, Colorado, United States of America. Poster 0-115.
4. Centers for Disease Control and Prevention (CDC). Emergence of *Mycobacterium tuberculosis* with extensive resistance to second-line drugs—Worldwide, 2000–2004. Morb Mortal Wkly Rep. 2006;55:301-5.
5. Centers for Disease Control and Prevention (CDC). Notice to readers: Revised definition of extensively drug-resistant tuberculosis. MMWR Morb Mortal Wkly Rep. 2006;55:1176.
6. Migliori GB, Loddenkemper R, Blasi F, Raviglione MC. 125 years after Robert Koch's discovery of the tubercle bacillus: The new XDR-TB threat: is "science" enough to tackle the epidemic? Eur Respir J. 2007;29:423-7.
7. Joshi JM. Preventing extremely drug resistant tuberculosis: Directly observed treatment is the only answer. Editorial. Indian J Chest Dis Allied Sci. 2008;50:183-5.
8. Sarita Shah N, Abigail Wright, Gill-Han Bai, Lucia Barrera, Fadila Boulahbal, Nuria Martín-Casabona, et al. Worldwide emergence of extensively drug-resistant tuberculosis. Emerg Infect Dis. 2007;13:380-7.
9. Kam KM, Yip CW. Surveillance of *Mycobacterium tuberculosis* susceptibility to second-line drugs in Hong Kong, 1995–2002, after the implementation of DOTS-Plus. Int J Tuberc Lung Dis. 2004;8:760-6.
10. Pardini M, Iona E, Varaine F, Karakozian H, Arzumanian H, Brunori L, et al. *Mycobacterium tuberculosis* drug resistance: Abkhazia [letter]. Emerg Infect Dis. 2005;11:501-3.
11. Gandhi NR, Moll A, Sturm AW, Pawinski R, Govender T, Lalloo U, et al. Extensively drug-resistant tuberculosis as a cause of death among patient coinfected with tuberculosis and HIV in a rural area in South Africa. Lancet. 2006;368:1575-80.

12. Masjedi MR, Farnia P, Sorooch S, Pooramiri MV, Mansoori SD, Zarifi AZ, et al. Extensively drug-resistant tuberculosis: 2 years of surveillance in Iran. Clin Infect Dis. 2006;43:841-7.
13. WHO/IUALTD Global Project on Anti-Tuberculosis Drug Resistance Surveillance (2002-2007), Fourth Global Report (2008).
14. Carole D, Mitnick C, et al. Comprehensive treatment of extensively drug-resistant tuberculosis. N Engl J Med. 2008;359:563-74.
15. Multidrug and Extensively Drug-resistant TB (M/XDR-TB) Global Report on Surveillance and Response. 2010, 2012.
16. Jain A, Dixit P, Prasad R. Pre-XDR and XDR in MDR and Ofloxacin and Kanamycin resistance in non-MDR Mycobacterium tuberculosis isolates. Tuberculosis. 2012; 92: 404-6.
17. Udwadia Z, Jain S, Rodrigues C, Mehta A. XDR-TB in India: What's in a name? The Lancet Infectious Diseases. 2007;7:441-2.
18. Mondal R, Jain A. XDR *Mycobacterium tuberculosis* isolates, India (letter). Emerg Infect Dis 2007. available from http:/www.cdc.gov/EID/content/13/9/ 1429.htm.
19. Thomas A, Ramachandran R, Rehman F, et al. Management of multi drug resistant tuberculosis in the field: Tuberculosis Research Centre Experience. Indian J Tuberc. 2007;54:117-24.
20. Jeon CY, Hwang SH, Min JH, et al. Extensively drug resistant tuberculosis in South Korea: risk factors and treatment outcomes among patients at a tertiary referral hospital. Clin.Infect. Dis. 2008;46:42-9.
21. Prasad R, Garg R. XDR-TB: An emerging threat. Chest. India. 2007;8:3-4.
22. Guidelines for the programmatic management of drug-resistant tuberculosis—WHO 2008, 2011.
23. Guidelines on programmatic management of drug-resistant tuberculosis, 2012. India.
24. Pfyffer GE, Welscher HM, Kissling P, et al. Comparison of the mycobacteria growth indicator tube (MGIT) with radiometric and solid culture for recovery of acid-fast bacilli. J Clin Microbiol. 1997;35:364-8.
25. Palomino JC. Non-conventional and new methods in the diagnosis of tuberculosis: feasibility and applicability in the field. Eur Respir J. 2005;26:339-50.
26. Furin J. The clinical management of drug resistant tuberculosis. Curr Opin Pulm Med. 2007;13:212-7.
27. Mitnick CD, et al. Comprehensive treatment of extensively drug-resistant tuberculosis. N Engl J Med. 2008;359:563-74.
28. Brossier F, Veziris N, Aubry A, Jarlier V, Sougakoff W. Detection by GenoType MTBD Rsl Test of Complex Mechanisms of Resistance to Second-Line Drugs and Ethambutol in Multidrug-Resistant Mycobacterium tuberculosis Complex Isolates. Journal Clinical Microbiology. 2010;48:1683-89.
29. Keshavjee S, Gelmanova IY, Farmer PE, Mishustin SP, Strelis AK, Andreev YG, et al. Treatment of extensively drug-resistant tuberculosis in Tomsk, Russia: A retrospective cohort study. Lancet. 2008;372:1403-9.
30. Gandhi NR, Moll A, Sturm AW, Pawinski R, Govender T, Lalloo U, et al. Extensively drug-resistant tuberculosis as a cause of death among patient co-infected with tuberculosis and HIV in a rural area in South Africa. Lancet. 2006;368:1575-80.
31. XDR-TB (extensively drug-resistant tuberculosis): what, where, how and action steps. Geneva, World Health Organization. 2007.
32. Migliori GB, et al. Extensively drug-resistant tuberculosis, Italy and Germany [letter]. In: Emerging Infectious Diseases [serial on the Internet], May 2007.
33. Francis RS, Curwen MP. Major surgery for pulmonary tuberculosis: final report. A national survey of 8232 patients operated on from April 1953 to March 1954 and followed up for five years. Tubercle. 1964;5:5-79.

34. Pomerantz M, Madsen LA, Goble M, Iseman MD. Surgical management of resistant mycobacterial pulmonary infection. Ann Thorac Surg. 1991;52:1108-12.
35. Wells CD, et al. HIV infection and multidrug-resistant tuberculosis: the perfect storm. Journal of Infectious Diseases. 2007;196 Suppl 1:S86-S107.
36. Swanson DS, Starke JR. Drug resistant tuberculosis in pediatrics. Pediatric Clinics of North America. 1995;42:553-81.
37. Mukherjee JS, et al. Clinical and programmatic considerations in the treatment of MDR-TB in children: A series of 16 patients from Lima, Peru. International Journal of Tuberculosis and Lung Disease. 2003;7:637-44.
38. Warren RW. Rheumatologic aspects of pediatric cystic fibrosis patients treated with fluoroquinolones. Pediatric Infectious Disease Journal. 1997;16:118-22.
39. Hampel B, Hullmann R, Schmidt H. Ciprofloxacin in pediatrics: worldwide clinical experience based on compassionate use—safety report. Pediatric Infectious Disease Journal. 1997;16:127-9.
40. Figueroa-Damián R, Arredondo-García JL. Neonatal outcome of children born to women with tuberculosis. Archives of Medical Research. 2001;32:66-9.
41. Brost BC, Newman RB. The maternal and fetal effects of tuberculosis therapy. Obstet and Gynec Clin of North America. 1997;24:659-73.
42. Duff P. Antibiotic selection in obstetric patients. Infectious Disease Clinics of North America. 1997;11:1-12.
43. The Global MDR-TB and XDR-TB Response Plan 2007–2008. Geneva, World Health Organization, 2007 (WHO/HTM/TB/2007.387).
44. Prasad R, Nautiyal RG, Ahuja RC, et al. Treatment of new pulmonary tuberculosis patients: what do allopathic doctors do in India? Int J Tuberc Lung Dis. 2002;6:895-902.

Chapter 32

Bacillus Calmette-Guerin (BCG)

INTRODUCTION

Bacillus Calmette-Guerin is named after two French scientists Albert Calmette (a bacteriologist) and Camille Guerine (a veterinarian). BCG is a live attenuated form of bovine tubercle bacilli, first isolated from a cow with tubercular mastitis, which had lost its power to produce progressive disease in human beings and most experimental animals.[1-3] This chapter aims to describe in detail about BCG.

BASIS OF GIVING BCG

In 90–95% of individuals, primary infection heals spontaneously under the influence of innate resistance of the host and leads to development of acquired resistance, but in 5–10% of all those infected, especially very young infants or in individuals with depressed immunity, the infection may assume progressive course and may lead to serious forms of tubercular disease.

BCG vaccination is done in those who have not been infected with tubercular bacilli and hence do not have acquired resistance. The vaccine is given to induce a harmless artificial primary complex, thus simulating real infection. Consequently, acquired resistance will be produced but due to its avirulence, BCG will not produce any progressive disease. Thus, BCG vaccine does not protect against infection or establishment of primary foci but rather protects against uncontrolled replication and dissemination of *M. tuberculosis* from primary foci to other parts of body and lung and thus protects against development of tubercular meningitis, miliary tuberculosis and other hematological lesions.[4-6]

TYPES OF BCG VACCINE

There are two types of BCG vaccine:—liquid and freeze dried. Liquid form is simple to prepare, provides better immunity than the freeze dried form as it has higher proportion of live to dead bacilli and does not need any reconstitution prior to use. But its shelf life even under best storage conditions is short as it is heat labile, sensitive to sunlight and requires quick transport because of its lability. The freeze dried vaccine is characterized by its higher stability both at 4°C and 37°C and therefore can be used in remote villages and has minimum wastage because of longer expiry and more stability.

DOSE AND SITE OF VACCINATION

0.1 mL to be given in left arm at the junction of upper 1/3rd and lower 2/3rd of upper half of deltoid region. 0.05 mL is the recommended dose for infants below 4 weeks of age.

ROUTES OF VACCINATION

BCG vaccine can be given by oral, subcutaneous and intracutaneous routes like intradermal, multiple puncture technique and scarification techniques. Intradermal method is the technique of choice in most of the countries for mass vaccination program because of the ease, speed, simplicity of technique and exact dose that can be administered. It is given by no. 27 gauge tuberculin syringe. Oral route was used previously but is not used nowadays due to low conversion rate, need for multiple doses, presence of more side effects like lymphadenitis, and because the quantity of vaccine absorbed from the intestine is unknown.[7]

EFFICACY AND SAFETY

Various controlled trials of the efficacy of BCG vaccine in humans have been carried out.[8] The first large field trial began in 1935 among eight North American Indian tribes. The protective efficacy against active tuberculosis was 75% and there was an 82% reduction in deaths resulting from tuberculosis. Similarly Rosenthal and colleagues[9] and the trial of Medical Research Council of Great Britain[6] also found BCG to be effective. Other controlled trials in Georgia and Albama found no protection after BCG vaccination.[10,11] Because of the variable results of the published trials of BCG efficacy and the concerns that the vaccines used in previous studies were so heterogeneous that they might not be of uniform potency, the largest controlled community trial to examine the efficacy of BCG vaccine was started. It was cosponsored by the Indian Council of Medical Research (ICMR) and US Public health service in Chingleput district earlier in Madras) in 1968. Studies in Chingleput

(South India) have revealed that BCG vaccine does not offer any protection against the infectious form of pulmonary tuberculosis casting doubt on the efficacy of BCG in India, but the trial had not elaborated on the prevalence of prevention of serious complications of primary tuberculosis, e.g. tubercular meningitis and miliary tuberculosis. Rather than resolving the issue of efficacy of BCG, Chingleput study brought forth even more questions. Various case-control trials later conducted[12-14] found varied results. The effectiveness of the vaccination programs ranged from 2 to 84 percent. Protection conferred by vaccination was highest against disseminated forms of tuberculosis, such as meningitis. Various hypotheses have been put forward to explain the variable efficacy of BCG in field trials including methodological biases, different strains and doses used, infection with environmental *Mycobacterium* and different virulence of strains of *M. tuberculosis*. Other factors like genetic factors, nutritional factors have also been proposed.

Clemens and colleagues[15] reviewed the eight major controlled trials of BCG and concluded that BCG can confer protection against tuberculosis and that the disparate results found in the controlled trials may have resulted, at least in part, from methodological differences in the studies. In a meta-analysis of BCG, Colditz and colleagues[16] found that the number of tuberculosis cases was reduced by 50% after BCG vaccination. BCG vaccination had a protective effect of 64% against tuberculous meningitis. There was a 78% percent protective effect against disseminated tuberculosis and a 71% protective effect from death due to tuberculosis. Extensive studies conducted so far have established the usefulness of BCG vaccination. The prevalence of tuberculosis in vaccinated group is lower than a similar group of persons who have not been vaccinated. WHO recommends the administration of BCG vaccine to children on a world wide basis to be given at birth or at the first contact of infant with the health system upto 1 year by direct and upto 5 years in tuberculin negative (by indirect vaccination). BCG vaccination was earlier under the NTP and is now administered in India under the expanded program of immunization. Routine BCG vaccination is not recommended as a means of preventing drug resistant TB in laboratory workers.[17]

CONTRAINDICATIONS TO BCG VACCINATION

The only absolute contraindication is in a child with symptomatic HIV infection or AIDS. BCG may be administered to asymptomatic HIV infected children. Adverse reactions are more in patients having generalized eczema, infective dermatitis, and hypogammaglobulinemia and may also be withheld in individuals on corticosteroids, antimetabolites and radiation therapy.

NORMAL REACTION AFTER BCG VACCINATION

When BCG is administered in correct dose, an immediate wheel of 7–8 mm diameter is formed which is then absorbed in 20–30 minutes. By 3rd–4th week, induration appears at the site of vaccination followed by papule at about 4th or 5th week. In many cases, crust appears by about 4th week which detaches leaving a small ulcer which heals by 3 months without any treatment. In a few cases, papule attains maximum size of 8–10 mm diameter by the 6th week, it then begins to regress leaving a round white scar by 3–4 months. Sensitivity to tuberculin testing appears by as early as 10 days and maximal response occurs by 12 weeks.[18]

COMPLICATIONS

Most of these so called complications are only an exaggeration of the normal reaction of vaccination and medically are of no significance. They are important only because of the unpleasantness associated and the possibility that BCG vaccination may loose its popularity among lay public. All such exaggerated reactions ultimately heal without causing any harm to individual, only 2 exceptions being lupoid reaction at vaccination site and progressive disease due to BCG. Complications are more common in revaccinated persons and in infants. Reactions can be divided into: Local, focal and generalized.

Local

Koch's Phenomenon

This is similar to what Koch had observed in infected animals after deliberately infecting them again with TB bacilli, but in a much lesser degree and in a modified form. This generally results from vaccinating tuberculin positives and is characterized by an immediate accelerated local reaction with some breakdown at the site of vaccination as against as 6 weeks in normal vaccination with quick healing. This phenomenon, however, is observed in actual practice only infrequently. No treatment is usually necessary. In occasional cases showing severe reaction it may be worthwhile taking chest X-ray to exclude the possibility of any existing lung focus.

Accelerated Reaction

This is a modified form of Koch's phenomenon, in the form of an exaggerated reaction observed between 3rd and the 7th day. No treatment is required.

Local Abscess

This generally takes place as a result of subcutaneous injection of vaccine because of faulty technique when breakdown takes place in the subcutaneous tissue, causing a local subcutaneous abscess by about 6 weeks. The abscess generally heals spontaneously but occasionally aspiration of the pus may be necessary. Generally, a simple aspiration and a short course of broad spectrum antibiotics is enough.

Large or Indolent Ulcer

Faulty technique of vaccination is generally responsible for this complication. Normally, the ulcer produced by vaccination should not exceed 10 mm in diameter and should heal by the 13th week. If the ulcer is larger in size or takes a longer time in healing this may be considered as complication. In younger children and with stronger dose of vaccine, generally the ulcers are larger. Treatment is the same as for any other ulcer.

Keloid

Keloid may take place at the site of vaccination after healing of the vaccination ulcer. This is usually not harmful but it has been observed that occasionally the keloid grows in size with the growth of the vaccinated child and is likely to effect the reputation of the vaccine. The cause of keloid formation is not precisely known yet. If a keloid tends to grow in size or worries the individual because of disfigurement, excision may be considered.

Tuberculids

Small satellite BCG tubercles may develop in the vicinity of the vaccination and resolve by self by about 2 months.

Confluent Reaction

This is a rare complication of multiple puncture technique. It may lead to plaque formation which may later ulcerate. No ATT is usually required.

Lupoid Lesions

Presents as local skin tuberculosis similar to lupus at the site of vaccination. They appear to occur only after multiple puncture technique and responds well to anti-tubercular treatment.

Focal

Enlargement of the Lymph Node

Enlargement of the lymph node draining the site of vaccination is the expected result of vaccination and is not a complication, as its development is consistent with the normal development of the BCG complex. Normally, this enlargement is discovered only by an examination as it does not cause any complaint and subsides by itself.

Abscess Formation in the Regional Lymph Node

Occasionally, the lymph node breaks down in the 3rd to 6th month or later and forms an abscess, the frequency of this complication being directly proportional to the strength of vaccine used and is noticed after intradermal vaccination, being very rare with vaccination by multiple puncture method. The larger the dose and the younger the child, the higher is the frequency of enlarged or supporting axillary lymph glands. In oral vaccination, it is possible to have suppuration of tonsillar or cervical lymph nodes because of bacilli remaining in the throat or tonsils while swallowing the vaccine.

Ultimately such cervical abscess may result in scarring. Treatment is the same as for local abscesses.

General

Fever

Low grade fever at the height of reaction, temporary check in weight curve of infants, general malaise, etc. may occur but such reactions are often too mild and transient to be observed and are of no significance. In fact such general reaction can be taken as a part of a normal vaccination.

Mediastinal Adenitis

Occasional cases showing enlargement of hilar lymph nodes with suggestion of atelectasis in X-rays taken between the 6th and the 12th week have been reported, but otherwise these are symptomless and later resolve completely, as such they are of no practical importance.

Erythema Nodosum

Very few cases of this condition at the time of development of allergy as result of vaccination have actually been reported. It develops less frequently than in case of natural infection.

Otitis Media

This condition is observed rarely with oral vaccination with certain strains only. It could be as a result of some bacilli contained in the vaccine passing into the middle ear along the Eustachian tube when oral vaccination is given and the nose of the baby is pinched to force swallowing.

Others

Isolated cases of there complications like benign BCG foci appearing in bones, phlyctenular conjunctivitis, urticarial rashes, etc. are reported in the medical literature from time to time.

Progressive Disease due to BCG

The only serious complication observed is disseminated BCG disease, seen in some children especially co-infected with HIV. While the documented risk of disseminated BCG disease in non-HIV-infected infants is < 5 per 1 million vaccinated and is associated with rare congenital immune deficiencies, it has been shown to be 1100 to 4170 per 1 million in HIV-infected infants routinely vaccinated at birth. Systemic or disseminated BCG disease may be clinically indistinguishable from tuberculosis and can only be confirmed through positive mycobacterial culture species identification, preferably by polymerase chain reaction (PCR) for the RD1 genetic region that is lost during attenuation of BCG.

VARIOUS STRATEGIES FOR THE DEVELOPMENT OF NEWER TUBERCULOSIS VACCINES

Despite the lack of a perfect understanding about protective immunity and effectors mechanisms involved in TB, there are several reasons to believe that a better TB vaccine is biologically possible. To out-perform *Mycobacterium tuberculosis,* a vaccine should induce a more potent immune response than the natural infection. The various vaccination strategies that have emerged in the last two decades are as follows:

Recombinant Bacilli Calmette-Guerin

It is well-acclaimed that BCG protects children against childhood TB. Hence, instead of replacing BCG with another vaccine, it would be wise to improve the current vaccine by expressing in it the immunodominant antigens involved in pathogenesis, persistence and immunomodulation. Alternatively, BCG can be employed in a prime boost strategy. Thus, without hampering the childhood immunization program, a recombinant BCG vaccine would help in improving the protective efficacy against adult pulmonary TB. Along with its potent immunoadjuvant property, high degree of safety for human use and the availability of expression systems that provide enhanced and stable expression of genes in mycobacteria, BCG became a very attractive vehicle for the development of new recombinant BCG vaccines. Apart from the restoration of the lost genes, like ESAT-6 and MPB-64, which are absent from BCG, several other antigens like major secretory 30–32 kDa protein, 38 kDa lipoprotein, etc. have been expressed in BCG and analyzed for their protective efficacy in mice and guinea pig models of TB.[19,20]

Recently, a rBCG strain expressing listeriolysin of *Listeria monocytogenes* which forms pores in the phagocytoplasm, thereby promoting antigen processing by class I pathway resulting in a greater cytotoxic T-cell response and a better protection against *Mycobacterium tuberculosis* infection.[21] This vaccine is now undergoing phase I clinical trial for its protective efficacy against TB.

Live Attenuated Mutants and Auxotrophs of *Mycobacterium tuberculosis*

The development of *Mycobacterium tuberculosis* mutants as vaccine candidates primarily relies upon the assumption that the vaccine strain should be antigenically as identical as possible to the disease-causing organism.[22] By comparative genomics, it has been revealed that in comparison to *Mycobacterium tuberculosis* 16 defined regions (RD1–RD16) are deleted from the currently used BCG strains.[23] Such strains can be developed by either: (i) producing auxotrophic mutants of *Mycobacterium tuberculosis* with limited replication capacity in immunocompromised subjects or (ii) by disrupting virulence genes necessary for host pathogen interaction.[24] A number of auxotrophic *Mycobacterium tuberculosis* mutant strains have been assessed for their protective efficacy in experimental animal models.[22] The methionone, tryptophan and proline auxotrophs of *Mycobacterium tuberculosis* have been found to be highly attenuated and confer protection equivalent (Proline) to or better (tryptophan) than BCG against *Mycobacterium tuberculosis* infection in DBA/2 mice.[25] A second approach relies on attenuation of *Mycobacterium tuberculosis* genes required for virulence. Till date several virulence genes have been identified, knocked out and the mutants assessed for their growth in vitro and in vivo.[26] These knockout strains were found to have differences in their virulence and growth characteristics.

Non-tuberculous Mycobacterial Vaccines

Non-tuberculous mycobacteria (NTM) that are closely related to *Mycobacterium tuberculosis* have been evaluated for their vaccine efficacy in various animal models and human trials. Apart from having the adjuvant-like property, these NTM are non-pathogenic even in immunocompromised individuals. *Mycobacterium microti* when used in a prophylactic mode conferred 77 percent protection (equivalent to BCG) against TB infection in infants.[27] Several studies have also been carried out with killed/ live or recombinant *Mycobacterium vaccae* in both prophylactic and immunotherapeutic modes resulting in protective efficacy comparable to BCG.[28] In a separate study, *Mycobacterium habana* exhibited improved protection as compared to BCG in the mouse model.[29] In another approach, killed *Mycobacterium wolinskyi (Mw)* caused reduction in the bacillary load in mice and prevented formation of granulomatous lesions in guinea pigs.[30] Furthermore, with the advent of comparative genomics, sequencing of these NTM would aid in the development of these viable or killed NTM as a vaccine against TB.

Subunit Vaccines

Subunit vaccines represent one of the most popular approaches for vaccine development. Subunit vaccines against *Mycobacterium tuberculosis* mainly comprise of secretory (culture filtrate proteins) and non-secretory proteins or lipids and carbohydrate antigens derived from *Mycobacterium tuberculosis* cell wall but also includes vaccines based on non-mycobacterial vectors like attenuated pox virus and adenovirus. Most of the vaccines included in this class have been identified by screening purified fractions or 2-D gels with antiserum collected from TB patients or by analyzing T-cell response against these antigens and are expected to be inherently safe. Lately, some new bioinformatic tools like MHC-I antigenic peptide processing prediction (MAPPP), Epimatrix, etc. have enabled MHC-I epitope identification.[31] *Mycobacterium tuberculosis* changes its antigenic repertoire when it shifts from an active state to a dormant non-replicating state. Indeed a vaccine that includes antigens from both the classes is most likely to protect individuals from various populations with different age groups and exposure levels. The apparent inability of the subunit vaccines to mount a strong T-cell response has accelerated the process of adjuvant discovery required to induce a potent Th1 response by these subunit vaccines and new adjuvants like DDA, MPL-A and AS02A of Glaxo Smith Kline, which are potent modulators of T-cell responses, have now been shown to better enhance the immunogenicity and protective efficacy of several subunit vaccines than traditional adjuvants.[32] The fusion protein 72f when used along with an adjuvant containing a saponin derivative from *Quillaja saponaria* [QS21] mixed with MPL-A exhibited very promising results in several animal models and now represents the first subunit vaccine to enter a clinical trial.

DNA Vaccines

The DNA vaccines, the latest entry in the field of vaccine development, have quickly emerged as one of the most promising advancements in the field of vaccine discovery. Intramuscular injection of a mammalian expression vector encoding a desired gene, results in the expression of corresponding protein, which subsequently induces a potent cellular immune response against the encoded antigen. The DNA vaccine allows continuous expression of a particular antigen, thereby exposing the immune system to the antigen for a prolonged time. Direct injection, electroporation or gene-gun based delivery into muscles, delivery to the respiratory mucosa using liposome encapsulated DNA vaccines, etc. are in common use for delivery of DNA vaccines these days. Expression of antigens by DNA vaccines and their subsequent processing and presentation along with the MHC class I molecules mimics the antigen-processing pathway followed by an intracellular pathogen. The DNA vaccination with genes encoding the members of Ag85 complex of *Mycobacterium tuberculosis* and 65 kDa heat shock protein of *Mycobacterium leprae* conferred protection equal to BCG.[33] Moreover, coexpression of costimulatory molecules, such as different cytokines and chemokines, inclusion of CpG motifs in the DNA vaccine backbone has helped in enhancing immunogenicity of DNA vaccines. Modifications in the mode of delivery would further improve the transfection ability of DNA vaccines, thereby enhancing the expression levels and consequently immunogenicity of the associated antigen.[34]

Epitope-based Vaccines

Strategies for exclusive delivery of immunodominant T-cell epitopes of a single or multiple proteins have emerged. Till date, many immunodominant proteins like 38 kDa,[35] 30–32 kDa antigens,[36] MPT51[37] and 16 kDa[38] protein of *Mycobacterium tuberculosis* have been screened for immunodominant T-cell epitopes and some of them have also been assessed for immunogenicity in vitro and in animal models, but protective efficacy of these epitope-based vaccines is yet to be confirmed.

Prime Boost Immunization Strategies

Repeated administration with the same vaccine (called homologous boosting) has proved to be relatively inefficient at boosting cellular immunity; instead it generates a very strong humoral response. In order to circumvent this problem, 'Heterologous boosting' came into being, which involves sequential administration of vaccines with appropriate intervals using different antigen-delivery system such that the immune system is primed to the antigen using one vector and is then boosted with the same antigen delivered through a different vector. With the emergence of new strategies involving adenovirus and poxvirus in heterologous prime boost vaccination schemes, synergistic effects can be achieved instead of an additive effect generally observed in case of homologous boosting.[39] The protective efficacy of this vaccination strategy is currently being evaluated for its efficacy in Cynomolgus monkeys. With these encouraging results, this vaccine became the first of the new generation TB vaccines to enter the human trials.[40]

Apart from the viral vectors, which have been highly recommended as boosting agents, subunit vaccines including both recombinant proteins and DNA vaccines are now being used to boost the immunity imparted by BCG.

Besides the use of BCG as the priming agent, several efforts to develop other heterologous prime boost immunization strategies are underway. Though these vaccination protocols need to be evaluated for conferring protective efficacy in various animal models, the promising subunit vaccines would definitely find their use in the immunocompromised individuals, where live vaccines based on viral or bacterial vectors pose problems.

CONCLUSION

Despite controversies BCG vaccination has stood the test of time. World Health Organization continues to recommend its use in infant immunization program in countries with heavy endemicity and where threatening HIV epidemic is an emerging problem. Adoption of a '5C' concept viz. case detection, chemotherapy short course, contact elimination, chemoprophylaxis and lastly control by BCG vaccine will be a desirable national approach in combating adult and childhood TB.

REFERENCES

1. Grange JM, Gibson J, Osborn TW. What is BCG? Tubercle. 1983;64:129-39.
2. Gardner LV. The history of the R1 strain of tubercle bacillus. Am Rev Tuberc. 1932;25: 577-90.

3. Crispen R. History of BCG and its substrains. In BCG in superficial bladder cancer. EORTC Genitourinary group Monograph. 1989;Vol 6:Pp 35-50.
4. Levy FM, Conge GA, Pasquier JF, Mauss H, Dubos R, Schaeder R. The effect of BCG vaccination on the fate of virulent tubercle bacilli in mice. Am Rev Respir Dis. 1961;84:28-36.
5. Smith DW, Mcmurray DN, Wiergerhaus EH, Grover AA, Harding GE. Host-parasite relationships in experimental tuberculosis IV. Early events in the course of infection in vaccinated and non-vaccinated guinea pigs. Am Rev Respir Dis. 1970;102:937-49.
6. Wunsch-Filho V, De Castilho Ea, Rodrigues LC, Hutly SRA. Effectiveness of BCG vaccination against tuberculosis meningitis: A case-control study in Sao Paulo, Brazil. Bull WHO. 1990; 68:69-74.
7. Hart Pd, Sutherland I. BCG and whole bacillus vaccines in the prevention of tuberculosis in adolescence and in early adult life. BMJ. 1977;2:293-5.
8. Aronson JD, Aranson CF, Taylor HC. A twenty year appraisal of BCG vaccination in the control of TB. Arch Intern Med. 1958;101:881-93.
9. Rosenthal SR, Loewinsohn E, Graham M, Liveright D, Thorne M, Johnson V. BCG vaccination against tuberculosis in Chicago. A 20 year study statistically analyzed. Paediatrics. 1961;28:622-41.
10. Comstock GW, Webster RG. Tuberculosis studies in Muscogee County, Georgia. VII. A twenty year evaluation of BCG vaccination in a school population. Am Rev Respir Dis. 1969;100:839-45.
11. Comstock GW, Woolpert SF, Livesay Vt. Tuberculosis studies in Muscogee County, Georgia. Twenty year evaluation of a community trial of BCG vaccination. Public Health Rep. 1976; 91:276-80.
12. Smith PG. Case-control studies of the efficacy of BCG against tuberculosis. Bull Int Union Tubercle Lung Dis. 1987;62:73-9.
13. Miceli I, De Kantor In, Colaiacovo Dk, et al. Evaluation of the effectiveness of BCG vaccination using the case-control method in Buenos Aires, Argentina. Int J Epidemiol. 1988;17:629-34.
14. Myint TT, Win H, Aye HH, Kyaw-Mint TO. Case-control study on evaluation of BCG vaccination of newborn in Rangoon, Burma. Ann Trop Paediatric. 1987;7:159-66.
15. Clemens JB, Chuong JJH, Fienstein AR. The BCG controversy: A methodological and statistical reappraisal. JAMA. 1983;249:2361-9.
16. Colditz GA, Brewer T, Berkey C, et al. Efficacy of BCG in the prevention of tuberculosis: Meta-analysis of the published literature. JAMA. 1994;271:698-702.
17. Guidelines for the programmatic management of drug-resistant tuberculosis—WHO. 2008.
18. Stewart CJ. Skin sensitivity to human, avian and BCG PPDs after BCG vaccination. Tubercle. 1968;49:8.
19. Harboe M, Wiker HG. Searching for the secreted proteins of *Mycobacterium leprae.* Indian J Lepr. 1999;71:19-35.
20. Horwitz MA, Harth G, Dillon BJ, Maslesa-Galic' S. Recombinant bacillus Calmette-Guerin [BCG] vaccines expressing the *Mycobacterium tuberculosis* 30-kDa major secretory protein induce greater protective immunity against tuberculosis than conventional BCG vaccines in a highly susceptible animal model. Proc Natl Acad Sci USA. 2000;97:138.
21. Hess J, Miko D, Catic A, Lehmensiek V, Russel DG, Kauffman SH. *Mycobacterium bovis* bacillus Calmette–Guerin strains secreting listeriolysin of *Listeria monocytogenes*. Proc Natl Acad Sci USA. 1998;95:5299-304.
22. Sampson SL, Dascher CC, Sambandamurthy VK, Russell RG, Jacobs WR Jr, Bloom BR, et al. Protection elicited by a double leucine and pantothenate auxotroph of *Mycobacterium tuberculosis* in guinea pigs. Infect Immun. 2004;72:3031-7.
23. Mahairas GG, Sabo PJ, Hickey MJ, Singh DC, Stover CK. Molecular analysis of genetic differences between *Mycobacterium bovis* BCG and virulent M.bovis. J Bacteriol. 1996;178: 1274-82.

24. Sambandamurthy VK, Jacobs WR Jr. Live attenuated mutants of *Mycobacterium tuberculosis* as candidate vaccines against tuberculosis. Microbes Infect. 2005;7:955-61.
25. Smith DA, Parish T, Stoker NG, Bancroft GJ. Characterization of auxotrophic mutants of *Mycobacterium tuberculosis* and their potential as vaccine candidates. Infect Immun. 2001;69: 142-50.
26. Singh A, Gupta R, Vishwakarma RA, Narayanan PR, Paramasivan CN, Ramanathan VD, et al. Requirement of the mymA operon for appropriate cell wall ultrastructure and persistence of *Mycobacterium tuberculosis* in the spleens of guinea pigs. J Bacteriol. 2005;187:4173-86.
27. Manabe YC, Scott CP, Bishai YR. Naturally attenuated, orally administered *Mycobacterium microti* as a tuberculosis vaccine is better than subcutaneous *Mycobacterium bovis* BCG. Infect Immun. 2002;70:1566-70.
28. Abou-Zied C, Gares MP, Inwald J, Jansen R, Zhang Y, Young DB, et al. Induction of a type 1 immune response to a recombinant antigen from *Mycobacterium tuberculosis* expressed in *Mycobacterium vaccae*. Infect Immun. 1997;65:1856-62.
29. Chaturvedi V, Srivastava A, Gupta HP, Srivastava BS. Protective antigens of *Mycobacterium habana* are distributed between peripheral and integral compartments of plasma membrane: a study in experimental tuberculosis of mouse. Vaccine. 1999;17:2882-7.
30. Singh IG, Mukherjee R, Talwar GP. Resistance to intravenous inoculation of *Mycobacterium tuberculosis* H37Rv in mice of different inbred strains following immunisation with a leprosy based vaccine on *Mycobacterium w*. Vaccine. 1991;9:10-4.
31. Hakenberg J, Nussubaum AK, Schild H, Rammensee HG, Kuttler C, Holzhutter HG, et al. MAPPP: MHC class I antigenic peptide processing prediction. Appl Bioinformatics. 2003;2:155-8.
32. Doherty TM, Anderson P. Vaccines for tuberculosis: novel concepts and recent progress. Clin Microbiol Rev. 2005;18:687-702.
33. Lozes E, Huygen K, Content J, Denis O, Montogomery DL, Yawman AM, et al. Immunogenicity and efficacy of a tuberculosis DNA vaccine encoding the components of secreted antigen 85 complex. Vaccine. 1997;15:830-3.
34. van Drunen Little, van den Hurk S, Babiuk SL, Babiuk LA. Strategies for improved formulation and delivery of DNA vaccines to veterinary target species. Immunol Rev. 2004;199:113-25.
35. da Fonseca DP, Joosten D, van der Zee R, Jue DL, Singh M, Vordermeier HM, et al. Identification of new cytotoxic T-cell epitopes on the 38-kilodalton lipoglycoprotein of *Mycobacterium tuberculosis* by using lipopeptides. Infect Immun. 1998;66:3190-7.
36. Silver RF, Wallis RS, Ellner JJ. Mapping of T-cell epitopes of the 30 kDa alpha antigen of *Mycobacterium bovis* strain bacillus Calmette-Guerin in purified protein derivative [PPD]-positive individuals. J Immunol. 1995;154:4665-74.
37. Suzuki M, Aoshi T, Nagata T, Koide Y. Identification of murine H2-Dd- and H2-Ab-restricted T-cell epitopes on a novel protective antigen, MPT51, of *Mycobacterium tuberculosis*. Infect Immun. 2004;72:3829-37.
38. Caccamo N, Meravigilia S, Dieli F, Romano A, Titone L, Salemo A. Th0 to Th1 switch of CD4 T-cell clones specific from the 16 –kDa antigen of *Mycobacterium tuberculosis* after successful therapy: lack of involvement of epitope repertoire and HLA-DR. Immunol Lett. 2005;98:253-8.
39. Woodland DL. Jump-starting the immune system: prime boosting comes of age. Trends Immunol. 2003;171:1602-9.
40. McShane H, Pathan AA, Sander CR, Goonetilleke NP, Fletcher HA, Hill AV. Boosting BCG with MVA85A: The first candidate subunit vaccine for tuberculosis in clinical trials. Tuberculosis [Edinb]. 2005;85:47-52.

Chapter 33

Chemoprophylaxis in Tuberculosis

INTRODUCTION

The term chemoprophylaxis implies prevention of infection or its complications with drugs. It has been attempted since a long time to prevent the occurrence of tuberculosis by treating infected persons before clinical expression of the disease. The lifetime risk is estimated to be 10%, is increased in children, presence of fibrotic lesions radiologically and immunocompromised conditions. It is maximal during the first 2 years after infection and wanes over time. If it can be provided to whole population with high rate of latent infection, this procedure can produce dramatic result in decreasing TB incidence in future. The current chapter aims to describe various important aspects of chemoprophylaxis in tuberculosis.

CHEMOPROPHYLAXIS IN TUBERCULOSIS

Chemoprophylaxis in tuberculosis can be of two types:

Primary Chemoprophylaxis

When chemoprophylaxis is administered in tuberculin negative subjects to avoid infection with *Mycobacterium tuberculosis*.

Chemoprophylaxis as a short-term measure is given for:

a. Breastfeeding child of an infectious pulmonary tuberculosis mother, as separation of child from mother is undesirable.
b. Tuberculin negative nurses and doctors posted in a tuberculosis hospital for short time.
c. Out break of local epidemic of tuberculosis in a school or closed community.

Secondary Chemoprophylaxis

Chemoprophylaxis to prevent serious complications of an already infected but healthy person. It is given in the following conditions:

a. Persons and children under 5 years of age who are household and other close contacts of smear positive patient.[1,2] Chemoprophylaxis has been strongly recommended for such individuals. However, it is not required for tuberculin-negative contacts in this situation and BCG vaccination must be offered.

b. Persons having positive tuberculin skin-test with an abnormal but suggestive of inactive disease on chest X-ray. The International Union Against Tuberculosis and Lung Disease (IUATLD) performed a European multi-center, double-blind, placebo-controlled trial of INH prophylaxis in patients with a positive PPD and an old fibrotic scar on chest X-ray.[3] Of the 27,830 patients enrolled (median age 50 years), 6,953 were randomized to receive INH for 12 weeks, 6,965 INH for 24 weeks, 6,919 INH for 52 weeks and 6,990 patients were randomized to placebo. Over the 5 years study, active pulmonary tuberculosis developed in 97 placebo recipients (14.3 per 1,000), 76 patients on INH for 12 weeks (11.3 per 1,000), 34 patients on 24 weeks of INH (5.0 per 1,000) and 24 patients on 52 weeks of INH (3.6 per 1,000). This represents a 60% reduction in cases for patients receiving a 6-month-course and approximately 90% reduction for patients receiving a 12-month-course of INH. Based on this study, it can be inferred that there is fair evidence to support the use of INH prophylaxis in this setting.

c. Persons under 35 years of age with tuberculin-positive skin test. It has been stated that treatment of 1000 tuberculin positive patients with no symptoms aged 35 years for one year with isoniazid would prevent 23 cases of TB or one case every two years.[4] Some authorities are not considering to be an essential indication reason being development of disease despite of chemoprophylaxis.

d. Persons infected with both HIV and *M. tuberculosis*. It has been observed that persons coinfected with HIV and tuberculosis have a 5–10% chance of developing TB every year.[5] Chemoprophylaxis in either of these categories can reduce the risk of developing active tuberculosis, increase life expectancy and reduce overall medical cost.[6] Whether the disease is due to reinfection or reactivation, it carries no significance since provision of chemoprophylaxis to all such persons having greater than 5 mm induration has been efficient in preventing the treatment of disease.

e. Tuberculin positive patients in special clinical situations such as those receiving steroid or immunosuppressive therapy, those with diabetes mellitus, those having malignancy such as leukemia and lymphoma undergoing chemoradiotherapy and undergoing surgical procedures such as gastrectomy or ileal bypass and also organ transplantation.

One of the studies has stated that chemoprophylaxis is not essential for patients receiving moderate doses of long-term corticosteroids for respiratory disease.[7] A high index of suspicion of development of tuberculous disease must always be kept in mind whether or not all of these patients receive chemoprophylaxis.

However, it is contraindicated in patients suffering from progressive tubercular disease, having previous adequate course of isoniazid treatment, past history of isoniazid hypersensitivity and previous history of drug induced hepatotoxicity or acute liver disease.

TREATMENT REGIMENS AND DURATION

Regimen of isoniazid for 6–12 months has been the mainstay of secondary chemoprophylaxis, though recently various shorter regimens as alternative to isoniazid have become popular (Table 33.1).

Prospective, randomized trials in HIV-negative person indicate that preventive treatment with isoniazid for 12 months is more effective than 6 months treatment. However, daily isoniazid regimen for 9 months is recommended in many countries as 12 months treatment gives little additional benefit.[8-11] Rifampicin given daily for 4 months is recommended in tuberculin positive patients with silicosis.[8] Emergence of multidrug resistant strains of tuberculosis has meant that preventive therapy with first line drugs such as isoniazid and/or rifampicin may not be appropriate so either pyrazinamide and ethambutol or pyrazinamide and ofloxacin can be used depending on drug sensitivity of the patient to whom exposed. These shorter regimens may be equally effective and improve the adherence to treatment making them more efficient.

CHEMOPROPHYLAXIS UNDER REVISED NATIONAL TUBERCULOSIS CONTROL PROGRAM

Close contacts of sputum smear positive pulmonary tuberculosis patients who are under 6 years and not having symptoms of tuberculosis and if

Table 33.1: Drug with duration and frequency used in chemoprophylaxis

Drugs	Duration	Frequency
Isoniazid	12 months	Daily/twice weekly
Isoniazid	9 Months	Daily/twice weekly
Isoniazid	6 months	Daily/twice weekly
Rifampicin + Pyrazinamide	2 months	Daily/twice weekly
Rifampicin + Isoniazid	3 months	Daily
Rifampicin	4 months	Daily
Pyrazinamide + Ethambutol	6–12 months	Daily
Pyrazinamide + Ofloxacin	6–12 months	Daily

tuberculin test is not available then the child should receive 6 months of isoniazid at 5 mg/kg body weight. If tuberculin test is available then it is done after 3 month of isoniazid therapy and if the test turns positive, isoniazid is continued for three more months, while if tuberculin test is negative then isoniazid is stopped and child is given intradermal BCG if not previously vaccinated.

CHEMOPROPHYLAXIS FOR DRUG RESISTANT TUBERCULOSIS

Since by definition MDR-TB is resistant to both of these drugs, it is unlikely that use of these drugs to treat latent infection caused by an MDR-TB strain will prevent the development of active TB disease.[12] Contacts of MDR-TB patients in whom latent infection is diagnosed may not be infected with the same strain; some may be infected with isoniazid susceptible strains, particularly in high-burden areas where many different strains of TB may circulate in homes, schools, workplaces, etc. Studies from high-burden TB areas have shown that approximately one-half to two-thirds of household members had the same strain of TB, as determined by genetic testing.[13-15] (The degree of strain concordance could be higher in contacts who are children aged under 5 years because they have less exposure to strains circulating outside the household.) Close contacts of DR-TB patients should receive careful clinical follow-up for a period of at least two years. If active disease develops, prompt initiation of treatment with a regimen designed to treat MDR-TB is recommended. On the basis of the currently available evidence, WHO does not recommend the universal use of second-line drugs for chemoprophylaxis in MDR-TB contacts.[16]

LIMITATIONS OF CHEMOPROPHYLAXIS

It should be practiced only after excluding active tuberculosis. For this reason, it cannot be practiced without strict medical supervision. In a developing country like ours, where it is even difficult to provide sufficient drugs to treat known active case of tuberculosis with complete supervision, giving important primary drugs like (R and H) for chemoprophylaxis is not feasible. So, it is not practiced in India in revised National Tuberculosis Control Program except in localized group.

PLACE OF SECONDARY CHEMOPROPHYLAXIS IN TUBERCULOSIS CONTROL[17]

A large scale use of this preventive measure for control of tuberculosis in this country will necessarily involve the routine tuberculin testing in mass scale to pick tuberculin positive children. Radiographic and clinical examination of all tuberculin positive children to find out those who have active tuberculosis.

The parents of these otherwise normal children will then have to be motivated for prolonged treatment. Drugs will have to be made available to them regularly and easily for that period. Adequate supervision will have to be provided to ensure regular administration of drugs. The magnitude of such a task for a country wide program like India is difficult to achieve. Considering all these points, it is obvious that chemoprophylaxis though theoretically a very sound measure for control of tuberculosis can be given a lower priority than BCG which is relatively simple, easier and more economically viable in the nationwide tuberculosis control program. So children who escape receiving BCG vaccination soon after birth and subsequently become tuberculin positive should be considered for chemoprophylaxis if the risk of tuberculosis in them is thought to be high.

CONCLUSION

Although theoretically, it appears very sound measure to control tuberculosis but it is not practiced in tuberculosis control except in localized group. It can be used by individual clinician in clinical situations where patient is tubercular positive and have high chance of getting active disease but it should be practiced only after excluding active tuberculosis disease. The debate about when and where to implement chemoprophylaxis will continue. There is no doubt that for all indications currently recommended for chemoprophylaxis such intervention is effective in reducing subsequent number of active TB cases but difficulty lies with that so many healthy people have to be treated to prevent so few cases, especially with a disease eminently curable by current chemotherapy should it develop.

REFERENCES

1. Preventive therapy against tuberculosis in people living with HIV. Policy statement. Weekly Epidemiological Record. 1999;74:385-400.
2. Starke JR, Jacobs RF, Jereb JA. Resurgence of tuberculosis in children. Journal of Pediatrics. 1992;120:839-55.
3. International Union Against Tuberculosis and Lung Disease Committee on Prophylaxis: Efficacy of various durations of isoniazid preventative therapy for tuberculosis: five years of follow-up in the IUATLD trial. Bull World Health Organization. 1982; 60:555-64.
4. Anon.Chemoprophylaxis for tuberculosis.Tubercle. 1981;62:69.
5. Selwyn PA, Hartel D, Lewis VA, et al. A prospective study of the risk of tuberculosis among intravenous drug users with HIV infection.N Engl J Med. 1989;320:545
6. Harries AD, et al. TB/HIV: a clinical manual. Geneva, World Health Organization, 2004 (document WHO/TB/04.220).
7. Bateman ED. Is TB chemoprophylaxis necessary for patients receiving corticosteroids for respiratory disease? Respir Med. 1993;87:485.
8. A double-blind placebo controlled trial of three antituberculosis chemoprophylaxis regimens in patients with silicosis in Hong Kong. Hong Kong Chest Service/Tuberculosis Research Center, Madras/British Medical Research Council. American Review of Respiratory Disease. 1992;145: 36-41.

9. Villarino ME, et al. Rifampin preventive therapy for tuberculosis infection: experience with 157 adolescents. American Journal of Respiratory and Critical Care Medicine. 1997;155: 1735-8.
10. Comstock GW. How much isoniazid is needed for prevention of tuberculosis among immuno-component adults? International Journal of Tuberculosis and Lung Disease. 1999;3:847-50.
11. Barnes PF, et al. Transmission of tuberculosis among the urban homeless. Journal of the American Medical Association. 1996;275:305-7.
12. Kritski AL, et al. Transmission of tuberculosis to close contacts of patients with multidrug-resistant tuberculosis. American Journal of Respiratory and Critical Care Medicine, 1996, 153(1):331-5.
13. Verver S, et al. Proportion of tuberculosis transmission that takes place in households in a high-incidence area. Lancet. 2004;363(9404):212-4.
14. Schaaf HS, et al. Evaluation of young children in household contact with adult multidrug-resistant pulmonary tuberculosis cases. Pediatric Infectious Disease Journal. 1999;18(6):494–500.
15. Steiner P, Rao M. Drug-resistant tuberculosis in children. Seminars in Pediatric Infectious Diseases. 1993;4:275-82.
16. Guidelines for the programmatic management of drug-resistant tuberculosis—WHO, 2008, 2011.
17. API Consensus Expert Committee. API TB Consensus Guidelines 2006: Management of pulmonary tuberculosis, extrapulmonary tuberculosis and tuberculosis in special situations. J Assoc Physicians India. 2006;54:219-34.

Chapter 34

Tuberculosis Control in India: DOTS

INTRODUCTION

Tuberculosis is a leading cause of death as an infectious disease in developing countries. India accounts for 1/5 global TB burden with 1.98 million developing disease each year and nearly 0.30 million dying due to tuberculosis each year. Epidemic of HIV-AIDS and MDR-TB are further worsening the condition of TB in India. Our country ranking third highest in HIV burden, had an estimated 2.31 million (0.36% of adult population in the country) people living with HIV/AIDS in 2007, emphasizing the enormous challenge ahead.[1,2] Tuberculosis control is the point of time when "reduction of the problem of tuberculosis in a community is reached so low a level that there is less then one percent of prevalence of specific natural reactors to standard tuberculin among children in the 14 years of age group" is defined as achievement of tuberculosis control. Elimination has been defined arbitrarily as no more than one new case per million populations per year or a prevalence of tuberculosis infection of below 1% in the general population.[3] Various TB related Millennium Development Goals has been set—To combat HIV/AIDS, malaria and other diseases (Goal 6), to halt and reverse the incidence of malaria and other major diseases including tuberculosis by 2015 (Target 8), to halve the prevalence and death rates associated with tuberculosis between 1990 and 2015 (Indicator 23) and to detect 70% of new smear positive TB cases arising annually and to successfully treat 85% of these cases by 2005 (Indicator 24). The Stop TB Partnership has set targets to reduce global burden of TB (per capita prevalence and death rates) by 50% relative to 1990 levels by 2015 and also reduction of the global incidence of active TB less than 1 case per million per year by 2050. The present chapter describes in detail about TB control in India.

LANDMARKS OF TUBERCULOSIS CONTROL IN INDIA

Prechemotherapy Era

Review of the history of tuberculosis showed that initial antitubercular measures implemented in India were unplanned confined mainly to hospital and sanatorium. It was because of lack of resources and more attention was given to other epidemics at that time. First open-air sanatorium was founded in 1906 at Tilounia in Ajmer. Many more sanatoria and TB dispensaries came into existence with object to educate the people about the cause and prevention. Tuberculosis Association of India (TAI)[4] was established on february 23, 1939. Recognizing the complexity of the TB and to meet the need of large number of TB patients, idea of domiciliary treatment was conceived as early as 1940. Tuberculosis division in Director General Health Services (DGHS) of Ministry of Health was established in 1947 for planning and execution of activities against tuberculosis. It was estimated that 4000 clinics and 500,000 beds were required to control tuberculosis in India but the cost of establishment was too high and therefore attention was directed to prevention of tuberculosis by way of BGG vaccination, a more economical and operatively feasible alternative option. BCG vaccination was introduced on a small scale in Madanpalli in 1948 and extended to mass scale in 1951.[5]

Postchemotherapy Era

National Sample Survey (1955–58)[6] conducted by Indian Council of Medical Research (ICMR) in six zones of the country covering both urban and rural population revealed that the prevalence of active and probably active tuberculosis varied from 13 to 25 per 1000 population in aged five years and more and bacteriologically positive cases varied from 2 to 8 per 1000 population. The prevalence of tuberculosis was similar in rural and urban area.

Tuberculosis Chemotherapy Center (TCC) presently known as Tuberculosis Research Center (TRC), established in 1956 in Chennai (Madras) under the auspices of the Indian Council for Medical Research (ICMR), with the assistance of British Medical Research Council (BMRC), World Health Organization (WHO) and Government of India (GOI), conducted a series of studies on the application of mass domiciliary chemotherapy and revealed that sanatorium based treatment measures were unimportant and specific potent and readily available anti-tubercular drugs given in combinations were proved to be the best and most effective treatment against tuberculosis as shown by New Delhi TB Center and Tuberculosis Research Center (TRC), Chennai.[7] These studies also prepared the base for organizing a comprehensive tuberculosis program with wide coverage.

National Tuberculosis Institute, (NTI) Bengaluru (Bangalore), was established in 1959, with an aim to initiate research for development of a program. Different studies by NTI Bengaluru observed that active case finding is not necessary as 95% of the infectious tuberculosis patients are conscious of symptoms and 50% contacted to nearest health center to seek medical aid within few weeks of their presentation of symptoms.[8] Initially, there were three major tools for tuberculosis control. BCG vaccination for prevention, sputum microscopy and chest X-ray for diagnosis and ambulatory domiciliary chemotherapy for treatment but the major problem was to organize them in the form of a program that would be feasible and applicable in both rural and urban areas and economically affordable and beneficial to the community.[9]

National Tuberculosis Control Program

National Tuberculosis Control Program (NTP) was pilot tested in Anantpur District of Andhra Pradesh in 1961 on the basis of studies conducted by NTI and implemented in phased manner throughout the country integrated with general health care system from 1962. By 1978 NTP had covered 81% of the country, using 12–18 months regimen for treatment of tuberculosis under the program. Initially monitored on a regional basis, after which NTI took up the monitoring of entire country, treatment compliance was observed as the significant problem. Availability of rifampicin and pyrazinamide provided a big support to change the chemotherapy from 12–18 months to short-course chemotherapy. TRC Chennai in 1983 tested the SCC in 18 districts that showed encouraging results and subsequently the Government of India (GoI) agreed to introduce the SCC in tuberculosis control. Short-course chemotherapy regimen costed higher and showed only a marginal improvement. NTP was evaluated by three independent agencies: the ICMR in 1975, Institute of Communication, Operations Research and Community Involvement (ICORCI) in 1988 and at last by Government of India, World Health Ogranization (WHO) and Swedish International Development Agency (SIDA)[10] in 1992. They explained the wide gap between expected and actual achievement of the program due to some programmatic deficiencies like managerial weakness, inadequate funding, over reliance on chest X-ray for diagnosis, interrupted supplies of drugs, poor compliance of patient. No appreciable change was observed in the epidemiological situation of tuberculosis in country during existence of NTP from 1962 to 1992. Epidemic of HIV and multidrug resistance tuberculosis (MDR-TB) were threatening further the status of tuberculosis in the country. To rectify these deficiencies government decided to boost up the NTP with the help of international agencies in 1993.

The Revised National Tuberculosis Control Program

The Revised National Tuberculosis Control Program (RNTCP) came in to existence by formulating and adopting the internationally recommended DOTS (Direct Observation Treatment Short-Course) strategy as most systemic and cost-effective approach to revive the TB control program in India with an objective to achieve at least 85 percent cure rate of the newly diagnosed sputum smear-positive tuberculosis patients and to detect at least 70 percent of new sputum smear-positive patients. The RNTCP was built on extensive infrastructure created by NTP for tuberculosis control, with the network of more than 446 district tuberculosis centers, 330 tuberculosis clinics and more than 47,600 tuberculosis beds[11,22] and this was further strengthened by adequate funds, staff and other essential inputs. The RNTCP was pilot tested in a population of 2.35 million in 1993 in five sites across different states in Delhi, Gujrat, Kerala, Maharashtra and West Bengal. It was expanded to cover 13.88 million people in 1995 and 16 million in 1996.

During 1996–97 after confirmation of technical and operational feasibility of the revised program, India planned to initially implement the RNTCP in 102 districts (271 million populations) in a phased manner. It was envisaged that another 447 million would be strengthened as a transitional step for introduction of revised strategy at a later stage. In 1998, another 100 million populations were covered under the program. By the end of 2001 RNTCP had made rapid strides, with a 25 folds expansion to cover a population of 450 million in 221 districts in 21 states/union territories of the country. By March 2006 coverage had increased to 1 billion. DOTS services are now available in 563 districts of 26 states/union territories.[12]

REVISED NATIONAL TUBERCULOSIS CONTROL PROGRAM STRATEGY

DOTS (Direct Observation Treatment Short course) are a WHO recommended comprehensive public health strategy, to control tuberculosis[13] is now in operation in 180 countries in the form of Revised National Tuberculosis Control Program (RNTCP). DOTS reliably increases cure rates, decreases the proportion of deaths due to tuberculosis and prevents the further emergence of drug resistance. RNTCP strategy is based on following five principles.The components of strategy are:

1. Political and administrative commitment at all levels ensuring the availability of adequate fund, staff and other key inputs. Since TB can be cured and epidemic reversed, it warrants the top most priority which has been accorded by Government of India (GoI).
2. Diagnosis through quality sputum microscopy primarily among chest symptomatic patients attending health facilities. Binocular microscopes are supplied to all RNTCP areas and regular quality services are assured.
3. Uninterrupted supply of SCC drugs, supplied in patientwise boxes (an innovation of the RNTCP) containing entire course of treatment for an individual patient, so that no patient can ever stop treatment for lack of medicines.
4. Direct observation of every dose of treatment in intensive phase and at least first dose of every week in continuation phase of treatment. This has been made possible through the involvement of peripheral health functionaries, NGOs, community volunteers and trained persons who are not a family member, watch the patient swallowing the anti-TB medicines in his/her presence. DOTS is not just a supervised swallowing but a service to the patient, develops a human bond between patient and

observer, increasing the probability of treatment completion to achieve a high cure rate. RNTCP shift the responsibility of cure from the patient to health system.

5. Systematic supervision, monitoring and evaluation of program at all level. RNTCP analyzes performance in every district, every state and country as a whole every quarterly. This is published and widely circulated and is available on RNTCP website (www.tbcindia.org).

REVISED NATIONAL TUBERCULOSIS CONTROL PROGRAM STRUCTURE

It comprises of five levels: National level, State level, District level, Sub-district level, Peripheral Health Institutions level. The Central Tuberculosis Division (CTD) is part of Ministry of Health and Family Welfare and responsible for tuberculosis control in the whole country. CTD is also responsible for developing technical policies, providing drugs, preparing training module, program and financial monitoring, quality assurance, advocacy, operational research and mobilizing funds. NTI Bengaluru, TRC Chennai and LRS Institute of Tuberculosis and Respiratory Diseases, New Delhi assists the CTD. Deputy Director General (DDG) supervises CTD and under his supervision an independent agency has been hired for drugs and logistics management. At State level RNTCP is integrated with the general healthcare delivery system. The states via state tuberculosis cells are now directly responsible for monitoring and supervising the work of district TB control societies.

District Tuberculosis Center (DTC) is the key organizational unit responsible for the implementation of the program in respect to district. DTC is supported by sub-district tuberculosis units (TU) established for every 5,00,000 population (2.5 lakh in tribles, desert, remote and hilly region) and serve as a link between district level and periphery. The TU is the lowest reporting unit under RNTCP and the nodal point for tuberculosis control activities in the sub-district. Medical Officer TB Control (MOTC) at the TU has over all responsibility of management of RNTCP and is assisted by the Senior Treatment Supervisor (STS) and Senior Tuberculosis Laboratory Supervisor (STLS). RNTCP designated microscopy centers have been established for every 100,000 population (0.5 lakh in tribal, desert, remote and hilly region) to further decentralize the diagnostic and treatment services. A vast network of DOTS center, all with trained DOTS providers have been established all over the areas for a better access to patient. Dispensaries, Primary Health Centers, Community Health Centers, referred hospitals, major hospitals, special clinics within the district come at the level of peripheral health institutions.

DIAGNOSIS UNDER REVISED NATIONAL TUBERCULOSIS CONTROL PROGRAM (RNTCP)

Nearly 70% of the cases diagnosed and put on treatment on the basis of chest X-ray alone did not have tuberculosis at all.[14] The International Union Against Tuberculosis and Lung Disease (IUATLD) international study on X-ray classification demonstrated high level of Inter and Intra reader variability among experts on chest radiographs.[15] Similarly, NTI demonstrated that laboratory technicians were able to perform sputum smear microscopy effectively in the periphery after giving minimal training and regular supervision.[16,17] These strategies made the basis for using sputum smear microscopy as primary diagnostic tool under the program and modular training is provided to all laboratory technicians involved in RNTCP diagnostic activities.

All chest symptomatic or other symptoms suggestive of tuberculosis are advised to undergo three sputum examinations (two spot and one overnight sample collected in two visits). Patients with two or three smear positive results are diagnosed as sputum positive pulmonary tuberculosis. Those with only one positive result, are advised to get a chest X-ray done, and if found to be compatable with tuberculosis, are treated as sputum positive pulmonary tuberculosis. Patients with all the 3 negative results are prescribed broad-spectrum antibiotics such as cotrimoxazole for 10–14 days. If not suffering from tuberculosis, patients improve with antibiotics. Persistent symptoms direct for re-evaluation of patient on the basis of sputum microscopy and chest X-ray (Fig. 34.1). Lastly, if treating physician have an opinion that

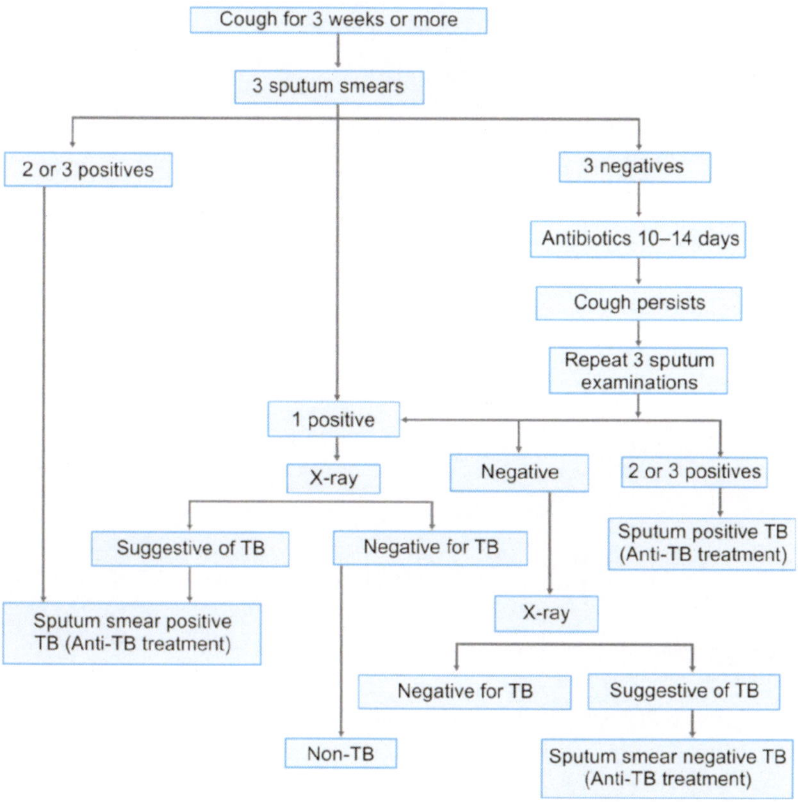

Fig. 34.1: Diagnostic algorithm for pulmonary tuberculosis

patient is suffering from pulmonary tuberculosis, treatment is initiated accordingly. However, RNTCP has launched recent guidelines in April, 2009 (Fig. 34.2) which recommends that the number of specimen required for diagnosis of smear positive pulmonary TB is two, with one of them being a morning sputum specimen. One specimen positive out of the two is enough to declare a patient as smear positive TB. Smear positive TB is further classified as a new or retreatment case based on their previous treatment history, and appropriate therapy is prescribed. Patients in whom both specimens are smear-negative should be prescribed symptomatic treatment and broad-spectrum antibiotics for 10–14 days. In such cases, antibiotics such as fluoroquinolones (ciprofloxacin, ofloxacin, etc.), rifampicin or streptomycin, which are active against tuberculosis, should not to be used. Most patients

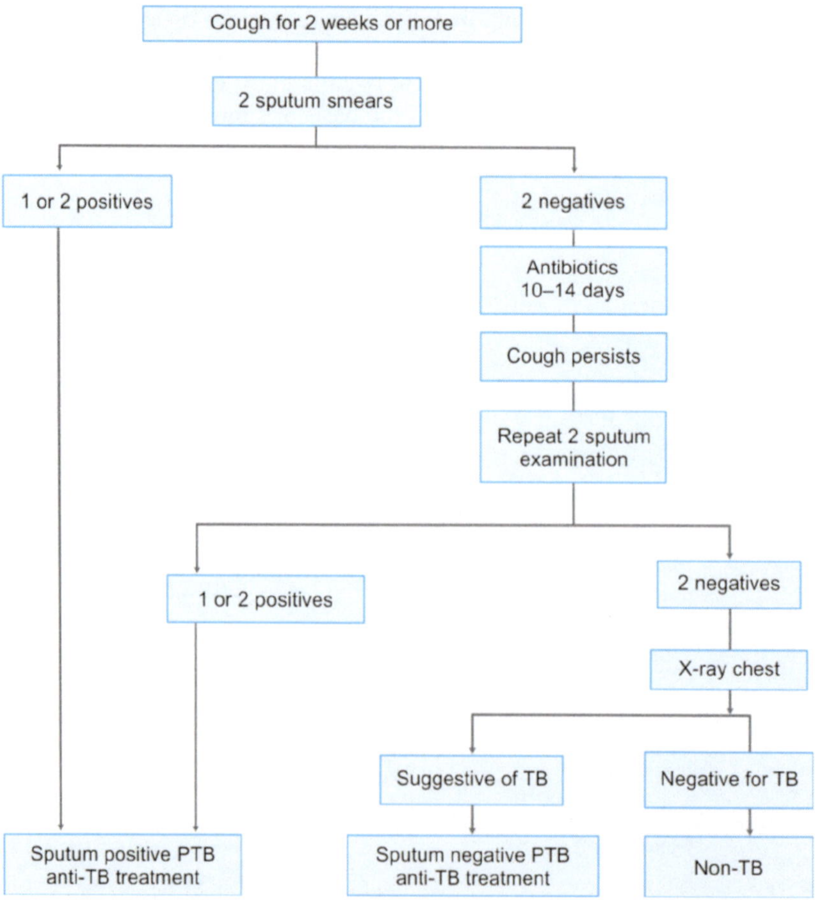

Fig. 34.2: Diagnostic algorithm for pulmonary tuberculosis revised in 2009

are likely to improve with antibiotics if they are not suffering from TB. If the symptoms persist after a course of broad spectrum antibiotics, repeat sputum smear examination (2 samples) must be done for such patients. If one or more smears are positive, the patient is diagnosed as having smear-positive pulmonary TB. If none of the repeat sputum specimens is positive, a chest X-ray is taken, and if findings of the X-ray are consistent with pulmonary tuberculosis, the patient is diagnosed by the physician as a case of sputum negative pulmonary TB.

The extrapulmonary tuberculosis (EPTB) is defined on the basis of international classification[18] including the tuberculosis of organs other then the lung, such as pleura, lymph node, abdomen, genitourinary tract, skin, joint, bones, tubercular meningitis, tuberculoma of the brain, etc.[19,20] Diagnosis of EPTB is based on one culture positive specimen from the extrapulmonary site or histological evidence or strong evidence consistent with active EPTB disease following which a medical officer can take a decision to treat a full course of anti-tuberculosis therapy. Sputum smear examination should be done in patients suspected of having EPTB.

TREATMENT REGIMEN USED IN REVISED NATIONAL TUBERCULOSIS CONTROL PROGRAM (RNTCP)

Since 1962, tuberculosis control in India is based on evidence based, scientifically and technically sound tuberculosis program. Self-administered domiciliary treatment daily for a long duration was not proved as effective treatment against tuberculosis. There was a large amount of concealed irregularity in drug intake and these finding highlighted the need for supervised treatment. Meanwhile, there was enough evidence that drugs given three times a week were as effective as that given daily. So a thrice weekly, directly observed short course chemotherapy was recommended in RNTCP.[21-23]

Categorization of patients for treatment is based on the severity of illness, bacillary load, the site of the disease and the duration of prior specific anti-tuberculosis chemotherapy received. Thus newly diagnosed patient with pulmonary tuberculosis are classified, depending on their sputum smear status and on the site and severity of the lesion.

Category I includes the newly diagnosed sputum smear-positive patients and seriously ill patients sputum smear-negative patients. Category I also include seriously ill new patients with extrapulmonary tuberculosis, e.g. tubercular meningitis, disseminated tuberculosis, tubercular peritonitis and intestinal tuberculosis, bilateral or extensive pleurisy, spinal tuberculosis with neurological complications, genitourinary tract tuberculosis. The treatment consists of two-month intensive phase of four drugs—rifampicin (R), isoniazid (H), ethambutol (E) and pyrazinamide (Z)- followed by a four-month continuation phase of rifampicin (R), isoniazid (H) ($2R_3H_3E_3Z_3/4R_3H_3$). Patient whose smears remains positive at the end of the intensive phase, are given another month of intensive phase treatment.

Category II includes patients who have been treated earlier and have developed smear-positive tuberculosis again, i.e. relapse, treatment after default and treatment failure. These patients need a longer duration of treatment and more drugs because their chances of harboring drugs resistant mutants are high. Hence, they receive an intensive phase of three months with five drugs for the first two months ($2S_3R_3H_3E_3Z_3/1R_3H_3E_3Z_3/5R_3H_3E_3$) and four drugs for the third month, with a continuation phase of three drugs for five months. Patients treated with category II regimen, whose smears are positive at the end of the intensive phase, are given another month of intensive phase treatment before being started on the continuation phase treatment.

Category III includes newly diagnosed smear-negative patient and less severe forms of extrapulmonary disease as lymph node and cutaneous tuberculosis, and minimal pleural effusion. These patients harbor fewer organisms, their chances of having drug resistant mutants are low, and hence they require fewer drugs. The treatment consists of a two-month intensive phase of three drugs ($2R_3H_3Z_3/4R_3H_3$), followed by a four-month continuation phase of two drugs.

Category IV includes chronic and multidrug resistant tuberculosis (MDR-TB) cases (still sputum positive after supervised re-treatment).These patients require more drugs especially second-line drugs as they display resistance to first-line drugs particularly to isoniazid and rifampicin. Therefore, they require daily supervised regimen for longer duration. The treatment consists of 6–9 months of intensive phase including Kanamycin (Km), Ofloxacin (Ofx), Ethionamide (Eto), Cycloserine (Cs), Pyrazinamide (Z), Ethambutol (E) followed by 18 months of continuation phase—Ofloxacin (Ofx), Ethionamide (Eto), Cycloserine (Cs), Ethambutol (E). Recently ofloxacin has been replaced with levofloxacin.

Recently, category I and category III has been merged together and all the new patients of tuberculosis will be treated with category I regimen, i.e. $2R_3H_3E_3Z_3/4R_3H_3$.

Case definitions, type of cases and treatment outcomes have been tabulated in Tables 34.1, 34.2, 34.3. Categorywise treatment in RNTCP is tabulated in Table 34.4.

During the intensive phase, each dose of medication is packed in blister packs containing one day's medication and is given under the direct observation of a DOT provider. During the continuation phase, medication is packed in weekly blister packs, with the first of the thrice-weekly doses being given under direct observation.

Table 34.1: Case definitions used in RNTCP

Case definitions
Pulmonary tuberculosis, smear-positive
TB in a patient with at least 2 initial sputum smear examinations (direct smear microscopy) positive for AFB **Or** TB in a patient with one sputum examination positive for AFB and radiographic abnormalities consistent with active pulmonary TB as determined by the treating MO **Or** TB in a patient with one sputum specimen positive for AFB and culture positive for *M. tuberculosis* However, recent RNTCP guidelines (2009) recommends that one specimen positive out of the two is enough to declare a patient as smear positive TB
Pulmonary tuberculosis, smear-negative
TB in a patient with symptoms suggestive of TB with at least 3 sputum examinations negative for AFB, and radiographic abnormalities consistent with active pulmonary TB as determined by a MO, followed by a decision to treat the patient with a full course of anti-tuberculosis therapy **Or** Diagnosis based on positive culture but negative AFB sputum examinations According to recent RNTCP guidelines (2009), TB in a patient with symptoms suggestive of TB with at least 2 sputum examinations negative for AFB, and radiographic abnormalities consistent with active pulmonary TB as determined by a MO, followed by a decision to treat the patient with a full course of anti-tuberculosis therapy **Or** Diagnosis based on positive culture but negative AFB sputum examinations for defining pulmonary tuberculosis smear-negative
Extrapulmonary tuberculosis
TB of organs other than the lungs, such as the pleura (TB pleurisy), lymph nodes, abdomen, genitourinary tract, skin, joints, tuberculoma of the brain, etc. Diagnosis should be based on one culture-positive specimen from an extrapulmonary site, or histological evidence, or strong clinical evidence consistent with active extrapulmonary TB followed by a MO's decision to treat with a full course of anti-TB therapy. Pleurisy is classified as extrapulmonary TB A patient diagnosed with both pulm and extrapulmonary TB should be classified as a case of pulmonary TB

Table 34.2: Type of cases in RNTCP

Types of cases
New case A TB patient who has never had treatment for tuberculosis or has taken anti-tuberculosis drugs for less than one month **Relapse** A TB patient who was declared cured or treatment completed by a physician, but who reports back to the health service and is found to be sputum smear positive **Transferred in** A TB patient who has been received into a Tuberculosis Unit/District, after starting treatment in another unit where he/she has been recorded Treatment after default A patient who received anti-tuberculosis treatment for one month or more from any source and who returns to treatment after having defaulted, i.e. not taken anti-TB drugs consecutively for two months or more **Failure case** Smear-positive patient who is smear-positive at 5 months or more after starting treatment. Failure also includes a patient who was treated with category III regimen but who becomes smear positive during treatment **Chronic case** A TB patient who remains smear-positive after completing a retreatment regimen **"Other" case** TB patients who do not fit into the above-mentioned categories. Reasons for putting a patient in this category must be specified

Table 34.3: Treatment outcomes in RNTCP

Treatment outcomes
Cured Initially smear-positive patient who has completed treatment and had negative sputum smears, on at least two occasions, one of which was at completion of treatment **Treatment completed** Sputum smear-positive case who has completed treatment, with negative smears at the end of the initial phase but none at the end of treatment **Or** Sputum smear-negative patient who has received a full course of treatment and has not become smear-positive during or at the end of treatment **Or** Extrapulmonary patient who has received a full course of treatment and has not become smear-positive during or at the end of treatment **Died** Patient, who died during treatment, regardless of cause **Defaulted** A patient who, at any time after registration, has not taken anti-TB drugs for 2 months or more consecutively **Transferred out** A patient who has been transferred to another Tuberculosis Unit/District and his/her treatment results are not known

Table 34.4: RNTCP—Category and treatment

TB diagnostic category	TB patients	TB treatment regimens*	
		Initial phase (3 times weekly)[b]	Continuation phase (3 times weekly)
I	• New smear positive patients; • New Smear negative PTB with extensive parenchymal involvement • Severe concomitant HIV disease • Severe forms of EPTB (Tuberculous meningitis, miliary, pericarditis, peritonitis,B/L or extensive pleural effusion, spinal disease with neurological complications, intestinal, genitourinary)	$2H_3R_3Z_3E_3$[c]	$4H_3R_3$
II	Previously treated sputum smear positive PTB: • Relapse • Treatment after interpretation • Treatment failure[d] • Others**	$2H_3R_3Z_3E_3S_3$/ $1H_3R_3Z_3E_3$	$5H_3R_3E_3$
III[a]	• New smear negative PTB (Other than in category I); • Less severe forms of EPTB (lymph node, U/L pleural effusion, bone excluding spine, peripheral joint, skin)	$2H_3R_3Z_3$[e]	$4\ H_3R_3$
IV	Chronic and MDR-TB cases (still sputum positive after supervised re-treatment)[f]	(6–9) Km Z E Eto Cs Levo	18 E Eto Cs Levo

[a]- Recently, category I and category III has been merged together and all the new patients of tuberculosis will be treated with category I regimen, i.e. $2R_3H_3E_3Z_3/4R_3H_3$.

[b] Direct observation of drug intake is required during the initial phase of treatment in smear-positive cases and always in treatment that includes rifampicin.

[c] Streptomycin may be used instead of ethambutol in meningeal TB. In tubercular meningitis (TBM), spinal TB with neurological complications and other hematogenous tuberculosis continuation phase is prolonged for 3 more months.

[d]Whenever possible, drug sensitivity testing is recommended before prescribing category II treatment in failure cases. It is recommended that patients with proven MDR-TB use category IV regimens.

[e]Ethambutol may be omitted during the initial phase of treatment for patients with non-cavitary, smear-negative PTB who are known to be HIV negative, patients known to be infected with fully drug-susceptible bacilli, and young children with primary TB.

[f]Contacts of patients with culture proven MDR-TB should be considered for early culture and sensitivity testing.

*The number before the letters refers to the number of months of treatment. The subscript after the letters refers to the number of doses per week. The dosage strengths are as follows: H: Isoniazid (600 mg), R: Rifampicin (450 mg), Z: Pyrazinamide (1500 mg), E: Ethambutol (1200 mg), S: Streptomycin (750 mg). Patients who weigh 60 kg or more receive additional Rifampicin 150 mg. Patients who are more than 50 years old receive Streptomycin 500 mg. Patients who weigh less than 30 kg receive drugs per body weight. Patients in categories I and II who have a positive sputum smear at the end of the initial intensive phase receive an additional month of intensive phase treatment.

**In rare and exceptional cases, patients who are sputum smear-negative or who have extrapulmonary disease can have relapse or failure. The diagnosis in all such cases should be made by the MO and should be supported by culture or histological evidence of current active TB. In these cases, the patient should be categorized as 'others' and given category II treatment.

ACHIEVEMENTS OF REVISED NATIONAL TUBERCULOSIS CONTROL PROGRAM

Since 1993, RNTCP has made a rapid strides to cover a population of 1 billion (90%) by March 2006. DOTS services are now available in 513 districts of 26 states/union territories. Over the 10 years analysis period, the population covered increased from 139 million to 1.16 billion population. As expected from service expansion, the absolute number of TB suspects examined by smear microscopy annually has increased manifold, from 0.96 million to 7.2 million. Over the same time period, the annual rate of TB suspect examination also increased by 50%, from 397 per 100,000 population covered by RNTCP services to 623 per 100,000 population covered. Similarly, the rate of sputum-positive cases diagnosed by microscopy has increased by 27%, from 62 to 80 per 100,000 population. According to RNTCP 2009 status report total patients initiated on treatment are 1,533,309. New smear positive patients initiated on treatment 825,397. Case detection rate of new smear positive is 71% and treatment success rate is 87% in new smear positive patient (2008). Treatment success rates have tripled from 25 to 87% and TB death rates have been cut seven-folds from 29% to less than 5% in comparison to the pre-RNTCP era. Death rate has been brought down seven-folds from 42/100,000 to 24/100,000. Since its inception, the program has initiated more than 11 million patients on treatment, thus saving more than 2 million additional lives. Among NSP cases, the treatment success rate has been > 85% since the year 2001. The death rate and failure rate has been about 5% and 2% respectively. During the period

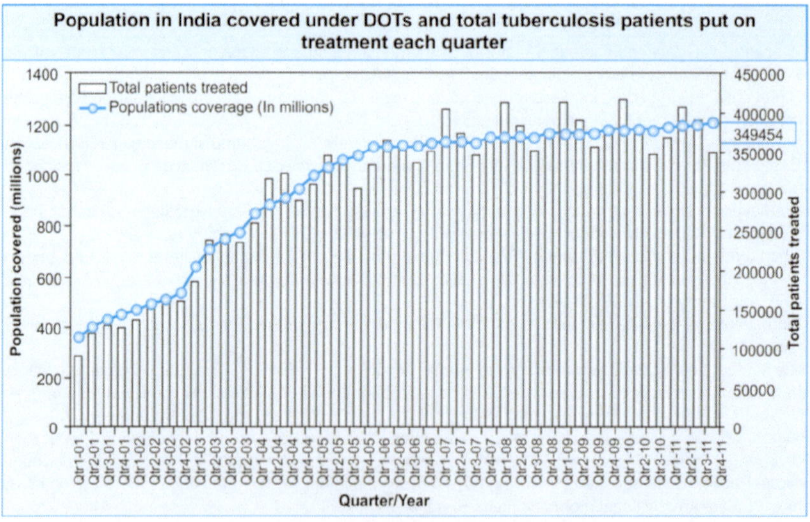

Fig. 34.3: Population in India covered under DOTs and total tuberculosis patients put on treatement each quarter

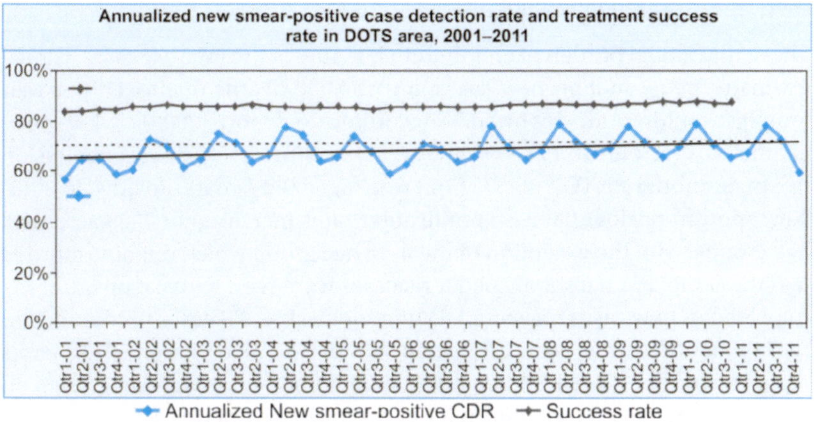

Fig. 34.4: Annualized new smear-positive case detection rate and treatment success rate in DOTs areas, 2000–2009

2006–2009, an average 1.4 additional NSP cases per 100,000 population were notified each year. The default rates has decreased from 9% for the cohort of TB patients registered in 1999 to 6% for the cohort of patients registered in 2008. The program has consistently maintained the treatment success rate > 85% and NSP case detection rate (CDR) close to the global target of 70%. In 2009, RNTCP has achieved the NSP-CDR of 72% and treatment success rate of 87% which is in line with the global targets for TB control (Figs 34.3 and 34.4).

OTHERS PRIORITY INITIATIVES IN REVISED NATIONAL TUBERCULOSIS CONTROL PROGRAM

Non-Government Organizations

The active role of Non-Government Organizations (NGOs) in health promotion in the community has been well-recognized. Community participation holds the key to the successful long-term implementation of the DOTS strategy in India. Government of India has released different schemes for the involvement of NGOs in the RNTCP. About 2,500 NGOs are associated with the program.[24]

Private Practitioners

India has the largest private health sector in the world, which is used by both rural and urban patients. Bulk of the tuberculosis patients are taking treatment from private practitioners, as they are often the first points of contact for people with tuberculosis. Their involvement in the program is essential for the future success of the RNTCP.[25-28] Various schemes have been formulated and approved by Government of India for this purpose and more than 19,000 private practitioners (PPs) and 150 corporate entities are involved in the RNTCP presently.

Pediatric Tuberculosis Guidelines

The actual global burden of childhood TB is 10% of the total TB cases. Global estimates of 1.5 million new cases and 130,000 deaths due to TB per year amongst children are reported.[29] According to report (2009), it has been estimated that out of 439,899 new smear positive PTB cases initiated on treatment under RNTCP, 86,532 (7%) were aged 0–14 years. Relative to 2001, New sputum positive TB case notification rates increased in 2009 across all age groups, with the exception of the 0–14 age group which remains more or less the same. From a survey pediatric cases were seen to make up 3% of the total load of new cases registered. Lymph node (LN) TB cases predominated (> 75%) amongst the pediatric Extrapulmonary Tuberculosis (EPTB) cases registered under RNTCP. About 40% of lymph node cases were diagnosed on clinical grounds with no confirmatory examinations performed. An almost comparable number of pediatric TB cases were being diagnosed in the same health facilities, but were not being registered under RNTCP. Of those pediatric cases treated under RNTCP, cure and completion rates were both above 90%. Comparative figures for those cases not treated under RNTCP were 80% and 70%, with default rates between 27–33%. Modified guidelines for diagnosis and treatment of pediatric TB were published in early 2004. Pediatric patientwise boxes have been completed and recommendation has been made. Staff already trained under RNTCP is being given updates on the revised diagnostic and treatment guideline and the recording and reporting format. This is a unique global achievement for RNTCP, as no other DOTS program in the world has such patients wise boxes (PWBs) for treatment of children with tuberculosis. Pediatric tuberculosis is part of RNTCP from 2006.

Medical Colleges

Medical colleges also play an important role in introducing the principles of DOTS as a part of the medical curriculum and as advocates of the program. The involvement of medical colleges in the RNTCP is considered important as large numbers of TB patients are treated at medical college hospitals. To define the structure and processes for effective involvement of medical colleges in the RNTCP workshops have been organized. National, zonal and state task forces have been established to monitor the involvement of medical colleges in the respective states. More than three hundred medical colleges are now implementing DOTS.[30]

IMA-GFATM-RNTCP-PPM Project

Government of India and Stop TB Partnership strongly feel that public private mix is reaquired to achieve the desired results of eliminating TB as a public health problem by 2050. IMA has accepted and adopted the DOTS strategy of RNTCP. The goal is to achieve to bring down the burden of TB in India till it ceases to be a public health problem. In this project, IMA has choosen to carry out intensified activities in five states and one union territory in India. With the idea, expected outcomes can be categorized at 3 levels—national, state and district. The individuals of IMA leadership will provide services on an honorary basis, so that the project can be best implemented in its truest sense. The RNTCP-PPM-IMA project supported by round-6 of the GFATM has completed two years. The project is being implemented in 167 districts in the six states of Andhra Pradesh, Chandigarh, Maharashtra, Haryana, Punjab and Uttar Pradesh. The project is being extended to another 10 states, under the Rolling Continuation Channel (RCC) Project of GFATM. Now this project has involved many more states.

TB/HIV Coordination Activities

The coordination between the RNTCP and the National AIDS Control Program has started in the eleven high HIV/AIDS prevalence state. Referral linkages between the Voluntary Counseling and Testing Centers (VCTCs) and RNTCP diagnostic sites are being established; and reporting of HIV-TB cases at the level of VCTCs is an ongoing activity.[31,32]

Training

Sound technical and training policies have been formulated and nearly 4,50,000 health workers have been trained in the RNTCP. RNTCP training modules were developed in 1997, and have been revised in 2005.

Quality Assurance of Sputum Microscopy

About 12,500 microscopy centers have been upgraded under the RNTCP. A protocol for quality assurance of the sputum smear microscopy network has been prepared by the RNTCP to maintain the quality of diagnostic services provided by the RNTCP. It has been pilot tested in five states in 2004, and is now being implemented in the country.

DOTS Plus

The RNTCP views the treatment of multidrug resistance tuberculosis (MDR-TB) patients a "Standard of Care" issue recognizing that the treatment of MDR-TB cases is very complex, treatment will follow the internationally recommended DOTS-Plus guidelines[33] and will be done in designated RNTCP DOTS-Plus sites. The DOTS-Plus sites will be initiated in a phased manner similar to that for the established of the culture and drug sensitivity testing (DST) laboratory network, and sites will be linked geographically to the establishment of the RNTCP accredited intermediate reference laboratories (IRLs). The framework is organized around the same five components of the DOTS strategy, as the underlying principals are the same. The core components are comprehensive, ensuring that all essential elements of the DOTS-Plus strategy are included, and are:

1. Sustained government commitment.
2. Acute, timely diagnosis through quality assured culture and drug susceptibility testing.
3. Appropriate treatment utilizing second-line drugs under strict supervision.
4. Uninterrupted supply of quality assured anti-TB drugs.
5. Standardized recording and reporting system.

(For further details about DOTS-Plus, refer to chapter 35)

IMPACT OF REVISED NATIONAL TUBERCULOSIS CONTROL PROGRAM

Since starting in 1993, RNTCP has passed almost 20 years and whole of the country is covered by 2006 and made a definite impact on the status of tuberculosis in the country. Cure rate has been consistently high and has exceeded global target of 85% (more than tripled in respect to National Tuberculosis Program), increasing trend in case detection in DOTS area is 66%, death rate is reduced 7 fold (29 to 4%) in new smear positive cases, deaths reduced from 1 per min to 2 per 3 min and from 500,000 to < 300,000/ years. As a rate, the NSP case notification rates in the population covered under RNTCP has been consistently increasing, with the exception of the year 2005. Case notification has been increasing since whole-country RNTCP coverage in 2006, though at a slower rate than during the DOTS expansion period. From 1999–2005, an average 3.2 additional NSP cases notified per 100,000 population each year. During the period 2006–2009, an average 1.4 additional NSP cases per 100,000 population were notified each year. From its starting till 2009, the program had initiated more than 11.6 million patients on DOTS, thus saving over 18,00,000 additional lives. Impact on incidence not yet documented, recent base line ARTI survey conducted and repeat survey at 4–5 years interval planned to document impact on incidence. The program is currently undertaking repeat Zonal ARTI survey and disease prevalence surveys to assess the impact of the program on TB control and additionally monitor the progress towards Millennium Development Goals.

CHALLENGES FOR REVISED NATIONAL TUBERCULOSIS CONTROL PROGRAM

Though the program has made admirable achievements, there are many challenges facing it at this point of time like maintain and sustain quality of services, further improvement in the quality of diagnostic and treatment services, uninterrupted supply of drugs, effective supervision, providing benchmark for universal standard of TB care, capacity building of laboratory network, providing DOTS services to slums, tribal, migrating population, etc. management of extrapulmonary tuberculosis, management of pediatrics tuberculosis, emergence and spread of HIV and drug resistant tuberculosis, maintaining the partnership with all care providing sectors, improve the management information system, strengthening coordination between the RNTCP and Medical Colleges activities, involvement of private practitioner and Non-Government Organizations as per their capacity and available infrastructure and at last the implementation of DOTS plus.

PROBLEMS OF REVISED NATIONAL TUBERCULOSIS CONTROL PROGRAM

RNTCP has passed more than 20 years since starting, in 1993. Though made creditable achievements, program is still facing some problems which are to be discussed and solved as early as possible to maintain the services and to achieve the targets. There is less involvement of private practitioner/ non-government organizations, practical difficulty in reaching DOTS center especially school children, old/sick/disabled persons, pregnant ladies, migrating population and providing drugs during festivals and functions, accidents, deaths in family and during flood, riots, curfew. Long-term follow-ups of patients is required to get the outcome of program.

REFERENCES

1. National AIDS Control (NACO)—estimation of HIV infection in India: http// www.nacoonline.org/facts_hivestimates.htm.
2. AIDS profile: India http://www.census.gov/ipc/www/hivctry.html.
3. Styblo K. Eradication of tuberculosis in developed countries in the HIV era. Bulletin of the International Union against Tuberculosis and Lung Disease. 1989;64:58-64.
4. Tuberculosis Association of India, New Delhi. Proceedings of the Tuberculosis Association of India, New Delhi, November 1939:171.
5. Proceeding of the VI All India BCG Conference, Bangalore, 1963: 20-30.
6. Indian Council of Medical Research: Tuberculosis in India: A national sample survey 1955-58. ICMR technical report series New Delhi, ICMR. 1959.
7. Tuberculosis Chemotherapy Centre, Madras: A concurrence comparison on home and sanatorium treatment of pulmonary tuberculosis in South India: Bull Wld Hlth Org. 1959; 21:51.
8. Benerji D, Anderson S. A sociological study of awareness of symptoms among persons with pulmonary tuberculosis. Bull World Health Organ. 1963;29:665-83.
9. National tuberculosis institute, organization and functions; website: http://ntiindia.kar.nic.in.
10. Tuberculosis Programme review-India, 1992; World Health Organization, Geneva. 1992. National Tuberculosis Institute, Summaries of NTI Studies, 1997:101.
11. Khatri GR, Frieden TR. The status and prospects of tuberculosis control in India, Int J Tuberc Lung Dis. 2000;4:193.
12. Central TB Division, Directorate General of Health Services, Ministry of Health and Family welfare, RNTCP performance report, India, first quarter. 2004.
13. Framework for Effective Tuberculosis Control. Geneva, WHO, 1994. WHO/TB/94. 179.
14. Gothi GD, Chakraborty AK, Banerjee GC. Interpretation of photofluorograms of active pulmonary TB patients found in epidemiological survey and their five year fate. Indian Journal of Tuberculosis. 1974;21:90-7.
15. Nyboe J. Results of the international study on X-ray classification. Bulletin of the International Union against Tuberculosis. 1968;41:115-24.

16. Raъ KP, et al. Assessment of diagnosis of pulmonary tuberculosis by sputum microscopy in a district tuberculosis programme. Inna Journal of Tuberculosis. 1971;18:10-21.
17. Nagpaul, DR, et al. Case-finding by microscopy. Bulletin of the International Union Against Tuberculosis. 1968;61:148-58.
18. World Health Organization (WHO), Treatment of Tuberculosis, Guidelines for National Programmes, 3rd ed. WHO/CDS/TB 2003.313 Geneva, Switzerland: WHO, 2003.
19. CTD. Revised National TB Control Programme. Technical guidelines for TB Control. New Delhi: CTD, 1997.
20. CTD, Managing the Revised National TB Control Programme in your area. A training course. Modules 1-4. New Delhi:CTD, 1998.
21. Canetti G, Grumbach F, Grosset J. Long-term, two-stage chemotherapy of advanced experiment murine tuberculosis with intermittent regimens during second stage. Tubercle. 1963; 44:236-40.
22. East Africa/British Medical Research Council. Controlled clinical treatment of short course (6 months) regime of chemotherapy for treatment of pulmonary tuberculosis. Third report. lancet. 1974;2:237-48.
23. Fox W, Ellard GA, Michison DA. Study on treatment of tuberculosis undertaken by British Medical Research Council tuberculosis unit,1946–1986, with relevant subsequent publications. Int J Tuberc Lung Dis. 1999;3:S231-S79.
24. Central TB Division, Directorate General of Health Services, Ministry of Health and Family Welfare, New Delhi; TB India 2003;16-46.
25. Uplekar M. Involving private health care providers in delivery of TB care: global strategy. Tuberculosis (Edinb). 2003;83:156-64.
26. Prasad R, Nautiyal RG, Mukherji PK, Jain A, Singh K, Ahuja RC. Treatment of new pulmonary tuberculosis patients: what do allopathic doctors do in India? Int J Tuberc Lung Dis. 2002;6: 895-902.
27. Uplekar M, Juvekar S, Morankar S, Rangan S, Nunn P. Tuberculosis patients and practitioners in private clinics in India. Int J Tuberc Lung Dis. 1998;2:324-9.
28. The Behavior and Interaction of TB Patients and Private for—Profit Health Care Provider in India: A review. Geneva, Switzerland: WHO; 1997.WHO/TB/97.223.
29. World Health Organization (WHO).WHO report on Tuberculosis epidemic:WHO;1996.
30. National Tuberculosis Institute, Bangalore. Report on national workshop on involvement of Medical Colleges in RNTCP. 14-15 September 2001.
31. Hargreaves N, Scano F. Guidelines for Implementing Collaborative TB and HIV Programme activities, World Health Organization, Geneva, 2003;7,9,11,13-5.
32. National AIDS Control Organization, Government of India. Programme implementation guidelines for a phased scale up of access to antiretroviral therapy for people living with HIV/AIDS, draft version, accessed via http://www.nacoonline. Org/guidelines/guideline_1. pdf, 2004.
33. Central TB Division, Directorate General of Health Services, Ministry of Health and Family Welfare, RNTCP DOTS-Plus Guidelines. 2006;14-6.

Chapter 35

Tuberculosis Control in India: DOTS-Plus

INTRODUCTION

The first WHO endorsed DOTS-Plus programs began in 2000. For this purpose, the Green Light Committee (GLC) was established to promote access to high quality second-line drugs for appropriate use in TB control Programs. DOTS-Plus is an integral component of RNTCP to manage MDR-TB which is to be implemented through program infrastructure of the DOTS program. The strategy is designed to manage MDR-TB and XDR-TB using second-line anti-TB drugs within the DOTS strategy in low- and middle-income countries like India. Therefore in every DOTS implementing unit of the country, DOTS would be prioritized above DOTS-Plus with the view that DOTS reduces the emergence of MDR-TB, and therefore the need for DOTS Plus over time. The present chapter aims to describe framework of DOTS-Plus program now known as programmatic management of drug resistant tuberculosis (PMDT) as integral component of Revised National Tuberculosis Control Program to manage MDR-TB and XDR-TB.

FRAMEWORK

The DOTS-Plus framework for the management of multidrug-resistant TB is organized around the same five components of the DOTS strategy, as the underlying principles are the same.

1. Sustained political and administrative commitment: It consists of a well functioning DOTS program, long-term investment of staff and resources, coordination efforts between community, local governments and international agencies and addressing the factors leading to the emergence of MDR-TB.

2. Diagnosis of MDR-TB through quality-assured culture and drug susceptibility testing: It should include proper triage of patients for culture and DST testing and management under DOTS-Plus and co-ordination with National and Supra-National Reference Laboratories.
3. Appropriate treatment strategies that utilize second-line drugs under proper management conditions: Emphasis given on rational standardized treatment design (evidence-based), treatment is directly observed therapy (DOT) ensuring long-term adherence, monitoring and management of adverse drug reactions and adequate human resources.
4. Uninterrupted supply of quality assured anti-TB drugs.
5. Recording and reporting system designed for DOTS-Plus programs that enable performance monitoring and evaluation of treatment outcome.

Each of these components involves more complex and costly operations than those for controlling drug sensitive TB. Accurate and timely diagnosis is the backbone of the DOTS-Plus activities. MDR-TB must be diagnosed correctly before commencement of treatment. Quality assured culture and DST is thus indispensable. Non-viable cultures, culture contamination, and unreliable DST results have major consequences for both individual patients and the TB control program as a whole. Therefore, internal quality control and external quality assurance will be in place, including a link for proficiency testing with a recognized reference laboratory such as one of the RNTCP National Reference Laboratories. The program is in the process of establishing a network of state level quality assured culture and DST laboratories. The RNTCP aims to have one such laboratory, known as the Intermediate Reference Laboratory (IRL), for culture and DST in each large state by 2009–10.[1]

CASE FINDING STRATEGY

The prevalence of multi-drug resistant TB (MDR-TB), defined as resistance to isoniazid and rifampicin with or without resistance to other drugs, is found to be at a low level in most of the regions. Data from studies conducted by TRC (TB research center) Chennai and NTI (National TB Institute) Bengaluru, have found MDR-TB levels of less than 1 to 3% in new cases and around 12% in re-treatment cases.[2,3] According to the WHO/IUATLD 4th global survey, the estimated prevalence of primary and acquired MDR-TB in India was 2.8% (95% CI, 2.3-3.4%) and 17.2% (95% CI, 15.0–19.7%) respectively.[4] According to the global tuberculosis report 2012, the prevalence of MDR-TB in India among notified pulmonary tuberculosis patients is 5.3% (3.6–6.2%). Among new tuberculosis cases, the prevalence of MDR-TB is 2.1% (1.5–2.7%) and is 15% (13–17%) among retreatment cases. The RNTCP DOTS-Plus strategy strives to identify and initiate adequate treatment for MDR-TB in a timely manner for confirmed cases of MDR-TB. Timely identification and prompt initiation of treatment prevent the patient from spreading the disease to others, developing a resistant strain to more drugs, and progressing to chronic state of permanent lung damage. RNTCP has undertaken state representative DRS surveys in order to obtain data for new and re-treatment patients, to further inform program planning and drug procurement. At present, RNTCP does not have sufficient quality assured laboratory capacity to do culture and DST in all patients. Hence, the program will use a strategy that enrols patients with a very high risk of MDR-TB into RNTCP DOTS-Plus activities and treatment with the RNTCP category IV regimen.

Patients who are defined as an "MDR-TB suspect" should be identified and investigated further for MDR-TB. RNTCP uses a strategy that screens patients with initially a very high risk of MDR-TB using DST. As laboratory and treatment capacity builds, the program will scale up to achieve universal access to quality assured DST. During scale-up, the criteria for referral of a specimen for DST will by necessity differ among the districts. The graded criteria for suspecting MDR-TB are as follows:

MDR Suspect Criteria

Criteria A

- All failures of new TB cases
- Smear positive previously treated cases who remain smear positive at 4th month onwards
- All pulmonary TB cases who are contacts of known MDR-TB case.

Criteria B—*in addition to Criteria A*

- All smear positive previously treated pulmonary TB cases at diagnosis
- All smear positive follow up result in new or previously treated cases.

Criteria C—*in addition to Criteria B*

- All smear negative previously treated pulmonary TB cases at diagnosis
- HIV TB co-infected cases at diagnosis.

ENROLMENT INTO DOTS-PLUS PROGRAM

Once the MO-PHI confirms that the patient is an MDR-TB suspect, he/she should arrange for sending two sputa samples, one of which is an early morning sample and the other a "supervised" spot sample, from the patient to the RNTCP certified C-DST laboratory along with the RNTCP Culture and DST request form. All attempts must be made to communicate the DST results to the district as soon as available, so that patient treatment decisions can be smoothly managed.

If results may be delayed more than 7 days of sample collection, the patient should be initiated on RNTCP DOTS treatment till the results are available. Such patients are classified according to the following definition:

CONFIRMED MDR-TB CASE

An MDR-TB suspect who is sputum culture positive and whose TB is due to *Mycobacterium tuberculosis* that are resistant in-vitro to at least isoniazid and rifampicin (the culture and DST result being from an RNTCP accredited laboratory).[1] Internal quality control and external quality assurance of the laboratory are required. Mishandling of a specimen or cross-contamination in the laboratory can result in erroneous reports. It is to be noted that rifampicin resistance is quite rare without isoniazid resistance. The great majority of DST results with rifampicin resistance will also be isoniazid resistance, i.e. MDR TB. Therefore RNTCP has taken the programmatic decision that patients who have any rifampicin resistance, should also be managed as if they are an MDR-TB case, even if they do not formally qualify as an MDR-TB case. Therefore, program and clinical actions will be driven primarily by rifampicin DST results. Once a patient has been confirmed as having MDR-TB, his category II treatment will be stopped and she/he will be placed on an RNTCP category IV treatment regimen after pre-treatment evaluation. These patients will have to be given a treatment outcome under category II. The treatment outcome will depend on the duration of category II treatment completed at the time of confirmation as MDR-TB cases. The outcome will be "Failure" if the patient has completed more than 5 months of category II treatment or "Switched to category IV" if the patient has completed less than 5 months of category II treatment.[5] However, some patients may have other outcomes, e.g. died on category II treatment or defaulted from category II treatment prior to culture and DST result being available. After the referral or transportation of sputa samples of an MDR-TB suspect to the RNTCP certified laboratory, the results of the smear, Culture and DST/LPA are entered in the Culture and DST Register held at the laboratory. The culture results are communicated to the DTO immediately by e-mail. In case the culture result is positive, this would be followed by the DST result when available. If the patient is confirmed as a case of MDR-TB, the culture and DST or LPA results are also communicated to the respective DRTB Center. If the culture result shows contamination, the same is informed to the DTO within 24 hours and she/he should arrange to send a repeat sample (one early morning and one spot) to the laboratory within 3 days. If rifampicin resistance—with or without INH resistance—is confirmed, the DTO will trace the patient, with help of the Medical Officer—TB control (MO-TC) and Senior Treatment Supervisor (STS) and bring them to the DTC where they will be counseled by the DTO. After counseling, the patient is referred to the concerned DR-TB Center with their DST result and PMDT referral treatment form, for pre-treatment evaluation and initiation of regimen for MDR-TB.

DRUG RESISTANT TUBERCULOSIS CENTER

Treatment is decentralized, but the complicated clinical care needs require a clinical expert resource center. This is the drug resistant TB center (DR-TB Center). These DR-TB centers is utilized to initiate treatment, follow-up case management, and manage complications. One DR-TB center is expected per 10 million populations roughly, and these sites are being scaled up nationwide in a phased manner. Once confirmed, the MDR-TB patient is referred to the DR-TB center, with their DST result and request for MDR-TB treatment form. The DR-TB center committee will review the patients details, including previous history, DST result and concurrent illnesses, and make a decision in relation to treatment under RNTCP with a category IV regimen. If the committee decides on treatment with an RNTCP category IV regimen, the patient is initially admitted at the designated DR-TB center, counseled in regards to their treatment, their treatment card is opened and treatment initiated. If the patient is able to tolerate the category IV drugs he/she can be discharged one week post-treatment initiation. In case a patient refuses for hospitalization all, efforts should be made to convince him/her. However, if despite all efforts the patient is still unwilling for hospitalization, treatment should not be denied and alternative local arrangements should be made for pre-treatment evaluation and initiation of treatment. The patient and/or the results of the pre-treatment evaluation done at the district level are sent to the DR-TB center Committee. The committee after reviewing the results will decide on starting category IV treatment. The decision is communicated to the DTO (District TB officer) who initiates the treatment with the first dose administered at the DTC (District TB center). DTO will open the treatment card and send a copy of the same to the DR-TB center for registration. On registration the DR-TB center will convey the DOTS Plus TB number to the DTO. Once the DR-TB center decides upon RNTCP category IV treatment for the patient, the patient is counseled, an RNTCP DOTS-Plus treatment card opened, a DOTS-Plus patient identity card issued to the patient, and category IV treatment initiated. Patients admitted at the DR-TB center, if clinically appropriate, may be discharged 7 days after treatment initiation to their district of residence with a maximum of 7 day supply of drugs and arrangement for injections in transit. This period of admission will allow for all necessary investigations to be undertaken, initiation of the category IV regimen, monitoring of patient tolerance of the category IV regimen, motivation, counseling and providing health education to the patient and their families, developing linkages with the services in the respective district where the patient resides (including identification and training of a local DOT provider and family treatment supporter) and contact assessment.

The patient should be discharged to the district that they reside in, with upto a maximum of one week's supply of drugs, arrangements for injections in transit, and a copy of the treatment card and referral form. The respective DTO should be informed by the attending physician of the patient's planned discharge 3 days prior to the actual date of discharge. The DTO will inform the respective MO-PHI and the identified DOT provider about the expected discharge of the patient. The 3 monthly drug box and the patient records will be passed on to the identified DOT Provider from the respective TU. Local arrangements will need to be made for daily injections during the intensive phase. After discharge, the patient goes to DOTS-Plus site (DR-TB center) facility for management of severe adverse reactions, change of regimen or dosage and at the end of treatment. It is not essential to send the patient to DOTS Plus site for change from IP (intensive phase) to CP (continuation phase). The respective DTO can switch the patient to CP after obtaining the approval of the DOTS-Plus site committee by e-mail.

PRE-TREATMENT EVALUATION

The patient should be hospitalized at the DR-TB Center for pre-treatment evaluation and treatment initiation. Pre-treatment evaluation should include a thorough clinical evaluation by a physician, chest radiograph, pregnancy test and relevant hematological (Complete blood count with platelets) and bio-chemical tests (blood glucose, liver functions, renal functions, TSH, urine) Since the drugs used for the treatment of MDR-TB are known to produce adverse effects, a proper pre-treatment evaluation is essential to identify patients who are at increased risk of developing such adverse effects.

COUNSELING

Patients should receive counseling on the nature and duration of treatment, need for regular treatment and possible side effects of these drugs and the consequences of irregular treatment or pre-mature cessation of treatment. It is advisable to involve close family members during the counseling, since family support is an essential component in the management. Patients should be advised to report if he/she experiences any unusual problem. Female patients should receive special counseling on family planning.

While the MDR-TB case is undergoing pre-treatment evaluation, the DTO should ensure an initial home visit to verify the address and meet the family members. A DOT provider (who can either be a health care worker, a community worker or a community volunteer), should be identified in consultation with the patient. The DOT center can be either at the sub-center of the health system or in the community. The DOT provider should be given training for drug administration and to identify possible adverse effects during treatment, and the frequency of follow up.

MONITORING PROGRESS DURING TREATMENT

Clinical Monitoring

Patients should be seen by the respective DTO for clinical evaluation at monthly intervals during the IP, after discharge from the state DOTS-Plus site (DR-TB center), and at 3-monthly intervals during the CP until the end of treatment. The DTO should screen patients for clinical improvement and possible adverse reactions. Body weight should be monitored by the DTO at every visit. The patient may need to be hospitalized during treatment for medical or sociological reasons.

Investigations During Treatment

Chest radiograph will be done during the pre-treatment evaluation, at the end of the IP, end of treatment and when clinically indicated.

Serum Creatinine is to be done every month for the first 3 months and every three months thereafter till the patient is receiving injection kanamycin.

Liver function tests and thyroid stimulating hormone (TSH) will be done as and when indicated clinically. These investigations can be done at the DOTS-Plus site or district hospitals/medical colleges as per the arrangement, however patients should not be charged for these investigations.

Smear and Culture Schedule During Treatment

Sputum specimens are to be collected and examined by smear and culture at least 30 days apart from the 3rd to 7th month of treatment (i.e. at the end of the months 3, 4, 5, 6 and 7) and at 3-monthly intervals from the 9th month onwards till the completion of treatment (i.e. at the end of the months 9, 12, 15, 18, 21 and 24). Category IV patients who after 9 months of treatment do not seem to be responding and the last available culture results (7th month culture) are positive are considered treatment failure and DST for second line drugs would be done at a National Reference Laboratory (NRL). As on 2012 three NRLs (NTI-Bengaluru, NIRT-Chennai and LRS-New Delhi) are performing the second line DST in solid and liquid culture. Two early morning sputum samples will be collected from such patients and sent for culture and DST for kanamycin, capreomycin and fluoroquinolones to these accredited laboratories. RNTCP has identified eight laboratories that includes few IRLs (Andhra Pradesh, Delhi, Gujarat, Kerala, Maharashtra-Nagpur, Rajasthan) and Medical College (SMS Jaipur and JJ Hospital, Mumbai) laboratories to initiate proficiency testing for second line DST.

Methods for Drug Susceptibility Testing

Presently, 3 technologies are available for diagnosis of MDR-TB viz. the conventional solid egg-based Lowenstein-Jensen (LJ) media, the liquid culture (MGIT), and the rapid molecular assays such as Line Probe Assay (LPA) and similar Nucleic Acid Amplification Tests like Xpert MTB/RIF. Conventional DST evaluates if *M. tuberculosis* grows in the presence of drug-containing media, and is also known as *phenotypic DST*. Molecular DST evaluates for the presence of genetic mutations that are highly associated with phenotypic resistance, and is also known as *genotypic DST*.

Phenotypic DST is available for more drugs, and is considered very reliable for isoniazid (H), rifampicin (R), and streptomycin (S), and somewhat less reliable for other drugs such as ethambutol (E). Molecular/genotypic DST is highly reliable for rifampicin, but has limited sensitivity for detection of isoniazid resistance.

Molecular/genotypic tests are much faster than phenotypic tests, as molecular tests do not require growth of the organism, and *M. tuberculosis* is notoriously slow growing. The turnaround time for C-DST results by Solid LJ media is around 84 days, by Liquid Culture (MGIT) is around 42 days, by LPA is around 72 hours and by CB-NAAT is around 2 hours.

Organization and Development of the Laboratory Network

RNTCP has a three tier laboratory network based on the designated microscopy centers (DMCs) covering one lakh populations and providing sputum smear microscopy services, and IRLs (undertaking training, external quality assessment (EQA) of sputum smear microscopy network in the districts and DMCs, and culture and DST for first line drugs for *M. tuberculosis*), and NRLs (undertaking training, EQA of sputum smear microscopy network in the states allotted to them, and culture and DST for first and second line drugs for *M. tuberculosis*).

CATEGORY IV REGIMEN

The RNTCP will be using a standardized treatment regimen (STR), comprising of 6 drugs (kanamycin, levofloxacin, ethionamide, cycloserine, pyrazinamide and ethambutol) during 6–9 months of the intensive phase and 4 drugs (levofloxacin, ethionamide, cycloserine and ethambutol) during the 18 months of the continuation phase. *p*-aminosalicylic acid (PAS) is included in the regimen as a substitute drug if any bactericidal drug (kanamycin, levofloxacin, pyrazinamide and ethionamide) or any 2 bacteriostatic (ethambutol and cycloserine) drugs are not tolerated. In case of intolerence/ resistance to kanamycin, capreomycin is used. In case of ofloxacin resistance moxifloxacin with combination of PAS is used.

DRUG DOSAGES AND ADMINISTRATION

Drug dosages for MDR-TB cases are decided according to the weight band as shown in Table 35.1

Table 35.1: Drug dosages for MDR-TB according to weight band

Sl.No.	Drugs	16–25 kg	26–45 kg	46–70 kg
1.	Kanamycin	500 mg	500 mg	750 mg
2.	Levofloxacin	250 mg	750 mg	1000 mg
3.	Ethionamide	375 mg	500 mg	750 mg
4.	Ethambutol	400 mg	800 mg	1200 mg
5.	Pyrazinamide	500 mg	1250 mg	1500 mg
6.	Cycloserine	250 mg	500 mg	750 mg
7.	Pyridoxine	50 mg	100 mg	100 mg
	Reserve/Substitute drugs			
	Na PAS (80% weight/vol)*	5 g	10 g	12 g
	Moxifloxacin (Mfx)	200 g	400 g	400 g
	Capreomycin (Cm)	500 g	750 g	1000 mg

*In case of PAS with 60% weight/volume the dose will be increased to 7 g (16–25 kg); 14 g (26–45 kg) and 16 gm (> 45 kg)

All drugs should be given in a single daily dosage under directly observed treatment (DOT) by a DOT Provider. All patients will receive drugs under direct observation on 6 days of the week. On the 7th day (Sunday) the oral drugs will be administered unsupervised whereas injection kanamycin will be omitted. If intolerance occurs to the drugs, ethionamide, cycloserine and PAS may be split into two dosages and the morning dose administered under DOT. The evening dose will be self-administered. The empty blister packs of the self-administered doses will be checked the next morning during DOT. Pyridoxine at a dose of 100 mg should be administered to all patients on an RNTCP category IV regimen. If a patient gains 5 kg or more weight during treatment and crosses the weight-bands range, the DOTS-Plus site committee may consider moving the patient to the higher weight-band drug dosages. Similarly if a patient loses 5 kg or more in weight during treatment and crosses the weight band the DR-TB center committee may consider moving the patient to the lower weight band. The new dosages are provided whenever the patient is due for the next supply of drugs in the normal course of treatment and not as soon as change of weight is noted. In deciding about the dosages, apart from the considerations mentioned above, it is also necessary to rule out the existence of medical illnesses or organ dysfunctions in the individual by conducting routine hematological investigations like full blood count, random blood sugar, liver and kidney function tests, etc. and of urine microscopy. Other investigations like skiagram, ultrasound, etc. may be appropriately carried out as required in a particular case.

TREATMENT DURATION

The treatment is given in two phases, the intensive phase (IP) and the continuation phase (CP). The total duration of treatment for regimen for MDR

TB is 24–27 months, depending on the IP duration. IP should be given for at least six months. After 6 months of treatment, the patient will be reviewed and the treatment changed to CP if the 4th or 5th month culture result in solid or liquid culture is negative respectively. If the 4th or 5th month culture result remains positive, the treatment is extended by 1 month. Extension of IP beyond 1 month will be decided on the results of sputum culture of 5th or 6th and 6th or 7th months. If the result of the 4th month culture is still awaited after 6 months of treatment, the IP is extended until the result is available, with further treatment being decided according to the culture result. The IP can be extended up to a maximum of 3 months after which the patient will be initiated on the CP irrespective of the culture result. The recommended duration for CP is 18 months.

REGIMEN FOR XDR-TB

All XDR-TB patients should also be subject to a repeat full pre-treatment evaluation, but also including consultation by a thoracic surgeon for consideration of surgery. Identification must be done for the site (tertiary centers) with such surgical facilities. MDR-TB patients diagnosed as XDR-TB would be given an outcome of "Switched to Regimen for XDR-TB". The decision and initiation of regimen for XDR-TB is to be taken by the concerned DR-TB center committee. The intensive phase (6–12 months) will consist of 7 drugs—capreomycin (Cm), PAS, moxifloxacin (Mfx), high dose-INH, clofazimine, linezolid, and amoxyclav. The continuation phase (18 months) will consist of 6 drugs—PAS, moxifloxacin (Mfx), high dose-INH, clofazimine, linezolid, and amoxyclav.

The dosage of the drugs would vary as per the weight of the patient (≤ 45 kg or > 45 kg) (Table 35.2). All drugs are to be given on a daily basis. Injections of capreomycin will be given for 6 days/week (not on Sundays). All morning doses are to be supervised by the DOT provider except on Sundays. After taking DOT for morning doses on Saturday, next day medicines would be given to the patient to be taken at home on Sunday. Empty blisters of medicines taken unsupervised in evening and on Sundays are to be collected by DOT provider.

DURATION OF REGIMEN FOR XDR-TB

The regimen for XDR TB would be of 24–30 months duration, with 6–12 months intensive phase (IP) and 18 months continuation phase (CP). The change from IP to CP will be done only after achievement of culture conversion, i.e. 2 consecutive negative cultures taken at least one month apart. In case of delay in culture conversion, the IP can be extended from

Table 35.2: Drug dosages for XDR-TB according to weight band

Drugs	Dosage/day	
	≤ 45 kg	> 45 kg
Injection Capreomycin (Cm)	750 g	1000 g
PAS	10 g	12 g
Moxifloxacin (Mfx)	400 g	400 g
High dose INH (High dose-H)	600 g	900 g
Clofazimine (CFz)	200 mg	200 mg
Linezolid (Lzd)	600 mg	600 mg
Amoxyclav (Amx/Clv)	875/125 mg BD	875/125 mg BD
Pyridoxine	100 mg	100 mg
Reserve/Substitute drugs*		
Clarithromycin (Clr)	500 mg BD	500 mg BD
Thiacetazone (Thz)[#]	150 mg	150 mg

*Reserve/Substitute drugs would be used in case the patient was already on PAS, unable to tolerated one are more of the drugs and is resistant to capreomycin

6 months up to a maximum of 12 months. In case of extension, the DR-TR center committee, which will be responsible for initiating and monitoring the Regimen for XDR-TB, can decide on administering capreomycin injection intermittently (3 times/week) for the months 7 to 12.

TREATMENT INTERRUPTION AND DEFAULT

All efforts should be made to ensure that category IV patients do not interrupt treatment or default. Action should be taken to promptly retrieve patient who fail to come for DOT.

The following situations may be seen in case of treatment interruption.

Category IV Patients in IP/CP Who Miss Doses

All the missed doses during IP must be completed prior to switching the patient to CP. Similarly all missed doses during CP must be completely administered prior to ending treatment.

Category IV Patients Who Interrupt Treatment for less than 2 months During IP

When the patient returns to resume treatment the IP will be continued, however the duration of treatment will be extended to complete IP. The follow up cultures will be done as per the revised schedule.

Category IV Patients Who Interrupt Treatment for less than 2 months During CP

When the patient returns to resume treatment, the CP will be continued, however the duration of treatment will be extended to complete the CP. The period of interruption shall not be included in the duration of treatment. The follow up cultures will be done as per the revised schedule.

Category IV Patients Who Default and Return Back for Treatment

These patients will be given an outcome of default in the existing cohort and thereafter reregistered for treatment.

TREATMENT OUTCOMES

Standardized treatment outcome definitions are to be used following treatment of an MDR-TB case and are as follows:

Cure

An MDR-TB patient who has completed treatment and has been consistently culture negative (with at least 5 consecutive negative results in the last 12 to 15 months). If one follow-up positive culture is reported during the last three quarters, patient will still be considered cured provided this positive culture is followed by at least 3 consecutive negative cultures, taken at least 30 days apart, provided that there is clinical evidence of improvement.

Treatment Completed

An MDR-TB patient who has completed treatment according to guidelines but does not meet the definition for cure or treatment failure due to lack of bacteriological results.

Death

An MDR-TB patient who dies for any reason during the course of MDR-TB treatment.

Treatment Failure

Treatment will be considered to have failed if two or more of the five cultures recorded in the final 12–15 months are positive, or if any of the final three cultures are positive.

Treatment Default

An MDR-TB patient whose MDR-TB treatment was interrupted for two or more consecutive months for any reasons.

Transfer Out

An MDR-TB patient who has been transferred to another reporting unit and for whom the treatment outcome is not known

Treatment Stopped Due to Adverse Drug Reactions

A patient on MDR-TB treatment who develops severe adverse reactions and could not continue the MDR-TB treatment in spite of the management of the adverse reactions as per the defined protocols and decision has been taken by the DOTS-Plus site committee to stop treatment.

Treatment Stopped due to Other Reasons

A patient on MDR-TB treatment who could not continue the MDR-TB treatment for any other medical reason (than adverse drug reactions), and a decision has been taken by the DOTS-Plus site committee to stop treatment.

Still on Treatment

An MDR-TB patient who, for any reason, is still receiving their RNTCP category IV treatment at the time of the submission of the RNTCP DOTS-Plus Treatment Outcome Report.

PROVIDING PATIENT AND FAMILY COUNSELING

Providing counseling and health education to the MDR-TB patient about the disease and about the necessity of taking regular and adequate treatment is of utmost importance, for they must clearly understand that by taking the drugs irregularly or inadequately, or by defaulting, they fell into a category that was difficult to treat and that required a prolonged therapy. It is vital for them to realize that this is their last chance of treatment. Hence, it is extremely essential to strictly adhere to the prescribed line of treatment, as well as, to the scheduled follow-up of sputum and other laboratory investigations. Health education and counseling is provided to all patients and family members at different levels of health care, right from one at the periphery to those at the DOTS-Plus site facility. It is started at the initial point of contact and carried on a continuous basis at all visits by the patient to a health facility. The counseling and motivation is required to be done not only of the patient but also of the family members. In addition to the emphasis on regular treatment, health education also attempts to cross check the manner and the number of drugs/injections being taken, the occurrence of side-effects like yellowish skin and/or eyes, pain and swelling of joints, imbalance, etc. if any, and the frequency of sputa examinations being performed.

MONITORING FOR EARLY DETECTION OF ADVERSE REACTIONS

Close monitoring of patients is necessary to ensure that the adverse effects of category IV anti-TB drugs are recognized early by the DOT provider. DOT makes it possible to closely monitor patients. Patients will not be asked any leading question to elicit any adverse reaction.[11] However, if the patient makes any spontaneous complaint, she/he will be interrogated in detail and the necessary action taken. Commonly, patients will volunteer if they experience any adverse effects. The DOT provider should be trained to recognize adverse reactions like nausea, vomiting, diarrhea, skin rash, ototoxicity, peripheral neuropathy, psychiatric symptoms and jaundice.[12-15] Training should also be provided on the management of minor reactions and when the patients should be referred to the medical officer. In addition to clinical monitoring, certain laboratory investigations may be required to detect certain occult adverse effects.

Common Adverse Reactions to the Drugs Used

Kanamycin: Toxicity includes ototoxicity,[6,7] nephrotoxicity, vertigo and electrolyte imbalance.

Ofloxacin/Levofloxacin:[8,9] Gastrointestinal symptoms includes: diarrhea, vomiting, and abdominal pain. Central nervous system (CNS): dizziness and convulsions, phototoxicity and photosensitivity, tendinopathy and tendonitis, nephrotoxicity, skin rash, cardiotoxicity, arthralgia.

Ethambutol: Visual disturbance.

Pyrazinamide: Arthralgia, hyperuricemia, hepatitis and pruritis with or without rash.

Ethionamide: Gastrointestinal: Epigastric discomfort, anorexia, nausea, metallic taste, vomiting, excessive salivation, and sulfurous belching, Psychiatric: hallucination and depression, hepatitis, hypothyroidism and goiter with prolonged administration, gynecomastia, menstrual disturbances, impotence, acne, headache, alopecia and peripheral neuropathy.

Cycloserine:[10] CNS: Dizziness, slurred speech, convulsions, headache, tremor, and insomnia, psychiatric: confusion, depression, altered behavior, and suicidal tendency, hypersensitivity reaction.

Para-aminosalicylic acid:[11] Gastrointestinal: anorexia, nausea, vomiting, and abdominal discomfort, skin rashes, hepatic dysfunction, hypokalemia, hypothyroidism and goiter with prolonged administration.

ROLE OF DR-TB COMMITTEE IN THE MANAGEMENT OF ADVERSE REACTIONS

Whenever a patient has serious adverse reactions necessitating hospitalization or reduction/withholding/termination of any drug in the treatment regimen, the DR-TB committee should meet and arrange for specialist consultation, if required. The committee also should arrange for the drugs to be given for managing these reactions. Timely and intensive monitoring for identifying and management of adverse reactions to category IV drugs are essential components of the DOTS-Plus program. This will help to improve patient adherence to treatment, reduce mortality and obtain better treatment outcomes. Ancillary drugs for the management of adverse reaction should be made available to the patient free of cost (pyridoxine will be supplied by RNTCP and the other ancillary drugs should be available through the general health system drug supplies). Proper training of staff and support to the patient are other important activities that are required. In most cases, management of the adverse effects can be accomplished using relatively simple and low-cost interventions without compromising the integrity of the MDR-TB treatment regimen.[12]

ADHERENCE

Patients with MDR-TB may be more likely to have had problems with non-adherence in the past.[13] In addition, adherence with MDR-TB therapy is made more difficult by its prolonged treatment regimens, with larger numbers of drugs that have more serious adverse effect profiles[14] Thus, MDR-TB patients are at risk of not being able to appropriately adhere with treatment, an essential element to prevent the generation of panresistant strains with the potential for community-wide spread and virtually no chance of cure for the patient.[15] MDR-TB treatment can be successful with high overall rates of adherence when adequate support measures are provided.[16] These measures include enablers and incentives for delivery of DOT to ensure adherence to treatment and may include the following: reimbursement of travel expenses to patient and attendants for visits to DTC and designated State level DOTS-Plus site in-door facility; emotional support; patient, family and peer's education on MDR-TB treatment; early and effective management of adverse drug reactions; and honorarium to the non-salaried DOT providers.

FOLLOW-UP OF THE NON-ADHERENT PATIENT

When a patient fails to attend a DOT appointment, a system should be in place that allows prompt patient retrieval. The DOT provider should visit the patient's home on the same day to find out why the patient has not appeared for his/her DOT, and ensure that treatment is resumed promptly and effectively. The situation should be addressed in a sympathetic, friendly, and non-judgmental manner. Every effort should be made to listen to reasons for why the patient missed a dose(s) and to work with patient and family to ensure treatment continuation.

DOTS-PLUS PLAN

The RNTCP PMDT Vision is to promptly diagnose and effectively treat all TB patients with drug-resistant TB, through decentralized DST and PMDT treatment services integrated into RNTCP. Given the complexity, scale and cost, a phased approach has been developed, focusing first on those most likely to have drug-resistant TB. PMDT has the following specific objective to realize this vision:

- By end 2012, complete nationwide geographical coverage of access to basic MDR-TB diagnostic and treatment services
- By 2012–13, expanded access to MDR-TB diagnosis and treatment for all smear positive re-treatment TB cases and new cases who have failed an initial first-line drug treatment
- By 2015, nationwide access to MDR-TB diagnosis and treatment for all smear positive TB (re-treatment or new) cases registered under RNTCP before or early during their treatment.
- RNTCP expects to treat about 1,60,000 MDR-TB and 4,100 XDR-TB cases over the next 5 years (2012–2017).

Recent technological advances in laboratory diagnostics have expanded the list of WHO recommended methods available for DST, and can significantly reduce the delay between detection of TB and diagnosis of first-line and second-line drug resistance. Rapid methods of DST allow for the timely design of appropriate treatment regimens based on patients' drug resistance profiles using diagnostics that can be feasibly implemented in settings worldwide. This increased capacity for DST also translates into increased capacity for surveillance. After comprehensive review, WHO has endorsed certain new DST methodologies, including molecular line probe assays and liquid culture systems. With liquid culture, confirmation of pulmonary TB can be obtained in less than two weeks, and DST results in an additional one to two weeks. Use of liquid culture methods is possible for susceptibility testing for both first-line and second-line drugs. Molecular line probe assays are a genotypic method of DST that are used to detect the most common mutations of *M. tuberculosis* DNA that confer resistance to anti-tuberculosis drugs especially for isoniazid and rifampicin. Line probe assays have the great advantage of being able to produce results within 24 to 48 hours, thus representing a revolutionary step forward in the ability to rapidly confirm or rule out MDR-TB. GeneXpert MTB/RIF system is another molecular method to determine rifampicin resistance which is considered to be a surrogate marker for MDR-TB. Xpert MTB/RIF system has been found to be highly sensitive (98%) and specific (98%) in detecting TB and rifampicin resistance directly from sputum, in less than two hours.

REFERENCES

1. DOTS PLUS guidelines, Revised National Tuberculosis Control Program, Central TB Divison Directorate General Health Services, Ministry of Health & Family welfare, Nirman Bhawan, New Delhi. Sep 2008;/Revised National Tuberculosis Control Program. Guidelines on Programmatic Management of Drug Resistant TB (PMDT) in India. Central TB Division, Directorate General of Health Services, Ministry of Health and Family Welfare, Nirman Bhavan, New Delhi. May 2012.
2. Mahadev B, Kumar P, Agarwal SP, Chauhan LS, Srikantaramu N. Surveillance of drug resistance to anti-tuberculosis drugs in districts of Hoogli in West Bengal and Mayurbhanj in Orissa. Indian J Tuberc. 2005:52;5-10.
3. Paramasivan CN, Venkataraman P, Chandrasekaran V, Bhat S, Narayanan PR. Surveillance of drug resistance in tuberculosis in two districts of South India. Int J Tuberc Lung Dis. 2002:6; 479-84.
4. WHO IUALTD Global Project on Anti-Tuberculosis Drug Resistance Surveillance (2002–2007), Fourth Global Report (2008)./World Health Organization (WHO). Global Tuberculosis Report 2012. WHO/HTM/TB/2012.6.
5. World Health Organization (WHO). Treatment of Tuberculosis: Guidelines for National Programs, 3rd edn. WHO/CDS/TB 2003.313 Geneva, Switzerland: WHO, 2003, 2009.
6. Moore RD, Smith CR, Lietman PS. Risk factors for the development of auditory toxicity in patients receiving aminoglycosides. J Infect Dis. 1984;149:23-30.
7. De Jager P, Van Altena R. Hearing loss and nephrotoxicity in long-term aminoglycoside treatment in patients with tuberculosis. Int J Tuberc Lung Dis. 2002;6:622-7.
8. Arora VK, Tumbanatham A. Severe arthropathy with ofloxacin in two cases of MDR tuberculosis. Int J Tuberc Lung Dis. 1998;2:941-3.
9. Yew WW, Chan CK, Chau CH, et al. Outcomes of patients with multidrug-resistant pulmonary tuberculosis treated with ofloxacin/levofloxacin-containing regimens. Chest 2000;117:744-51.
10. Akula SK, Aruna AS, et al. Cycloserine-induced Stevens-Johnson syndrome in an AIDS patient with multidrugresistant tuberculosis. Int J Tuberc Lung Dis. 1997;1:187-90.
11. Vega P, Sweetland A, Acha J, et al. Psychiatric issues in the management of patients with multidrug-resistant tuberculosis. Int J Tuberc Lung Dis. 2004;8:749-58.
12. Furin JJ, Mitnick CD, Shin SS, et al. Occurrence of serious adverse effects in patients receiving community-based therapy for multidrug-resistant tuberculosis. Int J Tuberc Lung Dis. 2001;5:648-55.
13. Mitchison D. How drug resistance emerges as a result of poor compliance during short course chemotherapy for tuberculosis. Int J Tuberc Lung Dis. 1998;2:10-5.
14. Chaulk C, Chaisson R, Lewis J, et al. Treating multidrug-resistant tuberculosis: compliance and side effects. Journal of the American Medical Association 1994;271:103-4.
15. Espinal M, Dye C, Raviglione M, et al. A rational "DOTS-Plus" for the control of MDR-TB. Int J Tuberc Lung Dis. 1999;3:561-3.
16. Mitnick CD, Bayona J, Palacios E, et al. Community-based therapy for multidrug-resistant tuberculosis in Lima, Peru. New England Journal of Medicine 2003; 348:119-28.

Chapter 36

Tuberculosis and HIV

INTRODUCTION

The human immunodeficiency virus (HIV) pandemic presents a massive challenge to the control of tuberculosis (TB) at all levels. Tuberculosis, being the most common opportunistic infection is one of the most common cause of morbidity and leading cause of mortality in People living with HIV/AIDS (PLHA). This chapter aims to review the effect of HIV on TB.

EPIDEMIOLOGY

It has been estimated that 25 million people have been killed by HIV since its introduction in 1981. The World Health Organization (WHO) reports 8.7 million new cases of TB in 2011 of whom 13% were HIV-infected. In addition, many of these patients are infected with significant proportion of drug resistant tuberculosis, including multi-drug (MDR-TB) and extensively drug resistant TB (XDR-TB), which are difficult to treat and contribute to increased mortality. In India, there were 2.31 million People living with HIV and AIDS (PLWHA) at the end of 2011 while the incidence of TB was approximately 1.8 million cases per year.[1] Considering estimated 40% of the Indian population is infected with *Mycobacterium tuberculosis*, an estimated 1 million persons are co-infected with *Mycobacterium tuberculosis* and HIV. The WHO reported HIV prevalence among tuberculosis patients as 13% in 2011 and prevalence of HIV among tuberculosis patients in India as 4.2% in 2011.[1] In a survey carried out among new tuberculosis patients by the Revised National TB control Program (RNTCP) in 2007, HIV sero-prevalence varied widely and ranged from 1 to 13.8% across the 15 districts.[2] An increasing trend has been observed in HIV seropositivity among tuberculosis cases, which has been found to vary between 0.4% and 28.8% in different studies conducted mostly at tertiary health care centers.[3,4] There has been a rising trend of HIV prevalence among tuberculosis patients reported from Mumbai (2.3% in 1989 to 8.9% in 1993),[5,6,7] Pune (3.2% in 1991 to 20% in 1996),[8] and Chennai (0.59% in 1996 to 8.89% in 1999)[9,10] and from the Northern Regions of India (0.5 to 4.38%).[11-14] In the year 2012, about 8,21,807 (56%) TB patients were tested for HIV and 44,063 (5%) were found to be HIV positive in India.[15] This diverse data shows us that different strategies need to be employed within the country to reach out to PLHA and address their needs for early diagnosis, treatment, care and support. The need of the hour is to establish an intensified package of services for TB-HIV for high HIV prevalence areas and a basic package for the rest of the country. TB can be easily cured through the DOTS strategy provided through RNTCP but there is still no cure for HIV. With ART being provided free through National AIDS Control Program, HIV is now a chronic manageable illness. The basic purpose of HIV-TB collaborative activity is to ensure synergy between the two programs for the prevention and control of both diseases.

IMPACT OF HIV ON TUBERCULOSIS

The HIV is the most powerful factor for progression from tuberculosis infection to tuberculosis disease. A HIV positive person infected with *Mycobacterium tuberculosis* has a 50–60% lifetime risk of developing tuberculosis whereas an HIV negative person infected with *M. tuberculosis* has 10% risk of developing tuberculosis.[16] HIV breaks down the immune system and makes patients highly susceptible to TB and once infected there is rapid progression to active tuberculosis. In patients with latent TB infection, the risk of developing active disease is higher among recently infected persons compared to those with chronic infection, but is several hundred-fold higher among persons who acquire HIV.[17] Further these patients can then spread tuberculosis to other people. HIV infection acquired after TB infection is a significant risk factor for development of active TB mainly due to its effects on the immune system. HIV is associated with decreased chemotaxis, defective granuloma formation and maintenance, impaired antigen processing and presentation as well as generalized loss of $CD4^+$ T cells and selective clonal depletion of *M-tuberculosis* specific $CD4^+$T lymphocytes.[18] As HIV progresses, there is cutaneous anergy as well as impaired tissue containment of mycobacteria leading to widespread dissemination of mycobacteria. Though, TB can develop at any CD4 count, as the CD4 declines the cascade of TB manifestations shift from pulmonary to extrapulmonary to serious extrapulmonary forms such as meningitis and finally disseminated TB.

IMPACT OF TUBERCULOSIS ON HIV

Tuberculosis may accelerate the progression of HIV, as observed by a six- to seven-fold increase in HIV viral load in tuberculosis patients.[19] Clinical studies have shown the detrimental effect of tuberculosis on the course of HIV infection. Tuberculosis shortens the survival of patients with HIV infection. The risk of death in HIV infected persons with TB is reported to be twice as high as that in HIV infected patients without tuberculosis and tuberculosis is the cause of death for one out of every three people with AIDS worldwide. The higher mortality rate is due to progressive AIDS rather than tuberculosis. *M. tuberculosis* probably increases viral replication by inducing macrophages to produce tumor necrosis factors, IL-1 and IL-6. The degree of immunosupression is the most important predictor of survival in HIV infected patients with tuberculosis.

DIAGNOSTIC DIFFICULTIES IN PERSONS WITH HIV/TB COINFECTION

Patients with HIV have frequent pulmonary infections. Each time such an infection occurs, the patient must be evaluated for tuberculosis. The causes of respiratory infections are *Pneumocystis carinii* (*jiroveci*) pneumonia, Bacterial pneumonia, suppurative lung and sinus disease, *Mycobacterium tuberculosis, Mycobacterium avium* complex and cytomegalovirus. *Mycobacterium tuberculosis* infection usually develops much earlier as compared to other infections which occur in HIV positive patients. Unlike other opportunistic infections which have a selective range of CD4 in which the disease occurs, TB occurs throughout the course of HIV.[20] It may therefore happen that tuberculosis is diagnosed much earlier than the HIV infection in such patients. The clinical, laboratory and radiographic picture of tuberculosis in an HIV infected person varies depending on the patient's degree of immunosuppression. A HIV positive individual with any of the following symptoms should be suspected of having TB and investigated further: cough of more than 2 weeks' duration, fever lasting more than 2–3 weeks, weight loss, fatigue, listlessness, unexplained dyspnea, chest pain, or hemoptysis. Accelerated weight loss defined as greater than 10% weight loss in a month in HIV has earned the name "slimming disease".[16] The following table shows the different diseases that can manifest in a person with HIV infection.

REVISED WHO CLINICAL STAGING OF HIV/AIDS FOR ADULTS AND ADOLESCENTS WITH CONFIRMED HIV INFECTION[21]

Clinical Stage 1

- Asymptomatic
- Persistent generalized lymphadenopathy

Clinical Stage 2

- Moderate unexplained weight loss (<10% of presumed or measured body weight)
- Recurrent respiratory infections (sinusitis, tonsillitis, otitis media and pharyngitis)
- Herpes zoster
- Angular cheilitis
- Recurrent oral ulceration
- Papular pruritic eruptions
- Seborrheic dermatitis
- Fungal nail infections.

Clinical Stage 3

- Unexplained severe weight loss (>10% of presumed or measured body weight)
- Unexplained chronic diarrhea for >1 month
- Unexplained persistent fever for >1 month (>37.6°C, intermittent or constant)
- Persistent oral candidiasis (thrush)
- Oral hairy leukoplakia
- Pulmonary tuberculosis (current)
- Severe presumed bacterial infections (e.g. pneumonia, empyema, pyomyositis, bone or joint infection, meningitis, bacteremia)
- Acute necrotizing ulcerative stomatitis, gingivitis or periodontitis
- Unexplained anemia (hemoglobin <8 g/dL)
- Neutropenia (neutrophils <500 cells/μL)
- Chronic thrombocytopenia (platelets <50,000 cells/μL).

Clinical Stage 4

- HIV wasting syndrome
- Pneumocystis pneumonia (*Pneumocystis jiroveci*)
- Recurrent severe bacterial pneumonia
- Chronic herpes simplex infection (orolabial, genital, or anorectal site for >1 month or visceral herpes at any site)
- Esophageal candidiasis (or candidiasis of trachea, bronchi or lungs)
- Extrapulmonary tuberculosis
- Kaposi sarcoma
- Cytomegalovirus infection (retinitis or infection of other organs)
- Central nervous system toxoplasmosis
- HIV encephalopathy
- Cryptococcosis, extrapulmonary (including meningitis)
- Disseminated nontuberculosis mycobacteria infection
- Progressive multifocal leukoencephalopathy

- *Candida* of the trachea, bronchi, or lungs
- Chronic cryptosporidiosis (with diarrhea)
- Chronic isosporiasis
- Disseminated mycosis (e.g. histoplasmosis, coccidioidomycosis, penicilliosis)
- Recurrent nontyphoidal *Salmonella* bacteremia
- Lymphoma (cerebral or B-cell non-Hodgkin)
- Invasive cervical carcinoma
- Atypical disseminated leishmaniasis
- Symptomatic HIV-associated nephropathy
- Symptomatic HIV-associated cardiomyopathy
- Reactivation of American trypanosomiasis (meningoencephalitis or myocarditis).

DIAGNOSIS OF PULMONARY TUBERCULOSIS

Pulmonary involvement occurs in about 75% of all HIV infected patients with TB.[16,20,22] Cough is generally reported less frequently, probably because there is less cavitation, inflammation and endo-bronchial irritation as a result of a decrease in cell-mediated immunity. Hemoptysis, which results from caseous necrosis of the bronchial arteries, is less common in HIV infected patients. In the early stages of HIV infection when the immune system is relatively intact, the clinical spectrum of tuberculosis, sputum smears and X-ray findings are similar to a non-HIV infected tuberculosis patient. Disease is generally localized to the lungs: sputum smears show presence of acid-fast bacilli (AFB) and X-rays will reveal typical apical infiltrates and cavitatory lesions.[38] Pulmonary TB can be sputum positive or sputum negative. The following are suggested case definitions for use in HIV-prevalent settings:[21,23]

- **Smear-positive pulmonary tuberculosis**
  - One sputum smear examination positive for AFB and
  - Laboratory confirmation of HIV infection

    OR
  - Strong clinical evidence of HIV infection
- **Smear-negative pulmonary tuberculosis**
  - At least two sputum specimens negative for AFB, and
  - Radiographical abnormalities consistent with active tuberculosis

    OR
  - Decision by a clinician to treat with a full course of antituberculosis chemotherapy

    OR
  - A patient with AFB smear-negative sputum which is culture-positive for *Mycobacterium tuberculosis,* and

- Strong clinical evidence of HIV infection, and
- Laboratory confirmation of HIV infection.

Sputum smears are more likely to be negative in the advanced stages. HIV-infected smear-positive patients also tend to excrete fewer organisms per mL of sputum than HIV-negative patients, which can lead to AFB being missed if the appropriate number of high power fields is not examined by microscopy.

Diagnosis of Tuberculosis in Ambulatory Patient in HIV-Prevalent Settings

The patient is said to be ambulatory when suspected for tuberculosis without the danger signs (Respiratory rate > 30/min, fever > 39° C, pulse rate > 120/min and unable to walk unaided). The diagnostic process should be expedited if the patient is HIV positive, or likely to be so. The total number of visits for separate evaluations from the time of initial presentation to a health facility to the time of diagnosis should not exceed four. Shortening the turn around time for sputum smear examinations is crucial. The following principles should be followed when applying the algorithms for the ambulatory patient in order to expedite the diagnosis of smear-negative pulmonary tuberculosis.

- **First visit:** HIV testing should be offered and AFB sputum examination should be performed. If AFB test is positive, treat for tuberculosis.
- **Second visit:** If the AFB examination is negative, the patient should be provided with all available investigations during the second visit. The second visit should ideally take place on the second day following first presentation at the health facility. The investigations include: repeated sputum AFB, sputum culture and chest X-ray. Clinical assessment is also important for deciding whether it is worth putting the patient on antituberculosis treatment at this stage. HIV assessment should also be performed and co-trimoxazole preventive therapy provided according to national guidelines.
- **Third visit:** Results of the second-visit investigations (except culture) should be available during the patient's third visit. Patients suspected of having tuberculosis after these investigations (e.g. compatible radiograph plus symptoms) should be treated for tuberculosis. Patients who are not treated for tuberculosis should receive either a broad based antibiotic (not a fluoroquinolone) to treat bacterial infection or treatment for PCP. HIV assessment should also be performed and co-trimoxazole preventive therapy provided according to national guidelines.
- **Fourth visit:** The patient's response is assessed and a clinical follow-up mechanism is established (in either the tuberculosis or the HIV services). For patients with immediate response to PCP or antibiotic treatment, continued vigilance is necessary to exclude superimposed

tuberculosis. Those patients with an unsatisfactory response to treatment for PCP or bacterial pneumonia should be reassessed both clinically and bacteriologically for tuberculosis.

Diagnosis of Tuberculosis in Seriously-ill Patient in HIV-Prevalent Settings

A seriously-ill patient with one of the danger signs should be immediately referred to a higher level health facility. When immediate referral is not possible, the following measures should be undertaken in the peripheral health facility.

- Immediately start with broad-spectrum parenteral antibiotics for bacterial infection and perform HIV test and sputum AFB examination. Safe injection practices should be strictly followed. If the indications laid down in national guidelines are present, PCP treatment should be considered. If the HIV test is negative or there is less clinical suspicion of HIV infection, or if the national or local guidelines do not classify the area as HIV-prevalent, continue management of the HIV-negative patient according to national practice and guidelines. If the HIV test is positive, or there is high clinical suspicion of HIV infection, follow the algorithm.
- If the diagnosis of tuberculosis is confirmed by AFB smear examination, start tuberculosis treatment. The antibiotic treatment should be continued and completed.
- If the AFB smear is negative, response to parenteral antibiotics should be assessed 3–5 days into treatment, and, if there is no improvement, tuberculosis treatment should be initiated. The initial antibiotic course should be continued and completed. HIV assessment and clinical staging should be performed. Patients should be referred to the next level of care to confirm the diagnosis of tuberculosis and for HIV care. If referral is not possible, tuberculosis treatment should be completed.
- If referral to a higher-level facility is possible, the patient should be managed as an emergency and all available investigations, including HIV testing, should be performed at one time for the diagnosis of tuberculosis.

EXTRAPULMONARY TUBERCULOSIS

As the immunity decreases in later stages of HIV infection, there is a atypical presentation of tuberculosis with more frequent extrapulmonary manifestations ranging from 46 to 79%.[24,25] Extrapulmonary disease has been reported in up to 70% of HIV-related tuberculosis cases when the CD4 lymphocyte count is less than 100 mm.[3] Extrapulmonary TB is the commonest cause of pyrexia of unknown origin (PUO) among HIV positive individuals in developing countries.[26,27] The most frequent extrapulmonary form of TB is involvement of the lymph nodes with cervical region being the commonest.[28]

Amongst extrapulmonary tuberculosis: Lymphadenitis, pleural effusion, pericardial disease, miliary tuberculosis and meningeal tuberculosis are seen to occur more frequently. The definitive diagnosis of extrapulmonary tuberculosis is often difficult because of the scarcity of diagnostic facilities.

Clinical Diagnosis of Extrapulmonary Tuberculosis

One specimen from an extrapulmonary site culture-positive for *Mycobacterium tuberculosis* or smear-positive for AFB

OR

Histological or strong clinical evidence consistent with active extrapulmonary tuberculosis

OR

A decision by a clinician to treat with a full course of antituberculosis chemotherapy, and

Laboratory confirmation of HIV infection

OR

Strong clinical evidence of HIV infection

High suspicion of tuberculosis should be kept if they are 2 cm or more in size, cervical location, painless swelling, asymmetrical/localized, firm/fluctuant/fistulated, and associated weight loss, night sweats, fever are present. Findings that suggest a non-tuberculosis diagnosis include symmetrical (probable lymphoma or HIV lymphadenopathy), Kaposi sarcoma in skin or mouth (probable Kaposi sarcoma nodes), tender, inflamed, purulent (bacterial or fungal) and site other than cervical location, i.e. intrathoracic lymphadenopathy is not a feature of primary HIV syndrome and should always the raise the suspicion of TB or lymphoma.[21] Essential investigations include a HIV test (rapid if possible), sputum smears if cough present and a 18–21 gauge needle aspirate for AFB and excision biopsy if the aspirate is non-diagnostic. Lymph node involvement in HIV is characterized by poor granuloma formation with abundant AFB picked up by Ziehl-Neelsen stain. While *Mycobacterium tuberculosis* accounts for most mycobacterial infections in India, a small proportion are due to non-tuberculous mycobacteria such as *M. avium* intracellulare, *M. fortuitum*, etc.[29]

The other forms of extrapulmonary TB include pleural effusion, pericardial effusion, TB meningitis and abdominal TB. Pleural effusion is usually unilateral and asymmetric, with parenchymal opacities. Tuberculosis is the cause of about 90% of HIV-related pericardial effusion, but a lower percentage (50–70%) of pericardial effusions in HIV-negative individuals.[30,31] High rates of undiagnosed disseminated tuberculosis have been consistently identified in febrile, HIV-positive inpatients and in postmortem series from several countries.[32,33] Mycobacteremia has been observed to be an important cause of PUO, particularly among patients with severe immunosuppression, but is difficult to diagnose as it requires facilities to perform blood culture using rapid culture techniques like BACTEC. Intracranial space occupying lesions are common in HIV-infected individuals: the differential diagnosis includes tuberculoma, cerebral toxoplasmosis, neurocysticercosis, cryptococcoma and lymphoma. In India, cryptococcal meningitis is the commonest form of meningitis followed by TB meningitis. Features of abdominal TB include hepatosplenomegaly with focal intra-abdominal lymphadenopathy. Ascitis and omental thickening are less common. Extrapulmonary tuberculosis is more strongly HIV-related than pulmonary tuberculosis, with a combination of the two being especially suggestive of underlying HIV-infection. In peripheral health facilities in HIV-prevalent settings, clinicians should initiate empirical antituberculosis treatment early in patients with serious illness thought to be due to extrapulmonary tuberculosis. Every effort should then be made to confirm the diagnosis of tuberculosis, including monitoring the clinical response of the patient, to ensure that the patient's illness is being managed appropriately. If additional diagnostic tests are unavailable, and if referral to a higher level facility for confirmation of the diagnosis is not possible, antituberculosis treatment should be continued and completed. Empirical trials of treatment with incomplete regimens of antituberculosis drugs should not be performed. If a patient is treated with empirical antituberculosis drugs, treatment should be with standardized, first-line regimens, which should be used for the entire duration of antituberculosis treatment. Empirical treatment should be stopped only if there is bacteriological, histological or strong clinical evidence of an alternative diagnosis.[21]

INVESTIGATIONS

Sputum Smear for AFB and Culture for *Mycobacterium tuberculosis*

Three sputum specimens should be collected for patients suspected to have TB, including at least one overnight collection. Starting from 1 April 2009, all the patients with cough that cannot be brought under control within 2 weeks should undergo two sputum tests, according to the new guidelines in India. The two sputum tests will help to confirm if the person with cough has TB in 85% of the cases.[34] Smear should be stained by Ziehl-Neelsen (conventional microscopy) or auramine-rhodamine (fluorescent microscopy). Fluorescent microscopy is advantageous over light microscopy for the detection of pulmonary TB. Studies have confirmed the finding that fluorescence microscopy yielded an average increase in sensitivity of 10% with no loss of specificity.[35] Culture (on Lowenstein-Jensen medium) is much more sensitive but takes 6–8 weeks and requires specialized laboratory facilities and trained staff. Newer culture systems that detect bacterial CO_2 production or O_2 consumption with radiometric (BACTEC), fluorescent (MGIT), colorimetric (MB/BACT system) or pressure sensors (ESP culture system II) roughly halve the time to detection and are being evaluated for use in resource-poor settings.[36,37] Molecular assays have been developed for rapid detection of growth as well as species identification and drug susceptibility testing. Most commonly polymerase chain reaction (PCR), transcription mediated amplification (Genprobe) and strand displacement amplification (Becton Dickinson) are used. They have good sensitivity and specificity. High cost and need of trained staff preclude their routine use in resource poor nations with high endemicity.

Chest Radiography

Chest X-ray is commonly done as an investigation since sputum smears are not always positive and typical features of TB are not present. X-ray findings are atypical with hilar adenopathy, diffuse pulmonary infiltrates/opacities/ military pattern (dominant radiological presentations) and absence of cavitations. It is important to note that HIV infected patients with pulmonary tuberculosis may have a normal chest X-ray (5–10% of HIV patients). Important HIV-related pulmonary diseases which may be confused with pulmonary tuberculosis include bacterial pneumonia, non-tuberculous mycobacteriosis, *Pneumocystis carinii* pneumonia, Kaposi's sarcoma, fungal infections, nocardiosis, lymphoma (mediastinal adenopathy) and cavitation is uncommon.

Tuberculin Skin (Mantoux) Test

HIV positive patients of TB are found to have less tuberculin positivity as compared to HIV negative patients of tuberculosis 26% vs 76.4%.[38] In HIV positive individuals tuberculin test is considered to be positive if reaction is more than 5 mm in response to 1TU of PPD-RT23. In a recent analysis, in India, with the cut off of 5 mm universally practiced for TB in HIV, the positive predictive value of a TST for TB was 48.8% for patients with CD4 < 200 cells/mm^3 and only 18.8% for patients with CD4 > 200 cells/mm^3.[39] Overall, tuberculin testing is not useful in routine practice either for diagnosis of TB or latent TB infection.

CT Scan of the Chest

For presence of enlarged lymph nodes or parenchymal lesions that are not visible on plain X-ray.

Induced Sputum/Gastric Lavage

Inhalation of nebulized hypertonic saline or salbutamol 2 mg given three times daily for a week are used in order to induce sputum production. Gastric lavage can be performed in patients unable to expectorate. These specimens are tested for AFB by smear and culture.

Fiberoptic Bronchoscopy with Lavage and Transbronchial Biopsy

Though BAL in itself is not better than sputum test for AFB; it may help to rule out other infections like *Pneumocystis carinii.*

Total Lymphocyte and CD4 Counts

The percentage and absolute number of CD4 cells in blood provide a good index of the stage of HIV disease and have a prognostic value, especially when considered with the extent of viral load. Tuberculosis also produces a decline in $CD4^+$ T cells, thereby worsening the immunologic status.

TREATMENT OF TUBERCULOSIS IN HIV POSITIVE PATIENTS

Delays in the diagnosis of tuberculosis have been associated with worse outcomes, so initiation of treatment as soon as tuberculosis is suspected is very important. The tuberculosis relapse rate is low in HIV infected tuberculosis patients who complete a full rifampicin containing short course treatment regimens. Extending the duration of treatment regimens from 6–12 months in such patients further reduces frequency of relapse,[40] however, this difference is marginal and given the expenses, toxicity, and difficulty of longer treatment most programs treat HIV infected patients for 6, or at most 9 months. Thus in general, anti-tuberculosis treatment is the same for HIV-infected and HIV-negative tuberculosis patients, with the exception of the use of thiacetazone. In India, under the RNTCP, patients with newly diagnosed TB whether pulmonary or extrapulmonary receive a 6-month thrice-weekly regimen (category I—2HREZ3/4RH3) while those with relapse, default or failure receive an 8-month regimen (category II—2SEHRZ3/1EHRZ3/5EHR3). The category III—2HRZ3/4RH3, regimen is avoided in persons with HIV infection. Thiacetazone is also avoided because it can cause severe cutaneous reactions, exfoliative dermatitis or Steven-Johnson syndrome and can be fatal in HIV positive patients. Ethambutol is therefore used instead in patients known or suspected of having HIV infection. Case fatality and relapse rate is lower in HIV-infected tuberculosis patients who complete a full course of directly observed rifampicin containing short-course treatment than with the standard 12-month treatment regimens using isoniazid and ethambutol during the continuation phase, which do not include rifampicin. This is partly because short-course treatment is more effective, but may also be related to the fact that rifampicin has broad-spectrum antibacterial activity.[41–45] This may decrease deaths due to HIV-related bacterial infections during antituberculosis treatment. Direct observation of treatment is even more important for HIV-infected tuberculosis patients, as self-administration of treatment is associated with higher case fatality rates.[16] WHO has currently recommended that TB patients with known positive HIV status and also living in HIV-prevalent settings (defined as countries, subnational administrative units, or selected facilities where the HIV prevalence among adult pregnant women is ≥1% or among TB patients is ≥ 5%) should receive daily TB treatment at least during the intensive phase as well as for the continuation phase. If a daily continuation phase is not possible for these patients, three times weekly dosing during the continuation phase is an acceptable alternative.[46] Patients who complete treatment show the same clinical, radiographic and microbiological response to short-course treatment irrespective of whether they are HIV positive or negative. HIV-infected patients have a much higher mortality during and after antituberculosis treatment compared with HIV negative patients. This is partly due to tuberculosis itself, but largely due to other HIV related problems. The Tuberculosis Research Center (TRC) found, in a pilot study of patients with advanced HIV and TB, a favorable response of 72% and an unfavorable response of 28% (including treatment failure and deaths) when treated with RNTCP category I regimen.[20] Further, 37% of patients had died within 24 months of completing ATT. Outbreaks of multi-drug resistant tuberculosis and extensively drug resistant tuberculosis have been reported in patients with HIV infection.[47] HIV itself does not cause drug resistant tuberculosis, but it fuels the spread of this dangerous condition by increasing susceptibility to infection and accelerating the progression from infection to disease. Adequate sterilization and safe disposal of syringes and needles should be ensured whenever streptomycin is administered.

ADJUVANT CORTICOSTEROIDS IN EXTRAPULMONARY TB

Corticosteroids started at the time of tuberculosis diagnosis and given for the first 2 months of treatment significantly improve survival from tuberculous meningitis in HIV-negative patients, and are now recommended for such patients.[48] For other forms of extrapulmonary tuberculosis and for HIV-related tuberculous meningitis, the effects of steroids are still uncertain. The results of small trials on tuberculous pericarditis are promising.[49] There appears to be no benefit in adding steroids to the treatment of tuberculous pleural effusion, with some suggestion of possible harm to HIV positive patients.[50] Recommendations may change when the results of larger randomized clinical trials become available within the next few years.

HIGHLY ACTIVE ANTI-RETROVIRAL THERAPY

Currently available antiretroviral agents fall in the following groups of drugs: nucleoside reverse transcriptase inhibitors (NRTIs), non-nucleoside reverse transcriptase inhibitors (NNRTIs), protease inhibitors (PI), integrase inhibitors, chemokine receptor antagonists and entry (fusion) inhibitors. Highly active antiretroviral therapy (HAART) refers to the use of a combination of at least 3 antiretroviral drugs to form a maximally suppressive regimen.

Table 36.1: Antiretroviral drug

Nucleoside reverse transcriptase inhibitors
1. ZIDOVUDINE (AZT)* 2. DIDANOSINE (ddI) 3. STAVUDINE (d4T)* 4. LAMIVUDINE (3TC) 5. ZALCITABINE (ddC) 6. ABACAVIR (ABC) 7. TENOFOVIR (TDF)**
Non-nucleoside reverse transcriptase inhibitors
1. EFAVIRENZ (EFV) 2. NEVIRAPINE (NVP) 3. DELAVIRDINE
Protease inhibitors
1. SAQUINAVIR (SQV) 2. INDINAVIR (IDV) 3. NELFINAVIR (NFV) 4. LOPINAVIR (LPV) 5. RITONAVIR (RTV)*** 6. AMPRENAVIR

*Zidovudine and Stavudine as HAART not used together due to antagonistic effect.

**Tenofovir is a nucleotide reverse transcriptase inhibitor but is included in this group.

***Ritonavir is recommended for use in combination with IDV/LPV/SQV as a booster and not as a drug in its own right.

Regimens recommended for use in India for patients with concomitant TB are a combination of two NRTIs with efavirenz or less commonly nevirapine.[51] Various antiretroviral drugs are tabulated in Tables 36.1 and 36.2.

INTERACTIONS OF ANTITUBERCULOSIS THERAPY AND ANTIRETROVIRAL THERAPY

Till date no cure is available for HIV/AIDS. It is only the opportunistic infections in HIV/AIDS, which can be treated. The antiretroviral drugs, which are used in HIV positive patients, are effective in slowing down the action of the virus and prolonging life. Nucleoside reverse transcriptase inhibitors like zidovudine, didanosine, stavudine, lamivudine and abacavir can be safely co-administered with antituberculosis drugs. Co-administration of rifampicin with any of the protease inhibitors (ritonavir, indinavir, nelfinavir) or non-nucleoside reverse transcriptase inhibitor (nevirapine, delavirdine, thioben) is contraindicated. Protease inhibitors and non-nucleoside reverse transcriptase inhibitors may inhibit or induce cytochrome P-450 isoenzymes and thus these drugs may alter the serum concentration of rifamycins. Rifamycins induce cytochrome P-450 and may substantially decrease blood levels of the antiretroviral drugs resulting in the potential development of resistance. Rifabutin is a less potent cytochrome-450 inducer than rifampicin, and thus can be used concurrently with the NNRTIs (e.g. nevirapine, efavirenz) or with certain protease inhibitors (e.g.

Table 36.2: Antiretroviral (ART) recommendations for individuals with tuberculosis and HIV co-infection[51,52*]

CD4 Cell Count	Recommended Regimen	Comments
CD4 < 200 cu mm	Start tuberculosis treatment. Start ART as soon as tuberculosis treatment is tolerated (between 2 weeks and 2 months)	Recommended ART[a] .
CD4 between 200–350/cu mm	Start tuberculosis treatment.	Consider ART after 2 months/ intensive phase of TB therapy. (can be initiated early if severely compromised, i.e. within 2 weeks)
CD4 > 350 cu mm	Start tuberculosis treatment[b]	Defer ART monitor CD4 counts. Re-evaluate patient at 8 weeks and at the end of treatment start ART when indicated
CD4 not available	Start tuberculosis treatment[c]	Start ART between 2 and 8 weeks after ATT initiation

*According to WHO 2012 guidelines on TB-HIV, ART should be started in all TB patients living with HIV irrespective of their CD4 counts. Antituberculosis treatment should be initiated first, followed by ART as soon as possible within the first 8 weeks of treatment. Those HIV-positive TB patients with profound immunosuppression (CD4 counts less than 50 cells/mm^3 should receive ART immediately within the first 2 weeks of initiating TB treatment)

[a]EFV containing regimens are preferred.Alternatively Nevirapine or triple NRTI (based on tenofovir or abacavir) can be considered. EFV is contraindicated in pregnant women or women of child bearing potential without effective contraception The regimens that can be used are:
Zidovudine (AZT)/Lamivudine (3TC)/Efavirenz (EFV)
Stavudine (d4T)/Lamivudine(3TC)/Efavirenz (EFV)
Zidovudine (AZT)/Lamivudine(3TC)/Abacavir(ABC)
Zidovudine (AZT)/Lamivudine(3TC)/Nevirapine(NVP)

[b]Start ART if non-tuberculosis stage III, IV conditions are present. Otherwise start ART upon completion of TB treatment.

[c]For some TB diagnoses that respond well to anti-TB therapy (Lymph node, uncomplicated pleural effusion) deferral of ART should be considered. If no other signs of immunodeficiency present and patients are improving on tuberculosis treatment, ART should be started upon completion of tuberculosis treatment. In case of extrapulmonary tuberculosis regardless of CD4 count, Start ATT first. Start ART as soon as TB treatment is tolerated after 2 weeks.

indinavir, nelfinavir). Neuropathy induced by isoniazid can be potentiated by NRTI's (didianosine, stavudine) which also cause neuropathy.[18] Isoniazid, ethambutol, pyrazinamide and streptomycin can be concurrently used with protease inhibitors or non-nucleoside reverse transcriptase inhibitors. If protease inhibitor or non-nucleoside reverse transcriptase inhibitor is to be started after giving rifampicin, then at least 2 weeks should elapse after the last dose of rifampicin. This time gap is necessary for reduction of the enzyme inducing activity of rifampicin prior to commencing of antiretroviral drugs. HIV infected who does not appear to be at a higher risk of dying, it may be preferred to defer ART until the intial phase of tuberculosis treatment has been completed. This decreases the risk of immune reconstitution syndrome and avoids the risk of drug interaction between rifampicin and a protease inhibitor. Initiating antiretroviral therapy (ART) together with tuberculosis therapy could reduce mortality risk among coinfected patients by 55%, according to interim findings from a large clinical trial in South Africa.[53]

IMMUNE RECONSTITUTION SYNDROME

Immune recovery usually occurs rapidly in HIV-infected adults who are started on antiretroviral treatment (ART). Occasionally, recovery of the immune system leads to clinical signs and symptoms of active tuberculosis. This may be because patients had subclinical tuberculosis before the ART began, or because a latent tuberculosis infection has been reactivated. The condition is known as immune reconstitution inflammatory syndrome (IRIS). It can also appear as a temporary exacerbation of symptoms and signs or radiological manifestations of tuberculosis after beginning anti-TB treatment (ATT), similar to the well-documented paradoxical reactions seen in some patients without underlying HIV infection. In one study, the incidence of IRIS in TB alone was 2%, with HIV coinfection it was 7%, and in those started on HAART it was 36%.[54] The median period of IRIS presentation is approximtely 4–6 weeks after starting ART, usually occurs within 3 months of initiation of ART. However, IRIS has been observed as early as 1 week after starting ART. Risk factors for TB–IRIS include a low baseline CD4 cell count, high baseline viral load, shorter interval between commencing ATT and ART, disseminated tuberculosis, greater increase in CD4 cell count and greater reduction in viral burden after initiation of ART.[44,55] This paradoxical reaction is thought to be due to immune restoration and includes a sharp amplification of interferon-gamma producing mycobacteria-specific T cells along with an acute outpouring of Th1 cytokines. It is likely that $CD4^+$ T cells are not the only mediators of IRIS; therefore an increase in CD4 cell count with HAART does not necessarily correlate with the development of IRIS.[56] IRIS is commonly associated with tuberculosis, although it can also occur with other pathogens.

Symptoms and signs may include high fever and lymphadenopathy, expanding central nervous system lesions and worsening of chest X-ray findings, development of respiratory failure along with other less common findings such as occurrence or worsening of serositis, epididymitis, hepatosplenomegaly, soft tissue abscesses and disseminated skin lesions. In TB-IRIS, fever is the most frequent symptom, along with worsening infiltrates on chest X-ray. An initially negative PPD may become positive when IRIS occurs and this has been suggested as a marker for IRIS.[57] Interferon-gamma secretion and cell mediated immune response to mycobacteria are restored leading to restoration of DTH skin test response to mycobacterial-antigens. Hypercalcemia is a strange but frequent manifestation in TB-related IRIS.

It is probably related to increased production of 1,25 dihydroxycholecalceferol in functioning granulomas. A thorough evaluation is necessary to exclude other causes before diagnosing a paradoxical reaction. The differential diagnoses include treatment failure/drug resistance, progression of TB, super added infections and drug reaction. WHO recommends that IRIS is not a reason to switch patients on to second-line ART, although adjustment to the treatment regimen may be needed to ensure compatibility with anti-TB treatment (ATT). Healthcare workers should be aware of paradoxical worsening of tuberculosis on starting ART, and both antiretroviral and antituberculosis treatments should be continued. For mild paradoxical reactions just symptomatic management like NSAID is effective, along with continuation of ART. For severe paradoxical reactions, prednisolone (1–2 mg/kg body weight for 1–2 weeks then gradually decreasing dose over 4–6 weeks) may help although there is no conclusive evidence. Thalidomide and pentoxifylline have also been tried as anti-inflamatory agents.[57] Rarely, ART needs to be terminated.

HIV AND DRUG RESISTANT TB

Reports have shown high mortality rates among HIV-infected patients with DR-TB[58,59] and alarming mortality rates in patients coinfected with XDR-TB and HIV.[47] Early diagnosis of DR-TB and HIV, prompt treatment with adequate regimens, sound patient support and strong infection control measures are all essential components in the management of DR-TB in HIV-infected people. HIV is a powerful risk factor for all forms of TB, and DR-TB outbreaks, including XDR-TB outbreaks in HIV-infected patients, appear to be common.[47,60] DR-TB is often associated with higher mortality rates in the HIV-infected compared with the non-infected; however, the use of ART in addition to treatment of DR-TB has been reported to improve outcomes of DR-TB in the HIV-infected.[61,62]

DRUG INTERACTIONS OF SECOND LINE DRUGS AND ART

Buffered didanosine contains an aluminium/magnesium-based antacid and, if given jointly with fluoroquinolones, may result in decreased fluoroquinolone absorption, so it should be avoided, but if it is necessary it should be given 6 hours before or 2 hours after fluoroquinolone administration.[63] Ethionamide/prothionamide is thought to be metabolized by the CYP450 system, although it is not known which of the CYP enzymes are responsible. Whether doses of ethionamide/protionamide and/or certain antiretroviral drugs should be modified during the concomitant treatment of DR-TB and HIV is completely unknown.[64] Clarithromycin is a substrate and inhibitor of CYP3A and has multiple drug interactions with protease inhibitors and NNRTIs. If possible, the use of clarithromycin should be avoided in patients coinfected with DR-TB and HIV because of both its weak efficacy against DR-TB and multiple drug interactions.[65]

RECURRENCE OF TUBERCULOSIS AFTER COMPLETION OF TUBERCULOSIS TREATMENT

Among TB patients who complete short course chemotherapy, the recurrence rate is higher in HIV-positive than in HIV-negative TB patients. Post-treatment prophylaxis (e.g. with isoniazid) can decrease the risk of TB reoccurrence. In HIV infected individuals, although it does not appear to prolong survival. Further studies are needed to confirm the benefit, establish the optimal regimens (drug and duration) and assess the operational feasibility, before treatment aimed at decreasing the risk of TB recurrence is widely recommended.

TREATMENT OF TB AND HIV—WHO RECOMMENDED COLLABORATIVE TB/HIV ACTIVITIES[52,65]

Since HIV fuels the tuberculosis epidemic, prevention of HIV should be a priority for tuberculosis control and tuberculosis control and prevention should be primary concern for HIV/AIDS program. The goal of collaborative TB/HIV activities is to decrease the burden of TB and HIV in people at risk of affected by both diseases. The objectives are: (1) To establish and strengthen the mechanisms of collaboration and joint management between HIV programs are TB and HIV services preferably at the same time and location; (2) To reduce the burden of TB in people living with HIV, their families and communities by ensuring the delivery of the "Three I's for HIV/TB" and the early initiation of ART in line with WHO guidelines. The "Three I's for HIV-TB" are: Intensify TB case-finding and ensure high quality anti-TB treatment, initiate TB prevention with isoniazid preventive therapy and early ART and ensure control of TB infection in health-care facilities and congregate settings (3) To reduce the burden of HIV in patients with presumptive and diagnosed TB, their families and communities by providing HIV prevention, diagnosis and treatment.

CONCLUSION

TB in HIV-infected patients is highly lethal and a growing problem in many parts of the world. The diagnosis of TB still relies on the age old technique of sputum smear microscopy, and chest radiography which lacks specificity. Extrapulmonary, disseminated and sputum smear negative manifestations are more common in patients with advanced immunosuppression. Newer diagnostic tests are urgently required that are not only sensitive and specific, but easy to use in resource poor nations like India. Treatment of HIV-TB coinfection is complex and associated with high pill burden, overlapping drug toxicities, risk of IRIS and challenges related to adherence. From a programmatic point of view, screening of all HIV-infected persons for tuberculosis and vice-versa will help identify coinfected patients who require treatment for both infections. As programs embark on TB and HIV control strategies, the activities should be strengthened, and where absent, implemented. Improved detection, timely and appropriate ART as well as ATT, close clinical monitoring, management of adverse effects and infection control measures are the essential components of a successful program. With increasing availability of ART across the country, diagnosis of HIV is beneficial to the individual as he/she can be referred to the nearest ART center for evaluation and initiation of ART if indicated. Tuberculosis clinics, form an important entry point for HIV diagnosis, care and support. Co-ordination and crosstalk between these two government health programs is crucial not only to improve the outcome of HIV-infected TB patients but also to control the burden of tuberculosis in India.

REFERENCES

1. World Health Organization. Global Tuberculosis in report 2012. WHO/HTM/TB/2012.6.
2. Intensified TB/HIV package Training Manual for Councellors. Central TB Division and National AIDS Control Organisation; Ministry of Health and Family Welfare. Government of India. New Delhi, 2008.
3. Williams BG, Granich R, Chauhan LS, Dharmshaktu NS, Dye C. The impact of HIV/AIDS on the control of tuberculosis in India. Proc Natl Acad Sci (USA). 2005;102:9619-24.
4. Mohanti KC, Nair S, Sahasrabudhe T. Changing trends of HIV infection in a Bombay area since 1998. Ind J Tub. 1994;41:147-9.
5. Mohanti KC, Sudhrani RM, Nair S. HIV infection in patients with respiratory diseases. Ind J Tub. 1993;40:5-6.
6. Behera D. RespiratoryMedicine in India in the 21st century. Editorial: Indian J Chest Dis Allied Sci. 2008;50:179-81.
7. Mohanti KC, Basher PMM. Changing trends of HIV infection and tuberculosis in a Bombay area since 1998. Ind J Tub. 1995;42:117.
8. Paranjape RS, Tripathi SP, Menon PA, Josh P. Increasing trend of HIV seroprevalence among pulmonary tuberculosis in Pune India. Ind J Med Res. 1997:106.
9. Solomon S, Anuradha S, Rajasekharan S. Trend of HIV infection in patients with pulmonary tuberculosis in South India. Tubercle Lung. Dis. 1995;76:17.
10. Rajasekharan S, Lima A, Kamakshi S, Jeyaganesh D, et al. Trends of HIV infection in patients with tuberculosis in rural South India Ind J Tub. 2000;47:223-4.
11. Jain SK, Agarwal JK, Rajpal S, et. al. Prevalence of HIV infection among tuberculosis patients. Ind J Tub. 1996;43:105.
12. Jain SK, Agarwal JK, Rajpal S, et. al. Prevalence of HIV infection among tuberculosis patients in Delhi. A sentinel Surveillance study. Ind J Tub 2000;47:21.
13. Kaur, et. al. HIV infection in tuberculosis patients in Ludhiana. Ind J Chest Dis allied Sci. 1997:21.
14. Prasad R, Saini JK, Kannaujia RK, Sarin S, et al. Trend of HIV infection in patients with pulmonary tuberculosis in Lucknow area. Ind J Tub. 2003;50:39-41.

15. TB India 2013. Revised National TB Control Program Annual Status Report. Central TB Division. New Delhi, 2013.
16. WHO/HTM/TB/2004.329: TB/HIV: a clinical manual, Second Edition. Stop TB Department, Department of HIV/AIDS.
17. Rieder HL. Epidemiological Basis of tuberculosis control. First edition (Internation Union against Tuberculosis and Lung Diseases (UNION) 1999;PP 50-2.
18. Lawn SD, Butera SB and Shinnick TM. Tuberculosis unleashed: the impact of HIV infection on the host granulomatious response to mycobacterium tuberculosis; Microbes Infection. 2002;4:635-46.
19. De Cock KM, Soro B, Coulibaly IM, Lucas SB. Tubeculosis and HIV infection in sub-saharan Africa; JAMA. 1992;268:1581-7.
20. Swaminathan S, Narendran G. HIV and tuberculosis in India; J. Biosci. 2008;33:527-37.
21. World Health Organization. Improving athe diagnosis and treatment of smear-negative pulmonary and extrapulmonary tuberculosis among adults and adolescents: recommendations for HIV-prevalent and resource-constrained settings WHO/HTM/TB/2007.379, WHO/HIV/2007.01.
22. Deivanayagam CN, Rajesekaran S, Senthilnathan V, Krishnarajasekhar R, Raja K, Chandrasekar C, et al. Clinicoradiological sprctrum of tuberculosis aong HIV sero-positives—a Tambaram study. Indian J. Tuber. 2001;48:123-7.
23. Treatment of tuberculosis: guidelines for national programmes, 3rd ed. Geneva, World Health Organisation, 2003 WHO/CDS/TB/2003.313).
24. Kumarasamy N, Vallabhaneni S, Flangian TP, Mayer KH, Solomom S. Clinical profile of HIV in India; Ind J Med Res. 2005;121:377-94.
25. Sharma SK, Mohan A, Kadhiravan T. HIV-TB coinfection: Epidemiology, diagnosis and management; Ind J Med Res. 2005;121:550-67.
26. Rupali P, Abraham OC, Zachariah A, Subramaanian S, Mathai D. Aetiology of prolonged fever in antiretroviral-naïve human immunodeficiency virus-infected adults;Natl Med J India. 2003;16:193-9.
27. Kejariwal D, Sarkar N, Chakraborti SK, Agarwal V, Roy S. Pyrexia of unknown origin: a prospective study of 100 cases; J Postgrad Med. 2001;47:104-7.
28. Arora VK, Kumar SV. pattern of opportunistic pulmonary infections in HIV sero-positive subjects: Observations from Poncicherry, India; Indian J Chest Dis Allied Sci. 1999;41:135-44.
29. Singh S, Gopinath K, Shadad S, Kaur M, Singh B, Sharma P. Nontuberculous mycobacteria infections in Indian AIDS patients detected by a novel ser of ESAT-6 polymerase chain reaction primers; Jpn. J. Infect. Dis. 2007;60:14-8.
30. Maher D, Harries AD. Tuberculous pericardial effusion:a prospective clilnical study in a low resurce setting- Blantyre, Malawi. Int. J Tubercu Lung Dis. 1997;1:358-64.
31. Reuter H, Burgess LJ, Doubell AF. Epidemiology of pericardial effusions at a large academic hospital in South Africa. Epidemological Infection. 2005;133:393-9.
32. Archibald LK, McDonald LC, Nwanyanwu O, Kazembe P, Dobbie H, Tokars J, et al. A hospital-based survey of bloodstream infections in febrile patients in Malawi: implications for diagnosis and therapy. Journal of Aquired Immune Deficiency Syndromes and Human retrovirology. 2000;181:1414-20.
33. McDonald, Archibald LK, Rheanpumikankit S, Tansuphaswadikul S, Eampokalap B, Nwanyanawu O, et al. Unrecognised *Mycobacterium tuberculosis* bacteraemia among hospital inpatients in less developed countries. Lancet. 1999;354:1159-63
34. Compulsory sputum AFB test in India for coughs lasting over 2 weeks. CTD-Directorate general health services, Ministry of Health and Family Welfare. Government of India. March 26, 2009. (http://www.dancewithshadows.com/pillscribe/compulsory-sputum-tb-test-in-india-for-cough-lasting-over-2-weeks).

35. Steingart KR, Henry M, Hopewell PC, Ramsay A, Cunningham J, Urbanczik R, et al. Fluorescence versus conventional sputum smear microscopy for tuberculosis: a systematic review; Lancet Infect Dis. 2006;6:570-81.
36. Gil-Setas A, Torroba L, Fernandez JL, Martinez-Aortola V, Olite J. Evaluation of the MB/BacT system compared with Middlebrook 7H11 and Lowenstein-Jensen media for detection and recovery of mycobacteria from clinical specimens; Clin. Microbol. Infect. 2004;10:224-8.
37. Lee JJ, Suo J, Lin CB, Wang JD, Lin TY, Tsai YC. Comparative evaluation of the BACTEC MGIT 960 system with solid medium for isolation of mycobacteria. Int J Tuber. Lung Dis. 2003;7:569-74.
38. Prasad R, Saini JK, Gupta R, Kannaujia RK, Sarin S, Suryakant, et al. A clinico-radiological spectrum of tuberculosis among HIV seropositive and HIV seronegative patients. Indian Journal of Chest Diseases and Allied Science. 2004;46:99-103.
39. Swaminathan S, Deivanayagam CN, Rajesekaran S, Padmapriyadarshini C, Menon PA, Ponnuraja C, Dilip M. Long-term follow-up of HIV-infected patients with tuberculosis treated with 6-month intermittent short course chemotherapy; Natl Med. J 2008;21:3-7.
40. Periens JH, St Louis ME, Mukadi YB, Brown C, Prignot J, Pouthier F, et. al. Pulmonary tuberculosis in HIV infected patients in Zaire. A controlled trial oftreatment for either 6 or 12 months. N E J M 1995;332:779-84.
41. Hawken M, Nunn P, Gathua S, Brindle R, Godfrey-Faussett P, Githui W, et al. Increased recurrence of Tuberculosis in HIV-1 infected patients in Kenya. Lancet. 1993;342:332-7.
42. Elliot AM, Halwiindi B, Hayes RJ, Luo N, Mwinga AG, Tembo G, et al. The impact of HIV virus on response to treatment and recurrence rate in patients treated for tuberculosis: Two year follow-up of a cohort in Lusaka, Zambia. Journal of tropical Medicine and Hygiene. 1995;98:9-21.
43. Jindani A, Nunn A, Enarson D A. Two 8-month regimens of chemotherapy for treatment of newly diagnosed pulmonary tuberculosis: international multicentre randomized trial: Lancet. 2004;364:1244-51.
44. Lawn SD, Meyer L, Bekker LG, Wood R. Tuberculosis associated immune reconstitution disease: incidence, risk factors and impact in an antiretroviral treatment service in South Africa. AIDS 2007;21:335-41.
45. Nahid P, Gonzalez LC, Rudoy I, De Long BC, Unger A, Kawamura LM. Treatment outcomes of patients with HIV and tuberculosis; Am J Respire Crit Care Med. 2007;175:1196-206.
46. World Health Organization. Treatment of TB Guidelines - 4th Edition. WHO/HTM/TB/2009.
47. Gandhi NR, Moll A, Sturm AW, Pawinski R, Govender T, Lalloo U, et al. Extensively drug-resistant tuberculosis as a cause of death in patients coinfected with tuberculosis and HIV in a rural area of South Africa Lancet 2006;368:1575-602.
48. Thwaites GE, Nguyen DB, Nguyen HD, Hoang TQ, et al. Dexamethasone for the treatment of tuberculous meningitis in adolescents and adults. N E J M. 2004, 351:1741-51.
49. Mayosi BM, Ntsekhe M, Volmink JA, Commerford PJ. Inteventions for treating tuberculous pericarditis. Cochrane Database of Systematic Reviews, 2002. (4):CD000526.
50. Elliot AM, Luzze H, Quigley MA, Nakiyingi JS, Kyaligonza S, Namujju PB, et. al. A randomized, double-blind, placebo-controlled trial of the use of prednisolone as an adjunct to treatment in HIV-1- associated pleural tuberculosis. Journal of Infectious Diseases. 2004;190:869-78.
51. World Health Organisation 2006, 2010, 2013 antiretroviral therapy for HIV-1 infection in adults and adolescents; Recommendations for a public health approach.
52. World Health Organization 2012. WHO policy on collaborative TB/HIV activities guidelines for national programs and other stakeholders. WHO/HTM/TB/2012; WHO/HIV/2012.1.
53. Important new research finding on treatment of HIV-TB coinfection. Durban, South Africa: CAPRISA- Centre for the AIDS Programme of Research in South Africa; Sep 19, 2008 (http://www.caprisa.org/joolma/index.php/memberaccess/95-pressrelease 170992008).

54. Narita M, Ashkin D, Hollender ES, et al. Paradoxical reaction with antiretrorival therapy and ATT Am J Respire Crit Care Med. 1998;158:157-61.
55. Lawn S, Myer L, Bekker L G, Wood R. Early mortality among patients with HIV associated TB in Africa: Implications for the time to initiate ART (Conference on Retroviruses and Opportunitic Infections:Abstract 81, 2007).
56. Manabe YC, Campbell JD, Syndor E, Moore RD. Immune reconstitution inflammatory syndrome: risk factors and treatment implications; J Acquir Immune Defici. Syndr. 2007;46: 456-62.
57. Lawn SD, Myer L, Bekker LG, Miller RF. Immune reconstitution disease associated with mycobacterial infections in HIV infected individuals receiving antiretrovirals. Lancet Infect Dis. 2005;5:361-73.
58. Park MM, Davis AL, Schluger NW, Cohen H, Rom WN. Outcome of MDR-TB patients, 1983–1993. Prolonged survival with appropriate therapy. Am J Respire Crit Care Med. 1996; 158:153:317-24.
59. Finlay AF. Treatment outcomes of patients with multidrug resistant tuberculosis in South Africa using a standardized regimen, 1999–2000 (Poster session 58, N_2101). In: Infectious Disease Society of America Boston, Massachusetts, September 2004.
60. Masjedi MR, Tabarsi P, Baghaei P, et al. Treatment outcomes of extensively drug-resistant tuberculosis: 2 years of surveillance in Iran. Clinical Infectious Disease. 2006;43:841-7.
61. Burgos M. Treatment of multidrug-resistant tuberculosis in San Francisco: an outpatient-based approach. Clinical Infectious Disease. 2005;40:968-75.
62. Waisman JL. Improved prognosis in HIV/AIDS related multi-drug resistant tuberculosis patients treated with highly active antiretroviral therapy, Medicina (B Aires), 2001;61: 810-4.
63. Sahai J. Cautions in the didanosine tabled reduce ciprofloxacin bioavailability. Clinical Pharmacology and Therapeutics. 1993;53:292-7.
64. Center for Disease Control and Prevention (CDC). Managing drug interactions in the treatment of HIV-related tuberculosis [online]. 2007 (available at http://www.cdc.gov/tb/TB_HIV_Drugs/default.htm; accessed may 2008).
65. Guidelines for the programmatic management of drug-resistant tuberculosis—WHO 2008.

Chapter 37

Interaction between Antitubercular and Antiretroviral Drugs

INTRODUCTION

Worldwide, tuberculosis (TB) is one of the most important infectious diseases in subjects with human immunodeficiency virus (HIV) infection. Rifamycin based antituberculosis therapy (ATT) can cure HIV related TB and, where available, the introduction of highly active antiretroviral therapy (HAART) has markedly reduced the incidence of acquired immunodeficency syndrome (AIDS) and death. Although effective therapy is available for both conditions, there are major problems in the concurrent treatment of HIV and TB co-infection. This chapter aims to describe antiretroviral therapy (ART) for the treatment of HIV-infection, pharmacokinetic issues in the treatment of HIV-related tuberculosis and interactions between antitubercular and antireroviral drugs.

ANTIRETROVIRAL THERAPY FOR THE TREATMENT OF HIV INFECTION

Rapid progress in developing ART led in 1996 the introduction of HAART. HAART is a combination of at least three antiretroviral drugs. HAART is the global standard of care in the treatment of HIV infection. Although not a cure for HIV infection, HAART usually results in near-complete suppression of HIV replication. Treatment has to be lifelong. ART results in dramatic reductions in morbidity and mortality in HIV-infected people. There are several requirements for successful use of ART. These include considerable efforts to maintain adherence to lifelong treatment and to monitor response to treatment, drug toxicities and drug interactions.[1]

Antiretroviral Drugs

Antirectroviral drugs belong to following classes:

1. Reverse transcriptase inhibitors (RTIs)
2. Protease inhibitors (PIs)
3. Fusion or entry inhibitors, and
4. Integrase inhibitors.

RTIs are further divided into three groups:

i. Nucleoside reverse transcriptase inhibitors (NsRTIs)
ii. Non-nucleoside reverse transcriptase inhibitors (NNRTIs)
iii. Nucleotide reverse transcriptase inhibitors (NtRTIs).

Nucleoside Reverse Transcriptase Inhibitors (NsRTIs)

NsRTI inhibit reverse transcription by being incorporated into the newly synthesized viral DNA and preventing its further elongation. Drugs available with their toxicities from this group are tabulated in Table 37.1.

Table 37.1: Nucleoside reverse transcriptase inhibitors with their toxicities

Drugs	Abbreviation	Toxicity	Food restriction
Zidovudine	(AZT, ZDV)	Anemia, granulocytopenia, myopathy, lactic acidosis, hepatomegaly with steatosis, headache and nausea	Taken with or without food
Didanosine	(ddl)	Pancreatitis, peripheral neuropathy, abnormalities in liver function tests, lactic acidosis, hepatomegaly with steatosis	Taken on an empty stomach 30 minutes before, or 2 hours after a meal
Stavudine	(D4T)	Peripheral neuropathy, pancreatitis, lactic acidosis, hepatomegaly with steatosis, ascending neuromuscular weakness and lipodystrophy	Taken with or without food
Lamivudine	(3TC)	Headache and dry mouth	Taken with or without food
Zalcitabine	(ddC)	Peripheral neuropathy, pancreatitis, lactic acidosis, hepatomegaly with steatosis and oral ulcers	Taken with or without food
Emtricitabine	(FTC)	Headache, nausea, insomnia, hypertrophy of palms and soles	Taken with or without food
Abacavir	(ABC)	Hypersensitivity reaction (can be fatal); fever, rash, nausea, vomiting, malaise or fatigue, and loss of appetite	Taken with or without food

Nucleotide Reverse Transcriptase Inhibitors

Mechanism of action is similar to NsRTIs, it undergoes diester hydrolysis to form the nucleoside monophosphate tenofovir. Drugs available with their toxicities from this group are tabulated in Table 37.2.

Table 37.2: Nucleotide reverse transcriptase inhibitors with their toxicities

Drug	Abbreviation	Toxicity	Food Restriction
Tenofovir	(TDF)	Potential for renal toxicity	Taken with or without food

Non-nucleoside Reverse Transcriptase Inhibitors

NNRTIs inhibit reverse transcriptase directly by binding to the enzyme and interfering with its function. Drugs available with their toxicities from this group are tabulated in Table 37.3.

Table 37.3: Non-nucleoside reverse transcriptase inhibitors with their toxicities

Drugs	Abbreviation	Toxicity	Food Restriction
Delavirdine	(DLV)	Skin rash, abnormalities in liver function tests	Taken with or without food
Efavirenz	(EFV)	Rash, dysphoria, elevated liver function tests, drowsiness, abnormal dreams, depression	Taken on empty stomach
Nevirapine	(NVP)	Skin rash, hepatotoxicity	Taken with or without food
Etravirine	(ETR)	Elevation in liver function tests	Taken following a meal

Protease Inhibitors

Protease Inhibitors (PTs) target viral assembly by inhibiting the activity of protease, an enzyme used by HIV to cleave nascent proteins for final assembly of new virions. Drugs available with their toxicities from this group are tabulated in Table 37.4.

Fusion or Entry Inhibitors

It interfere with binding, fusion and entry of HIV to the host cell by blocking one of several targets. Drugs available with their toxicities from this group are tabulated in Table 37.5.

Integrase Inhibitors

It inhibit the enzyme integrase, which is responsible for integration of viral DNA into the DNA of the infected cell. Drugs available with their toxicities from this group are tabulated in Table 37.6.

Table 37.4: Protease inhibitors with their toxicities

Drugs	Abbreviation	Toxicity	Food Restriction
Amprenavir	(APV)	Nausea, vomiting, diarrhea, rash, oral paresthesias, elevated liver function tests, hyperglycemia, fat redistribution, lipid abnormalities	Taken with or without food; avoid high fat meals.
Fosamprenavir	(FOS-APV)	Vomiting, elevated liver function tests, hyperglycemia, fat redistribution	Taken with or without food
Atazanavir	(ATV)	Hyperbilirubinemia, PR prolongation, nausea, vomiting, hyperglycemia, fat maldistribution	Taken with food
Darunavir	(DRV)	Diarrhea nausea, headache	Taken with food
Indinavir	(IDV)	Nephrolithiasis, hyperglycemia,fat redistribution, lipid abnormalities, indirect hyperbilirubinemia	Taken on an empty stomach 60 minutes before, or 2 hours after a meal. Avoid taking within an hour of taking didanosine
Lopinavir/Ritonavir	(LPV/RTV)	Diarrhea, hyperglycemia, fat redistribution, lipid abnormalities	
Nelfinavir	(NFV)	Diarrhea, loose stools, hyperglycemia, fat redistribution, lipid abnormalities	Taken with food
Ritonavir	(RTV)	Nausea, abdominal pain, hyperglycemia, fat redistribution, lipid abnormalities, may alter levels of many other drugs, including saquinavir	Taken with food
Saquinavir	(SQV)	Diarrhea, nausea, headaches, hyperglycemia, fat redistribution, lipid abnormalities	Taken within two hours of food
Tipranavir	(TPV)	Nausea, vomiting, diarrhea, elevation in liver function tests, increased total cholesterol and triglyceride, rash and intracranial hemorrhage	Taken with or without food

Table 37.5: Fusion or entry inhibitors with their toxicities

Drugs	Abbreviation	Toxicity	Food Restriction
Maraviroc	(MVC)	Diarrhea, nausea, fatigueness, cough, headache, joint pain, muscle pain, hepatitis	Must be prepared from a powder and injected into thigh, arm or abdomen
Enfuvirtide	(T-20)	Local injection reactions, hypersensitivity reactions, increased rate of bacterial pneumonia	Taken with or without food

Table 37.6: Integrase inhibitors with their toxicities

Drug	Abbreviation	Toxicity	Food Restriction
Raltegravir	RAL	Nausea, diarrhea, elevation in amylases, dizziness, pruritis and rash	Taken with or without food

PHARMACOKINETIC ISSUES IN THE TREATMENT OF HIV-RELATED TUBERCULOSIS

Two pharmacokinetic issues complicate the treatment of HIV-related tuberculosis: the possibility of malabsorption of antituberculosis drugs, and the complex drug-drug interactions. There are conflicting data on whether patients with HIV-related tuberculosis are more prone to malabsorption of antituberculosis drugs than are HIV-uninfected patients. It appears that serum drug concentrations, particularly of rifampin, are somewhat lower in tuberculosis patients with HIV infection and very low CD4 cell count.[2]

INTERACTION BETWEEN ANTIRETROVIRAL AND ANTITUBERCULAR DRUGS

Treatment of TB in the presence of HIV infection is complicated by drug-drug interactions between the rifamycin class of antimycobacterial drugs (rifampin, rifabutin and rifapentine), and the PI and the NNRTI classes of drugs used to treat HIV infection.[3,4] Both PIs and NNRTIs are metabolized by hepatic CYP3A, specifically the CYP3A4 isozyme. Rifamycins are inducers of the CYP3A family of enzymes, which includes the CYP3A4 isozyme. This will adversely affect the ability of the antiretroviral regimen to adequately suppress the virus, which is the goal of antiretroviral treatment regimen.

Rifamycins and Nucleoside/Nucleotide Analogues

Rifamycins are inducers of the CYP3A system but rifampin is not metabolized by this system. Of the three available rifamycins, rifampin is the most potent inducer of CYP3A and rifabutin is the least potent, with rifapentine falling somewhere in between. Rifapentine should not be used for the treatment of TB in HIV-infected individuals because of the increased rate of acquired rifamycin resistance. Rifabutin has been used extensively in the developed world as a substitute for rifampin in the treatment of active TB, outcomes are similar with rifampin or rifabutin. Rifabutin is metabolized by the CYP3A system and there is significant interactions when rifabutin is coadministred with PIs and NNRTIs. Rifabutin dosing has to be adjusted according to the choice of the coadministered antiretroviral.

Rifamycins and Protease Inhibitor

Protease inhibitors (PIs) and the rifamycins have opposite effects on CYP3A family of enzymes in the liver. This causes the following types of drug-drug interactions when PIs are taken together with rifamycins: PI serum concentrations and overall bioavailability may decrease to subtherapeutic levels because rifamycins accelerate the metabolism of PIs by inducing the CYP3 enzymes. Rifampin levels are not affected since it is not metabolized by the CYP3A and rifabutin bioavailability may increase to toxic levels because PIs decrease its metabolism. Rifampicin causes a 75–95% reduction in serum concentrations of PI other than ritonavir. Such reductions lead to loss of antiretroviral activity of PI-containing regimens and consequently can result in the emergence of resistance to one or more of the other drugs in the HAART regimen. Currently, most patients are given combinations of PI, which includes low dose ritonavir (usually 100 mg per dose) in order to take advantage of its enzyme inhibiting properties. In effect ritonavir boosts the concentrations of the other PI allowing easier and more tolerable dosing. Rifabutin can be used with single (unboosted) PI except saquinavir. However, because of the balance between rifabutin induction and protease inhibition of CYP3A4, when this combination is used a modification in the dose of the PI may be required and the dose of rifabutin should be decreased by half to 150 mg.

Rifamycins and Non-nucleoside Reverse Transcriptase Inhibitors

The NNRTIs are all metabolized by the hepatic CYP3A. Therefore, NNRTI levels are adversely affected by the rifamycins. The effect of NNRTIs on the CYP3A is less uniform; delavirdine inhibits the CYP3A, whereas nevirapine and efavirenz induce the CYP3A. Delavirdine should not be used with either rifampin or rifabutin because both rifamycins greatly diminish the levels of delavirdine. Rifampin modestly decreases the efavirenz activity. Therefore, it is probably safe to use rifampin concomitantly with efavirenz at a slightly higher dose (800 mg of efavirenz instead of the usual 600 mg). Efavirenz effectiveness is not significantly affected by rifabutin, but efavirenz does decrease rifabutin bioavailability. Therefore, the rifabutin dosage must be increased (from the usual dosage of 300 mg to a daily dose of 450–600 mg) when it is given with efavirenz. Bioavailability of nevirapine is reduced by rifampin. Rifabutin decreases bioavailabilty of nevirapine and nevirapine also slightly decreases rifabutin bioavailability. Therefore, nevirapine can be used with rifabutin, both at their usual doses.

Rifamycins and Nucleoside Reverse Transcriptase Inhibitors

There is a slight decrease in the level of zidovudine and probably abacavir when coadministered with rifampin. The other NRTIs do not interact significantly with rifamycins. Rifamycins can therefore be included in the anti-TB regimen if a PI- or NNRTI-sparing antiretroviral regimen is chosen. The fusion inhibitor enfuvirtide, is not known to be a substrate for the CYP450 enzymes or to have any effect on the levels of these enzymes and can be used with all anti-TB drugs.

Isoniazid and Antiretroviral Drug Interactions

Pharmacokinetic or clinical interactions between isoniazid and antiretroviral agents have not been extensively studied. In-vitro studies have shown that isoniazid, at clinically relevant concentrations, is a reversible inhibitor of CYP3A4 and CYP2C19, and that it mechanistically inactivates CYP1A2, CYP2A6, CYP2C19 and CYP3A4 in human liver microsomes.[5] Isoniazid, co-administered with drugs such as PI and NNRTI, which are metabolized by these isoforms, may result in significant drug-drug interactions. These interactions might be significant when isoniazid is given alone to treat latent TB infection in an HIV co-infected patient who is receiving PI or NNRTI.

DRUG-DRUG INTERACTIONS IN THE TREATMENT OF HIV AND DRUG RESISTANT-TB (DR-TB)

Currently, little is known about drug-drug interactions between second-line antituberculosis agents and ART. Buffered didanosine contains an aluminium/magnesium-based antacid and, if given jointly with fluoroquinolones, may result in decreased fluoroquinolone absorption; it should be avoided, but if it is necessary, it should be given 6 hours before or 2 hours after fluoroquinolone administration. The enteric coated formulation of didanosine can be used concomitantly without this precaution. Ethionamide/protionamide is thought to be metabolized by the CYP450 system, although it is not known which of the CYP enzymes are responsible. Whether doses of ethionamide/protionamide and/or certain antiretroviral drugs should be modified during the concomitant treatment of DR-TB and HIV is completely unknown.[6] Clarithromycin is a substrate and inhibitor of CYP3A and has multiple drug interactions with protease inhibitors and NNRTIs. If possible, the use of clarithromycin should be avoided in patients coinfected with DR-TB and HIV because of both its weak efficacy against DR-TB and multiple drug interactions.

CONCLUSION

With non-rifamycin containing regimens, drug-drug interactions might be fewer but a non-rifamycin regimen is inferior to a rifampicin-based regimen for the treatment of HIV-related tuberculosis. These should be only contemplated in patients with serious toxicity to rifamycins, where desensitization/reintroduction has failed, or in those with rifamycin-resistant isolates. The various options to reduce drug-drug interactions are: (1) to postpone antiretroviral therapy, (2) to use no PI or NNRTI containing antiretroviral combinations, (3) to use certain PI/ and/or NNRTIs with modification in doses, (4) Efavirenz (EFZ) or saquinavir with ritonavir, without the need to adjust the doses, (5) to use non-rifamycin regimens, e.g. 2SHEZ+10HE.

REFERENCES

1. TB/HIV Clinical manual. second edition. WHO/HTM/TB/2004.329.
2. Corbett EL, Watt CJ, Walker N, et al. The growing burden of tuberculosis: global trends and interactions with the HIV epidemic. Arch Intern Med. 2003;163:1009-21.
3. UNIADS/WHO. AIDS epidemic update: December 2003. UNAIDS/WHO 2003. http://www.unaids.org/wad/2003/epiupdate2003.
4. Sahai J, Gallicano K, Swick L, Tailor S, Garber G, Seguin I, et al. Reduced plasma concentrations of antituberculous drugs in patients with HIV infection. Ann Intern Med. 1997; 127:289–93.
5. Desta Z, Soukhova NV, Flockhart DA. Inhibition of cytochrome P450 (CYP450) by isoniazid: potent inhibition of CYP2C19 and CYP3A. Antimicrob Agents Chemother. 2001;45:382-92.
6. Centers for Disease Control and Prevention (CDC). Managing drug interactions in the treatment of HIV-related tuberculosis. 2007 (available at http :// www .cdc. Gov /tb/ TB_ HIV_ Drugs/default.htm.

Chapter 38

Tuberculosis and Diabetes

INTRODUCTION

Tuberculosis (TB) and diabetes frequently coexist together. Situation becomes precarious for India, where tuberculosis is a public health problem and now also facing the epidemic of diabetes. Diabetic patients are not only more susceptible to tuberculosis but when it occurs, it tend to be more severe. Persons with diabetes mellitus have a risk for developing active TB two to four times greater than persons without diabetes mellitus, and this risk is likely greater in persons with insulin-dependent or poorly controlled diabetes. Also patients with tuberculosis have higher prevalence of diabetes.[1] WHO has projected that the maximum increase in diabetes would occur in India.[2] This chapter aims to describe the diagnosis and treatment of tuberculosis in diabetes.

EPIDEMIOLOGY

Diabetics are at higher risk for tuberculosis, especially insulin dependent patients, in whom risk is about 38 times higher than the general population under 40 years age.[3] The global figure of people with diabetes is projected to rise from the current estimate of 150 million to 220 million in 2010 and 300 million in 2025. The diabetic epidemic, although apparent across the world, has been most pronounced in non-European populations, as evidenced by studies in the native American and Canadian communities, Pacific and Indian Ocean island populations, groups in India and Australian aboriginal communities. The potential for increase in the number of cases of diabetes is greatest in Asia. The 10 years actual risk of acquiring tuberculosis was 24.2% for 116 type I diabetes patients and 4.8% for the rest in one study from Chile.[3] In patients even above 40 years of age, the prevalence of tuberculosis in diabetics is higher. Diabetes accounts for 14.8% (7.1–23.8%) of pulmonary tuberculosis and 20.2% (8.3–41.9%) of smear-positive tuberculosis. Type-2 diabetes in children, teenagers, and adolescents is a serious new aspect to the epidemic and is an emerging public health problem of significant proportions. Prevalence of type 2 diabetes in the adult population of India has been steadily increasing, especially in urban areas from a low of 2.15% reported in early seventies to 13.2% reported in 2000. Prevalence of pulmonary tuberculosis in diabetics was 5.9% in a study conducted in 1989. According to recent study, in 2002 prevalence was 27% (mostly patients were more than 40 years of age). Diabetes makes a substantial contribution to the burden of tuberculosis in India, and the association is particularly strong for the infectious form of tuberculosis. Prevalence of diabetes in patients with pulmonary tuberculosis in India is 9.7% and in males above 40 years of age, it was 17.8% compared with 5.1% in those below 40 years.[4] Onset of diabetes occurs at younger age in India, as well as prevalence of impaired glucose tolerance test is also increasing in India.[4] In Mumbai, tuberculosis was found to be the most common complicating illness (5.9%) in patients with diabetes.[5] The current diabetes epidemic may lead to a resurgence of tuberculosis in endemic regions, especially in urban areas. This potentially carries a risk of global spread with serious implications for tuberculosis control and the achievement of the United Nations Millennium Development Goals.

EFFECT OF DIABETES ON PULMONARY TUBERCULOSIS

It has been observed that rate of infection with *Mycobacterium tuberculosis* is not different though relative risk for developing the disease is 3.5 times higher in patients with diabetes as compared to controls.[6] Prevalence of tuberculin skin test reactivity is almost similar in both diabetics as well as non-diabetics.[7,8] Sputum acid-fast bacilli (AFB) positivity has been variably reported to be higher than usual in patients with diabetes mellitus. The bacteriological conversion rates as well as relapse rates after antitubercular treatment have been found to be similar for TB patients with and without diabetes. The cause of an increased susceptibility of diabetic patients to develop TB is still not known. It has been postulated that Human Leukocyte Antigen HLA-DRB[1]*09 allele was found to increase the susceptibility towards pulmonary TB whereas HLA-DQB[1]*05 allele was observed to be protective for TB in patients with diabetes mellitus. Various factors has been attributed for the high association of diabetes with tuberculosis, e.g. low opsonic index, decreased bactericidal activity, decreased synthesis of collagen, impaired defensive function of reticulo endothelial cell, increased availability of glycerol in tissue that act as substrate for growth of *Mycobacterium tuberculosis* bacilli, lack of adequate substrate for antibody formation due to disturbed protein metabolism and lowered production of IL-1 β and TNF-α by peripheral blood monocytes. It can be the non-enzymatic glycosylation of tissue proteins inducing an alteration in connective tissue in diabetes mellitus. Diabetic autonomic neuropathy leading to abnormal basal airway tone due to an alteration in vagal pathways and thus cause a reduced bronchial reactivity and bronchodilation is also considered as one of the probable causes. However, a recent study[9] on rats, shown that there is no significant difference in phagocytosis of tuberculosis bacilli by alveolar macrophages in diabetic and non-diabetic rats, but in diabetic rats alveolar macrophages were not fully activated by *M. tuberculosis* infection.

EFFECT OF PULMONARY TUBERCULOSIS ON DIABETES

While diabetics are at increased risk of developing tuberculosis, a converse association has also been observed, i.e there is a high prevalence of diabetes mellitus and impaired glucose tolerence test in patients with tuberculosis and after antitubercular treatment, normalization of glucose intolerance occur up to 50%.[10] Various studies have been conducted in order to establish this association but the results were not comparable due to variability in diagnostic criteria of diabetes mellitus in earlier decades. However, after introduction of standard diagnostic criteria for diabetes mellitus by World Health Organization (WHO), it became approachable to estimate prevalence of the disease in patients suffering from tuberculosis. One study performed in over 506 tuberculosis patients reported a prevalence rate of 4% for diabetes mellitus and 16.2% for impaired glucose tolerance which are respectively two times and four times higher as compared to that of general population.[11] Another study reported glucose intolerance in 49% of TB patients of which 29% were having impaired glucose tolerance and remaining 20% were having diabetes mellitus.[10] Approximately half of these patients were having normal blood glucose levels after antituberculosis treatment (ATT). No association has been established with age, family history, ethnicity and duration of treatment. Many postulates have been suggested to explain the increased prevalence of diabetes in tubercular patients such as malnutrition and low body mass index (BMI) in developing countries. Occult glucose intolerance predisposes to TB infection. Tuberculosis of pancreas can be another reason though it is a rare phenomenon. Stress can induce diabetes mellitus in patients suffering from chronic illnesses such as tuberculosis. Abnormalities of glucose intolerance in TB patients can be corrected with ATT.

CLINICAL FEATURES AND COURSE OF TUBERCULOSIS IN DIABETICS

Tuberculosis in diabetics are more often due to reactivation of old foci rather than through fresh infection, with a risk of 2–6 times higher than in patients without diabetes. Clinical symptoms and presentation of pulmonary TB are similar in patients with and without diabetes mellitus. Effectively treated diabetics are no more liable for tuberculosis infection than non-diabetics.

Patients with diabetes who develop tuberculosis have higher blood glucose level and higher complication rates such as coma and microangiopathy. It has been suggested that TB occurs predominantly in lower lobes with frequent cavitary lesions in diabetic patients. On the other hand, patients with tuberculosis who develop diabetes have greater clinical severity at the time of onset, a greater degree of lung involvement and residual changes. However, presenting features of pulmonary tuberculosis are not affected by diabetes. Greater severity and poor prognosis in tuberculosis patients with diabetes can be attributed to delay in diagnosis as both diseases share common symptoms such as anorexia, lassitude and weight loss. There is no evidence that treatment of active tuberculosis in patients with diabetes is less effective than it is in patients without diabetes.[12]

ROENTGENOGRAPHIC ASPECTS OF TUBERCULOSIS IN DIABETICS

Radiographic findings have been described as both typical and atypical in patients with concomitant tuberculosis and diabetes. While there are some studies that have shown that lower lung field involvement is an uncommon location of pulmonary tuberculosis in diabetics.[13-15] Most of studies suggest, there is increased frequency of lower and lower plus upper lung field lesion, cavitation, multiple cavitations, and lower zone cavitations in diabetics as compared with patients with tuberculosis alone[16] (Figs 38.1 and 38.2). Evaluation of CT features of TB in immunocompromized and diabetics when compared with patients having no underlying disease, revealed similar results regarding cavitation but not for lower lung field involvement,[17] i.e. unusual location including basal segment of lower lobe, anterior segment

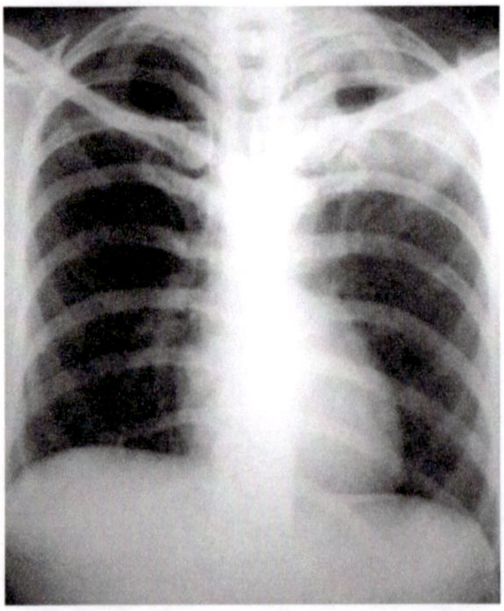

Fig. 38.1: Chest X-ray showing pulmonary tuberculosis (Sputum positive) with diabetes mellitus

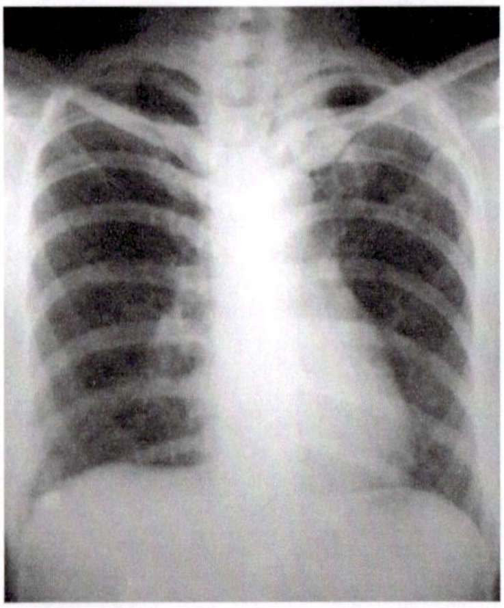

Fig. 38.2: Chest X-ray showing response after ATT and antidiabetic treatment

of upper lobe or right middle lobe occurred equally in both the group (17% and 18%), but a higher prevalence of cavitation (44%) has been reported. Another detailed study in India has shown that CT findings in pulmonary tuberculosis in diabetics differ from those without diabetes. Patients with diabetes have a higher incidence of consolidation with associated loss of volume, nonsegmental distribution of disease and multiple small cavities in any given lesion.[18]

MULTIDRUG RESISTANT TUBERCULOSIS (MDR-TB) AND DIABETES

Earlier study had shown that the proportion of cases of MDR-TB was significantly higher in patients with coexisting diabetes,[17] however recent study revealed that diabetic tuberculosis patients do not have an increased risk of mycobacterial drug resistance and drug resistance to first-line antitubercular drugs was not found to be associated with diagnosis or duration of diabetes.[19]

EFFECT OF ANTITUBERCULOSIS DRUGS ON BLOOD GLUCOSE LEVEL AND OHA IN TUBERCULAR DIABETICS

Rifampicin, a powerful enzyme inducer of hepatic microsomal enzyme system and frequently interact with antidiabetic drugs, i.e. it lowers the serum level and plasma half life of sulfonylureas and biguanides.[20] Rifampicin can also cause early hyperglycemia in non-diabetic patients with or without tuberculosis. Isoniazid, another primary line drug, antagonizes sulfonylureas and impair insulin release and INH rarely causes pancreatitis and may interfere with carbohydrate absorption. Overdose of INH may also cause hypoglycemia. Biguanides and sulfonylureas are contraindicated in hepatic disease, which is a common side effect of antitubercular therapy. Rarely diabetes may be difficult to control in patients on pyrazinamide. Ethionamide may cause hypoglycemia on rare occasions. The side effects of antitubercular treatment do not differ in patients with and without diabetes except peripheral neuropathy which is more common in diabetics.

PRINCIPLES OF MANAGEMENT[21,22]

Because of higher prevalence of diabetes or impaired glucose tolerance test (GTT), few authors argue that all patients of pulmonary tuberculosis should be subjected for screening for diabetes. In case of diabetes, however it is clear that every diabetic patient with chest symptoms, increased insulin requirement or increased weight loss should be evaluated for pulmonary tuberculosis. All diabetics require regular medical examination and preferably bi-annual chest radiograph. This should be followed more rigorously in patients who are more than 40 years of age or with weight less than 10% of the ideal body weight. Any diabetic who suddenly develops cough, loss of weight, abnormal chest radiograph or needs increasing doses of insulin to control blood glucose should be investigated for presence of tuberculosis. Patients with poor diabetic control should be hospitalized for stabilizing their blood sugar level. Glycemic equilibrium is essential for the success of ATT and must be achieved in every patient having pulmonary tuberculosis with diabetes mellitus. The goals of therapy are to maintain fasting plasma glucose < 120 mg% and glycosylated Hb < 7%. In moderate and severe diabetes, ideally insulin should be used to control blood glucose level along with high calorie and high protein diet (if not otherwise contraindicated) to counteract negative nitrogen balance and also carbohydrates should not be unduly restricted. It has been shown by various studies that diet does not play an important part as an adjunct in the treatment of tuberculosis as it was in the prechemotherapy period. Higher caloric nourishing diet is still advocated by some of the physicians usually because of the traditional belief. Diet being an important feature in the treatment of diabetes and should be based on the caloric requirement of the individual depending upon the nature of his work. Diet should not be liberal even though containing all the nutrients. Oral hypoglycemics should be used only in cases of mild diabetes. It is stated that physician should ensure that diabetes is effectively controlled by oral antidiabetic drugs failing which, insulin should be used. Biguanides as well as sulfonylureas are contraindicated in hepatic disease, which is a common adverse effect of antitubercular therapy. Marked weight loss, increasing age, longer duration of diabetes mellitus, higher insulin and caloric needs in tuberculosis are other important indications for withholding oral antidiabetic therapy in diabetes mellitus. Drug interaction with rifampicin should be kept in mind. Insulin requirements may be increased in patients of tuberculosis with diabetes mellitus taking rifampicin. Rifampicin accelerates the metabolism of oral hypoglycemic agents, as it is a potent hepatic enzyme-inducing agent. It was also known to cause early hyperglycemia in non-diabetic patients with or without pulmonary tuberculosis, and also to augment intestinal absorption of glucose. Isoniazid antagonizes sulfonylureas and impairs insulin release and action, and rifampicin shortens the plasma half-life of sulfonylureas. Vigorous and good chemotherapy is essential. Monitoring for adverse effects, particularly of hepatic and nervous systems should be done. Use of potentially neuropathic agents such as isoniazid in patients with peripheral neuropathy demands special consideration with mandatory administration of pyridoxine. Duration of chemotherapy is entirely dependent upon the control of diabetes and response of the patient to treatment. A longer treatment course may be needed. Tuberculosis Research Center in Chennai has reported encouraging results in the treatment of new smear-positive pulmonary tuberculosis patients with concomitant type II non-insulin dependent diabetes mellitus and have shown that the category

I regimen is adequate for the treatment of such patients.[23] Supportive therapy for diabetes must be actively pursued. Uncontrolled diabetes may be indirectly responsible for the spread of tuberculosis.

REFERENCES

1. Nicols GP. Diabetes among young tuberculosis patients. Am Rev Tuber 1957;76:10-6.
2. King H, Aubert RE, Herman WH. Global burden of diabetes, 1995–2025: prevalence, numerical estimates, and projections. Diabetes Care.1998;21:1414-31.
3. Olmos P, Donoso J, Rojas N, Landeros P, Schurmann R, Retamal G, et al. Tuberculosis and diabetes mellitus: a longitudinal-retrospective study in a teaching hospital Rev Med Chil. 1989;117:979-83.
4. Ramachandran A, Snehalatha C, Viswanathan V. Burden of type-2 diabetes and its complications-the Indian scenario.Current Science. 2002;83;1471-6.
5. Patel JC. Complications in 8793 cases of diabetes mellitus 14 years study in Bombay Hospital. Ind J Med Sci. 1989;43:177-83.
6. Kim SJ, Hong YP, Lew WJ, Yang SC, Lee EG. Incidence of pulmonary tuberculosis among diabetics. Tuber Lung Dis. 1995;76:529-33.
7. Garcia PH, Cruz MF, Martinez CT. PPD and chemoprophylaxis in diabetes mellitus. Aten Primaria. 1992;9:106-8.
8. Kameda K, Kawabata S, Masuda N. Follow-up study of short course chemotherapy for Tuberculosis complicated with Diabetes mellitus. Kekkaku. 1990;65:791-803.
9. Sugawara I, Yamada H, Mizuno S. Pulmonary tuberculosis in spontaneously diabetic Go to Kakizaki Rats. Tohoku J. Exp. Med. 2004;204:135-45.
10. Jawad F, Shera AS, Memon R, Ansari G. Glucose intolerance in pulmonary tuberculosis. J Pak Med Assoc. 1995;45;237-8.
11. Mugusi F, Swai AB, Alberti KB, Mclarty DG. Increased prevalence of diabetes mellitus in patients with pulmonary tuberculosis in Tanzania. Tubercle. 1990;71:271-6.
12. Rose DN, Silver AL, Schecter CB. Tuberculosis chemoprophylaxis for diabetics: Are the benefits worth the risk? Mt Sinai J Med. 1985;52:253-6.
13. Berger H. Lower lung field tuberculosis. Chest. 1974;65:522-6.
14. Morris JT, Seaworth BJ, McAllister CK. Pulmonary tuberculosis in diabetics. Chest. 1992;102: 539-41.
15. Prasad R, Verma SK, Pathak SK, Agarwal CG, Ahuja RC. Clinicoradiological study of pulmonary tuberculosis in diabetes mellitus: A comparative study. JIMA 2006;9:99-103.
16. Ezung T, Devi NT, Singh NT, Singh TB. Pulmonary tuberculosis and Diabetes-a study. J Indian Med Assoc. 2002;100:376,378-9.
17. Bashar M, Alcabes P, Rom W, Condos R. Increased incidence of multidrug-resistant tuberculosis in diabetic patients on the bellevue chest service, 1987 to 1997. Chest. 2001;120;1514-9.
18. Khanna S, Sharma VK. CT findings in active pulmonary tuberculosis: comparison between diabetic and non-diabetic patients. Indian journal of Radiology and Imaging. 1997;7:87-90.
19. Subhash HS, Ashwin I, Mukundan U, et al. Tuberculosis and diabetes mellitus; a problematic association. India Trop Doct. 2003;33:154-6.
20. Acocella G, Canti R. Interaction of rifampicin with other drugs. Tubercle. 1980;61:171-7.
21. Shah A. Tuberculosis and diabetes. Ann Indian Med Assoc. 1991;554-5.
22. Report of the Expert Committee on the diagnosis and classification of diabetes mellitus. Diabetes Care. 1997;20:1183-97.
23. Clinical research: Overview of the activities of chemotherapy division. Annual report: Tuberculosis Research Center, Chennai. 2003–2004.

Chapter 39

Tuberculosis and Pregnancy

INTRODUCTION

The diagnosis of tuberculosis in pregnancy is of utmost importance to both the mother and fetus since untreated disease carries much greater risk to both, and represents a greater hazard to a pregnant woman and her fetus than does its treatment. Tuberculosis is a major health problem all over the world. One third of the world's population and approximately 50% of Indian adults are infected with *Mycobacterium tuberculosis.*[1,2] Considering the high prevalence of this disease in many developing countries including India, a large number of pregnant women can be expected to suffer from tuberculosis. There is no national statistics available regarding incidence of TB in pregnant women. It is expected that the incidence of tuberculosis among pregnant women would be as high as in general population. The clinical and laboratory diagnosis, and therapy during pregnancy and post-partum period, deserve special attention. Untreated pulmonary tuberculosis in pregnant women would be a definite risk for transmission of disease to the newborn. Limitations in the diagnosis of tuberculosis during pregnancy, safety of antituberculosis therapy (ATT) and the need for prophylaxis must be in the knowledge of all the physicians giving care to pregnant women. This chapter aims to describe effect of tuberculosis on pregnancy, diagnosis and treatment of tuberculosis in pregnancy and postpartum period.

EFFECT OF PREGNANCY ON TUBERCULOSIS

Before the age of effective chemotherapy, the role of pregnancy in the reactivation and progression of TB was intensely debated. Schaefer, in 1975, demonstrated that the rate of progression of TB was not significantly different in pregnant women as compared to non-pregnant controls.[3] By the middle of the twentieth century, there was an increased concern regarding the progression of TB in the postpartum period. It was thought that the descent of the diaphragm after parturition leads to changes in the intrathoracic pressure accompanied by hormonal fluctuations, nutritional deprivation and altered immunity leading to increased susceptibility to pulmonary tuberculosis.[4,5]

EFFECT OF TUBERCULOSIS ON PREGNANCY AND CHILDBIRTH

With the advent of effective chemotherapy, most studies have demonstrated that tuberculosis does not increase complications of childbirth.[6,7] There is no statistically significant increase in congenital malformations in children born to mothers with tuberculosis though prematurity, fetal growth retardation, low birth weight and increased perinatal mortality have been commonly reported.[8] The clinical presentation of tuberculosis in the pregnant women is similar to that in the non-pregnant patients. Cough, weight loss, fever, fatigue and hemoptysis are the usual features. Other features such as lethargy, abdominal distension, irritability and skin lesions may also be seen.[9] Extrapulmonary tuberculosis is also fairly common and has been observed in 20% of cases.[10] Lymphadenitis is the most common form of extrapulmonary tuberculosis reported and has no adverse effect on the maternal and fetal outcome. Other forms of extrapulmonary tuberculosis such as intestinal, spinal, endometrial and meningeal tuberculosis are associated with an increased frequency of maternal disability, fetal growth retardation and infants with low apgar scores.[11] Patients coinfected with HIV have a greater incidence of extrapulmonary tuberculosis. HIV-infected pregnant women who are suspected of having TB should be treated without delay. Multidrug resistant tuberculosis (MDR-TB) should be as common during pregnancy as in the nonpregnant patients although this is not documented. However, pregnant mothers with MDR-TB have increased risk of neonatal complications and the mother herself has more advanced disease with more extensive radiographic changes and longer sputum conversion times.

DIAGNOSIS OF TUBERCULOSIS IN PREGNANT WOMAN

A careful history is mandatory in high-risk cases in the antenatal period. History of exposure and symptoms should be obtained and in case of suspicion a tuberculin skin test should be carried out. If tuberculin skin test is greater than 10 mm of induration, a chest radiograph should be obtained in a symptomatic patient with proper abdominal screening (shielding). In an asymptomatic patient, the chest radiograph should be delayed until the 12th week of gestation. Routine screening with radiography is not indicated because of low yield and possible hazards. There has been some debate in literature about the sensitivity of tuberculin test during pregnancy and earlier reports suggested that tuberculin sensitivity might be diminished in pregnancy.[12] However, well-controlled trials have found no significant difference.[13] Tuberculin test is deemed a safe and useful method for screening tuberculosis infection in pregnancy and should be used in women with symptoms and signs of tuberculosis. Pregnant women with diabetes or HIV, women employed in hospitals, old age homes, prisoners and those belonging to low socioeconomic status are other candidates for tuberculin test. Women who are infected with HIV may have a diminished or negative tuberculin reaction and therefore an area of 5 mm or greater induration in an HIV positive patient is considered positive.[14]

TREATMENT OF PREGNANT WOMAN WITH ACTIVE TUBERCULOSIS

The indications for treatment of active tuberculosis in pregnant women are the same as for a non-pregnant woman. Treatment should be initiated without delay. Review of published data reveals that INH is safe during pregnancy. Although, it crosses the placental barrier, it is not teratogenic even when administered in the first trimester.[15] Only 1% incidence of abnormalities was reported in infants of mothers treated with INH, which falls below the 1.2–6% incidence of fetal malformations cited in the population at large. The rate of congenital malformations in infants who received rifampicin was 3.35% in a study and included limb reduction, CNS lesions and hemorrhagic complications postulated to be due to inhibition of DNA dependent RNA polymerase.[15] However, the incidence falls within the safety limits and hence rifampicin is also considered to be safe. Ethambutol is the next commonly used drug in pregnancy with an incidence of malformations reported at two percent. Although, it was feared that ethambutol might interfere with ophthalmological development, this was not observed in doses of 15–25 mg/kg body weight/day.[15] Pyrazinamide, the bactericidal drug used in most first-line regimens, does not have sufficient studies to ensure its safety during pregnancy. Although some international organizations recommend its use, it may be avoided due to inadequate data on teratogenecity.[14] Streptomycin has been proved to be potentially teratogenic throughout pregnancy causing fetal malformations and eighth nerve paralysis with deficits ranging from mild hearing loss to bilateral deafness. Other aminoglycosides including kanamycin, amikacin and capreomycin are also contraindicated during pregnancy. TB treatment regimens for HIV-infected pregnant women should include a rifamycin. Although, the routine use of PZA during pregnancy is not recommended in the United States, the benefits of a TB treatment regimen that includes PZA for HIV-infected pregnant women outweigh the undetermined potential risks to the fetus.

Treatment of multidrug-resistant tuberculosis (MDR-TB) in pregnancy is controversial. Little is known, about the safety of the drugs used to treat MDR-TB during pregnancy. There were no existing guidelines for the treatment of pregnant women with drug resistant tuberculosis and it has been suggested that elective abortion may be considered while treating a pregnant women with MDR-TB.[16] Some recent studies have evaluated the treatment of MDR-TB during pregnancy with second line drugs and found no evidence of significant late-presentation toxicity among the children. Other studies have also found that neither obstetrical complications nor perinatal transmission of MDR-TB was observed. The results suggest that aggressive management of MDR-TB may benefit both mother and child.[17] Under certain circumstances, MDR-TB can be successfully treated during pregnancy.[18] Currently, pregnancy is no longer considered to be a contraindication for treatment of active drug resistant TB, which poses great risks to the lives of both mother and fetus. However, birth control is strongly recommended for all non-pregnant women receiving therapy for drug resistant TB because of the potential consequences for both mother and fetus resulting from frequent and severe adverse drug reactions. Pregnant patients should be carefully evaluated, taking into consideration gestational age and severity of the MDR-TB. The treatment should be initiated in second trimester or sooner if condition of patient is severe as majority of teratogenic effects occur in first trimester. When therapy is started, three or four oral drugs with demonstrated efficacy against the infecting strain should be used and then an injectable agent and possibly other drugs must be added immediately postpartum. Injectable agents should be avoided to prevent fetal ototoxicity but capreomycin can be used if an injectable agent cannot be avoided.Ethionamide should be avoided in pregnancy because of high emetogenic property in pregnancy and risk of teratogenicity.

TREATMENT OF TUBERCULOSIS IN LACTATING WOMAN

The safety of breastfeeding is an important issue. Several studies have measured the concentration of ATT drugs in breast milk.[19-22] There is consensus that breastfeeding should not be discouraged. ATT drugs should be taken preferably after breastfeeding and the next feed could be replaced with a bottle feed. Drug concentration in breast milk is low and has no therapeutic value and is not an effective treatment for TB disease or latent infection in a nursing infant. If both the mother and infant are taking isoniazid (INH), the drug may reach supratherapeutic doses and in such circumstances bottle-feeding is recommended. Supplemental pyridoxine should be administered to an infant on INH or if the breastfeeding mother is taking INH because pyridoxine deficiency may cause seizures in the newborn. A woman who is breastfeeding with active MDR-TB should receive a full course of antituberculosis treatment timely and properly as it is the best way to prevent transmission of tubercle bacilli to her baby. The mother and her baby should not be completely separated. However, if the mother is sputum smear-positive, the care of the infant should be left to family members until she becomes sputum smear-negative, if this is feasible. When the mother and infant are together, this common time should be spent in well-ventilated areas or outdoors.

ISONIAZID PROPHYLAXIS IN PREGNANT WOMAN

Preventive therapy with INH is highly effective and there is no teratogenic risk in pregnant women treated with standard dosages (Maximum dose 300 mg/day) for 6–12 months. However, there is a significant risk of hepatotoxicity, which is more during the postpartum period.[23] In view of the same, all the pregnant women to be put on INH prophylaxis should have baseline liver function tests before starting prophylactic therapy and the same should be repeated every month and as when symptoms suggestive of hepatitis develop. Pyridoxine should be given to these women to decrease the risk of INH induced neuropathy.[24] It is recommended that in pregnant women with positive tuberculin test, therapy with INH should be delayed until after delivery if the chest radiograph is normal. However in certain situations, it is advisable to give INH prophylaxis during pregnancy. These include: (a) Recent converters: If there is documented tuberculin conversion within preceeding 2 years. This is based on the fact that chances of a person with tuberculin conversion developing active tuberculosis are maximum during the first 2 years. (b) Close contacts of person with active tuberculosis. (c) If the woman is immunocompromized (e.g. HIV seropositivity). In the areas with high endemicity for tuberculosis, the tuberculin positivity in general population is high. For example, in India approximately 50% of adult population is tuberculin positive. Therefore, in such areas tuberculin positivity should not be taken as indication for INH prophylaxis. However, in the event of a documented recent tuberculin conversion and/or a recent exposure to close contact with active tuberculosis and immunosuppression would be indications for INH prophylaxis. The usual dose of INH is 5 mg/kg body weight with a maximum dose of 300 mg/day.

ISONIAZID PROPHYLAXIS FOR INFANT BORN TO WOMAN WITH ACTIVE TUBERCULOSIS

Tuberculin positive mother without active tuberculosis does not pose any risk to the newborn. Also, if a pregnant woman with active pulmonary tuberculosis is sputum negative during the last 3 months of gestation, the risk to infant is negligible. However, if the mother is not documented to be sputum negative or if she is sputum positive, then the infant needs evaluation for active tuberculosis with chest radiograph and examination of gastric aspirate or sputum for AFB. If there is no evidence of active tuberculosis, the infant should receive INH prophylaxis for 3 months until after the mother's sputum becomes negative for AFB and the baby is tuberculin negative. If the infant is tuberculin positive then INH prophylaxis should be given for a total period of 6 months after ruling out active tuberculosis.[25] There is a recommendation that if the mother is suffering from MDR-TB, then INH prophylaxis has no role and hence should not be given. In such cases, the infant should receive BCG vaccination. BCG vaccination has been shown to have a protective effect.[26-28] In countries with high TB prevalence, WHO recommends a policy of routine BCG immunization for all neonates. WHO recommended policy depends on the TB prevalence in a particular country. In a country with high TB prevalence, the possible benefits of BCG immunization outweigh the possible disadvantages. WHO has recommended BCG vaccination for all children except those having symptoms of HIV disease in countries with high TB prevalence whereas it should not be given to HIV-infected children in countries with low prevalence of TB.

CONCLUSION

Thus, it is important to make an early diagnosis of tuberculosis infection and disease in a pregnant woman. Tuberculosis in pregnancy is as common as in the non-pregnant women. Better results are obtained in women known to have tuberculosis before the onset of pregnancy and who have been treated, as compared to untreated patients with active tuberculosis. The poorest results have been shown to occur in patients in whom tuberculosis is first discovered in the puerperium, since it has been unsuspected and untreated during pregnancy and the disease is generally well-advanced. If tuberculosis is diagnosed and treated appropriately, the prognosis for both the mother and child is excellent.

REFERENCES

1. World Health Organization. WHO report 2009. Global tuberculosis control: epidemiology, strategy, financing. WHO/HTM/ TB/2009.411. Geneva:World Health Organization; 2009.
2. Chakraborty AK. Epidemiology of tuberculosis: current status in India. India J Med Res. 2004;120:248-75.
3. Schaefer G, Zervoudakis I, Fuchs F, et al. Pregnancy and pulmonary tuberculosis. Obstet Gynaecol. 1975;45:706-15.
4. Cohen JD, Patton EA, Badger TL. The tuberculous mother. Am Rev Respir Dis. 1952;65:1-23.
5. Rosen bach LM, Gangemi CR. Tuberculosis and pregnancy. JAMA 1956;161:1035-8.
6. Lowe C. Congenital defect among childrenborn to women under supervision or treatmentfor pulmonary tuberculosis. Br J Prev Soc Med. 1964;18:14-6.
7. Greeneville-Mathers R. Tuberculous primary nfection in pregnancy and its relation to congenital tuberculosis. Tubercle. 1960;41:181-5.

8. Jana N, Vasista K, Jindal SK, Khunnu B, Ghosh K. Perinatal outcome in pregnancies complicated by pulmonary tuberculosis. Int J Gynaecol Obstet 1994;44:119-24.
9. Good JT (Jr), Iseman MD, Davidson PT, Lakshminarayan S, Sahn SA. Tuberculosis in association with pregnancy. Am J Obstet Gynaecol 1981;140:492-8.
10. Wilson E. Thelin T, Dilts P. Tuberculosis complicated by pregnancy. Am J Obstet Gynaecol. 1972;115:526-31.
11. Jana N, Vasishta K, Saha SC, Ghosh K. Obstetrical outcomes among women with extrapulmonary tuberculosis. N Engl J Med. 1999;341:645-9.
12. Finn R, St Hill C, Grovan A, et al. Immunological responses in pregnancy and survival of fetal homograft. BMJ. 1972;3:150-2.
13. Present P, Comstock GW. Tuberculin sensitivity in pregnancy. Am Rev Respir Dis. 1975;112:413-6.
14. Bass JB (Jr), Farer LS, Hopewell PC, et al.Treatment of tuberculosis and tuberculosis infection in adults and children. Am J Respir Crit Care Med. 1994;149:1359-74.
15. Snider DE (Jr), Layde P, Johnson M, et al. Treatment of tuberculosis during pregnancy. Am Rev Respir Dis. 1980;122:65-79.
16. Good J, Iseman M, Davidson P, et al. Tuberculosis in association with pregnancy. Am J Obstet Gynecol. 1981;140:492-8.
17. Drobac PC, del Castillo H, Sweetland A, Anca G, Joseph JK, Furin J, et al. Treatment of multidrug-resistant tuberculosis during pregnancy: long-term follow-up of 6 children with intrauterine exposure to second-line agents. Clin Infect Dis. 2005;40(11):1689-92.
18. Shin S, Guerra D, Rich M, Seung KJ, Mukherjee J, Joseph K, et al. Treatment of multidrug-resistant tuberculosis during pregnancy: a report of 7 cases. Clin Infect Dis. 2003;36(8):996-1003.
19. Berlin C, Lee C. Isoniazid and acetyl isoniazid disposition in human milk, saliva and plasma. Fed Proc. 1979;38:426.
20. Vorherr H. Drug excretion in breast milk. Postgrad Med J. 1974;56:97-104.
21. Fujimori H, Imai S. Studies on dihydro-streptomycin administered to the pregnant and transferred to their fetuses. Jpn Obstet Gynecol Soc. 1957;4:133-49.
22. Snider DE (Jr), Powell K. Should women taking antituberculous drugs breast feed? Arch Intern Med. 1984;144:589-90.
23. Moulding TS, Redeker AG, Kanel GC. Twenty isoniazid associated deaths in one state. Am Rev Respir Dis. 1989;140:700-5.
24. Snider DE L (Jr), Caras CJ. Isoniazid-associated hepatitis deaths: A review of available information. Am Rev Respir Dis. 1992;145:494-7.
25. Central TB Division, New Delhi. Tuberculosis: A Guide for Practicing Physicians. Revised National Tuberculosis Control Programme. Central TB Division, Directorate General of Health Services, Nirman Bhawan, New Delhi.
26. Kendig E. The place of BCG vaccination in the management of infants born of tuberculous mothers. N Engl J Med. 1969;281:520-3.
27. Curtis H, Leck I, Bamford F. Incidence of childhood tuberculosis after neonatal BCG vaccination. Lancet 1984;1:145-8.
28. Young T, Hershfield E. A case-control study to evaluate effectiveness of mass neonatal BCG vaccination among Canadian Indians. Am J Public Health. 1986;76:783-6.

Chapter 40

Tubercular Pleural Effusion

INTRODUCTION

It is an inflammatory condition of visceral as well as parietal pleura due to presence and growth of *Mycobacterium tuberculosis*. In all cases, effusion is due to actual infection of the pleura by tubercle bacilli, though tuberculin hypersensitivity probably plays a part in potentiating the reaction. It is characterized by the formation of fluid in pleural cavity and associated with local or constitutional symptoms. The diagnosis of tuberculous effusion should be considered in any patient with an exudative pleural effusion, especially in regions where tuberculosis is endemic. A pleural effusion as an isolated manifestation of tuberculosis (TB) is self-limiting and of little immediate concern, but may lead to serious disease many years later. Almost, all case are caused by *M. tuberculosis*, but a few cases have been reported to be caused by MOTT (mycobacteria other than tuberculosis) and *M. bovis*.[1] This chapter aims to describe pathogenesis, diagnosis and treatment of tubercular pleural effusion.

EPIDEMIOLOGY

Incidence of tubercular pleural effusion is increasing in West due to the HIV epidemic.[2] It is the most common cause of exudative pleural effusion in India. Though earlier considered to be a disease of children and young adults, there is an upward shift in age spectrum. Both sexes are equally affected.

PATHOGENESIS

Pleural effusion occurs as a manifestation of TB in four situations. It can occur as part of primary tuberculosis in children, when a peripheral foci or caseous lymph node ruptures into pleural cavity. This usually occurs 3–6 months after primary infection. This disease is usually self-limiting leaving only the evidence of primary complex. It can also occur in adolescents and young adults with acute pleuritic pain and fever. This presentation is also self-limiting without treatment, but upto two third of them develop active pulmonary tuberculosis in 5 years. A third manifestation is due to rupture of tubercular cavity in a patient with post-primary tuberculosis. This usually leads to a tuberculous pyopneumothorax. Another cause of tubercular effusion is disseminated tuberculosis in patients with AIDS. Spread from tubercular osteitis of ribs or from paravertebral abscess associated with TB of thoracic spine can also cause effusion.[3]

In tubercular effusion, there is a significant decrease in lymphatic outflow from pleura which leads to accumulation of proteins in the pleural fluid.[4-5] Inflammatory response is thought to obstruct the lymphatic outflow. Delayed hypersensitivity plays a large role in the pathogenesis of tuberculous pleural effusion. The hypersensitivity reaction is initiated when tuberculous protein gains access to the pleural space. The neutrophil appears to play a key role in the development of experimental tuberculous effusion. The neutrophils in the pleural space appear to secrete a monocyte chemotaxin that recruits monocytes to the pleural space and thereby contributes to the formation of granulomas.[6] Macrophages predominate in the pleural fluid from day 2–5 days.[6] It has been shown that mesothelial cells stimulated with BCG or interferon-gamma produce macrophage inflammatory protein and monocyte chemotactic peptide.[7] These two proteins account for more than 75% of the mononuclear chemotactic factor in tuberculous pleural fluid.[7] After this period, lymphocytes are the predominant cells in the pleural fluid.[8] Probably delayed hypersensitivity also plays a large role in the development of tuberculous pleural effusions in humans. The mycobacterial cultures of the pleural fluid from most patients with tuberculous pleural effusions are negative.[9-11] T lymphocytes specifically sensitized to tuberculous protein are present in the pleural fluid.[12] There is an increased percentage of specifically sensitized lymphocytes in the pleural fluid.[12] Tuberculous pleural effusions are enriched with many potentially immunoreactive cells and substances that comprise the vigorous local cell-mediated immune response.[13] Compared with peripheral blood, pleural fluid is enriched with T lymphocytes. The CD4 (helper-inducer) to CD8 (suppressor/cytotoxic) ratio is 3:4 in pleural fluid, compared with 1:7 in blood.[13] Pleural fluid lymphocytes from patients with tuberculous effusion show greater responsiveness to tuberculin than do peripheral blood lymphocytes.[14]

CLINICAL MANIFESTATIONS

Although TB is usually considered a chronic illness, tuberculous effusion most commonly manifests as an acute illness. Upto 62% patients have an acute onset of symptoms.[15] In one study, 35% had initial symptoms of less than 1 week in duration, whereas 70% had been symptomatic for less than a month.[16] Most patients have a cough, usually nonproductive, and most have chest pain, usually pleuritic in nature.[15,17,18] If both cough and pleuritic chest pain are present, the pain usually precedes the cough. Most patients are febrile, but a normal temperature does not rule out the diagnosis. Occasionally, the onset of TB is less acute, with only mild chest pain, perhaps with a low-grade fever and a non-productive cough, weight loss, and easy fatigability. In general, patients with tuberculous effusion are younger than patients with parenchymal TB. The mean age is 28 years.[19] Patients with pleural effusions secondary to reactivation tend to be older than those with post-primary pleural effusion.[17]

CLINICAL MANIFESTATIONS IN HIV POSITIVE PATIENTS

The clinical manifestations of pleural TB tend to be somewhat different in the HIV-positive patient. One might anticipate that the incidence of tuberculous effusion would be relatively low in patients with AIDS and TB because the patient with AIDS has a compromised immunologic system, and pleural TB is thought to be due to hypersensitivity. However, overall it appears that the incidence of pleural effusions is higher in patients with AIDS. One possible explanation for this apparent paradox is that the pleural effusion in patients with AIDS is related to pleural invasion by the mycobacteria rather than to delayed hypersensitivity.[20] The fact that smears and cultures are more often positive in the HIV patient lends support to this hypothesis. Patients with HIV tend to have a longer duration of illness and a lower incidence of chest pain.[21] Systemic signs and symptoms such as night sweats, fatigue, diarrhea, hepatomegaly, splenomegaly, and lymphadenopathy are significantly more common in HIV-infected patients.[22] Patients with HIV are more likely to have concomitant parenchymal lesions.[23] Their pleural fluid is more likely to be smear positive for acid-fast bacilli (AFB) and culture positive for *M. tuberculosis*.[24,25] If the CD4 count is less than 100, approximately 50% have a positive smear for AFB on their pleural fluid.[24] HIV patients have significantly lower lymphocyte counts.[25] Interestingly, the viral load per mL was higher than that in simultaneously obtained serum in each of eight patients in one study.[21]

DIAGNOSIS

Radiology

Tuberculous effusion are usually unilateral and can be of any size. Less than 10% tubercular effusions are bilateral and usually indicate disseminated or miliary tuberculosis. In one series, the effusions occupied more than two-thirds of the hemithorax in 18%, between one-third and two-thirds of the hemithorax in 47%, and less than one-third of the hemithorax in 34%.[26] In approximately 20% of patients with pleural effusions secondary to TB, coexisting parenchymal disease is radiologically visible.[26] Some series have reported the co-existence of parenchymal lesions to be as high as 30–50%.[27] In such patients, the pleural effusion is almost always on the side of the parenchymal infiltrate and invariably indicates active parenchymal disease. On rare occasions, pleural TB can present with pleural-based nodules and thickening.[28] Tuberculosis is the most common cause of encysted effusion in India.[29] Encystment usually occurs during antitubercular therapy and involves the costoparietal region of posterior pleura. It may mimic a mass lesion of pleura, mediastinum or chest wall. Ultrasound can be useful in detecting minimal fluid and for accurate localizing. Ultrasound in tubercular effusion demonstrates delicate septa, regular pleural thickening and occasional nodularity.[30,31]

Tuberculin Test

In the past, the tuberculin skin test was an important diagnostic aid in patients suspected of having tuberculous effusion. Although delayed hypersensitivity to tuberculous protein is probably responsible for most clinical manifestations of tuberculous effusion, many patients when first evaluated have a negative tuberculin skin test. This negative skin test does not rule out the diagnosis of tuberculous effusion. In one series from Spain, the tuberculin was positive in only 66.5% of 254 patients with tuberculous effusion.[26] Many of these patients will become tuberculin reactive after 6–8 weeks. Therefore, in patients with an undiagnosed exudative pleural effusion, a negative tuberculin skin test performed 8 weeks after the development of symptoms can be used to exclude the diagnosis of tuberculous effusion. However, if the patient is markedly immunosuppressed with HIV infection or is severely malnourished, the tuberculin may remain negative.

Pleural Fluid Analysis

Pleural fluid analysis is useful in the diagnosis of tuberculous effusion. Usually, fluid is clear or yellow in color although it can be cloudy or serosanginous. The fluid is invariably a serous exudate. Frequently, the pleural fluid protein level is above 5 g/dL, and this finding suggests tuberculous effusion. In most patients, the pleural fluid differential white blood cell (WBC) count reveals more than 50% small lymphocytes.[15,26,32,34] In patients with symptoms of less than 2 weeks' duration, the pleural fluid differential WBC may reveal predominantly polymorphonuclear leukocytes.[16] If serial thoracenteses are performed, the differential WBC reveals a change to predominantly small lymphocytes.[15] The separation of the lymphocytes into T lymphocytes and B lymphocytes is not useful diagnostically. If eosinophils are found in the pleural fluid in significant numbers (>10%), one can virtually exclude the diagnosis of tuberculous effusion, unless the patient has a pneumothorax or has had a previous thoracentesis leading to entry of blood in pleural space.[35,36] A useful study for ruling out tuberculous effusion is analysis of the pleural fluid for mesothelial cells. Several studies have confirmed that pleural fluid from patients with TB rarely contains more than 5% mesothelial cells.[33,34,37,38] Unfortunately, the absence of mesothelial cells is not diagnostic of TB because with any condition in which the pleural surfaces are extensively involved by an inflammatory process, mesothelial cells are not found in the pleural fluid. It has been suggested that HIV-infected patients with tuberculous effusion may have significant numbers of mesothelial cells in their pleural fluid.[39]

Adenosine Deaminase

The diagnosis can also be established with reasonable certainty by demonstrating elevated levels of adenosine deaminase (ADA). ADA is the enzyme of purine metabolism that catalyzes the conversion of adenosine to inosine. It is seen in most human tissues especially in lymphoid tissues. Its level is 10 times higher in activated T cells and its plasma activity is high in diseases in which cellular immunity is stimulated.[40] Demonstration of an elevated pleural fluid ADA level is useful in establishing the diagnosis of tuberculous effusion. In an early study, Ocana et al.[55] measured the pleural fluid ADA levels in 221 pleural or peritoneal effusions. All patients with a pleural fluid ADA level above 70 U/L had TB, whereas no patient with a pleural fluid ADA level below 40 U/L had tuberculous effusion.[41] This has been confirmed in subsequent studies.[42-46] Different authors have used various cutoff levels for the pleural fluid ADA between 30–70 U/L for the diagnosis of pleural TB. The higher the pleural fluid ADA level, the more likely the patient is to have tuberculous effusion. In a meta-analysis of 40 studies, the sensitivity and specificity of pleural fluid ADA levels in the diagnosis of pleural TB were both 92%.[47] ADA level is elevated also in empyema, rheumatoid effusion, chronic lymphoid leukemia, lymphoma, mesothelioma, parpneumonic effusion, Q fever or brucellosis.[48-50] However, it should be easy to differentiate diseases from tuberculous effusion by the clinical picture and the fact that the first two diseases do not have pleural fluid lymphocytosis. Indeed, if the diagnostic criteria for tuberculous effusion includes a pleural fluid lymphocyte-to-neutrophil ratio of 0.75 or more, the specificity of the test is increased.[51,52] This increase in specificity is due to excluding the cases with rheumatoid effusion or empyema. The levels of ADA in patients with and without AIDS are comparable.[45] Renal transplant patients who develop a pleural effusion have elevated pleural fluid ADA levels.[53] The pleural fluid ADA level can be used to exclude the diagnosis of tuberculous pleural effusions in patients with undiagnosed pleural effusions. There are two molecular forms of ADA, ADA1 and ADA2. ADA1 is found in all cells, but has its greatest activity in lymphocytes and monocytes.[54] ADA2 is found only in monocytes, and most of the ADA in tuberculous pleural fluid is ADA2, whereas most of the ADA in other pleural fluids is ADA1.[54] Although, the use of a ratio of the ADA1 to total ADA of less than 0.42 will slightly increase the sensitivity and specificity of the ADA in diagnosing tuberculous effusion, the separation of ADA into its isoenzymes is not necessary in the vast majority of cases.[54,55] When preservatives are added to pleural fluid, the pleural fluid ADA levels remain stable during transportation. However, if pleural fluid is maintained at ambient temperatures without preservatives, the ADA levels will linearly decrease. The ADA levels remain stable for long periods in pleural fluid frozen at -70°C.[50]

Interferon-Gamma

Another test that is useful in the diagnosis of tuberculous effusion is the level of interferon-gamma in the pleural fluid.[44,56-59] Interferon-gamma is produced by the CD4⁺ lymphocytes from patients with tuberculous effusion.[58] Patients with tuberculous effusion tend to have higher pleural fluid interferon-gamma levels than do patients with pleural effusions of other etiologies. Villena et al.[60] reported that a cutoff level of 3.7 IU/mL yielded a sensitivity of 0.98 and a specificity of 0.98. Most of the false positives in this study occurred in patients with hematologic malignancies. Comparable results have also been reported in other studies,[56-59] but comparison of the series is difficult because the units have differed from one study to another. Patients with empyema frequently have elevated pleural fluid levels of interferon-gamma.[44]

Adenosine Deaminase Versus Interferon-Gamma

Which is the better test for the diagnosis of tuberculous effusion ADA or interferon-gamma? Greco et al.[61] performed a meta-analysis comparing ADA and interferon-gamma for the diagnosis of tuberculous effusion and they reported that the summary receiver operating characteristic curve yielded a maximum joint sensitivity and specificity of 93% for ADA and 96% for interferon-gamma.[61] They concluded that both ADA and interferon-gamma are reasonably accurate at diagnosing tuberculous effusion. Measurement of the pleural fluid ADA level is preferred to measurement of the pleural fluid interferon-gamma level in evaluating patients suspected of having pleural TB, because the ADA measurement is less expensive.[62]

Polymerase Chain Reaction

Polymerase chain reaction (PCR) is certainly not superior to either the pleural fluid ADA or interferon-gamma levels in establishing the diagnosis of tuberculous effusion. Querol et al.[63] reported that the sensitivity and specificity of PCR for the diagnosis of tuberculous effusion were 81% and 100%, respectively. In the same patients, the sensitivity and specificity for an ADA level of 45 U/L were nearly identical (86% and 98% respectively).[63]

Currently, PCR of the pleural fluid should not be considered to be a clinically useful test until there is more data available regarding its sensitivity and specificity.

Pleural Fluid Tuberculous Proteins or Antibodies

In recent years, the possibility of establishing the diagnosis of tuberculous effusion by the demonstration of tuberculous antigens or specific antibodies against tuberculous proteins in the pleural fluid has been investigated. None of these tests have proved to be of use in the diagnosis of tuberculous effusion. The presence of antituberculous antibodies in the pleural space appears to result from their passive diffusion from the serum rather than local antibody production.[64] Therefore, it is unlikely that measurement of such antibodies in the pleural fluid will be diagnostically useful.

Other Chemical Tests

Other chemical analyses of the pleural fluid are of limited value in establishing the diagnosis of tuberculous effusion. Although in the past, it was believed that the pleural fluid glucose level was reduced in most cases of tuberculous effusion,[65] more recent studies show that most patients with tuberculous effusion have a pleural fluid glucose level above 60 mg/dL.[15,21] A low pleural fluid pH level was once thought to be suggestive of tuberculous effusion,[66] subsequent studies,[67,68] however indicate that the pleural fluid pH has approximately the same distribution in malignant as in tuberculous pleural effusions. The mean level of C-reactive protein (CRP) is higher in tuberculous effusions than in other exudative effusions. Chierakul et al. reported that the optimal cut-off level for the pleural fluid CRP level was 30 mg/dL and this level had a sensitivity of 72% and a specificity of 93%.[69] Garcia-Pachon et al. reported that a CRP level greater than 50 mg/L had a 95% specificity for TB, whereas a CRP level less than 30 mg/L had a 95% sensitivity for excluding tuberculous effusion.[70] The mean level of lysozyme in the pleural fluid from patients with tuberculous effusion is higher than it is in other exudative pleural fluids.[71,72] A value of 1.2:1 for the ratio of the pleural fluid to the serum lysozyme has been proposed as a good test for diagnosing tuberculous effusion.[72] But the lysozyme ratio is distinctly inferior[42] to ADA. Measurement of the levels of tumor necrosis factor alpha (TNF-α) in the pleural fluid or the ratio of the pleural fluid to the serum TNF-α is inferior to measurements of the pleural fluid ADA in making the diagnosis of tuberculous effusion.[73] There have been many other studies on cytokine levels in the pleural fluid and although the mean cytokine levels in tuberculous effusions differ significantly from those in pleural fluids of other etiologies, there is always so much variation in the levels that their measurement has not proved as diagnostically useful as that of ADA or interferon-gamma.

Pleural Fluid Smears and Cultures

The diagnosis of tuberculous effusion depends on the demonstration of tubercle bacilli in the sputum, pleural fluid, or pleural biopsy specimen, or the demonstration of granulomas in the pleura. For non-immunosuppressed patients, routine smears of the pleural fluid for acid-fast bacilli (AFB) are not indicated because they are usually negative, unless the patient has a tuberculous empyema.[26,74] If the patient is HIV positive, the smears may be positive in more than 20%.[21] Cultures for mycobacteria should be obtained. In most series of patients with tuberculous effusion, the pleural fluid cultures are positive for mycobacteria in fewer than 40%.[15,26] Culture positivivity is reported in 13–70% cases. In reports giving 70% culture positivity, it was done by guinea pig innoculation and the average yield in solid medium inoculation is 30%. Yield is higher with bedside innoculation. Use of a BACTEC system provides faster results than do conventional methods. In one study, the median time for the BACTEC cultures to become positive was 18 days (range 3–40 days), whereas the median time for conventional cultures was 33.5 days (range 21–48 days).[75] In a second study, the pleural fluid cultures were positive by the BACTEC system in 24% of HIV-negative and 75% of HIV-positive individuals, whereas the cultures were positive by the Lowenstein-Jensen medium in 12% of HIV-negative patients and 56% of HIV-positive patients.[24] The mean time to positive culture with the BACTEC system was 3.5 weeks compared with 4.7 weeks with the Lowenstein-Jensen medium.[24]

Sputum Smears and Cultures

Examination of the sputum for mycobacteria is frequently ignored in the diagnostic workup of patients with a pleural effusion. Conde et al. prospectively evaluated the diagnostic yield of AFB smear and culture of the sputum in 84 patients with tuberculous effusion. They reported that the sputum studies were positive in 44 of the 84 patients (52%). In 10 of the 44 patients, sputum smears were positive, whereas cultures were positive in all 44.[76] Study of the peripheral blood is not useful as most patients do not have leukocytosis.[15]

Pleural Biopsy

For the last 40 years, the diagnosis of tuberculous effusion has been most commonly made with needle biopsy of the pleura. Biopsy is diagnostic in 50–80% of cases. The demonstration of granuloma in the parietal pleura suggests tuberculous effusion; caseous necrosis and AFB need not be demonstrated. Although other disorders including fungal diseases, sarcoidosis, tularemia,[77] and rheumatoid effusion may produce granulomatous effusion, more than 95% of patients with granulomatous effusion have TB. Even when granulomas are not demonstrated in the pleural biopsy, the biopsy specimen should be examined for AFB because organisms are occasionally demonstrated when no granulomas are present in the biopsy. In one study, needle biopsy of the pleura, showed granulomas in 80% whereas the acid-fast stain of the biopsy was positive in 25.8%, the culture of the biopsy tissue was positive in 56%, and at least one of the preceding three tests was positive in 91%.[26] Ultrasound guided biopsy can increase the yield to upto 86% as it helps in localizing the involved area of pleura and thus decreases false negative biopsies due to nonuniform involvement.[78,79] Thoracoscopy is a useful method for diagnosing pleural disease that has been missed by pleural fluid cytology and closed needle pleural biopsy. Thoracoscopy reveals yellow or white miliary tubercles on parietal pleura and reddening of the pleura. It can also help in obtaining guided biopsy from the involved pleural site.

In recent years, the availability of tests on the pleural fluid, such as the ADA, which are at least as sensitive in diagnosing tuberculous effusion as is needle biopsy of the pleura, have resulted in a decreased use of needle biopsy of the pleura.[80] A possible criticism of relying on the pleural fluid tests rather than the pleural biopsy is that with pleural fluid markers, no culture results are obtained. Accordingly, the sensitivities of the organisms cannot be determined. It should be noted that although the cultures of the biopsy are positive in approximately 55%, cultures of the fluid itself are positive in 35%. Therefore, the culture of the biopsy itself provides additional positive cultures in only 20% of the patients. A recent study has demonstrated that multidrug resistance occurs in only approximately 1% of patients with pleural TB and that any first line drug resistance occurs in less than 10%.[81]

Recommended Diagnostic Approach in Patients with Undiagnosed Exudative Pleural Effusion

When a patient is seen with an exudate pleural effusion, the diagnosis of tuberculous effusion should always be considered. When the initial thoracentesis is performed, the pleural fluid should be analyzed for the ADA level and differential cell count, and the fluid should be cultured for mycobacteria. If the pleural fluid ADA is above 70 U/L and the pleural fluid has a lymphocyte-to-neutrophil ratio of more than 0.75, the diagnosis of TB is virtually established. If the pleural fluid ADA level is between 40 and 70 U/L and the patient has a lymphocyte-to-neutrophil ratio of more than 0.75, a presumptive diagnosis of TB can be made. In this situation, consideration can be given to further studies (thoracoscopy or needle biopsy of the pleura) if the patient's clinical picture is not typical for tuberculous. If the patient's pleural fluid ADA level is below 40, the diagnosis of TB is unlikely. However, if the patient has a clinical picture typical of TB and, particularly, if the pleural fluid has a high percentage of lymphocytes, the possibility of TB can be further evaluated with thoracoscopy or needle biopsy of the pleura.

NATURAL HISTORY OF UNTREATED TUBERCULOUS EFFUSION

Without treatment, tuberculous effusion usually resolves spontaneously, only to return as active tuberculosis at a later date. Patiala followed up for at least 7 years all 2,816 members of the Finnish Armed Forces who developed pleural effusions between 1939 and 1945 and reported that 43% of this large group of young men developed TB during the follow-up period. Even in the 1-year observation period 5 years following the initial episode, 5% of the total population studied developed active TB.[82] Roper and Waring followed up 141 military personnel first seen from 1940 to 1944 with a pleural effusion and a positive tuberculin test and reported that in most patients, the effusions resolved and all the other symptoms disappeared within 2–4 months. Nevertheless, 65% of them subsequently developed some form of active TB. Manifest TB did not develop in the lung or elsewhere in any of the patients within 8 months of the onset of the original pleurisy. The incidence of subsequent TB was 60% in those with initially negative pleural fluid cultures for TB and 65% in those with initially positive pleural fluid cultures. In addition, the size of the original effusions and the presence or the absence of small radiologic residual pleural disease were not correlated with the subsequent appearance of active TB.[83] Because the administration of antituberculous chemotherapy reduces the incidence of subsequent TB,[15,84] it is important to establish the diagnosis of tuberculous effusion and initiate proper treatment. Moreover, patients in whom the diagnosis cannot be established but is considered likely should also be treated.

TREATMENT

The treatment of tuberculous effusion has three goals: (a) To prevent the subsequent development of active TB, (b) To relieve the patient symptoms, and (c) To prevent the development of a fibrothorax. If the patient is dyspneic from a large pleural effusion, a therapeutic thoracentesis should be performed.

Chemotherapy

The recommendations for the treatment of all tubercular pleural effusion consists of a 6-month regimen consisting of a 2-month initial phase of isoniazid (INH), rifampin, and pyrazinamide. Ethambutol should be included in the initial regimen until the results of drug susceptibility studies are available, unless there is little possibility of drug resistance. The second phase of the treatment should be INH and rifampin given for 4 months. Directly observed therapy (DOT) is recommended.[85,86] RNTCP gives category III to patients of tubercular effusion without parenchymal lesions. Category I is given for massive effusions, bilateral effusions. However, there is recommendation to give category I to all cases of newly diagnosed tubercular effusion. In recent multicentric study, category III treatment was found to be safe and effective for treatment of uncomplicated unilateral TB pleural effusion in immunocompetent patients.[86]

Nine-month regimens using INH and rifampin are also effective when the organisms are fully susceptible to the drug. When patient cannot tolerate rifampicin or pyrazinamide coventional treatment using 2SHE/10HE or HE for 1 year may be used. One study demonstrated that the penetration of INH into pleural fluid was excellent, but the penetration of pyrazinamide was very poor, whereas the penetration of rifampin was intermediate.[87] The clinical significance of these findings remains to be determined.

Corticosteroids

The role of oral corticosteroids in the treatment of tuberculous pleural effusion is controversial. There were no benefits with systemic corticosteroids in two controlled studies in which therapeutic thoracentesis was also performed.[88,89] In a third study, however, the duration of fever and the time required for fluid resorption were decreased; but in this study, no therapeutic thoracentesis was performed.[90] In none of studies did the administration of corticosteroids influence the degree of residual pleural thickening at 6 or 12 months after therapy was initiated. In one randomized controlled study with HIV-associated pleural TB, the administration of prednisolone was associated with an increased risk of Kaposi sarcoma.[91] In view of these factors, if the patient is more than mildly symptomatic with tuberculous effusion, a therapeutic thoracentesis is recommended. It should be noted, however, that although previous studies suggested a beneficial effect of therapeutic thoracentesis, study by Large and Levick[92] was unable to demonstrate any difference in the clinical courses of patients who had serial therapeutic thoracenteses and those of patients who had only a single diagnostic thoracentesis. If the patient continues to have severe systemic symptoms such as fever, malaise, pleuritic chest pain after a therapeutic thoracentesis, and a definite diagnosis has been established, the administration of corticosteroid is recommended.

Fibrinolytics

In patients with loculated tuberculous pleural effusions, the intrapleural administration of a fibrinolytic may decrease the degree of residual pleural thickening. Kwak et al. randomized 43 patients to receive only antituberculous chemotherapy or antituberculous chemotherapy plus 100,000 IU urokinase daily administered through a pigtail catheter starting when the amount of pleural fluid drainage was less than 100 mL/day and finishing when the amount of pleural fluid was less than 50 mL/day. Patients received a mean of 3.8 urokinase instillations. After the cessation of treatment the width of the pleural thickening was 0.46 cm in the urokinase group and 1.86 cm in the control group.[93]

Surgery

Surgery should not be performed early for pleural thickening. Although, the pleura may be thickened when the patient's disorder is first diagnosed, the thickening decreases with treatment, so decortication should not be considered until the patient has undergone treatment for at least 6 months. After this period of observation, decortication is rarely necessary. At this time, decortication should only be performed if the patient's quality of life is diminished by dyspnea.

RESPONSE TO TREATMENT

With treatment, the patient's symptoms and radiologic abnormalities gradually abate. The average patient becomes afebrile within 2 weeks, but temperature elevations may persist for as long as 2 months.[94] If a therapeutic thoracentesis is performed at the same time that antituberculous therapy is initiated, most patients become afebrile within 5 days.[88,89] The mean duration for complete resorption of the pleural fluid is approximately 6 weeks, but it can be as long as 12 weeks.[94] The incidence of pleural thickening at 6–12 months after beginning treatment is approximately 50%.[95] In one study,[96] 10% patients had a forced vital capacity (FVC) less than 80% of predicted at the end of the follow-up period for their TB treatment. In this study, there was only a weak correlation between the degree of pleural thickening and the reduction in the FVC.[96] The incidence of residual pleural thickening is not closely related to the initial pleural fluid findings; patients with a low glucose, high lactate dehydrogenase (LDH) and high cytokine levels are only slightly more likely to have residual pleural thickening.[95,97] One study demonstrated that the intrapleural administration of 2.5 mL of a hyaluronate-based gel resulted in significantly faster fluid absorption and significantly less pleural thickening at 3 months (0.57 cm vs 1.14 cm).[98] Residual pleural thickening is more common if the pleural effusion is initially loculated.[99] Residual pleural thickening will continue to improve for at least 18 months after the antituberculous therapy is completed.[99] It appears that complete removal of the pleural fluid does not decrease the amount of residual pleural thickening. Lai et al. randomized 61 patients to receive pigtail drainage until the drainage was less than 50 mL/day or no drainage. The degree of residual pleural thickening was basically identical in both groups.[100]

An occasional patient will develop paradoxical worsening of their disease after antituberculous therapy is initiated. Al-Majed[101] serially studied 61 patients with tuberculous pleural effusion who were started on a standard regimen of rifampin, INH, pyrazinamide, and ethambutol for the first 2 months. He reported that the size of the effusion worsened in 17% patients after the initiation of antituberculous therapy. Six of the patients developed increasing dyspnea and were treated with pleural aspiration and oral prednisolone with complete resolution of the pleural effusion. Other studies suggested that such paradoxical responses might be due to INH-induced lupus effusion.[102] An occasional patient with tuberculous effusion will also develop a peripheral lung nodule while being treated for the effusion. The nodules represent pulmonary TB and disappear when the antituberculous therapy is continued.[103] An occasional patient will also develop a pleural effusion during antituberculous chemotherapy. Gupta et al.[104] reported 29 patients who developed pleural effusions while receiving chemotherapy for pulmonary (16 cases) or extrapulmonary TB. The pleural effusion developed between the 5th and 8th week of starting chemotherapy in 13 and between the 9th and 12th week in 9 and between the 13th and 24th week in 5. The pleural fluid was exudative in all cases and the culture was positive for *Mycobacterium tuberculosis* in four. Most patients had a good response to the same chemotherapeutic regimen without any interruption.

REFERENCES

1. Sauret J, Jolis R, Ausina V, Castro E, Cornudella R. Human tuberculosis due to *Mycobacterium bovis:* Report of 10 cases. Tuber Lung Dis. 1992:73;388-91.
2. Tuberculosis in New York City 1992. New York: Bureau of Tuberculosis Control, New York City Department of Health. 1993.
3. Seaton A. Diseases of the Pleura. In Anthony, douglas seaton, Leitch A Gordon (editors). Crofton And Douglas's Respiratory Disaeses. 2002. p 1158.
4. Apicella MA, Allen JC. A physiologic differentiation between delayed and immediate hypersensitivity. J Clin Invest. 1969;48:250-9.
5. Leckie WJH, Tothill P. Albumin turnover in pleural effusions. Clin Sci. 1965;29:339-52.
6. Antony VB, Sahn SA, Antony AC, et al. Bacillus Calmette-Guerin-stimulated neutrophils release chemotaxins for monocytes in rabbit pleural space in vitro. J Clin Invest. 1985;76:1514-21.
7. Mohammed KA, Nasreen N, Ward MJ, et al. *Mycobacterium*-mediated chemokine expression in pleural mesothelial cells: role of C-C chemokines in tuberculous pleurisy. J Infect Dis. 1998;178:1450-6.
8. Widstrom O, Nilsson BS. Pleurisy induced by intrapleural BCG in immunized guinea pigs. Eur J Respir Dis. 1982;63:425-34.
9. Ong A, Creasman J, Hopewell PC, et al. A molecular epidemiological assessment of extrapulmonary tuberculosis in San Francisco. Clin Infect Dis. 2004;38:25-31.
10. Bueno CE, Clemente G, Castro BC, et al. Cytologic and bacteriologic analysis of fluid and pleural biopsy specimens with Cope's needle. Arch Intern Med. 1990;150:1190-4.
11. Chan CH, Arnold M, Chan CY, et al. Clinical and pathological features of tuberculous pleural effusion and its long-term consequences. Respiration. 1991;58:171-5.
12. Fujiwara H, Tsuyuguchi I. Frequency of tuberculin-reactive T-lymphocytes in pleural fluid and blood from patients with tuberculous pleurisy. Chest. 1986;89:530-2.
13. Ellner JJ, Barnes PF, Wallis RS, et al. The immunology of tuberculous pleurisy. Semin Respir Infect 1988;3:335-42.
14. Mehra V, Gong JH, Iyer D, et al. Immune response to recombinant mycobacterial proteins in patients with tuberculosis infection and disease. J Infect Dis 1996;174:431-4.
15. Berger HW, Meha E . Tuberculous Pleurisy. Chest. 1973:63:88-92
16. Levine H, Szanto PB, Cugell DW. Tuberculous pleurisy: an acute illness. Arch Intern Med 1968;122:329-32.

17. Moudgil H, Sridhar G, Leitch AG. Reactivation disease: the commonest form of tuberculous pleural effusion in Edinburgh, 1980–1991. Respir Med. 1994;88:301-4.
18. Richter C, Perenboom R, Mtoni I, et al. Clinical features of HIV-seropositive and HIV-seronegative patients with tuberculous pleural effusion in Dar es Salaam, Tanzania. Chest 1994;106:1471-5.
19. Aho K, Brander E, Pahala J. Studies for primary drug resistance in tuberculous pleurisy. Scand J Resp Dis. 1968;63 (Supp1):111-4.
20. Hodsdon WS, Luzze H, Hurst TJ, et al. HIV-1-related pleural tuberculosis: elevated production of IFN-gamma, but failure of immunity to *Mycobacterium tuberculosis.* AIDS. 2001;15: 467-75.
21. Heyderman RS, Makunike R, Muza T, et al. Pleural tuberculosis in Harare, Zimbabwe: The relationship between human immunodeficiency virus, CD4 lymphocyte count, granuloma formation and disseminated disease. Trop Med Int Health. 1998;3:14-20.
22. Richter C, Perenboom R, Mtoni I, et al. Clinical features of HIV-seropositive and HIV-seronegative patients with tuberculous pleural effusion in Dar es Salaam, Tanzania. Chest. 1994;106:1471-75.
23. Qiu L, Teeter LD, Liu Z, et al. Diagnostic associations between pleural and pulmonary tuberculosis. J Infect. 2006;53:377-86.
24. Luzze H, Elliott AM, Joloba ML, et al. Evaluation of suspected tuberculous pleurisy: clinical and diagnostic findings in HIV-1-positive and HIV-negative adults in Uganda. Int J Tuberc Lung Dis. 2001;5:746-53.
25. Collins KR, Quinones-Mateu ME, Wu M, et al. Human immunodeficiency virus type 1 (HIV-1) quasispecies at the sites of *Mycobacterium tuberculosis* infection contribute to systemic HIV-1 heterogeneity. J Virol. 2002;76:1697-706.
26. Valdes L, Alvarez D, San Jose E, et al. Tuberculous pleurisy: a study of 254 patients. Arch Intern Med. 1998;158:2017-21.
27. Seibert AF, Haynes J Jr, Middleton R, Bass JB. Tuberculous pleuarl effusion. Twenty year expereience. Chest. 1991;99:883-6.
28. Ariyurek OM, Cil BE. Atypical presentation of pleural tuberculosis: CT findings. Br J Radiol 2000;73:209-10.
29. Parischa P, Suri JC. Goel A, Chauhan S. Clinical and roentgenological profiles and etiological correlations of encysted pleural effusion. Respiration. 1990;20:461-5.
30. Akhan O, Demirkazik FB, Balkanci F, Ozmen MN, Ozakara S, Coplu L, et al. Tuberculous pleuarl effusion: Ultrasonic diagnosis. J Clin Ultrasound. 1992:20:461-5.
31. Carazo Martinez O ,Vargas Sarrano B, Rodriguez Romero R. Real-time ultrasound evaluation of tuberculous pleural effusion. J Clin Ultrasound. 1989;17:407-10.
32. Yam LT. Diagnostic significance of lymphocytes in pleural effusions. Ann Intern Med. 1967;66:972-82.
33. Light RW, Erozan YS, Ball WC. Cells in pleural fluid: their value in differential diagnosis. Arch Intern Med. 1973;132:854-60.
34. De Oliveira HG, Rossatto ER, Prolla JC. Pleural fluid adenosine deaminase and lymphocyte proportion: clinical usefulness in the diagnosis of tuberculosis. Cytopathology. 1994;5: 27-32.
35. Adelman M, Albelda Sm, Gottileb J, Haponik EF. Diagnostic utility of pleural fluid eosinophilia. Am J Med. 1984;77:915-20.
36. Light RW. Clinical manifestation and useful tests. In: Pleural Diseases. 2nd edition. Philaldelphia: Lea and Febirger. 1990. p 39-73.
37. Spriggs AI, Boddington MM. The cytology of effusions, 2nd ed. New York: Grune and Stratton, 1968.
38. Hurwitz S, Leiman G, Shapiro C. Mesothelial cells in pleural fluid: TB or not TB? S Afr Med J. 1980;57:937-39.

39. Jones D, Lieb T, Narita M, et al. Mesothelial cells in tuberculous pleural effusions of HIV-infected patients. Chest. 2000;117:289-91.
40. Nishida Y, Okwdaire K, Tanimoto K Akaoka I. The differences in purine metabolism between T and B lymphocytes. Exp Hematol. 1980;8:593-8.
41. Ocana I, Martinez-Vazquez JM, Segura RM, et al. Adenosine deaminase in pleural fluids: test for diagnosis of tuberculous pleural effusion. Chest. 1983;84:51-3.
42. Valdes L, San Jose E, Alvarez D, et al. Diagnosis of tuberculous pleurisy using the biologic parameters adenosine deaminase, lysozyme, and interferon gamma. Chest. 1993;103: 458-65.
43. Burgess LJ, Maritz FJ, Le Roux I, et al. Use of adenosine deaminase as a diagnostic tool for tuberculous pleurisy. Thorax. 1995;50:672-4.
44. Valdes L, Alvarez D, San Jose E, et al. Value of adenosine deaminase in the diagnosis of tuberculous pleural effusions in young patients in a region of high prevalence of tuberculosis. Thorax. 1995;50:600-3.
45. Riantawan P, Chaowalit P, Wongsangiem M, et al. Diagnostic value of pleural fluid adenosine deaminase in tuberculous pleuritis with reference to HIV coinfection and a Bayesian analysis. Chest. 1999;116:97-103.
46. Prasad. Tripathi RP, Mukerji PK, Singh M, Srivastava VML. Adenosine deaminase activity in pleural fluid – adiagnostic test of tuberculous pleural effusions. Indian J Chest Dis Allied Sci. 1992;34:123-6.
47. Goto M, Noguchi Y, Koyama H, et al. Diagnostic value of adenosine deaminase in tuberculous pleural effusion: a meta-analysis. Ann Clin Biochem. 2003;40:374-81.
48. Esteban C, Oribe M, Fernandez A, et al. Increased adenosine deaminase activity in Q fever pneumonia with pleural effusion. Chest. 1994;105:648.
49. Dikensoy O, Namiduru M, Hocaoglu S, et al. Increased pleural fluid adenosine deaminase in brucellosis is difficult to differentiate from tuberculosis. Respiration. 2002;69:556-9.
50. Lee YC, Rogers JT, Rodriguez RM, et al. Adenosine deaminase levels in nontuberculous lymphocytic pleural effusions. Chest. 2001;120:356-61.
51. Burgess LJ, Maritz FJ, Le Roux I, et al. Combined use of pleural adenosine deaminase with lymphocyte/neutrophil ratio. Increased specificity for the diagnosis of tuberculous pleuritis. Chest. 1996;109:414-9.
52. Diacon AH, Van de Wal BW, Wyser C, et al. Diagnostic tools in tuberculous pleurisy: a direct comparative study. Eur Respir J. 2003;22:589-91.
53. Chung JH, Kim YS, Kim SI, et al. The diagnostic value of the adenosine deaminase activity in the pleural fluid of renal transplant patients with tuberculous pleural effusion. Yonsei Med J. 2004;45:661-4.
54. Perez-Rodriguez E, Castro DJ. The use of ADA and ADA isoenzymes in the diagnosis of tuberculous pleuritis. Curr Opin. 2000;6:259-66.
55. Valdes L, San Jose E, Alvarez D, et al. Adenosine deaminase (ADA) isoenzyme analysis in pleural effusions: diagnostic role, and relevance to the origin of increased ADA in tuberculous pleurisy. Eur Respir J. 1996;9:747-51.
56. Shimokata K, Saka H, Murate T, et al. Cytokine content in pleural effusion. Chest. 1991;99: 1103-7.
57. Ribera E, Ocana I, Martinez-Vazquez JM, et al. High level of interferon gamma in tuberculous pleural effusion. Chest. 1988;93:308-11.
58. Barnes PF, Mistry SD, Cooper CL, et al. Compartmentalization of a CD4+ve T lymphocyte subpopulation in tuberculous pleuritis. J Immunol. 1989;142:1114-9.
59. Villena V, Lopez-Encuentra A, Echave-Sustaeta J, et al. Interferon-gamma in 388 immunocompromised and immunocompetent patients for diagnosing pleural tuberculosis. Eur Respir J. 1996;9:2635-9.

60. Villena V, Lopez-Encuentra A, Pozo F, et al. Interferon gamma levels in pleural fluid for the diagnosis of tuberculosis. Am J Med. 2003;115:365-70.
61. Greco S, Girardi E, Masciangelo R, et al. Adenosine deaminase and interferon gamma measurements for the diagnosis of tuberculous pleurisy: a meta-analysis. Int J Tuberc Lung Dis. 2003;7:777-86.
62. Sharma SK, Banga A. Pleural fluid interferon-gamma and adenosine deaminase levels in tuberculosis pleural effusion: a cost-effectiveness analysis. J Clin Lab Anal. 2005;19:40-6.
63. Querol JM, Minguez J, Garcia-Sanchez E, et al. Rapid diagnosis of pleural tuberculosis by polymerase chain reaction. Am J Respir Crit Care Med. 1995;152:1977-81.
64. Levy H, Wayne LG, Anderson BE, et al. Anti-mycobacterial antibody levels in pleural fluid reflect passive diffusion from serum. Chest. 1990;97:1144-7.
65. Barber LM, Mazzadi L, Deakins DD, et al. Glucose level in pleural fluid as a diagnostic aid. Dis Chest. 1957;31:680-1.
66. Holton K. Diagnostic value of some biochemical pleural fluid examinations. Scand J Respir Dis Suppl. 1968;63:121-5.
67. Chavalittamrong B, Angsusingha K, Tuchinda M, et al. Diagnostic significance of pH, lactic acid dehydrogenase, lactate and glucose in pleural fluid. Respiration. 1979;38:112-20.
68. Good JT Jr, Taryle DA, Maulitz RM, et al. The diagnostic value of pleural fluid pH. Chest 1980;78:55-9.
69. Chierakul N, Kanitsap A, Chaiprasert A, et al. A simple C-reactive protein measurement for the differentiation between tuberculous and malignant pleural effusion. Respirology. 2004;9:66-9.
70. Garcia-Pachon E, Soler MJ, Padilla-Navas I, et al. C-reactive protein in lymphocytic pleural effusions: a diagnostic aid in tuberculous pleuritis. Respiration. 2005;72:486-9.
71. Fontan Bueso J, Verea Hernando H, Garcia-Buela JP, et al. Diagnostic value of simultaneous determination of pleural adenosine deaminase and pleural lysozyme/serum lysozyme ratio in pleural effusion. Chest. 1988;93:303-7.
72. Verea Hernando HR, Masa Jimenez JF, Dominguez Juncal L, et al. Meaning and diagnostic value of determining the lysozyme level of pleural fluid. Chest. 1987;91:342-5.
73. Ugurman F, Gozu A, Akkalyoncu B, et al. Tumour necrosis factor-alpha in comparison to adenosine deaminase in tuberculous pleuritis. Respiration. 2003;70:270-4.
74. Bueno CE, Clemente G, Castro BC, et al. Cytologic and bacteriologic analysis of fluid and pleural biopsy specimens with Cope's needle. Arch Intern Med. 1990;150:1190-4.
75. Maartens G, Bateman ED. Tuberculous pleural effusions: increased culture yield with bedside inoculation of pleural fluid and poor diagnostic value of adenosine deaminase. Thorax. 1991;46:96-9.
76. Conde MB, Loivos AC, Rezende VM, et al. Yield of sputum induction in the diagnosis of pleural tuberculosis. Am J Respir Crit Care Med. 2003;167:723-5.
77. Schmid GP, Catino D, Suffin SC, et al. Granulomatous pleuritis caused by *Francisella tularensis:* possible confusion with tuberculous pleuritis. Am Rev Respir Dis. 1983;128:314-6.
78. Chang DB, Yang PC, Luh KT, Kuo SH, Yu CJ. Ultrasound guided pleural biopsy with tru-cut needle. Chest. 1991;100:1328-33.
79. Canto A, Rivas J, Saumench J, Morena R, Moya J. Points to consider when choosing a biopsy method in cases of pleurisy of unknown origin. Chest. 1983;84:176-9
80. Light RW. Closed needle biopsy of the pleura is a valuable diagnostic procedure. Con closed needle biopsy. J Bronchol. 1998;5:332-6.
81. Baumann MH, Nolan R, Petrini M, et al. Pleural tuberculosis in the United States: incidence and drug resistance. Chest. 2007.
82. Patiala J. Initial tuberculous pleuritis in the Finnish Armed Forces in 1939–1945 with special reference to eventual post pleuritic tuberculosis. Acta Tuberc Scand Suppl. 1954;36:1-57.
83. Roper WH, Waring JJ. Primary serofibrinous pleural effusion in military personnel. Am Rev Respir Dis. 1955;71:616-34.

84. Patiala J, Mattila M. Effect of chemotherapy of exudative tuberculous pleurisy on the incidence of post pleuritic tuberculosis. Acta Tuberc Scand. 1964;44:290-6.
85. Blumberg HM, Burman WJ, Chaisson RE, et al. American Thoracic Society/Centers for Disease Control and Prevention/Infectious Diseases Society of America: treatment of tuberculosis. Am J Respir Crit Care Med. 2003;167:603-62.
86. Sharma SK, Solanki R, Mohan A, Jain NK, Chauhan LS. Outcomes of Category III DOTs treatment in immunocompetent patients with tubercular pleural effusion. Int J Tuberc Lung Dis. 2012;16:1505-9.
87. Jutte PC, Rutgers SR, Van Altena R, et al. Penetration of isoniazid, rifampicin and pyrazinamide in tuberculous pleural effusion and psoas abscess. Int J Tuberc Lung Dis. 2004;8:1368-72.
88. Galarza I, Canete C, Granados A, et al. Randomised trial of corticosteroids in the treatment of tuberculous pleurisy. Thorax. 1995;50:1305-7.
89. Wyser C, Walzl G, Smedema JP, et al. Corticosteroids in the treatment of tuberculous pleurisy. A double-blind, placebo-controlled, randomized study. Chest. 1996;110:333-8.
90. Lee CH, Wang WJ, Lan RS, et al. Corticosteroids in the treatment of tuberculous pleurisy: a double-blind, placebo-controlled, randomized study. Chest. 1988;94:1256-9.
91. Elliott AM, Luzze H, Quigley MA, et al. A randomized, double-blind, placebo-controlled trial of the use of prednisolone as an adjunct to treatment in HIV-1-associated pleural tuberculosis. J Infect Dis. 2004;190:869-78.
92. Large SE, Levick RK. Aspiration in the treatment of primary tuberculous pleural effusion. Br Med J. 1958;1:1512-4.
93. Kwak SM, Park CS, Cho JH, et al. The effects of urokinase instillation therapy via percutaneous transthoracic catheter in loculated tuberculous pleural effusion: a randomized prospective study. Yonsei Med J. 2004;45:822-8.
94. Tani P, Poppius H, Makipaja J. Cortisone therapy for exudative tuberculous pleurisy in the light of the follow-up study. Acta Tuberc Scand. 1964;44:303-9.
95. Barbas CSV, Cukier A, de Varvalho CRR, et al. The relationship between pleural fluid findings and the development of pleural thickening in patients with pleural tuberculosis. Chest. 1991; 100:1264-7.
96. Wong P-C. Management of tuberculous pleuritis: can we do better? Respirology 2005;10:144-8.
97. Candela A, Andujar J, Hernandez L, et al. Functional sequelae of tuberculous pleurisy in patients correctly treated. Chest. 2003;123:1996-2000.
98. Zhou A, Guo L, Tang L. Effect of an intrathoracic injection of sodium hyaluronic acid on the prevention of pleural thickening in excess fluid of tuberculous thoracic cavity. Clin Exp Pharmacol Physiol. 2003;30:203-5.
99. Han DH, Song JW, Chung HS, et al. Resolution of residual pleural disease according to time course in tuberculous pleurisy during and after the termination of antituberculosis medication. Chest. 2005;128:3240-5.
100. Lai YF, Chao TY, Wang YH, et al. Pigtail drainage in the treatment of tuberculous pleural effusions: a randomized study. Thorax. 2003;58:149-51.
101. Al-Majed SA. Study of paradoxical response to chemotherapy in tuberculous pleural effusion. Resp Med 1996;90:211-4.
102. Hiraoka K, Nagata N, Kawajiri T, et al. Paradoxical pleural response to antituberculous chemotherapy and isoniazid-induced lupus. Review and report of two cases. Respiration. 1998;65:152-5.
103. Choi YW, Jeon SC, Seo HS, et al. Tuberculous pleural effusion: new pulmonary lesions during treatment. Radiology. 2002;224:493-502.
104. Gupta RC, Dixit R, Purohit SD, et al. Development of pleural effusion in patients during anti-tuberculous chemotherapy: analysis of twenty-nine cases with review of literature. Indian J Chest Dis Allied Sci. 2000;42:161-6.

Chapter 41

Tubercular Empyema

INTRODUCTION

The word 'empyema' is used to denote the presence of pus in a natural body cavity. Empyemas are sometimes described as acute or chronic but the division between the two is indistinct and arbitrary, the latter usually being reserved for those cases that have passed through the early exudative stage to reach a stage of organization in which a pleural rind has formed. Tubercular empyema thoracis complicates post-primary tuberculosis when caseous matter from superficial lung cavity or an adjacent parenchymal focus, paratracheal glands or paravertebral abscess secondary to Pott's spine erodes directly into pleural cavity. It still remains a major problem in developing countries despite availability of potent antitubercular drugs and improved surgical techniques. This chapter aims to review the clinical features, diagnosis and management of tubercular empyema.

ETIOPATHOGENESIS

Tuberculous empyema can occur after following events such as therapeutic pneumothorax leading to trapped lung, a progressive large tuberculous effusion leading to a trapped lung, extension of infection from thoracic lymph nodes or a paravertebral abscess secondary to Pott's spine, hematogenous spread and post-pneumonectomy. Once infected by pathogenic organisms, the connective tissue layers within the pleural membranes become edematous and produce an exudation of proteinaceous fluid that starts to fill the pleural cavity. At this early exudative stage the pleural fluid is thin with a relatively low white cell count (WCC) and the visceral pleura and underlying lung remain mobile.[1] If the infection proceeds unchecked by antimicrobial agents, the inflammatory process continues, so that newly formed layers of fibrin is laid down on the epithelial surface within the pleural cavity, particularly on the parietal pleura. The empyema fluid now becomes thicker and more turbid, containing a higher WCC. With the deposition of fibrin on both pleural surfaces, lung movement in this later fibrinopurulent stage may become increasingly restricted.[1] Depending upon the nature of the infecting organism and whether or not antibiotics and drainage procedures have been employed, these thickened fibrinous layers organize as collagen and become vascularized by an ingrowth of capillaries. This organizational stage may begin within 2 weeks[2], but usually takes 4–6 weeks to develop to a point at which the empyema cavity becomes surrounded by a cortex, 'peel' or 'rind' that may be more than 2 cm thick.[3] By this time the empyema contains frank pus, which may be viscid. The inner layers of the thickened empyema cortex continue to show a considerable inflammatory cell infiltrate and the fibrous outermost layers exert an increasingly restrictive effect both compressing the underlying lung (the so called 'trapped lung' effect) and also tending to draw the overlying ribs together, ultimately producing a chest deformity with a dorsal scoliosis that is concave towards the affected side. An empyema may become localized to one part of the pleural cavity or it may involve the whole of it. Such large empyemas may become loculated into smaller collections by the development of septate fibrinous bands, making the work of percutaneous aspiration difficult or impossible. Ultimately an inadequately treated empyema may become obliterated and its rind may calcify, producing a so called fibrothorax, particularly in the case of old tuberculous pleural effusion.

CLINICAL FEATURES

The clinical manifestations of an empyema vary widely depending on both the nature of the infecting organism and the competence of the patient's immune system. The spectrum ranges from an almost complete absence of symptoms to a severe illness with all the usual manifestations of systemic toxicity. The presenting features may vary according to the way in which the empyema has arisen. In patients with chronic tuberculous empyema; the infection may be present for years with a paucity of clinical symptoms. The prolongation of the asymptomatic period is explained by the marked pleural thickening that isolates the tubercle bacilli to the empyema cavity. Patients often come to clinical attention on evaluation of a routine chest radiograph or following the development of complications, such as bronchopleural fistula, or empyema necessitans. Some patients may have insidious constitutional symptoms such as fatigue and weight loss but also manifest low grade fever and night sweats. Physical examination may reveal chest wall tenderness, stony dullness to percussion and digital clubbing. Dyspnea may result from compression of underlying lung by the empyema or from primary disease involving the lung itself. A cough is frequent and in the presence of a bronchopleural fistula variable quantities of purulent sputum may be produced. The suppurative process, if undrained, and uncontrolled may extend beyond the pleural cavity, with pointing occurring in an intercostal space often close to the sternum where the chest wall is the thinnest.

DIAGNOSIS

The typical chest x-ray in chronic tuberculous empyema shows a moderate to large loculated pleural effusion with pleural calcification and overcrowding of overlying ribs. The diagnosis is virtually assured by finding a thick, calcific, pleural rind and rib thickening surrounding loculated pleural fluid on CT scaning. In contrast to serous tuberculosis effusions, it is characterized by grossly purulent fluid that is smear positive for acid-fast bacilli (AFB) and cultures. Tubercular empyema usually have >100,000 nucleated cells/microliter that are virtually all neutrophils, pH is < 7.2, the glucose concentration is < 20 mg/dL and LDH is >1000 IU/L. As there is often concomitant bacterial and mycobacterial infection, anaerobic and aerobic pleural fluid cultures should also be obtained. The pleural fluid is generally thick and cloudy and may look like frank pus or chyle (pseudochylous effusion) due to high levels of cholesterol in the fluid. The sensitivity of tuberculin skin test in patients having tubercular empyema varies between 73–93%, but its usefulness is limited by its inability to differentiate latent infection from active disease. Other investigations such as sputum for AFB, histopathological examination by pleural biopsy, or by suggestive radiological appearances can have diagnostic value. Direct microscopy of smears and mycobacterial cultures are usually positive, making pleural biopsy unnecessary. Other findings, such as a mild normocytic normochromic anemia, neutrophil leukocytosis and hypoalbuminemia, are common and non-specific.

TREATMENT

Tuberculous empyema is treated with same principles as other empyemas-drainage and antimicrobial chemotherapy. Problems specific to chronic tubercular empyema include the inability to re-expand the trapped lung spontaneously with drainage and to achieve therapeutic pleural fluid drug levels. It is important to secure adequate pain relief and also consider the fluid and nutritional needs of the usually toxic ill patient. Adequate short course chemotherapy should be given for 6–9 months. It is essential to provide anti-TB therapy (ATT) at their maximal tolerated dosages in order to prevent development of resistance. This is probably because the antituberculous drugs frequently do not reach their normal levels in the pleural space owing to the thick, fibrous, and often calcified pleura.[21]

Closed Drainage

Drainage of an empyema may be closed or open. Closed drainage may be either 'intermittent' in which repeated aspiration (thoracocentesis) is carried out, or 'continuous', in which an intercostal tube is connected to an underwater seal (closed-tube thoracostomy). Closed drainage is preferred provided that the pus is accessible and not too viscid to permit adequate removal by these methods or is loculated. These conditions are more likely to be present in the exudative stage but can be continued into the fibrinopurulent stage in some cases. Such medical treatment with antitubercular treatment and repeated thoracocentesis is appropriate for many individuals with pleural empyema and these patients may have a shorter and less complicated stay than those treated by tube drainage.[4] Recent studies reported complete resolution of empyema after daily or alternate day ultrasound-guided thoracocentesis with an average hospitalization of 31 days.[5,6]

Closed-tube thoracostomy is preferred by some clinicians from the start once the diagnosis of empyema has been confirmed.[4,7] It has the advantages that drainage is continuous and that it is more likely to be successful when the infected material is too viscid to be removed by manual aspiration, but with the disadvantage of greater discomfort and immobility for the patient; furthermore introduction of new infection at the drainage site is a possibility. When underwater seal drainage through a conventional large-bore intercostal tube becomes slight, the residual sinus is small or bronchopleural fistula closed and drainage minimal (< 50 mL daily for three consecutive days) the tube is clamped for three consecutive days. Further ultrasonographical evaluation is mandatory before the drain is removed as chest radiography does not allow sensitive differentiation between residual pleural fluid, pleural thickening and underlying parenchymal disease, still it is advised to exclude the presence of residual pneumothorax after removal of drain. Although relatively large (28–36F) chest tubes have been recommended by most in belief that smaller tubes would become obstructed with the thick fluid, such large tubes are probably not necessary. In one recent study, patients treated with 8–12F pigtail or 10–14F mallecot catheters inserted under ultrasound or CT guidance, resulted as the definitive treatment in 78% of patients.[8] The correct positioning of tube is probably more important than the size of tube.[9]

Closed drainage, whether by thoracocentesis or intercostal tube, is likely to be successful if the empyema is small[10] and if treatment of the empyema is started in the acute exudative or early fibrinopurulent stages of infection, in which case the wall of the empyema cavity gradually becomes reabsorbed allowing re-expansion of underlying lung and obliteration of the pleural space. This process can be expected to take several weeks in adult patients. The techniques outlined above may fail to cure an empyema if the pus is too thick to drain by thoracocentesis or tube, if a bronchopleural fistula has developed or if pockets of pus become loculated and inaccessible. There are reports of successful non-surgical treatment of tuberculous empyema with serial, space emptying thoracocentesis and long-term chemotherapy. 60–80% response rates have been reported in various studies with conservative measures.[10] It is recommended that needle aspiration, a simple procedure, should be used initially in all cases of simple empyema and intercostal drainage should be given as the first line of treatment in empyema cases with bronchopleural fistula (BPF). Negative pressure suction should be used in all patients, particularly those with BPF.[11] When closed drainage has failed to enable the lung to re-expand fully, a more invasive surgical procedure has to be employed. Surgical options include standard decortication, decortication limited to the parietal sides of the pleural sac, thoracoplasty, parietal wall collapse, open drainage and myoplasty and omentoplexy. If closed drainage does not result in prompt re-expansion of the lung and especially if loculi have been identified ultrasonically, a decision to intervene relatively early using video-assisted thoracoscopic surgery (VATS) with debridement and drainage is sometimes made, provided that the empyema is in the fibrinopurulent stage, with the thickened rind caused by fibrin rather than the mature scar tissue that forms when an empyema has become chronic. VATS enables the operator to achieve adequate debridement, breaking down loculi, evacuating pus and debris and freeing the lung. This may then result in prompt re-expansion of the lung and obliteration of the pleural cavity, avoiding the need for repeated or prolonged attempts at drainage.[12,13] The surgical procedures achieve the best drainage in gross empyema, but are limited by cost, operative risk and local availability.

Open Surgical Drainage

Surgical drainage is used if an empyema persists both clinically and radiographically in a patient in whom closed drainage has proved unsuccessful, when VATS is unavailable, unsuccessful or in patients who are debilitated to undergo the more invasive procedure of thoracotomy and decortication. It involves resection of the lowest rib above and below which pus can be aspirated. The surgeon makes an incision large enough to allow adequate drainage, cleans the inside of the empyema cavity and places a wide-bore tube surrounded by gauze in the unsutured wound. Daily dressing under surgical supervision with sterilization and replacement of the tube is recommended. Successful open drainage results in gradual obliteration of the empyema space, which allows ultimate removal of the tube and cure. Thoracotomy and decortication may still be recommended if, during open drainage, the patient's general condition improves sufficiently.

Decortication and Thoracotomy

This is an elective surgical procedure, in which the fibrous wall of the empyema cavity, referred as the cortex, rind or peel, is exposed at thoracotomy and stripped off the adjacent visceral and parietal pleura, which may be left intact.[14] It is carried out in patients in whom closed drainage and/or thoracoscopic methods have been unsuccessful, provided that they are fit enough to undergo this major procedure. It may also be used in the patient whose condition has stabilized following open drainage but who has entered a chronic phase in which the underlying lung does not expand because of failure of the cortex or rind to become reabsorbed. There is no consensus about the optimal time at which to perform a decortication, some surgeons arguing for early intervention and others adopting a more conservative approach.[15-17] In the early stage of organization the empyema cortex is poorly demarcated and friable, making decortication difficult. In intermediate stages of formation, it is rather vascular so that decortication is best delayed for 2 or 3 months in order to reduce morbidity.

Thoracoplasty

Thoracoplasty is now used only rarely in order to either obliterate an empyema space following pneumonectomy or to manage a persistent empyema cavity in patients where extensive ipsilateral parenchymal lung disease would prevent re-expansion after decortication and in whom extrapleural pneumonectomy would be unacceptably hazardous. Thoracoplasty is a mutilating procedure that produces a chest wall deformity which is not acceptable cosmetically but is nevertheless still sometimes used as a last resort.

Role of Fibrinolytics

Intrapleural streptokinase[18] and urokinase[19] appears to be a useful strategy to preserve lung function and reduce need for surgery in patients with late stage of empyema thoracis[20] when pleural fluid becomes loculated and drainage of pus is difficult. This procedure resulted in increase of drainage of pleural fluid in all patients. Mean hospital stay as well as the number of patients who required decortication was reduced. The usual dose of urokinase is 100,000 IU, and the usual dose of streptokinase is 150,000 IU. Both agents are administered intrapleurally in a total volume of 50–100 mL. But both the agents are quite expensive.

REFERENCES

1. American Thoracic Society. Management of non tuberculous empyema. Am Rev Respir Dis. 1962;85:935-6.
2. Shields TW. General thoracic surgery. Philadelphia: Lea and Febiger, 1972.
3. Spencer H. Pathology of the Lung. London: Pergamon Press, 1985.
4. Moores DWO. Management of acute empyema. Chest. 1992;102:1316-7.
5. Storm HK, Krasnik M, Bang K, et al. Treatment of pleural empyema secondary to pneumonia: thoracocentesis regimen versus tube drainage. Thorax. 1992;47:821-4.
6. Simmers TA, Jie C, Sie B.Minimally invasive treatment of thoracic empyema. Thorac Cariovasc Surg. 1999;47:77-81.

7. Light RW, Girard WM, Jenkinson SC, George RB. Parapneumonic effusions. Am J Med. 1980;69:507-12.
8. Shanker S, Gulati M, Kang M, et al. Image- guided percutaneous drainage of thoracic empyema: can sonography predict the outcome? Eur Radiol. 2000;10:495-9.
9. Light RW. Pleural diseases, 4th edn. Baltimore, Lippincott, Williams & Wilkins, 2001.
10. Ferguson AD, Prescott RJ, Selkon JB et al. The clinical course and management of thoracic empyema. Q J Med. 1996;89:285-90.
11. Sharma TN, Jain NK, Madan A, Sarkar SK and Durlabhji P. Tubercular empyema thoracis: A diagnostic and therapeutic problem. Indian J Chest Dis & All. Sci. 1982;11:127-31.
12. Lawrence OR, Ohri SK, Moxon RE, et al. Thoracoscopic debridement of empyema thoracis. Ann Thorac Surg. 1997;64:1448-50.
13. Mark JBO. New technology in the treatment of an old disease. Chest. 1997;111:1.
14. Thurer RJ.Decortication in thoracic empyema. Indications and surgical technique. Chest Surg Clin N Am. 1996;6:461-90.
15. Hoover EL, Hsu HK, Ross MJ. Reappraisal of empyema thoracis. Surgical intervention when the duration of illness is unknown. Chest. 1986;90:511-5.
16. Mayo P. Early thoracotomy and decortication for nontuberculous empyema in adults with and without underlying disease. A twenty-five year review. Am J Surg. 1985;51:230-6.
17. Frimodt-Moller L, Vejilsted H. Early surgical intervention in non-specific pleural empyema. Thorac Cardiovasc Surg. 1985;33:41.
18. Bouros D, Schiza S, Patsourakis G. et al. Intrapleural streptokinase versus urokinase in the treatment of complicated parapneumonic effusions: a prospective, double-blind study. Am J Respir Crit Care Med. 1997;155:291-5.
19. Temes RT, Follis F, Kessler RM, et al. Intrapleural fibrinolytics in management of empyema thoracis. Chest. 1996;110:102-6.
20. Banga A, Khilnani GC, Sharma SK, Dey AB, Wig N, Banga N. A study of empyema thoracis and role of intrapleural streptokinase in its management. BMC Infect Dis. 2004;29:4-19.
21. Iseman MD, Madsen LA. Chronic tuberculous empyema with bronchopleural fistula resulting in treatment failure and progressive drug resistance. Chest. 1991;100:124-7.

Chapter 42

Tubercular Lymphadenitis

INTRODUCTION

Tubercular lymphadenitis has been known to humanity since ancient times. Tuberculosis of the peripheral lymph nodes is one of the most common forms of extrapulmonary tuberculosis. Cervical lymph nodes are the most common site of involvement, with or without associated disease of other lymph nodes such as axillary, inguinal and mediastinal lymph nodes. The causes of tubercular lymphadenitis include *Mycobacterium tuberculosis, M. bovis* and atypical mycobacteria. Various atypical mycobacteria known to cause lymphadenitis are *Mycobacterium scrofulaceum, Mycobacterium avium*-intracellular complex, and *Mycobacterium kansasii*. This chapter aims to illustrate the epidemiology, diagnosis and treatment of tubercular lymphadenitis.

EPIDEMIOLOGY

There is variation in tubercular lymphadenitis prevalence in various geographical areas. Tuberculosis is responsible for approximately 43% of peripheral lymphadenopathy in the developing world whereas in developed countries like USA, about 20% of patients with tuberculosis have extrapulmonary disease of which lymphadenitis was reported in about 30–40% of cases. In developing and underdeveloped countries, tubercular lymphadenitis is most commonly caused by *Mycobacterium tuberculosis*[1,2] and non-tubercular mycobacteria is rare cause while in developed countries non-tubercular mycobacteria is the most common cause of lymphadenitis.[3,4] Several studies from different regions of India have reported that *Mycobacterium tuberculosis* has been the most common pathogen isolated from patients with lymphadenitis accounting for almost all the cases whereas in studies from Australia and British Columbia, non-tuberculous mycobacteria have been detected ten times more frequently than *Mycobacterium tuberculosis*. The HIV epidemic has been associated with an increase in the total incidence of tuberculosis and an increased proportion of miliary, disseminated and extrapulmonary tuberculosis cases including lymphadenitis.[5]

PATHOGENESIS

Lymph nodes can be infected via lymphatics as a part of primary complex. Cervical lymph nodes are involved as part of primary involvement of adenoids, tonsils, due to small tuberculous lesion (ulcer/granuloma) in gingival or oropharyngeal mucosa and scalp. Axillary and inguinal lymph nodes are involved due to granulomatous lesions in the drainage area in upper and lower limbs. Mediastinal and mesenteric lymph nodes are involved as a part of pulmonary and abdominal infection. They can be less commonly infected via blood borne route. Invasion of blood vessel by tuberculous focus presents with widespread involvement of lymph nodes.

Site of lymph node involvement most commonly in descending order are cervical, mediastinal/hilar, mesenteric, axillary and inguinal lymph nodes. Glands are first discrete and firm when periadenitis occur they become matted. Enlarged glands may become caseous and may lead to cold abscess which can perforate into deep fascia and present as fluctuant swelling on the surface as collar stud abscess. This can further progress and breakdown on overlying skin and lead to formation of tubercular sinus which has thin bluish undermined edges with watery discharge and is non-healing type. When tuberculous process reach the surface the skin gets involved to give typical thickened sinus ridden appearance of tubercular dermatitis or scrofuloderma. When immunity is more, hyperplastic type of lymphadenitis (essentially cellular reaction without caseation) can occur which results in matted firm, enlarged lymph nodes without abscess formation.

CLINICAL FEATURES

Tuberculous lymphadenitis is generally thought to be a local manifestation of a systemic disease. *M. tuberculosis* generally enters the human body via the respiratory tract and undergoes lymphohematogenous dissemination. Given to pulmonary route of organism entry, the first lymphoid tissue encountered are presumably hilar and mediastinal lymph nodes. Peripheral lymph nodes, especially in the cervical regions, are the most common sites of lymphadenopathy caused by *M. tuberculosis*. Classically presenting symptoms can be systemic and local. Patient may present with systemic symptoms such as fever, weight loss, and fatigue and somewhat less frequently with night sweats and cough. Systemic symptoms are not a prominent feature. Local symptoms can be manifested as painless swelling in the region, sinus formation. It commonly involves the jugular, posterior triangle, or supraclavicular lymph nodes. Surrounding pressure symptoms due to enlarging lymph nodes can also be a presenting symptoms, e.g. mediastinal lymphadenitis presenting as dysphagia, hoarseness of voice or superior vena cava obstruction. In contrast, lymphadenitis owing to non-tubercular *Mycobacterium* appears to be the result of a local infection in which the pathogens enter via oropharyngeal mucosa, salivary glands, tonsils, gingivae and conjunctiva. Lymph nodes may enlarge rapidly and may be associated with fistula formation. Physical examination may most commonly reveal enlarged multiple matted non-tender lymph nodes, occasionally patient may present with a single, discrete lymph nodes rubbery in consistency, cold abscess, discharging sinus fix to underlying lymph nodes, collar stud abscess, non-healing tubercular sinus with undermined edges and scrofuloderma (Figs 42.1–42.4). Jones and Campbell[6] had classified peripheral tubercular lymphadenopathy into five stages as described in Table 42.1.

Table 42.1: Staging of tubercular lymphadenitis

Stage 1	Enlarged, firm, mobile, discrete nodes showing non-specific reactive hyperplasia
Stage 2	Larger rubbery nodes fixed to surrounding tissue owing to periadenitis
Stage 3	Central softening due to caseation necrosis and abscess formation
Stage 4	Collar-stud abscess formation
Stage 5	Sinus tract formation

There are numerous causes of peripheral lymphadenopathy which should be excluded. The list include reactive lymphadenitis secondary to bacterial or viral infections, lymphomas, sarcoidosis, secondary carcinomas and uncommon causes such as fungal infections, toxoplasmosis. Three main clinical features such as multiplicity, matting, and caseation help in diagnosis of tubercular lymphadenitis. Tubercular lymphadenitis can be seen in HIV patients with multifocal involvement, more additional local signs such as sinus formation, tenderness and cold abscess formation, increased suppuration and non-reactivity as compared to HIV-negative individuals.

DIAGNOSIS

History and detailed physical examination is very important which should followed by other investigations to confirm the diagnosis of tubercular lymphadenitis. Tuberculin test is positive in about 75% of patients with lymph node tuberculosis while it is often non-reactive in non-tubercular mycobacteria lymphadenitis. However, a negative tuberculin test does not rule out the possibility. Chest X-ray should be done as a routine as there is reported incidence of paratracheal, hilar and mediastinal, lymphadenopathy

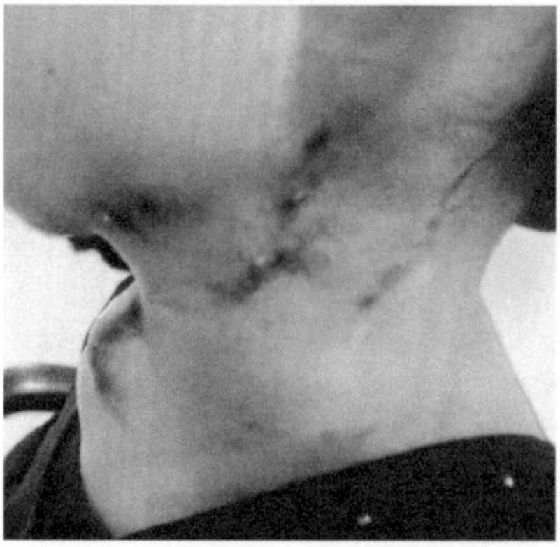

Fig. 42.1: Tuberculous lymphadenitis in the neck with multiple healed sinuses (For color version, see Plate 4)

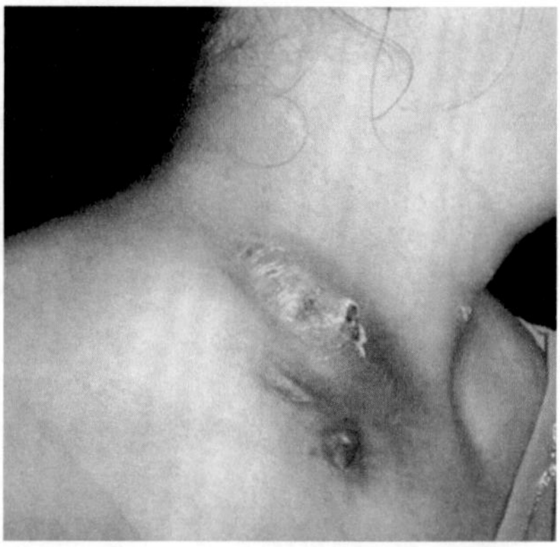

Fig. 42.2: Tuberculous lymphadenitis in the neck showing caseation with abcess formation (For color version, see Plate 4)

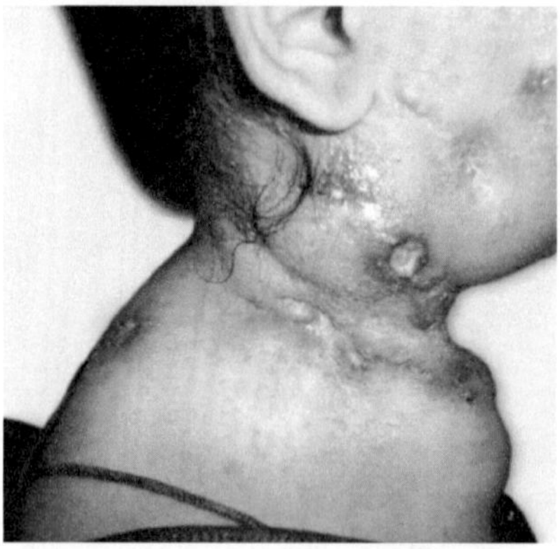

Fig. 42.3: Tubercular cervical lymphadenitis with ulceration in the neck (For color version, see Plate 5)

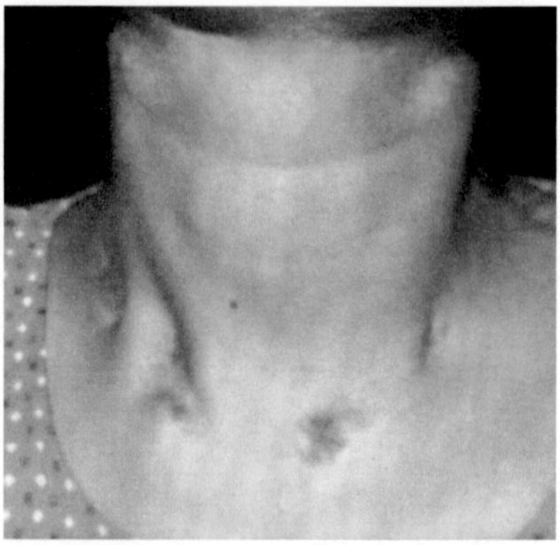

Fig. 42.4: Tuberculous lymphadenitis in the neck showing scarring after treatment (For color version, see Plate 5)

in patients with peripheral lymphadenitis, also there may be associated pulmonary tuberculosis. Diagnosis can be confirmed by smear examination for acid-fast bacilli, culture for *Mycobacterium* in the discharging pus. Fine-needle aspiration cytology (FNAC) is a rapid, reliable, safe and economical diagnostic tool for tubercular lymphadenitis and accuracy of 91.5% in diagnosis of tubercular lymphadenitis has been reported.[7-9] When FNAC of lymph node is inconclusive, biopsy of lymph node and histopathology, can be done for the diagnosis of tubercular lymphadenitis. Other investigations sometimes may be required for diagnosis, e.g. plain X-ray and ultrasound of abdomen, CT of the thorax and abdomen to rule out any gland. Ultrasound and CT guidance may be advised in order to perform biopsy of gland from difficult areas. Sometimes transtracheal/transbronchial needle aspiration or biopsy may be required to diagnose mediastinal gland. Newer technique such as endobronchial ultrasound and transesophageal route may be required to confirm the diagnosis. Polymerase chain reaction (PCR) may be of diagnostic value in some cases when other conventional methods are inconclusive.

TREATMENT

Medical Treatment

Various studies have clearly established the efficacy of short-course treatment in both children and adults with intermittent regimen as effective as daily regimen.[2,10] A 6-month anti-TB treatment (ATT) schedule comprising of 2RHEZ/4RH daily or thrice weekly supervised regimen has been recommended for management of tubercular lymphadenitis. Under the Revised National Tuberculosis Control Program (RNTCP) tubercular lymphadenitis is considered as extrapulmonary tuberculosis not seriously ill and is treated under category-III.[11-13] Recently, in a multicenter operational study in six Indian states, It was shown that 6-month thrice-weekly DOT for peripheral tubercular lymphadenopathy was satisfactory and there was no evidence of additional benefits of prolonging treatment of 9 months.[13] With revised WHO treatment guidelines 2009, all new cases of extrapulmonary tuberculosis including tubercular lymphadenitis are treated with category I regimen.[14]

Transitory appearance of new group of enlarged lymph nodes or increase in size of same lymph nodes during chemotherapy has been observed in one-third of cases and should not be taken as failure of therapy and the same drug should be continued. The decision to consider tubercular lymphadenitis as multidrug resistant needs demonstration of resistance to rifampicin and isoniazid from the culture and drug susceptibility test (DST) of lymph node aspirate. It is very difficult to isolate mycobacteria in cultures in most of the instances as the disease is paucibacillary. Chemotherapy at the most may cause only minor reduction in the size of lymph node. This fact should be made clear to the patients before initiating the therapy. Even after complete chemotherapy small shotty lymph node may persist. Occasionally for suppression of lymph node enlargement during chemotherapy, e.g. when mediastinal lymph nodes are causing bronchial obstruction, corticosteroids may need to be added to the therapy. It is speculated that caseation in peribronchial lymph nodes makes it difficult for drugs to reach all of the infected tissue. This condition may therefore merit the use of corticosteroids to help control the inflammatory response and resulting bronchial compression. The recommended corticosteroid regimen is usually given in the dose of 1–2 mg/kg/day for 4–6 weeks.

A phenomenon known as "paradoxical reaction" has been observed in about 2–23% of treated TB patients without HIV infection but it occurs more frequently in patients with HIV coinfection.[15] A confirmed case with paradoxical reaction can be defined as a patient who meets the following three criteria—radiological examinations showing worsening or emergence of intrathoracic lymphadenopathy, pulmonary infiltrates, pleural effusions, abdominal lymph nodes, hepatosplenomegaly, a good virological response and/or an increased CD4 lymphocyte count, and/or conversion of tuberculin skin test from negative to positive and/or adequate adherence to Antiretroviral therapy as well as TB treatment and a clear exclusion of other conditions that could explain the clinical manifestations of the patient, such as TB treatment failure or other concomitant infections, tumors or allergic reactions.

Surgical Treatment

Surgery is rarely required as tubercular lymphadenititis responds well to ATT. The main indications for surgery in tubercular lymphadenitis are difficulty in clinical diagnosis or inconclusive FNAC report, localized mass of lymph node persisting or increasing in size even after the chemotherapy and occurrence of collar stud abscess under deep fascia. Surgical techniques include aspiration, excision and drainage, complete surgical examination of affected lymph node and overlying skin and selective nodal and functional neck dissection when required. In all cases where local excision is possible, a transverse skin incision can be used. In extensive excisions, it is usually necessary to add to this an incision parallel to the posterior border of the sternomastoid in order to reach the apex of the posterior triangle. Although every effort can be made to preserve cutaneous branches of the cervical plexus and internal juglar vein, in many cases these are involved in the gland mass and are sacrificed.

Cold abscess must be evacuated either by antigravity aspiration or be drained. Block dissection of lymph nodes is rarely indicated now in this era of effective chemotherapy. Moreover, what may look like a few glands on superficial palpation, will turn out to be involvement of the entire chain on opening leading to extensive mutilating surgery. In very chronic lymphadenitis, limited surgery is indicated to remove the superficially located lymph nodes for cosmetic reasons. Nontubercular lymphadenitis is treated primarily by surgical excision.

REFERENCES

1. Dandapat MC, Mishra BM, Dash SP, Kar PK. Peripheral lymph node tuberculosis: a review of 80 cases. Br J Surg. 1990;77:911-2.
2. Jawahar MS, Sivasubramaniam S, Vijayan VK, Ramakrishnan CV, Paramasivan CN, Selvakumar V, et al. Short-course chemotherapy for tuberculous lymphadenitis in children. BMJ. 1990;301:359-62.
3. Pransky SM, Reisman BK, Kearans DB, Seid AB, Collins KL, Krous HF. Cervicofacial mycobacterial adenitis in children: endemic to San Diego. Laryngoscope. 1990;100:920-5.
4. Bailey WC. Treatment of atypical mycobacterial disease. Chest. 1983;84:625-8.
5. Hill AR, Premkumar S, Brustein S, et al. Disseminated tuberculosis in the AIDS era. Am Rev Respir Dis. 1991;144:1164-70.

6. Jones PG, Campbell PE. Tuberculous lymphadenitis in childhood; the significance of anonymous mycobacteria. Br J Surg. 1962;50:302-14.
7. Prasad R, Garg SK, Mukerji PK, Agarwal PK. Role of fine needle aspiration cytology in the diagnosis of lymphadenopathy; Indian J Chest Dis Allied Sci. 1993;35:27-9.
8. Narang RK, Pradhan S, Singh RP, Chaturvedi S. Place of FNAC in the diagnosis of lymphadenopathy. Indian J Tuber. 1990;37:29-31.
9. Malankar D, Jajoo UN, Swarup K, Gupta OP, Jain AP, Poflee VW. A clinical evaluation of FNAC in the diagnosis of lymphadenopathy. Indian J Tuber. 1991;38:17-9.
10. Balasubramanian R, Ramchandran R. Management of non-pulmonary forms of tuberculosis: review of TRC studies over two decades Indian Journal of Pediatrics 2000;67:S34-S40.
11. Kabra SK, Lodha R, Seth V. Category based treatment of tuberculosis in children. Indian Pediatr. 2004;41:927-37.
12. World Health Organization. Treatment of tuberculosis. Guidelines for national programmes. Third edition. Revised June 2004. WHO/CDS/TB/2003.313.
13. Jindal SK, Aggarwal AN, Gupta D, Ahmed Z, Gupta KB, Janmeja AK, et al. Tuberculous lymphadenopathy: a multicentre operational study of 6-month thrice weekly directly observed treatment. Int J Tuberc Lung Dis. 2013;17:234-9.
14. World Health Organization. Treatment of TB Guidelines. 4th Edition. WHO/HTM/TB/2009.420.
15. Colebunders R, John L, Huyst V, Kambugu A, Scano F, Lynen L. Tuberculosis immune reconstitution inflammatory syndrome in countries with limited resources. Int J Tuberc Lung Dis. 2006;10(9):946–53.

Chapter 43

Tuberculosis in Children

INTRODUCTION

Pulmonary tuberculosis was reported to be less of a problem in the pediatric population as compared to those aged 15 years and over.[1,2] Usually source of infection in children is from an adult family member or close contact of sputum smear positive pulmonary tuberculosis. Extrapulmonary tuberculosis is generally 3 times more common than pulmonary tuberculosis in children. Children rarely have sputum positive tuberculosis and so they are unlikely source of transmission of tuberculosis but tuberculosis in children represent failure of tuberculosis control in adult. Chances of developing disease are greatest shortly after infection and steadily decreases with time. This chapter aims to review the epidemiology, diagnosis and treatment of childhood tuberculosis.

EPIDEMIOLOGY

Children younger than 15 years contribute 15–20% of the global tuberculosis burden, although accurate data are scarce due to challenges in case ascertainment and lack of surveillance in this age group.[3] Knowledge regarding the extent of tuberculosis among children particularly in 0–4 years is based only on impression from hospital and clinic practices and it is generally believed that tuberculosis infection and disease in children is high and tuberculosis constitutes a common disease of pediatric age group. This could be a true reflection of the tuberculosis problem among sick children who attend clinics and hospitals, but it cannot be representative of the overall tuberculosis problem of childhood in the entire community.

Incidence of bacteriologically positive case among children was 1/5 of prevalence, whereas it was 1/3 in those aged 15 years and above. Of the 9 million annual tuberculosis cases, about 1 million (11%) occur in children under 15 years of age. Of these childhood cases, 75% occur annually in 22 high burden countries. Fewer studies have been conducted in various parts of our country in order to estimate burden of tuberculosis among children. Prevalence of tuberculosis infection obtained through tuberculin testing in children over a period of time is recognized to be a reliable indicator for defining tuberculosis burden and its trend in the community. Annual rate of infection (ARI) expresses the overall impact of various factors influencing the transmission of tubercle bacilli. In the Nicobar study, the best estimate of all forms of tuberculosis in children was 0.6%, including histopathologically confirmed glandular tuberculosis (smear positive case prevalence 0.4%).[4] One study conducted among school children in Bangaluru city reported 11.0% prevalence of infection with ARI 1.7%.[5] It is estimated that in developing countries, the annual risk of tuberculosis infection in children is 2.5%. In India, the overall estimates of average annual risk of infection in children 1–9 years of age was computed as 1.5%. It was higher in urban areas, at 2.2%, than in rural areas, at 1.3%. The prevalence of infection ranged from 4–12% in various other studies.[5-8] A high prevalence of tuberculosis infection was observed among urban slum children in Ahmedabad with observed prevalence of 20.5% and ARI of 5.4%.[9] A high rate of ARI (3%) was also observed in the study conducted among urban slum children of Chooli in Chennai.[7] It appears that considerable differences exist in the infection rate among children from area to area within the country. This could be a manifestation of the prevailing socioeconomic conditions in the population. Infants and young children under 5 years of age are at a particular risk after infection and many present with disease within 1 year of infection, probably due to immature cellular immunity. Children under 5 years of age are at higher risk of developing disseminated forms of TB, including miliary TB and TB meningitis, which are frequently associated with greater morbidity and mortality. Further, prevalence of disease between 5–12 years of age is generally low and then increase again in adolescent. For infants, generally, the most common source is mother. So if suspicion of tuberculosis in infant mother should be investigated for pulmonary tuberculosis. Infected children can develop tuberculosis at any time as various immunosuppressive disease and illnesses may trigger the progression from infection to disease such as HIV infection, measles, whooping cough and malnutrition. Rajnarain et al. considerably reported higher annual mortality rate in his study on a Chennai urban slum population group aged 1–4 years old having annual mortality rate 239 per 100,000 as compared to 52–55 per 100,000 in the rural areas under BCG-Trial in Tamil Nadu and Longitudinal Survey in Bangluru.[10] Nearly 8–20% of deaths caused by tuberculosis occur in children.[11,12]

CLINICAL PRESENTATION OF TUBERCULOSIS

Tuberculosis can present either as unilateral hilar or mediastinal lymphadenopathy without lung abnormality (most common presentation) or primary lesion of 3–10 mm size lung opacity with hilar or mediastinal lymphadenopathy, it is less common and classified as pulmonary tuberculosis. Rarely there can be large opacity (lobar or segmental) with lymphadenopathy. Lymphadenopathy can lead to compression of bronchi causing collapse. Acute disseminated post-primary tuberculosis (seen in children less than 5 years age) present as military tuberculosis with or without meningitis classified as severe extrapulmonary tuberculosis. BCG vaccination has been found to be more effective in preventing against disseminated tuberculosis.

Sputum negative pulmonary tuberculosis is commonest in children below 5 years of age because children have primary tuberculosis rather than post-primary tuberculosis and secondly at this age children do not produce sputum. Post-primary pulmonary tuberculosis is seen in older children. It is generally non-cavitatory smear negative pulmonary tuberculosis. Prevalence of pulmonary tuberculosis is low between 5–12 years of age and then increase in adolescents. In adolescents pulmonary tuberculosis is similar in presentation as adult pulmonary tuberculosis often with cavitations and smear positive for acid-fast bacilli (AFB).

POST-PRIMARY EXTRAPULMONARY TUBERCULOSIS

Common forms of extrapulmonary tuberculosis in children are lymphadenopathy, miliary tuberculosis, pleural effusion, pericardial effusion and spinal tuberculosis.

DIAGNOSIS OF CHILDHOOD TUBERCULOSIS

Diagnosis of pulmonary tuberculosis in children is difficult because child under 6 years rarely cough up sputum and there is generally non-cavitatory sputum smear negative pulmonary tuberculosis.[13] Gastric suction and laryngeal swab are generally not useful unless facilities for mycobacterial culture are available. There are no specific features on clinical examination that can confirm that the presenting illness is due to tuberculosis. Respiratory symptoms and disease are extremely common during childhood especially before 5 years of age so diagnosis of pulmonary tuberculosis in children is difficult and thus is commonly over diagnosed. Therefore, diagnosis should be based on a combination of clinical presentation, bacteriological as well as radiological examination, Mantoux test and history of contact. Diagnostic clues for tuberculosis in children are:

- Contact with sputum positive pulmonary tuberculosis is a step to identify source of infection and history for pulmonary tuberculosis should be sought for each contact in last 2 years

- Failure to thrive or weight loss is a good indicator of chronic disease in children and tuberculosis may be the cause
- Clinical symptoms such as fever and/or cough for more than 2–3 weeks not responding to broad spectrum antibiotics
- Positive tuberculin test indicate presence of infection while a negative test does not rule out tuberculosis as immunosuppression or severe infection can cause negative tuberculin test
- Neurological manifestations such as refusal to feed, irritability, headache, projectile vomiting or altered sensorium in suspected cases of tubercular meningitis.

In absence of these clues, tuberculosis is less likely and look for symptoms of other diseases such as whooping cough, asthma, bacterial pneumonias, HIV infection, cardiac failure due to congenital heart disease, rheumatic heart disease, bronchiectasis, cystic fibrosis.[14] Chest X-ray is investigation for suspected tuberculosis or miliary tuberculosis. Most consistent feature on chest X-ray is nodal enlargement and will be present in many children with pulmonary tuberculosis. Cavitation is seen in older children and adolescent who will be sputum smear positive. Normal chest X-ray may be used to exclude pulmonary tuberculosis or miliary tuberculosis in children but usefulness of chest X-ray is reduced in malnourished or immunocompromized child. Extra-pulmonary tuberculosis in comparison can be diagnosed by typical features like spinal deformity, scrofula, painless ascites and simple investigation can lead to confident diagnosis of tuberculosis even though not confirmed microbiologically.

As per Revised National Tuberculosis Control Program (RNTCP) guidelines all suspected pediatric TB cases having chest symptomatic or other symptoms suggestive of tuberculosis are advised to undergo three sputum examinations (two spot and one overnight sample collected in two visits). Patients with two or three smear positive results are diagnosed as sputum positive pulmonary tuberculosis. Those with only one positive result, are advised to get a chest X-ray done, and if found to be compatable with tuberculosis, are treated as sputum-positive pulmonary tuberculosis. Patients with all the three negative results are prescribed broad-spectrum antibiotics such as cotrimoxazole for 10–14 days. If not suffering from tuberculosis, patients improve with antibiotics. Persistent symptoms direct for re-evaluation of patient on the basis of sputum microscopy and chest X-ray (Fig. 43.1). Lastly, if treating physician have an opinion that patient is suffering from pulmonary tuberculosis, treatment is initiated accordingly. However, RNTCP has launched recent guidelines in April, 2009 which recommends that the number of specimen required for diagnosis of smear positive pulmonary TB is two, with one of them being a morning sputum specimen. One specimen positive out of the two is enough to declare a patient as smear positive TB. If none of the repeat sputum specimens is positive, a chest X-ray is taken, and if findings of the X-ray are consistent with pulmonary tuberculosis, the patient

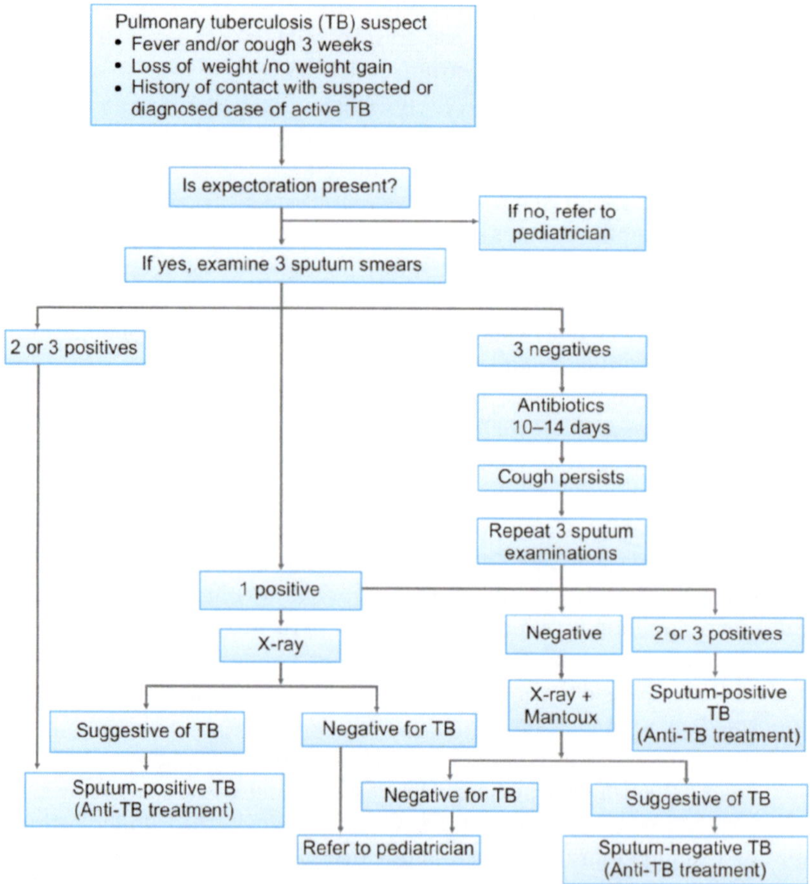

Fig. 43.1: RNTCP diagnostic algorithm for pediatric tuberculosis

is diagnosed by the physician as a case of sputum negative pulmonary TB (Fig. 43.2).

TREATMENT OF TUBERCULOSIS IN CHILDREN

WHO has recommended following strategy for management of pediatric patients with tuberculosis (Table 43.1).[15,16]

Management of childhood tuberculosis under Revised National Tuberculosis Program (RNTCP) with DOTS as the recommended strategy as in case of adults in order to prevent confusion and improve overall compliance. Intermittent short-course chemotherapy given under direct observation should be used in children (Table 43.2). The metabolism of drug varies with age and researches have not proved efficacy of 6 months of ethambutol and

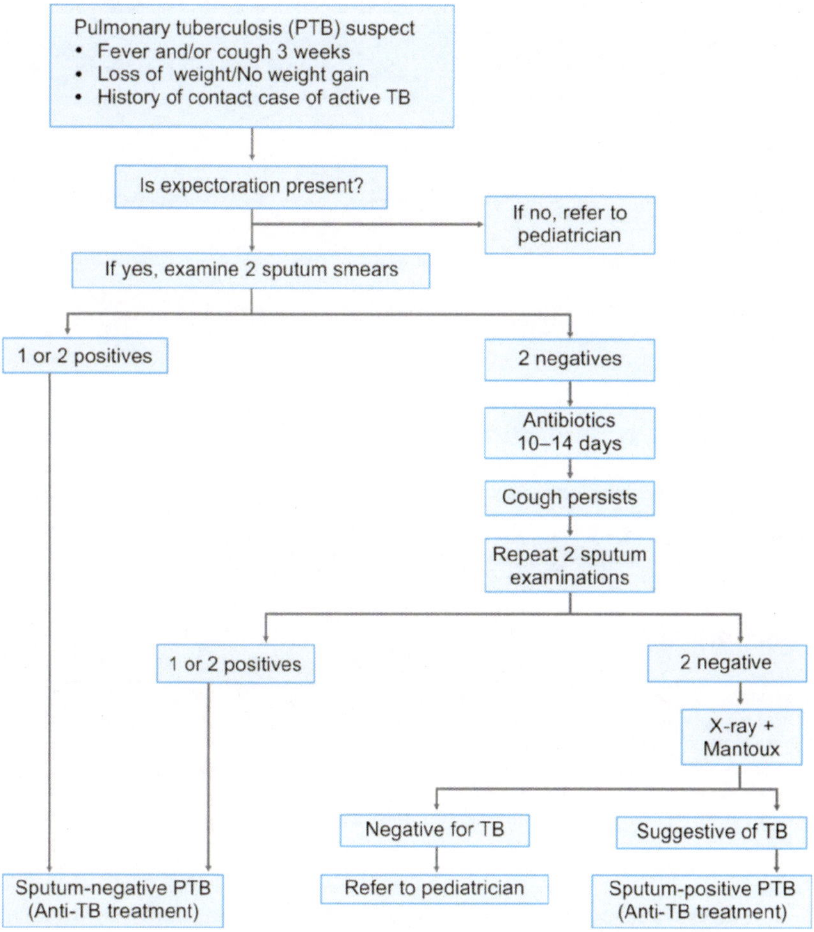

Fig. 43.2: Revised diagnostic algorithm for pediatric tuberculosis

isoniazid in continuation phase in children so 4 months of rifampicin and isoniazid is recommended.[17] The recommended dosages for intermittent therapy in case of children are: Isoniazid (10–15 mg/kg), rifampicin (10 mg/kg), pyrazinamide (30–35 mg/kg), ethambutol (30 mg/kg) and streptomycin (15 mg/kg).

The regimen recommended for treating the pediatric cases had been $2R_3H_3Z_3/4R_3H_3$ for children less than 6 years of age since introduction of DOTS in 1997. For all children above 6 years, the same regimen was recommended as for adults. In early 2004, in consultation with Indian Academy of Pediatrics, the recommendations were revised whereby ethambutol was included for treatment of pediatric cases even under 6 years of age. Tubercular meningitis is severe form of tuberculosis with high mortality and long-term complications. Streptomycin has greater cerebrospinal fluid (CSF)

Table 43.1: WHO treatment categories and regimen for children 2010, modified in 2011.

TB cases and diagnostic category	Anti-TB drug regimens	
	Intensive phase	Continuation phase
New Patient Regimen New smear-positive PTB Smear-negative PTB with extensive parenchymal involvement Severe forms of EPTB other than TB meningitis	2HRZE	4HR
New Patient Regimen Smear-negative PTB without extensive parenchymal involvement Less severe forms of EPTB (e.g TB cervical adenitis)	2HRZ	4HR
New Patient Regimen TB meningitis	2HRZS[a]	4HR
Retreatment regimen Previously treated smear-positive PTB (relapse, treatment after interruption or treatment failure) *If low risk for MDR-TB or risk unknown: continue with retreatment regimen* *If high risk for MDR-TB: use MDR-TB regimen below*	2HRZES/1HRZE	5HRE
MDR Regimen MDR-TB	Individualized regimens	

E, ethambutol; H, isoniazid; R, rifampicin; S, streptomycin; Z, pyrazinamide.

[a]: Other regimens are recommended for treatment of TB meningitits that include replacing streptomycin with ethionamide and treating for 9–12 months.

Recently, guidelines have been changed. The main changes are that all TB types (except TBM and OA TB) in HIV endemic setting should receive a fourth drug in intensive phase 2RHZE/4RH: TBM and osteo-articular TB should receive 2 RHZE/10RH and that streptomycin is no longer recommended as first-line in children.

penetration so ethambutol should be replaced with streptomycin in such cases. In tubercular meningitis spinal TB with neurological complications and other hematogenous tuberculosis continuation phase is prolonged for 3 more months. WHO currently recommends that children with suspected or confirmed tuberculous meningitis and osteoarticular tuberculosis should be treated with a four-drug regimen (HRZE) for 2 months, followed by a two-drug regimen (HR) for 10 months; the total duration of treatment being 12 months. The doses recommended for the treatment of tuberculous meningitis and osteoarticular tuberculosis are the same as those described for pulmonary tuberculosis. Children with proven or suspected pulmonary tuberculosis or tuberculous meningitis caused by multidrug resistant bacilli (MDR-TB) can be treated with a fluoroquinolone in the context of a well-functioning MDR-TB control program and within an appropriate MDR-TB regimen. The decision to treat should be taken by a clinician experienced in managing pediatric tuberculosis. Steroids are recommended during the early

Table 43.2: RNTCP treatment categories and regimens for children

Treatment Category	Type of Patients	Treatment Regimen***	
		Intensive phase	Continuation phase
Category I	• New sputum smear-positive pulmonary TB • New sputum smear-negative pulmonary TB, seriously ill* • New extrapulmonary TB, seriously ill*	2 $H_3R_3Z_3E_3$ ***	4 H_3R_3
Category II	• Sputum smear-positive relapse • Sputum smear-positive treatment failure • Sputum smear-positive treatment after default	2 $H_3R_3Z_3E_3S_3$ + 1 $H_3R_3Z_3E_3$	5 $H_3R_3E_3$
Category III****	• New sputum smear-negative, not seriously ill** • New extrapulmonary TB, not seriously ill**	2 $H_3R_3Z_3$	4 H_3R_3
Category IV	Chronic and MDR-TB	(6–9) Km Eto Cs LevoZE	18 Eto Cs Levo E

*In children, seriously ill sputum smear-negative pulmonary TB includes all forms of sputum smear-negative pulmonary TB other than primary complex such as TB meningitis, disseminated TB, Tubercular pericarditis,Tubercular peritonitis and intestinal TB, Bilateral extensive pleurisy, Spinal TB with or without neurological complications, Genitourinary TB and Bone and Joint TB.

**Not seriously ill sputum smear pulmonary TB includes primary complex. Not seriously ill. Extra-pulmonary TB includes Lymph node TB and unilateral pleural effusion.

***Prefix indicates month and subscript indicates thrice weekly.

****Recently, category I and category III has been merged together and all the new patients of tuberculosis will be treated with catogary I regimen, i.e. $2R_3H_3E_3Z_3/4R_3H_3$.

part of the treatment of TB meningitis, TB pericarditis and segmental/lobar collapse due to thoracic lymphadenopathy, with the doses being tapered off over 6–8 weeks. All children should be examined by pediatrician or an expert on TB if possible before initiating on catogary II treatment. As per current recommendation of WHO and in view of growing evidence that the use of ethambutol in young children is safe, it is to be used as per RNTCP regimens for all age groups. Monitoring of treatment is obtained in a similar way as in case of adults. Asymptomatic children under 6 years of age, exposed to a patient with infectious (smear-positive) TB from the same household, need to be given 6 months of daily isoniazid (5 mg/kg) as chemoprophylaxis against the disease. BCG vaccination is given at birth to provide benefit against the childhood forms of TB especially against meningitis TB and tubercular mengitis.

REFERENCES

1. Gothi GD, Nair SS, Pyarelal. Some epidemiological aspects of tuberculosis disease and infection in paediatric age group in a rural community. Indian Paediatrics. 1971;8:186-94.
2. Gothi GD, Isaac B, Chakraborty AK, Rajalakshmi R, Singh S.Tuberculosis in a slum community. Ind J Tuber. 1977;24:68-74.
3. Marais BJ, Gupta A, Starke JR, El Sony A. Tuberculosis in women and children. Lancet. 2010;375:2057-9.
4. Directorate of Health Services A & N Administration. Intensified TB control programme in the isolated tribal population of Car-Nicobar. WHO-HSR GOI Project No. IND/HSR 001/D.1989;p1-64.(unpublished).
5. Chadha VK, Jagannatha PS, Savanur SJ. Annual risk of tuberculosis infection in Bangalore city. Indian J Tubercul. 2001;48:63.
6. Chakraborty AK. Tuberculosis in India. Pediatrics Today. 1999;1:47-53.
7. Chakraborty AK, Ganapathy KT, Gothi GD. Prevalence of infection among unvaccinated children for tuberculosis surveillance. Indian J Med Res. 1980;72:7-12.
8. Chadha VK, Suryanarayana HV, Krishna-murthy MK, Jagnath PS, Shashidhara AN. Prevalence of undernutrition among peri-urban children and its influence on the estimation of annual risk of tuberculosis infection. Indian J Tubercul. 1997;44:67-71.
9. Bhagyalaxmi A, Kadri AM, Lala MK, et al. Prevalence of tuberculosis infection among children in slums of Ahmedabad. Indian Pediatrics. 2003;40:239-43.
10. Rajnarain, Dwakara AM. Mortality due to tuberculosis in children in India. Indian Paediatrics. 1975;12:529-37.
11. Munoz FM, Starke JR. Tuberculosis in children. In: Tuberculosis: A comprehensive international approach, 2nd edition New York: Marcell Dekker Inc. 2000:553-95.
12. Mukherjee A, Lodha R, Kabra SK. Changing trends in childhood tuberculosis.Indian J Pediatr. 2010. [Epub ahead of print].
13. Osborne CM. The challenges of diagnosing childhood tuberculosis de'enfant [ADD English translation of title of book]. Paris, Srinagar-Verlag, 1999.
14. Schaff HS, et al. Respiratory tuberculosis in childhood: the diagnostic value of clinical features and special investigations. Paediatric infections Disease Journal. 1995;14:189-94.
15. World Health Organization. Guidelines for national tuberculosis programs on the management of tuberculosis in children. WHO/HTM/ TB/2006.371.
16. World Health Organization. Guidance for National Tuberculosis and HIV Programs on the management of tuberculosis in HIV-infected children: recommendations for a public health approach. Geneva: World Health Organization; 2010.
17. Graham SM. Treatment of Paediatric TB: revised WHO Guidelines. Paediatric Respiratory Reviews. 12(2011) 22-6.

Chapter 44

Tuberculosis in Elderly

INTRODUCTION

Average age of the world population is increasing, due to the increasing life expectancy and decreasing birth rate. As per year 2000 data, they constitute 7.6% of Indian population. Tuberculosis (TB) is reported to be more frequent in elderly population. Almost half of the cases of TB identified at necropsy did not have the opportunity to receive treatment as diagnosis was not made when the patient was alive. There is controversy on whether elderly subjects present with different clinical or radiological features. This write-up reviews the challenges in diagnosis and management of tuberculosis in this age group.

EPIDEMIOLOGY

There is a difference in the epidemiological pattern of tuberculosis in high incidence and low incidence countries. In high incidence countries the peak of epidemic is in young adults while in low incidence countries there is an increase in the burden of tuberculosis with age.[1] In countries that have effectively fought against tuberculosis in past decades, early diagnosis and treatment of most TB cases has been achieved, thereby shortening the epidemiological chain of the disease and eliminating the infectious sources in the community. Thus, people born in the last four to five decades have had low community infection risks and very few infections have resulted. In such countries, TB is essentially found in the older age groups, where there is a persistent presence of individuals with *M. tuberculosis* infection—due to the poor social conditions, they had endured during their childhood when effective treatment measures were not yet available. In India, persons aged 65 years and above constituted 8% of sputum smear positive patients.[2]

In these elderly individuals, source of infection can be exogenous (reinfection) or endogenous reactivation. Though these are difficult to differentiate, it is generally believed that endogenous reactivation is the predominant mechanism.[3,4]

REASONS FOR REACTIVATION

That the oldest segment of the population suffers TB, the most can be attributed to two reasons. First, the elderly have the highest prevalence of *M. tuberculosis* infection, since the prevalence is cumulative in the course of a lifetime. Thus, the older the individual, the greater the probability of infection. Second, immune defects in cellular immunity tend to be found with advancing age, with a reduction in the number and function of the T-helper lymphocytes and an increase in the presence of T-suppressor cells, thereby augmenting the possibility of endogenous reactivation of TB disease.[5] Other risk factors that may exist in elderly are malnutrition, diseases such as malignancy, diabetes mellitus, HIV infection, immunosuppressive treatments such as corticosteroid, tobacco smoking, gastrointestinal surgery such as gastrectomy or jejunoileal byepass.

CLINICAL FEATURES

The immune deficiency characterizing the elderly population might alter the growth and multiplication of *M. tuberculosis* and the clinical and radiological presentations. Many studies have reported an increased frequency of disseminated forms of the disease; with a clinical presentation in which syndromes of systemic involvement tend to predominate.[6] Some of the difficulty in diagnosis is due to the inability to obtain a proper history due to factors such as dementia, deafness or impairment of speech. Sometimes pre-existing diseases, both diagnosed and undiagnosed, may mask the symptomatology of tuberculosis. A paucity of respiratory symptoms is observed in elderly. Sometimes pyrexia with progressive wasting mimicking a malignancy may occur.

Pulmonary Tuberculosis in Elderly

Most cases of pulmonary tuberculosis in elderly are due to reactivation of old lesions. The typical sites are apical segments of both upper and lower lobes and posterior segments of upper lobes. Pleural effusion or pneumothorax can also be a presentation. Tuberculosis should be included in the differential diagnosis of any illness in an elderly patient with pleuropulmonary symptoms and signs or with pulmonary infiltrates. Reactivation tuberculosis usually present with fever, cough with expectoration and hemoptysis.[7] X-ray shows fibronodular lesions in the upper zones with or without cavitation. Hilar and perihilar lesions may also be present and should be differentiated from other opportunistic infections, bronchogenic carcinoma and lymphoma. Primary tuberculosis infection in elderly present with constitutional symptoms and cough.[7] Chest radiography abnormalities are often seen in mid and lower zones and may lead to a missed diagnosis and transmission of infection.[8]

Extrapulmonary Tuberculosis in Elderly

Extrapulmonary tuberculosis in elderly results from reactivation of lesions that were the result of hematogenous spread of bacilli in the primary phase of infection. This is relatively more common in elderly than pulmonary tuberculosis. The common sites affected are bones and joints, urogenital, abdominal and meningeal. They may present with disseminated tuberculosis with involvement of two or more noncontiguous organs.

Tubercular Lymphadenopathy

It usually presents as slowly enlarging lymphadenopathy. Cervical nodes are the most commonly involved. Fever and other systemic symptoms may not be evident. Rarely axillary and inguinal lymphadenopathy may be present. Cold abscess, chronic non-healing TB sinus and ulcer may also be seen.

Pleural Effusion

Elderly patients with pleural effusion present with insidious onset of symptoms. Pleuritic pain and non-productive cough are the usual presenting symptoms. Fever and other systemic symptoms may also be evident. However, many may be asymptomatic.

Tuberculosis of Bones and Joints

This tends to affect weight bearing joints such as the vertebrae, hip or knee causing a combination of osteomyelitis and arthritis. It should be suspected in any elderly patient with unexplained unifocal inflammation or destruction of bone or joint.

Genitourinary Tuberculosis

It is often a reactivation of dormant hematogenous foci in kidneys. Most common symptoms are dysuria and urinary frequency caused by tubercular cystitis. It should be suspected in anybody with sterile pyuria.

Tubercular Meningitis

It is more commonly seen in elderly. They present with non-specific symptoms of headache, dizziness, confusion and the classical signs of meningitis may be absent. Severe hyponatremia due to SIADH (Syndrome of inappropriate secretion of ADH) may lead to confusional states. CT-scan of the brain and cerebrospinal fluid (CSF) analysis should be done.

Miliary Tuberculosis

It is increasingly being seen in elderly and can be difficult to diagnose.[9] The symptoms are often nonspecific such as fever, weakness, weight loss, and physical examination is often non-contributory. Sometimes lymphadenopathy or hepatosplenomegaly may be the only finding. A slowly progressive wasting syndrome with low grade or absent fever, without localizing symptoms or signs and without a miliary pattern on X-ray may also be seen.[10] Another variety of tuberculosis in elderly is 'areactive' in which the tubercle consists of caseous and necrotic material containing large numbers of tubercle bacilli with notable absence of inflammatory cells. This is due to the declining cell mediated immunity.[11]

DIAGNOSIS

A characteristic of tuberculosis in elderly TB patients is the increased diagnostic delay. The fact that elderly subjects often suffer from other concomitant diseases with symptoms that are similar to those of tuberculosis constitutes the main cause of diagnostic delay. Comorbid conditions such as COPD frequently coexist and delay sputum smear examination in those with productive cough. Sometimes congestive cardiac failure may mimic pleural effusion. Delays in establishing a diagnosis can also be attributable to many other reasons, such as memory problems, mental confusion, isolation due to partial loss of the senses (hearing, sight) and even the inability to communicate. It is evident that a high index of suspicion is essential to make a diagnosis of various forms of tuberculosis in elderly.

INVESTIGATIONS IN TUBERCULOSIS IN ELDERLY

Some diagnostic techniques are less sensitive in the elderly. For example, tuberculin testing clearly loses its utility in both diagnosing disease and identifying infection—a deficit that is related to the onset of age-related immune defects. For this reason, American Thoracic Society and Center for Disease Control and Prevention have recommended a two stage tuberculin skin testing in elderly (spaced 1 week apart) if previous results are negative.[12,13] The aim here is to identify the possible booster effect that these tuberculin doses may exert upon immune memory loss—a procedure that has been shown to be effective in all studies involving elderly persons.

Regarding the performance of microbiological tests in the elderly, the results seem to be similar to those obtained in younger patients, provided the same types of lesions are involved. In studies showing an increased frequency of non-typical forms, with a greater presence of infiltrations versus cavitary lesions, the performance of smear microscopy and culture may decrease. Performance is thus related to the bacillary population of the lesions. However, elderly people have insufficient strength to expectorate and may not be able to provide an adequate sputum sample for testing. If the clinical suspicion is high and the sputum smear is negative, more invasive methods such as laryngeal swab, fiberoptic bronchoscopy and examination of various bronchoscopic secretion and gastric aspirate can be undertaken.

In patients with extrapulmonary tuberculosis all effort should be made to obtain appropriate specimen for microbiological and/or histopathological diagnosis. Some studies have described a different presentation of tuberculous granulomas in some forms of TB in the elderly, including the repercussions, this may have for the histopathological study of biopsy specimens. Thus, a variant described in elderly patients is referred to as "a reactive" TB, often with a miliary presentation. Here, the classic caseous granuloma is not surrounded by the usual abundant inflammatory cells, but instead by numerous bacilli. This form of presentation, attributed to an inadequate immune response, is most frequently seen with fever and weight loss, but without the typical pathological signs.[11]

TREATMENT

Tuberculosis in the elderly is treated with the same treatment regimens indicated for younger patients, although some studies have described decreased efficacy of such treatments in the elderly. Other studies have described a longer time to negative culture conversion, again possibly due to the diminished immune support found in the elderly, although it is not known if a comparatively lesser effect of treatment could also be involved. Elderly patients pose increased treatment adherence problems because of the possibility of memory lapses (difficulty remembering the prescribed dosage), mental confusion, a decreased ability to comprehend the scope of the disease and the precise drug doses required, and even eyesight problems that make it difficult to recognize which tablet to take. Some of them become apathetic and lack the determination to complete a treatment that may last 6-months or longer. So treatment supervision is required.

Another important consideration in the treatment of tuberculosis in the elderly is the interactions of antituberculosis medication, especially rifampicin and isoniazid, with some medications that they may be already taking. Rifampicin increases the metabolic degradation of corticosteroids, digoxin, oral anticoagulants and hypoglycemic agents and the dosage of these may have to be adjusted. Similar to other medications adverse reactions are more common to antituberculous drugs in the elderly. The risk of liver toxicity, largely associated with isoniazid, is much greater in elderly patients, as a result of which periodic liver function tests may be advisable.[14] Similarly, nephrotoxicity is a consideration when streptomycin is used—a situation requiring monitoring of renal function and dose reduction.[15] Ethambutol may cause retrobulbar neuritis which may be difficult to detect in elderly patients with some impairment of vision or cataract.

CONCLUSION

In view of the above considerations, an increased diagnostic suspicion of TB is indicated in people over the age of 60–65 years. This is the age group with the highest TB disease rates, in whom the clinicoradiological presentation, associated diseases, and different performances or yields of the diagnostic techniques imply an increased delay in diagnosis. This delay is not only of great importance in terms of public health (related to increased infectious periods), but also for the patient, which explains why TB is found with some frequency in necropsy-based studies. Such studies have reported a considerably greater frequency of TB among older population groups. On the other hand, the most important finding possibly is that almost half of these TB cases identified at necropsy did not have the opportunity to receive treatment because the disease had not been diagnosed when the patient was alive.

REFERENCES

1. Doherty MJ, Spence DP, Davies PD. Trends in the mortality from tuberculosis in England and Wales: effect of age from non-respiratory disease. Thorax. 1995;50:976-9.
2. Central TB Division. Directorate General of Health Service, Ministry of Health and Family Welfare, Government of India. TB India. 2007. RNTCP Status Report. New Delhi.
3. Nagami P, Yoshikawa TT. Aging and tuberculosis. Gerontology. 1984;30:308-15.
4. Anonymous. Tuberculosis in old age. Leading Article. Tubercle. 1983;33:517.
5. Aspinall R. Age-related changes in the function of T cells. Microsc Res Tech. 2003;62: 508-13.
6. Liaw YS, Yang PC, Yu CJ, et al. Clinical spectrum of tuberculosis in older patients. J Am Geriatr Soc. 1995;43:256-60.
7. Van den Brande P, Vijgen J, Demedts M. Clinical spectrum of pulmonary tuberculosis in older patients: Comparison with younger patients. J Gerontol. 1991;46:M204-9.
8. Stead WW, Lofgren JP, Warren E, Thomas C. Tuberculosis as an endemic and nosocomial infection among the elderly in nursing homes. N Engl J Med. 1985;312:1483-7.
9. Stead WW, Dutt AK. Tuberculosis in the elderly. Semin Respir Infect. 1989;4:189-97.
10. Proudfoot AT, akhtar AJ, Douglas AC, Horne NW. Miliary tuberculosis in adults. BMJ. 1969:7:186-90.
11. Sahn SA, Neff TA. Miliary tuberculosis. Am J Med. 1974;56:495-505.
12. American Thoracic Society. Diagnostic standards and classification of tuberculosis. Am rev Respir Dis. 1990;142:725-35.
13. Centers for Disease Control. Prevention and control of tuberculosis in facilities providing long-term care to elderly. Morb Mortal wkly Rep MMWR. 1990;39 [No.RR-10].
14. Van den Brande P, Van Steenbergen W, Vervoort G, Demedts M. Aging and hepatotoxicity of isoniazid and rifampin in pulmonary tuberculosis. Am J Respir Crit Care Med. 1995;152: 1705-8.
15. Yoshikava TT. Tuberculosis in aging adults. J Am Geriatr Soc. 1992:40.

Chapter 45

Tuberculosis Abdomen

INTRODUCTION

Tuberculosis (TB) can involve any part of the gastrointestinal (GI) tract from mouth to anal canal, the peritoneum and pancreatic-biliary system. Autopsies conducted on patients with pulmonary tuberculosis before the era of effective antitubercular drugs revealed intestinal involvement in 55-90% cases, with the frequency related to the extent of pulmonary involvement. Pimparkar found evidence of abdominal tuberculosis (bowel, peritoneum and liver) in 3.72% of 11,476 autopsies carried out in KEM Hospital, Mumbai between 1964 to 1970.[1] TB of GI tract is the six most frequent form of extrapulmonary site after, lymphatic, genitourinary, bone and joint, miliary and meningeal tuberculosis.[2] In India most common pathogen is *M. tuberculosis* not *M. bovis*.[3,4] This chapter aims to describe the pathogenesis, clinical features, diagnosis and treatment of abdominal tuberculosis.

PATHOGENESIS

The postulated mechanisms by which the tubercule bacilli reach the GI tract are: hematogenous spread from the primary lung focus in childhood, with later reactivation; ingestion of bacilli in sputum from active pulmonary focus; direct spread from adjacent organs and through lymph channels from infected nodes. The most common site of involvement is the ileocecal region, possibly because of the increased physiological stasis, increased rate of fluid and electrolyte absorption, minimal digestive activity and an abundance of lymphoid tissue at this site. Tuberculous granulomas are initially formed in the mucosa or the Peyer's patches. These granulomas are of variable size and characteristically tend to be confluent, in contrast to those in Crohn's disease. Granulomas are often seen just beneath the ulcer bed, mainly in the submucosal layer. Submucosal edema or widening is inconspicuous. Tubercular ulcers are relatively superficial and usually do not penetrate beyond the muscularis. They may be single or multiple, and the intervening mucosa is usually uninvolved. These ulcers are usually transversely oriented in contrast to Crohn's disease where the ulcers are longitudinal or serpiginous. Cicatricial healing of these circumferential 'girdle ulcers' result in strictures. Occlusive arterial changes may produce ischemia and contribute to the development of strictures. Endarteritis also accounts for the rarity of massive bleeding in cases of intestinal tuberculosis.

CLINICAL FEATURES

Abdominal tuberculosis is predominantly a disease of young adults. Most of the patients are within age group of 21–40 years and is almost equal in both sexes, although some of the studies have suggested a slight female predominance. The spectrum of disease in children is different from adults, in whom adhesive peritoneal and lymph nodal involvement is more common than gastrointestinal disease. The clinical presentation of abdominal tuberculosis can be acute, chronic or acute on chronic. Most patients have constitutional symptoms of fever (40–70%), pain (80–95%), diarrhea (11–20%), constipation, alternating constipation and diarrhea, weight loss (40–90%), anorexia and malaise. Pain can be either colicky due to luminal compromise, or dull and continuous when the mesenteric lymph nodes are involved. Other clinical features depend upon the site, nature and extent of involvement.

Tuberculosis of the Esophagus

Esophageal tuberculosis is a rare entity, constituting only 0.2% of cases of abdominal tuberculosis.[2] Till 1997, only 58 cases had been reported in the English literature.[5] Esophageal involvement occurs mainly by extension of disease from adjacent lymph nodes. The patient usually presents with low grade fever, dysphagia, odynophagia and an ulcer most commonly midesophageal. The disease usually mimics esophageal carcinoma and extraesophageal focus of tuberculosis may not be evident.[6]

Tuberculosis of Stomach

Stomach and duodenal tuberculosis each constitute estimated 1% cases of abdominal tuberculosis. Male are more affected than females. Generally' tuberculosis of stomach is usually secondary to pulmonary tuberculosis. The first case is said to be reported by Barkhausen in year 1824. The incidence of tuberculosis of stomach varied between 0.13–0.52% in different studies.[7-12] The reason for relative rarity is attributed to bactericidal properties of gastric acidity, scarcity of lymphoid tissue in gastric wall and intact gastric mucosa of the stomach. These patients commonly mimic peptic ulcer or malignancy in clinical presentation.

Although there is no well-defined site for gastric tuberculosis but majority of cases reported in the lesser curvature and pyloric antrum. The cardiac end appears to be relatively immune to tuberculosis lesions. Tuberculosis in stomach manifested as multiple erosions or ulcers of the mucosa or as the infiltrating hypertrophic form or as sclerosing inflammatory type or as acute miliary type. Of these ulcerative lesions are most common. The ulcer is usually shallow and of small size. The surrounding mucosa is thickened, edematous and hyperemic. There is greater chance of fistula formation. Most common manifestations are having hypo or achlorhydria, pain in epigastrium after food ingestion, vomiting and progressive loss of weight. Fifty percent of patients with stomach tuberculosis, have palpable mass. The vomitus may be dark in color, suggestive of gastric hemorrhage. Diarrhea if present is due to simultaneous involvement of intestine. The differential diagnosis includes, peptic ulcers, gastritis and gastric carcinoma.

Intestinal Tuberculosis

Intestinal tuberculosis, though rare in developed countries but more common among developing countries. But exact data are not known. Incidence of isolated intestinal tuberculosis in unselected autopsy series from India has been reported to vary from 0.02–5.1%.[13,14] In Delhi, 0.8% of all hospital admission were reported to be due to intestinal tuberculosis.[15] In India, tuberculosis has been reported to be cause in 3–20% of patients with intestinal obstruction.[16] About 5–7% of all gastrointestinal perforations have been reported to be due to tuberculosis.[17] Most common site for this type of tuberculosis are ileocecal region. Intestinal tuberculosis occurs in two forms—primary intestinal tuberculosis and secondary intestinal tuberculosis which includes ulcerative and hyperplastic type. Though an uncommon disease in the Western world, while the primary tuberculosis of ileocecal region are quite common in India. It usually occurs by ingestion of unpasteurized cow's milk infected with *M. bovis*. But nowadays due to control of tuberculosis in cattle and pasteurization of milk, virtually all cases of intestinal tuberculosis are caused by *M. tuberculosis*. The predominant changes are in the mesenteric lymph node without any significant intestinal lesion. Grossly, the affected lymph nodes are enlarged, matted and caseous (tabes mesentrica). Healing occurring by fibrosis and calcification. Microscopically, initially there is primary complex or Ghon's complex in the intestinal mucosa, as occurs in primary tuberculosis, following infection later mesenteric lymph nodes are also enlarged and showing typical granulomatous reaction with caseative necrosis. Ulcerative type variety of secondary intestinal tuberculosis occurs following swallowing of sputum in patient with active pulmonary tuberculosis and may cause secondary intestinal tuberculosis. It involves most commonly terminal ileum and rarely colon. Intestinal lesions are more prominent than in regional lymph node. The lesion typically begins in the Peyer's patches or the lymphoid follicles with formation of small ulcers that spread through the lymphatics to form large ulcers which are transverse to the long axis of bowel, but perforation is rare. These ulcers may be coated with caseative material. In advanced cases, transverse fibrotic stricture and intestinal obstruction are also seen. Another type of secondary intestinal tuberculosis known as hyperplastic variety occurs secondary to pulmonary tuberculosis. Most common site is cecum or ascending colon. It becomes thickened with mucosal ulceration. This condition is often mistaken for carcinoma/crohn's disease but differentiated by granuloma with caseative necrosis. Factors contributing to infection in ileocecal junction are due to abundance of lymphoid tissue, relative physiological stasis because of presence of ileocecal valve, increased rate of absorption and prior contact of the bacillus with the intestinal mucosa. Other less common varieties of secondary intestinal tuberculosis are—ulcerative hypertrohic type characterizing both forms, diffuse colitis which is a less common variant, endoscopically very similar to ulcerative colitis and the sclerotic form which is generally associated with stricture that can be solitary or multiple. Fistula can also occur particularly enteroenteric, enterovesical and entrerocutaneous in this last variety. Diarrhea is a predominant symptom and there is also loss of weight. The stool has a fetid odor and contained pus and occult blood. Predominant symptoms are recurrent abdominal pain, intermittent diarrhea and constipation. Partial obstruction is also common usually above the ileum leading to stasis and consequent infection which are responsible for producing steatorrhea, anemia and loss of weight. Some time, the presenting picture is that of a mass in right iliac fossa, these findings should raise the possibility of an appendicular mass, carcinoma of cecum, and Crohn's disease.

Tuberculosis of Peritoneum

Tubercular peritonitis is more common in young adults in between 20–40 years and more common in females. It constitutes 4–10% of all patients with extrapulmonary tuberculosis and has been estimated to occur in 0.1–3.5% of patients with pulmonary tuberculosis.[18-20] Peritoneal involvement occurs most commonly by hematogenous route. Primary foci in peritoneum may be reactivated years after the infections. In about 30% cases, old healed lesions may be seen on X-ray. In about 30% cases, peritoneal tuberculosis may coexist with active tuberculosis and also involved in miliary tuberculosis and contiguous spread from ileocecal tuberculosis or fallopian tubes can also occur. The mode of infection occurs by four ways—from tuberculous mesentric lymphnode, from ulceration of bowel, in female from tuberculous pyosalpinx and as a part of disseminated tuberculosis. There are four pathological types which are described below:

Acute tubercular peritonitis: It may present as acute abdomen in an emergency condition, it is more prevalent in first few years (1–25 years) of life. On laparotomy, tubercles are distributed as minute gray tubercle and widely studded. Sometimes ascites may appear.

Subacute tubercular peritonitis: Condition may present as intermediate form. Peritoneum is studded with pinhead to pea sized tubercle. Bowel loops are also inflammed. It may resolve or may progress to chronic form.

Chronic tubercular peritonitis: It is more prevalent in between 25–45 years of age with female preponderance. Most common presenting symptoms are recurrent abdominal pain and lump in abdomen along with tubercular toxemia such as fever, loss of appetite and loss of weight, anemia.

Chronic peritoneal tuberculosis: It includes three pathological types: ascites form, that is usually seen in children of school going, adolescent or young female. Fluid may be small or large in amount. Fluid is typically straw colored, with high protein, more than 3 g/dL with lymphocyte predominance; encysted form having presentation similar to that of ascites form. Patient usually present as loculated lump along with tubercular toxemia. Occasionally, patient may present as intestinal obstruction in later stage; fibrotic/plastic form which usually develops following widespread adhesion especially in the iliac region along with matting and distension. These matted coils may act as blind loop leading to development of steatorrhea, malabsorption and abdominal pain. The disease may present as acute/subacute intestinal obstruction and purulent form which is of rare type. It usually occurs secondary to tubercular salpingitis in which cold abscess develops between mass of adherent intestinal and omentum. Common presentations are abdominal pain, distension and weight loss is seen in most of the patients. Per abdomen examination reveals tenderness and in few cases a mass may be palpable. The feel of abdomen has been described as doughy and is due to peritoneal involvement with caseating glands, adherent loops of bowel and caseating thickening of omentum.

Mesenteric Tubercular Lymphadenitis

More common in infants, school going children or adolescent. Lymph nodes are situated along with mesentery of small intestinal, mesoappendix, transverse mesocolon, and sigmoid mesocolon. Lymphadenitis clinically present as palpable mass along with tubercular toxemia. But sometimes, it is causing compression of portal vein leading to ascites and sign of partial obstruction. Obstruction of thoracic duct leading to chylous ascites and enlarged pancreatic lymph node can lead to chylous right sided pleural effusion. In case of tubercular abdominal lymphadenitis, common presenting symptoms are fever, abdominal pain, and loss of appetite, weight loss and palpable mass. Sometimes, it may produce sign of intestinal obstruction.

Rectal and Anal Tuberculosis

Clinical presentation of rectal tuberculosis is different from more proximal disease. Fresh bleeding per rectum is the most common symptom (88%) followed by constitutional symptoms (75%) and constipation (37%).[21] The high frequency of rectal bleeding may be because of mucosal trauma caused by scybalous stool traversing the strictured segment. Digital examination reveals an annular stricture. The stricture is usually tight and of variable length with focal areas of deep ulceration. It is usually within 10 cm of the anal verge. Associated perianal disease is very rare. Excessive fibrosis associated with the rectal inflammation results in an increase in presacral space. Overall rectal tuberculosis is rare and may occur in the absence of other lesions in the chest and small and large bowel.[22,23] Anal tuberculosis is less uncommon and has a distinct clinical presentation. Tubercular fistula are usually multiple. Dandapat et al. reported that 13 out of 15 multiple fistulas were of tubercular origin, as compared to only 4 out of 61 solitary perianal fistula.[24] Shukla et al. reported that in India, tuberculosis accounted for up to 14% of cases of fistula-in-ano. Anal discharge was present in all cases and perianal swelling in one-third. Constitutional symptoms were not present in any patient.[25] Anal tuberculosis is also seen in pediatric patients.[26]

INVESTIGATIONS

Hematological

Anemia, leukopenia with relative leukocytosis is commonly reported manifestations.[18-20] The raised ESR is reported in 50–100% patients with abdominal tuberculosis. Serum albumin levels tend to be lower. All these investigations are supportive to the diagnosis but not confirmatory.

Mantoux Test

This test has been reported positive in 50–100% patients with abdominal tuberculosis.[18-20] A positive tuberculin test only can support the diagnosis.

Imaging Technique

(a) **Chest X-ray:** It is mandatory to rule out pulmonary disease because it is abnormal in 24–28% cases. Sharma et al. studied 70 cases of abdominal tuberculosis and found evidence of active or healed lesions on chest X-ray in 22 (46%).[27] In other study of 300 patients, none had active pulmonary tuberculosis but 39% had evidence of healed tuberculosis.[28] Tandon et al. found X-ray to be abnormal in only 25% of their patients.[29]

(b) **Plain X-ray abdomen:** It may show calcified lymph node, calcified granuloma in the spleen, liver and pancreas. Other features include dilated bowel loops with fluid levels, dilatation of terminal ileum and ascitis.

(c) **Barium studies:** Barium contrast study seems to be most useful for diagnosis of abdominal tuberculosis till recently. Although features are non-specific but several of them are highly suggestive of the disease. Barium enema is the best protocol for evaluation of intestinal tuberculosis. Increased transit time with hypersegmentation and flocculation of barium is one of the earliest signs of intestinal involvement. Localized areas of irregular thickened folds, mucosal ulceration, dilated segments and stricture may also be seen. Ulcers may be linear or stellate and are situated along the circumference of the wall. Rarely, there may be deep ulcers with fistula. The ileocecal valve may be thickened initially and gives a broad appearance with base towards the cecum called as 'inverted umbrella sign'. "Stierlin's sign" is a manifestation of acute inflammation superimposed on a chronically involved segment and is characterized by lack of barium retention in the inflammed segments of the ileum, cecum and variable length of the ascending colon, with a normal configured column of barium on either side. It appears as a narrowing of the terminal ileum with rapid empyting into a shortened, rigid or obliterated cecum. String sign is a persistent narrow stream of barium in the bowel due to stenosis. Both Stierlin's sign and String's sign are also seen in Crohn's disease. Barium meal follow through findings in intestinal tuberculosis divided into four groups.[30]

Group I: Highly suggestive of intestinal tuberculosis if one or more of the following features are present such as deformed ileocecal valve with dilatation of terminal ileum, contracted cecum with an abnormal ileocecal valve and/or terminal ileum and stricture of the ascending colon with shortening and involvement of ileocecal region.

Group II: suggestive of intestinal tuberculosis if one or more of the following features are present such as contracted cecum, ulceration or narrowing of the terminal ileum, stricture of the ascending colon and multiple areas of dilatation, narrowing, and matting of small bowel loops.

Group III: Non-specific changes such as features of matting, dilatation and mucosal thickening of small bowel loops.

Group IV: Normal-study as no findings are visualized.

(d) **Abdominal ultrasonography (UCG):** It is very useful for imaging of peritoneal tuberculosis as barium studies though accurate for intrinsic bowel disease but is unable to detect lesions in peritoneum. Features suggestive of abdominal tuberculosis are 1-free or loculated intra-abdominal fluid which may be clear or complex (with debris and septae), can mimic as ovarian cysts. Two-club sandwitch or 'sliced bread' sign is due to localized collection of fluid in radially oriented bowel loops and due to exudation from the inflamed bowel (interloop ascites). Three-visualization of bowel wall thickening especially in the ileocecal regions which is uniform and concentric as compared to Crohn's disease where it is eccentric. Four-occurrence of pseudokidney sign suggesting involvement of the ileocecal region which is pulled up-to a subhepatic position.[31] USG is also very useful in case of mesenteric lymphadenitis. Lymphadenopathy may be discrete or conglomerate (matted). The echotexture is mixed and heterogenous in contrast to the homogenously hypoechoic nodes of lymphomas. Small discrete anechoic areas representing zones of caseation which may be with in the nodes. Calcification in healing lesions is seen as discrete reflecting lines. Both calcification and caseation are highly suggestive of tubercular etiology.

(e) **Abdominal CT-Scan:** CT scan of abdomen can evaluate Ileocecal tuberculosis that is usually hyperplastic. In early disease, there is slight symmetric circumferential thickening of cecum and terminal ileum. Later, the ileocecal valve and adjacent medial wall of the cecum is asymmetrically thickened. In more advanced disease gross wall thickening, adherent loops, large regional nodes and mesenteric thickening can together from a soft tissue mass centered around the ileocecal junction. CT scan can also pick up ulceration or nodularity within the terminal ileum, along with narrowing and proximal dilatation. Other areas of small and large bowel involvement manifest as circumferential wall thickening, narrowing of the lumen and ulceration. In the colon, involvement around the hepatic flexure is common. Complications of perforation, abscess, and obstruction are also seen. Tubercular ascitic fluid is of high attenuation value (24–45 HU) due to its high protein content. Strands, fine septae and debris within the fluid are characteristic, but are better appreciated on ultrasonography. Thickened peritoneum and enhancing peritoneal nodules may be seen. Mesenteric disease on CT scan is seen as a patchy or diffuse increase in density, strands within the mesentery, and a stellate appearance. Lymph nodes may be interspersed. Omental thickening is well-seen often as an omental cake appearance. A fibrous wall can cover the omentum, developing from long-standing inflammation and is called omental line. An omental line is less common in malignant infiltration. Caseating lymph nodes are seen as having hypodense centers and peripheral rim enhancement. Along with calcification, these finding are highly suggestive of tuberculosis. In tuberculosis the mesenteric, mesenteric root, celiac, porta hepatis and peripancreatic nodes are characteristically involved reflecting the lymphatic drainage of the small bowel. The retroperitoneal nodes (i.e. the periaortic and pericaval) are relatively spared, and are almost never seen in isolation, unlike lymphoma.[32,33]

Ascitic Fluid Examination

Ascitic fluid in tuberculosis is typically straw colored and exudative in nature with protein > 3 g/dL and total cell count of 150–4000 cells/mm,^{3} consisting predominantly of lymphocytes (70%), the ascites to blood glucose ratio is less than 0.96 and serum ascites albumin gradient is less than 1.1 g/dL. The yield of organism on smear and culture is low. Staining for acid-fast bacilli (AFB) is positive in less than 3% of cases. A positive culture is obtained in less than 20% of cases and it takes 6–8 weeks for mycobacterial colonies to appear. However, Singh et al. reported culture of 1 liter of ascitic fluid after centrifugation and obtained 83% culture positivity. Adenosine deaminase (ADA) is an enzyme and its activity is more in T than B lymphocyte. ADA is increased in tubercular ascitic fluid due to stimulation of T cells by mycobacterial antigens. However, definitive diagnosis done by biopsy material from granuloma and/or caseation by AFB staining and cultures. A peritoneal biopsy along with examination of ascitic fluid is diagnostic in 90% of the patients.

Stools for AFB

In immunocompetent patients suffering by pulmonary tuberculosis, AFB in stools may be positive even without intestinal involvement. But in case of immunocompromized patients AFB detected in stools most likely due to involvement by non-tuberculous mycobacteria (NTM).

Polymerase Chain Reaction

Polymerase chain reaction (PCR) has been evaluated for the diagnosis of abdominal tuberculosis. However, diagnostic accuracy of PCR as a single test still remains questionable. PCR testing has been advocated for peritoneal fluid analysis. It can be utilized in the diagnosis of intestinal tuberculosis where histopathology remains inconclusive.[34] The overall sensitivity, specificity, positive predictive value and negative predictive value of PCR were 97.87%, 100%, 100%, and 94.73% respectively.[35] One study reported the utility of PCR as a diagnostic aid to endoscopy for treatment of abdominal tuberculosis in a patient with chronic diarrhea.[36] It was concluded that maximum sensitivity and specificity can be achieved by the combined use of clinical diagnosis, histopathology and PCR. PCR has a potentially important role in improving the diagnostic accuracy of abdominal tuberculosis. In a case series of 11 patients with histologically confirmed TB peritonitis, all were positive for *M. tuberculosis* by PCR of ascetic fluid specimens.[37] Another study was conducted for evaluation of PCR as a diagnostic tool in abdominal tuberculosis and reported it to be a useful as it not only detected 60% of total cases but also additional six samples that were proven negative by histopathology.[38]

PCR of mucosal biopsy specimens diagnosed colonic tuberculosis in 45 to 64% of cases.[39,40] The *M. tuberculosis* genome has been demonstrated in the mucosal biopsies of two-thirds of patients with colonic tuberculosis. PCR amplification of IS6110 for *M. tuberculosis* in fecal samples was evaluated for the diagnosis of abdominal tuberculosis with the sensitivity and specificity of 88% and 100%, respectively. In comparison, the sensitivity for histopathology was 50% and culture was 33%. The PCR test had the advantage of using a non-invasive sample, which is subject to less sampling error in comparison to mucosal biopsy.

Colonoscopy

Colonoscopy is an excellent tool to diagnose colonic and terminal ileal involvement but is still often underutilized.[21,41,42] Mucosal nodules of variable sizes (2–6 mm) and ulcers in a discrete segment of colon, 4–8 cm in length are pathognomonic. The nodules have a pink surface with no friability and are most often found in the cecum especially near the ileocecal valve. Large (10–20 mm) or small (3–5 mm) ulcers are commonly located between the nodules. The intervening mucosa may be hyperemic or normal. Areas of strictures with nodular and ulcerated mucosa may be seen. Other findings are pseudopolypoid edematous folds, and a deformed and edematous ileocecal valve. Diffuse involvement of the entire colon is rare (4%), but endoscopically can look very similar to ulcerative colitis. Lesions mimicking carcinoma have also been described.

Most workers take up to 8–10 colonoscopic biopsies for histopathology and culture. Biopsies should be taken from the edge of the ulcers. However, there is a low yield on histopathology because of predominant submucosal involvement. Granulomas have been reported in 8–48% of patients and caseation in a third (33–38%) of positive cases. The yield of acid-fast bacilli stains has been variable in studies. Culture positivity is not related to the presence of granuloma. Bhargava et al. reported positive culture in 40% of patients and concluded that routine culture of biopsy tissue increase the diagnostic yield.[41] A combination of histology and culture of the biopsy material can be expected to establish the diagnosis in over 60% of cases. Biopsy may be usefull in diagnosis but there is usually a low yield of tubercular granuloma from the intestinal walls. Laparotomy may reveal thickened and inflamed bowel walls. The intestinal mucosa may be studded with tubercles. Regional lymph nodes may be increased in size and showing caseous necrosis.

Fine-needle Aspiration Cytology (FNAC)

FNAC of palpable abdominal mass in patients with tuberculosis showing a high diagnostic accuracy. LJ Medium culture of the material increasing diagnostic yields.[43,44]

Peritoneal Biopsy

Blind and open peritoneal biopsies under local anesthesia are also useful tool for confirming the diagnosis of abdominal tuberculosis. Shukla et al. carried out open peritoneal biopsy by a grid incision in right iliac fossa under local anesthesia and reported 80% diagnostic accuracy.[45]

Gastroscopy

Diagnosis of stomach tuberculosis can be made by gastroscopy and histopathlogical examination. Gastroscopy is an important tool for diagnosis of stomach tuberculosis. There are four peculiarities with gross manifestation-undermined edge of the ulcers, typical serpiginous nature of ulcer, multiple fistulous opening, and presence of superficial tubercle in the lesions.

Laproscopy

Direct inspection and biopsy of the peritoneum are perhaps the most effective method for diagnosing tubercular peritonitis. It alone will facilitate an accurate presumptive diagnosis in 80–95% of patients. Bhargava et al. studied 87 patients with high protein ascites, of which 38 were diagnosed as having tuberculosis.[46] They found appearance to be more helpful (95% accurate) than either histology, culture or guinea pig inoculation (82%, 3% and 37.5% sensitivity respectively). Caseating granulomas may be found in 85–90% of the biopsies. The laparoscopic findings in peritoneal tuberculosis can be grouped into three categories: 1—thickened parietal peritoneum with tubercles consisting of multiple, yellowish white, uniform sized (about 4–5 mm) tubercles diffusely distributed which is also hyperemic and lacks its usually shiny luster. The omentum, liver and spleen can also be studded with tubercles, 2—thickened peritoneum without tubercles. 3—fibro adhesive peritonitis with markedly thickened peritoneum and multiple thick adhesions fixing the viscera.

Serological Tests

Enzyme linked immunosorbent assay (ELISA) and soluble antigen fluorescent antibody (SAFA) can be used as an adjunct diagnostic tool for diagnosis of abdominal tuberculosis. ELISA can be useful in the establishment of diagnosis with accuracy of 84%, sensitivity of 81% and specificity of 88%.[47] However, presence of few limitations such as variable response to mycobacteria, poor reproducibility and persistence of positive result even after therapy suggests that it still remains undefined in clinical practice.[48] WHO and Government of India has banned various serological test for the diagnosis of tuberculosis.[49]

Diagnostic Criteria: Diagnosis of abdominal tuberculosis is essentially established on the basis of four criterias:

1. Histopathological evidence of caseating granulomas/acid-fast bacilli.
2. Presence of *M. tuberculosis* in sputum/tissue/ascitic fluid.
3. Clinical sign and symptoms/radiological/operative evidence of proven tuberculosis elsewhere with good therapeutic response.
4. Good therapeutic response to antituberculosis chemotherapy in suspected cases of abdominal tuberculosis.[50]

TREATMENT OF ABDOMINAL TUBERCULOSIS

Medical Treatment

All patients should receive conventional antitubercular therapy for at least 6 months including initial 2 months of rifampicin, isoniazid, pyrazinamide and ethambutol followed by 4 months of rifampicin and isoniazid given on daily or also thrice weekly under DOTS (Category I) under Revised National Tuberculosis Program (RNTCP). A randomized comparison of a 6-month short-course chemotherapy with a 12-month course of ethambutol and isoniazid (supplemented with streptomycin for the initial 2 months) was conducted by Balasubramanium et al. at Tuberculosis Research Center, Chennai, in 193 adult patients.[51] Cure rate was 99 and 94% in patients given short-course and the 12 months regimen respectively. However, many physicians extend the treatment duration to 12–24 months. Steroids can be prescribed which can help in healing of ulcers, prevent formation of stenosis, absorption of ascitic fluid and resolution of glands.

Surgical Treatment

The surgical treatment of intestinal tuberculosis has gone through three phases. Bypassing the stenosed segment by enteroenterostomy or by ileotransverse colostomy was practiced when effective antitubercular drugs were unavailable, as any resectional surgery was considered hazardous in the presence of active disease. This practice however, produced blind loop syndrome, and fistulae and recurrent obstruction often occurred in the remaining segments. With the advent of antituberculous drugs, more radical procedures became popular in an attempt to eradicate the disease locally. These included right hemicolectomy with or without extensive removal of the draining lymph nodes and wide bowel resections. These procedures were often not tolerated well by the malnourished patient. Moreover, the lesions are often widely spaced and not suitable for resection. The recommended surgical procedures today are conservative. Strictures which reduce the lumen by half or more and which cause proximal hypertrophy or dilation are treated by strictureplasty.[52] This involves at least 5–6 cm long incision along the antimesenteric side which is closed transversely in two layers. A segment of bowel bearing multiple strictures or a single long tubular stricture may merit reection. Resection is segmental with a 5 cm margin. Tubercular perforations are usually ileal and are associated with distal strictures. Surgery is best performed under the cover of adequate chemotherapy, preferably after the patient has taken 4 months of therapy. Resection and anastomosis is preferred as simple closure of the lesions is associated with a high incidence of leak and fistula formation.

REFERENCES

1. Pimparkar BD. Abdominal tuberculosis, J Assoc Physicians India. 1977;25:801-11.
2. Paustian FF. Tuberculosis of the intestine. In: Bockus HL editor. Gastroenterology, Vol. 11. 2nd ed. Philadephia W.B. Saunders Co. 1964;p.311-34.
3. Wig KL, Chitkara NK, Gupta SP, Kishore K. Ileocaecal tuberculosis with particular reference to isolation of *Mycobacterium tuberculosis*. Amm Rev Respir Dis. 1961;84:169-78.
4. Vij JC, Malhotra V, Choudhary V, Jain NK. A Clinicopathological study of abdominal tuberculosis. Indian J Tuberc. 1992;39:213-20.

5. DiFebo G, Calabrese C, Areni A, Savastio G, Grazia M, Miglioli M. Oesophageal tuberculosis mimicking secondary oesophageal involvement by mediastinal neoplasm. Ital Gastroenterol Hepatol. 1997;29:564-8.
6. Tassios P, Iadas S, Giannopoulos G, Iarion K, Katsogridakis J, Chalerelakis G, et al. Tuberculous esophagitis, Report of a case and review of modern approaches to diagnosis and treatment. Hepatogastroenterology. 1995;42:185-8.
7. Good RW. Tuberculosis of stomach, analysis of cases recently reviewed, Arch. Surg. 1931;22:415-25.
8. Crawford M, sawyer HP, Intestinal tuberculosis in 1400 autopsies. Am Rev, Tuberc. 1934;30:568-83.
9. Sullivan RC, Fancona NT, Kirshbaum JD. Tuberculosis study, Ann. Surg. 1940;112:225-33.
10. Cullen JH. Intestinal tuberculosis—A clinical pathological study. Quarl Bull Sea View Hosp. 1940;5:143-60.
11. Hardt IL, Cohen JJ. Gastrointestinal complications in pulmonary tuberculosis. Am Rev Tuberc. 1941;43:628-36.
12. Browne DC, McHardy G, wilen CJW. Gastric mucosal changes of tuberculosis. Am J Digest Dis. 1942;9:407.
13. Tribedi BD, Gupta DM. Intestinal tuberculosis in Bengal. J Indian Med Assoc. 1941;11:41.
14. Ukil AC. Early diagnosis of intestinal tuberculosis. Indian Med Gazette. 1942;77:613.
15. Chttani HK. Intestinal tuberculosis. In: Card WI, Creamer B, (eds). Modern trends in gastroenterology. London: Butterworth. 1970;p.309-27.
16. Bhansali SK, Sethna JR. Intestinal obstruction: A clinical analysis of 348 cases. Indian J Surg. 1970;32:57-70.
17. Bhansali SK. Gastrointestinal perforations: Clinical study of 96 cases. J Postgrad Med. 1967; 13:1-12.
18. Marshal JB. Tuberculosis of the gastrointestinal tract and peritoneum. Am J Gastroenterol. 1993;88:989-99.
19. Sohocky S. Tuberculous peritonitis: A review of 100 cases. Am Rev Respir Dis. 1967;95: 398-401.
20. Aguado JM, Pons F, Casafont F, San MiguelG, Valle R. Tuberculous peritonitis: A Study compairing cirrhotic and non cirrhotic patients. J Clin Gastroenterol. 1990;550-5.
21. Puri AS, Vij JC, Chaudhary A, Kumar N, Sachdev A, Malhotra V, et al. Diagnosis and outcome of isolated rectal tuberculosis. Dis colon Rectum. 1996;39:1126-9.
22. Chaudhary A, Gupta NM. Colorectal tuberculosis. Dis Colon Rectum. 1986;29:738-4.
23. Gupta OP, Dube MK. Tuberculosis of gastrointestinal tract: With special reference to rectal tuberculosis. Indian J Med Res. 1970;58:979-84.
24. Dandapat MC, Mukherjee LM, Behra AN, Fistula in ano. Indian J Surg. 1990;52:265-8.
25. Shukla HS, Gupta SC, singh C, Singh PA. Tubercular fistula in ano. Br J Surg. 1988;75:38-9.
26. Wadhwa N, Agarwal S, Mishra K. Reappraisal of abdominal tuberculosis. J Indian Med Assoc. 2004;102:31-2.
27. Kapoor VK, Chattopadhyay TK, Sharma LK. Radiology of abdominal tuberculosis, Australas Radial. 1988;32:365-7.
28. Prakash A. Ulcerative-constrictive tuberculosis of the bowel. Int Surg. 1978;63:23-9.
29. Tandon RK, Sarin SK, Bose SL, Berry M, Tandon BN. A Clinico-radiological reappraisal of intestinal tuberculosis-changing profile? Gastroenterol JPn. 1986;21:17-22.
30. Suri S, Kaur H, Wig JD, Singh KCT. In: Abdominal Tuberculosis–comparison with barium studies. Indian J Radiol. 1993;3:227-42.
31. Kedar RP, Shah PP, Shivde RS, Malde HM. Sonographic findings in gastrointestinal and peritoneal tuberculosis. Clin radiol. 1994;49:24-9.
32. Gulati MS, Sarma D, Paul SB. CT appearance in abdominal tuberculosis. A Pictorial assay. Clin Imaging. 1999;23:51-9.

33. HK Ha, Ji Jung, MS Lee, Choi BG, Lee MG, Kim YH. CT differentiation of tuberculosis peritonitis and peritoneal carcinomatosis. AM J Roentgenol. 1996;167:743-8.
34. Moatter T, Mirza S, Siddiqui MS, Soomro IN. Detection of *Mycobacterium tuberculosis* in paraffin embedded intestinal tissue specimens by PCR characterization of IS6110 element negative strains. J Pak Med Assoc. 1998;48:174-8.
35. Kesarwani RC, Pandey Anjana, Misra Ashutosh, Singh Anupam Kumar. Polymerase chain reaction (PCR). Its comparison with conventional techniques for diagnosis of extra-pulmonary tubercular diseases. Indian J Surg. 2004;66:84-8.
36. Anand BS, Schneider FE, El-Zaatari FA, Shawar RM, Clarridge JE, Graham DY. Diagnosis of intestinal tuberculosis by PCR on endoscopic biopsy specimens. Am J Gastroenterol. 1994;89:2248-9.
37. Uzunkoy A, Harma M, Harma M. Diagnosis of abdominal tuberculosis: experience from 11 cases and review of the literature. World J Gastroenterol. 2004;10:3647-9.
38. Kulkarni S, Vyas S, Supe A, Kadival G. Use of PCR in the diagnosis of abdominal tuberculosis. J Gastroenterol Hepatol. 2006;21:819-23.
39. Gan HT, Chen YQ, Ouyang Q, Bu H, Yang XY. Diferentiation between intestinal tuberculosis and Crohn's disease in endoscopic biopsy specimens by polymerase chain reaction. Am J Gastroenterol. 2002;97:1446-51.
40. Balamurugan R, Venkataraman S, John KR, Ramakrishna BS. PCR amplification of IS6110 insertion element of *Mycobacterium tuberculosis* in fecal samples from patients with intestinal tuberculosis. J Clin Microbiol. 2006;44:1884-6.
41. Bhargava DK, Tandon HD, Chawla TC, Shriniwas, Tandon BN, Kapur BM. Diagnosis of ileocecal and colonic tuberculosis by colonoscopy. Gastrointest endose. 1985;31:68-70.
42. Singh V, Kumar P, Kamal J, Prakash V, Vaiphei K, Singh K. Clinicocolonoscopic profile of colonic tuberculosis. Am J Gastroenterol. 1996;91:565-8.
43. Radhika S, Gupta SK, Chakrabarti A, Rajwanshi A, Joshi K. Role of culture for mycobacterium in fine needle aspiration diagnosis of tubercular lymphadenitis. Diagn Cytopathol. 1989;5: 260-2.
44. Rajwanshi A, Bhambhani S, Das SK. Fine needle aspiration cytology diagnosis of tuberculosis. Diagn Cytopathol. 1987;3:13-6.
45. Shukla HS, Bhatia S, Naitrani YP, Das P, Gupta SC. Peritoneal biopsy for the diagnosis of kochs abdomen. Postgrad Med J. 1982;58:226-8.
46. Bhargava DK, Shrinivas, Chopra P. Peritoneal tuberculosis:laproscopic pattern and its diagnostic accuracy. Am J Gastroenterol. 1992;87:109-12.
47. Bhargava DK, Dasarathy S, Shriniwas MD, Kushwaha AKS, Duphare H, Kapoor BML. Evaluation of enzyme linked immunosorbent assay using mycobacterial saline extracted antigen for the serodiagnosis of abdominal tuberculosis. Am J Gastroenterol. 1992;87: 105-8.
48. Steingart KR, Henry M, Laal S, Hopewell PC, Ramsay A, Menzies D, et al. A systematic review of commercial serological antibody detection tests for the diagnosis of extrapulmonary tuberculosis. Postgrad Med J. 2007;83:705-12.
49. Steingart KR, Ramsay A, Dowdy D, Pai M, et al. Serological tests for the diagnosis of active tuberculosis: relevance for India. Indian J Med Res. 2012;135:695-702.
50. Lingenfelser T, Zak J, Mark S. Abdominal tuberculosis. Still a potentially lethal disease. Am J Gastroenterol. 1993;88:744-9.
51. Balasubramanian R, Naraya M, et al. Randomised,controlled trial of short-course chemo-therapy in abdominal tuberculosis: a five-year report. Int J Tuberc Lung Dis. 1997;1:44-51.
52. Anand BS, Nanda R, Sachdev GK. Response of tuberculous stricture to antituberculous treatment. Gut. 1988;29:62-9.

Chapter 46

Tuberculosis of Kidney and Urinary Tract

INTRODUCTION

Genitourinary tuberculosis remains to be a major problem in the developing countries and constitutes at least 30% of all cases of extrapulmonary tuberculosis.[1-3] Early diagnosis and treatment of genitourinary tuberculosis is essential because undiagnosed and untreated disease can result in renal failure and death. This current chapter aims to describe the epidemiology, pathogenesis, clinical features, diagnosis and management of tuberculosis of kidney and urinary tract.

EPIDEMIOLOGY

Urogenital tuberculosis observed in 3-4% of all cases of pulmonary tuberculosis. It is usually the result of hematogenous dissemination of tubercle bacilli from a primary complex. The various clinically evident forms of primary tuberculosis usually appear within 3 years of initial infection, but an exception is renal tuberculosis which generally develops after 8 or more years. Medlar found bilateral renal cortical lesions in patients with pulmonary tuberculosis.[4] Cobalwala in a multicentric Indian study reported the incidence of 10- 34% with various urogenital diseases.[5] In India, BMRC reported incidence of 10.7% based on microbiological and histopathological examinations.[6] It has been observed that renal manifestations of TB are relatively more frequent in immunocompromized patients especially HIV and has caused a worldwide resurgence of tuberculosis.

PATHOPHYSIOLOGY

Tuberculosis of the kidney and urinary tract is like other forms of the disease. The most common causative organism is the human tubercle bacillus, *Mycobacterium tuberculosis* but, occasionally the bovine tubercle bacillus, *Mycobacterium bovis*, can be responsible. The vaccine strain, Bacille Calmette-Guérin (BCG), also has been the cause of renal lesions as a complication of intravesical instillation of BCG for the treatment of superficial bladder cancer. Environmental mycobacteria occasionally cause human disease, particularly in immunosuppressed individuals, including recipients of renal transplants.[7] The kidney may be involved when environmental mycobacteria causes disseminated disease, such as that caused by *M. avium* in AIDS patients. Renal disease caused by environmental mycobacteria in non-immunosuppressed individuals is exceedingly rare.[8] However, as environmental mycobacteria occur in water; they readily contaminate the lower urethra and external genitalia and thus often are isolated from urine samples. Tuberculosis of the kidney usually spreads by a hematogenous route from pulmonary disease, although it may be secondary to tuberculosis of the GI tract or bone too. By the time renal tuberculosis is diagnosed, the primary source of pulmonary infection may be inactive or calcified. True prevalence of renal tuberculosis is underestimated since radiologic signs may be absent. Moreover, tubercle bacilli are found in 7–29% of urine samples in patients with extra renal tuberculosis. The initial renal focus is usually a small tubercle in the glandular and cortical arterioles. With the passage of time, these lesions progress to form necrotizing lesions. The disease spreads to the renal tubules and renal medulla in which further tubercles develop, usually at the turn of the loop of Henle, coalescing into larger necrotic irregular cavities. The cavities usually communicate with the renal collecting system, generally a calyx, with formation of fistulae and strictures. Eventually, the kidney may become fibrotic and scarred. The course of renal tuberculosis may be indolent. Presentation is usually late and symptoms usually occur as a result of non-specific urinary tract infection. Constitutional symptoms usually do not occur or are sparse. Renal tuberculosis is bilateral although radiologic findings are asymmetric and unilateral in 25% of patients. Ultimately, the kidney becomes atrophic, scarred, densely calcified, and nonfunctioning (auto-nephrectomy) if not appropriately treated.

CLINICAL FEATURES

Classical Renal Tuberculosis

Tuberculosis of the urinary tract is easily overlooked. Many patients present with lower urinary tract symptoms typical of "conventional" bacterial cystitis, and suspicion of tuberculosis is aroused only when there is no response to the usual antibacterial agents or when urine examination reveals pyuria in the absence of a positive culture on routine media. Other symptoms that may occur include back, flank, and suprapubic pain; hematuria; increased frequency and nocturia. These symptoms are not pathognomonic of tuberculosis; they might also suggest conventional bacterial urinary tract infection. Renal colic is uncommon, occurring in fewer than 10% of patients and constitutional symptoms such as fever, weight loss, and night sweats also are unusual. Only one-third of the patients have an abnormal chest X-ray. The classical features of TB such as fever, night sweats, general malaise, anorexia and weight loss are unusual but their occurrence suggest the foci of TB elsewhere. In one study, 18 of 25 physicians with renal tuberculosis presented only after advanced cavitating disease had developed.[9] Indeed; the diagnosis is sometimes made for the first time at operation table or at postmortem. Another study reported that 9% of 200 consecutive cases of bacteriologically proven pulmonary tuberculosis were having clinical features of renal tuberculosis.[10] Prevalence of renal tuberculosis was higher in patients who had genitourinary symptoms dysuria being the most common and also associated findings of far advanced lesions and giant cavities in chest radiography. Chronic tuberculosis sometimes is complicated by amyloidosis, which, in India, is an important cause of renal disease.[11] There are a number of case reports of tuberculosis associated with various forms of glomerulonephritis but no firm associations have been established. There also is a case report of miliary tuberculosis complicated by focal proliferative glomerulonephritis; immune deposits were present but there were no granulomas.

Tuberculous Interstitial Nephritis

It is now clear that tuberculosis can insidiously affect the kidney more. In one report, three patients with advanced renal failure, in whom imaging showed equal sized smooth kidneys, were described.[12] In none of them tubercle bacilli were found in the urine. Renal histology revealed chronic tubulo-interstitial nephritis with granuloma formation in all three and caseation in two patients. In two patients, acid-fast bacilli (AFB) were identified with appropriate stains. Two of the three patients had evidence of tuberculosis on chest X-ray and one had tuberculous peritonitis.

End-Stage Renal Disease

Tuberculosis, although an uncommon cause of progressive renal failure, is an important one because unlike many renal conditions, it is potentially preventable and easily treatable. Worldwide evidence that tuberculosis can cause end-stage renal failure, is scanty.

Hemodialysis and Peritoneal Dialysis

There are a number of reports of tuberculosis developing in patients on regular hemodialysis. Commonly, the patient manifests with fever, anorexia, and weight loss and usually either is known to have had pulmonary or other forms of tuberculosis or is a member of a high-risk ethnic or social group. Often the recrudescence is extrapulmonary, so it is likely that, in most cases, the disease is due to reactivation of past disease rather than a primary infection. In a study of more than 300 hemodialysis patients in St Louis, Missouri, it was found that 48 of 307 patients tested had positive tuberculin skin test. Chest radiographs were done, but no new cases of tuberculosis were found.[13] There are fewer reports of tuberculosis in chronic ambulatory peritoneal dialysis (CAPD) patients, but there is no reason to suspect that the risk is different from patients on hemodialysis. There are a number of reports of tuberculous peritonitis,[14,15] which is easier to detect in patients on CAPD than in those on hemodialysis. In Turkey, a region with a high incidence of tuberculosis, 4 of 70 children on CAPD developed tuberculosis—affecting the lung in 3 and the bone in 1.[16] Disease caused by environmental mycobacteria also occurs in hemodialysis patients; it usually becomes apparent as pulmonary or disseminated disease or sometimes as skin lesions. Some infections have occurred as the result of contamination of the dialysis machine by environmental mycobacteria.

Transplant Patients

Tuberculosis is a serious complicating factor in renal and other forms of transplantation, with an incidence of 0.35–15.0%[17] depending on geographic region. In most cases, the disease involves the lung, but the disease is disseminated in one-third of the cases. Patients who have had tuberculosis while on dialysis are at increased risk, and it should be remembered that immunosuppression can obscure the diagnosis by producing false-negative tuberculin tests.[14] A retrospective study of 520 renal transplant patients from Turkey revealed that tuberculosis was diagnosed in 22 patients, a mean of 44.4 months after transplantation.[18] The pleuropulmonary form was the most common (54%). Despite treatment, six of the patients died, one due to isoniazid toxicity. In contrast, 23 patients who were at risk of developing tuberculosis had been given isoniazid prophylaxis for 1 year. None of the 23 developed tuberculosis none of them showed signs of toxicity.

TB of Ureter

Ureteric involvement occurs as a descending infection secondary to kidney infection. Tubercles may involve the transitional epithelium, causing mucosal granulomas that project into the ureteric lumen. Eventually, fibrosis occurs in the ureter. These pathologic processes can be demonstrated radiologically by the appearance of a beaded, saw-toothed, corkscrew or pipe stem ureter depending on the stage of disease. Usually, the upper and/or lower third of the ureters are involved. The vesicoureteric junction may become fixed and patulous, allowing vesicoureteric reflux. The kidneys are always involved when ureteric tuberculosis is present.

TB of Urinary Bladder

TB of bladder is always secondary to the renal tuberculosis. The earliest lesions of tuberculosis of bladder occur near one of the ureteric opening or in the neighborhood of the trigone and is characterized by pallor at the mucosa due to surrounding submucosal edema. Later on tubercle may be seen. If the disease progresses further, the inflammatory process spreads more deeply leading to replacement of bladder muscle by fibrosis. Later on due to development of fibrosis, the capacity of bladder is reduced. This form of tuberculosis of bladder is termed as thimble bladder.

HIV-Positive Individuals and Renal Tuberculosis

Approximately 10% of all cases of tuberculosis worldwide in 1999 were HIV related but in sub-Saharan Africa, the percentage was much higher, as high as 60% in some regions. The incidence is expected to rise in Africa and also in Asia. Tuberculosis was the cause of death in approximately 30% of the 3 million patients who were dying of AIDS in 1999. In those who are only mildly immunosuppressed, the disease resembles that in HIV-negative individuals. In the more profoundly immunosuppressed, particularly those with $CD4^+$ T-cell counts of 50/cu-mm or lower, a high viral load and a negative tuberculin test, the disease often is disseminated, and the kidney is involved incidentally with various pathologic manifestations; including granulomatous interstitial nephritis. The incidence of renal involvement may be higher than currently believed. In an autopsy study in India, 24 of 35 kidneys from patients who died of AIDS showed evidence of infection, including 17 cases of tuberculosis.[19] In a similar study in Mexico City, renal disease was demonstrable in 87 of 138 (63%) autopsies on AIDS patients. Infection was the cause of the renal disease in 36 cases, with 19 being due to *M. tuberculosis*.[20]

DIAGNOSIS OF TUBERCULOSIS OF KIDNEY AND URINARY TRACT

Urine Examination

The urine may be examined microscopically (for the presence of red cells, white cells, bacteria, crystals and casts), biochemically and bacteriologically. The early morning specimen should be cultured for detection of *M. tuberculosis*. Most specific therapy should never be started until a positive culture has been obtained. A patient with a positive urine culture for *M. tuberculosis* should not be dismissed even in the face of absent genitourinary symptoms, normal urinalysis and normal pyelogram but always be considered as a case of renal tuberculosis.[10]

Microbiological Examination

Since urinary bacillary excretion is intermittent so preferably five consecutive early morning specimens of urine should be cultured, each on the two slopes (1) L-J medium, (2) A pyruvate egg medium containing penicillin to identify *M. bovis*. Urine smears for Ziehl-Neelson staining are also negative and culture takes 6–8 weeks due to slow growth of mycobacteria. The microscope demonstrates the tubercle bacilli in 72% cases and culture positivity seen in about 90–98% of cases. A study detected renal tuberculosis in 14% of 100 consecutive osteoarticular tuberculosis patients with urine microbiological examination in correlation to clinicoradiological findings.[21]

Intravenous Urography

Intravenous urography has been mainstay investigation since 1930. A laxative is usally given prior to the investigation and patients requested not to drink for 6–8 hours prior to the study. The contrast (urograffin or niopam 370) is then injected into a suitable forearm vein. Careful observation for the presence of reaction should be maintained during the circulation of the first few milliliters injected. Early films may be taken to demonstrate the nephrogram phase. Here comparison between two kidneys can be made, a delay on one side signify the presence of perhaps renal artery stenosis or presence of unilateral obstructive uropathy. After a few minute contrast is excreted into the collecting system, appearing in the calyces and renal pelvis. Later films demonstrate ureter and bladder. At the end of study patient is asked to micturate and final film is taken of the bladder area. Changes in urogram start with loss or dysfunction of one or more calyces and irregular density in the nephrogram. Spasm or edema may obliterate a calyceal neck and if this becomes severe hydrocalyx will develop. Complete obstruction leads to an abscess displacing adjacent calyces and the appearance of a space-occupying lesion.

A variety of abnormalities may be demonstrated, including smudged papillae due to surface irregularity of the papillae, a moth-eaten calyx (early sign), irregular tract formation from the calyx to the papilla and large irregular cavities with extensive destruction secondary to papillary necrosis. Changes may be detected on intravenous urography, retrograde pyelography and on some CT scan and MRI.[22-24] Changes of renal tuberculosis are unilateral in 75% of patients. Dilated calyces often are associated with infundibular strictures and may be demonstrated radiologically. If tuberculous infection extends directly to the rest of the kidney, the entire kidney becomes a bag of caseous necrotic pus. Intravenous urography usually shows absence of function, although a faint nephrogram may be demonstrated if some function remains. Associated renal calculi are found in as many as 20% of patients with renal tuberculosis. The final outcome of renal tuberculosis is autonephrectomy, which represents a small, shrunken, scarred, non-functioning kidney and is often associated with dystrophic calcification. Although ureteral involvement is usually unilateral, bilateral changes are asymmetric when they occur. The most common site of involvement is the lower third of the ureter.[25] Mucosal ulceration is difficult to depict radiologically but rarely may show as irregularity in the contrast-filled ureter. The involved ureter may appear beaded or with a corkscrew configuration as a result of alternating dilatations and strictures. Ultimately, the ureter may form a rigid, aperistaltic, shortened tube. When tuberculosis involves the bladder, progressive thickening of the bladder wall occurs with increasing diminution of bladder volume. Trabeculation may develop. The bladder tends to become round and spastic when involved and ulceration may produce spasm and flattening of the bladder area. The ureteric fibrosis leads to loss of natural curves of ureter and a wider, straighter and shorter line between kidney and bladder. In late cases the contralateral ureter also gets dilated. The vesicoureteric junction orifice may become fixed and patulous, resulting in vesicoureteric reflux. The vesicoureteric junction may be affected by progressive narrowing, causing stenosis and resulting in bilateral hydroureters and hydronephrosis.

Cytoscopy

Cystoscopy is an important tool to evaluate the capacity of bladder and to identify any obvious growth and nature of efflux from both the ureters. By this procedure, biopsy can be taken for histopathological diagnosis.

Retrograde Pyelography

Retrograde pyelography is rarely done nowadays. It is usually done to locate the stricture of ureter at the lower end, extent of stricture, amount of obstruction and dilatation above the stricture. It is also valuable to obtain urine samples for culture of *M. tuberculosis*.

Percutaneous Antegrade Pyelography

Percutaneous antegrade pyelography is usually done in patients with gross hydronephrotic obstructed kidneys. It can also visualize non-functioning kidneys or condition of excretory pathway above the obstruction.

Voiding Cystourethrogram

Voiding cystourethrogram is a very valuable investigation to determine irregularities of the bladder walls because tuberculosis can produce cicatrisation/hyperplastic inflammatory lesions. Fibrosis in the region of the trigone produces gaping ureteric orifices which may show vesicoureteric reflux on voiding cystourethrogram.

Polymerase Chain Reaction (PCR)

In recent years, nucleic-acid amplification techniques, such as PCR, have been investigated extensively for the detection of *M. tuberculosis* and other mycobacteria in clinical specimens. PCR is a rapid tool to detect *M. tuberculosis* in urine samples in genitourinary TB patients.[26] Relatively few studies have specifically evaluated PCR for detection of genitourinary tuberculosis, and these show the technique to be sensitive and specific, although some urine specimens contain inhibitory substances. In addition, PCR has been used to detect mycobacterial DNA in urine in cases of HIV-related disseminated tuberculosis.[27–29] There have been a few reports of the successful use of PCR to detect organism in urine but needs further assessment as it displayed negative response in some culture-positive patients.

Plain Radiograph

Plain X-ray abdomen may show calcification in the renal areas of varying patterns (curvilinear, amorphous, speckled). Ureteric calcification is rare. Renal calcification is present in as many as 50% of patients and may appear as an amorphous granular opacification associated with active granulomatous infection and dense punctate calcification, which is associated with healed tuberculomas. Shell-like calcification within the renal collecting system and a thinned-out renal cortex are more a feature of autonephrectomy. Ureteric calcification more commonly occurs in patients with schistosomiasis but differentiation from ureteric tuberculous calcification is fairly reliable. In schistosomiasis, calcification is first observed in the bladder and then extends up the ureter. Ureteric calcification without bladder calcification is most unusual. In tuberculosis, calcification is more amorphous and patchy and extends down the ureter and the bladder is seldom calcified. Bladder wall calcification is also rare. Calcification may occur within bladder tumors, or calcium may be encrusted on the surface of bladder tumors, which need to be differentiated from bladder tuberculosis. A shrunken bladder may be neurogenic but the clinical presentation is not that of urinary tuberculosis. Signs of extrarenal active or inactive tuberculosis may be apparent, such as osseous or paraspinal changes of tuberculosis and old healed calcified splenic, hepatic, lymph node, and adrenal granulomas. Chest radiographs may show evidence of active or healed tuberculosis in 50% of patients. The remaining patients have normal chest studies.[30,31]

CT-sacn in Genitourinary Tuberculosis

While intravenous urography is the primary modality for imaging renal tuberculosis, CT-scans clearly reveal changes of renal tuberculosis, particularly in advanced disease. Changes such as calcification, calyceal dilatation without a hydropelvis, parenchymal loss and extrarenal spread are well-depicted. While CT-scans clearly demonstrate changes of advanced disease, sensitivity in early disease may be low because scans do not demonstrate the detailed calyceal anatomy.[32,33] Early disease may be missed on CT-scans. Mimics of renal tuberculosis include schistosomiasis, diabetes mellitus, fungal infections, brucellosis and focal papillary necrosis of other causes.

MRI in Genitourinary Tuberculosis

MRI is good at depicting tuberculous cavities, sinus tracts, fistulous communications and extrarenal and extraprostatic spread. MRI is also useful in the evaluation of peritonitis and adnexal masses. MRI is an excellent modality at depicting extra-organ spread and discharging sinuses and fistulae but calcification is not readily demonstrated. Sensitivity of MRI in the diagnosis of early genitourinary tract tuberculosis is low and changes of more advanced disease demonstrated on MRI scans are non-specific.[34,35]

Ultrasonography

Sonography is not as sensitive as intravenous urogram or CT scanning because of problems with identifying calyceal, pelvic, or ureteric abnormalities. The kidney may appear entirely normal in both early or later stages of renal tuberculosis; later, hypoechoic/cystic masses communicating with the collecting system may be observed, representing "excluded" calyces without dilatation of the renal pelvis. Large abscesses may distort the renal contour and may mimic tumors or cysts. Usually, renal tuberculomas appear as a solid mass however, a diffuse infiltrative type of renal tuberculosis has been described in which the kidney may appear normal on ultrasound images.[30] Fibrosis and scarring may appear identical to chronic pyelonephritis or multiple renal infarcts. Calcification is common in the late stages and varies from punctate foci to dense calcification of the entire kidney, which is associated with hydronephrosis or atrophy. Bacille Calmette-Guérin (BCG) delivered intravesically in the treatment of superficial bladder cancer may be complicated by a renal granuloma, probably as a result of vesicoureteric reflux. The granulomas have been reported as small intrarenal hypoechoic masses. Bladder tuberculosis causes fibrosis and mucosal thickening, leading to a thick-walled small-volume bladder with vesicoureteric reflux. Condition mimicking renal tuberculosis include conditions such as focal compensatory hypertrophy, focal non-tubercular hydronephrosis, acute focal bacterial nephritis, focal or global xanthogranulomatous pyelonephritis, BCG granulomas, and chronic pyelonephritis. Tuberculous autonephrectomy may resemble renal hydatid disease. Bladder tuberculosis may mimic bladder papilloma/transitional cell tumors.

TREATMENT

Medical Treatment

Modern short-course antituberculosis drug regimens are effective in all forms of tuberculosis. They are based on an initial 2 months intensive phase of treatment in which, usually, four drugs—rifampicin, isoniazid, pyrazinamide and ethambutol are given. This is followed by a 4-month continuation phase in which only rifampicin and isoniazid are given. For success, all doses must be taken, and because failure to comply with therapy is the major cause for treatment failure, the World Health Organization (WHO) has stressed the importance of direct supervision of therapy. To render such observation easier for both patient and supervisor, the drugs may be given thrice weekly. Under the Revised National Tuberculosis Control Program (RNTCP), this form of tuberculosis is treated with category I regimen.

In patients of tuberculosis with renal insufficiency, isoniazid and rifampicin are eliminated by biliary excretion, so no change in dosing is necessary. There is significant renal excretion of ethambutol and metabolites of pyrazinamide, and doses should therefore be adjusted. Three times per week administration of pyrazinamide (25 mg/kg), and ethambutol (15 mg/kg) is recommended.[36] While receiving isoniazid, patients with severe renal insufficiency or failure or on hemodialysis should also be given pyridoxine in order to prevent peripheral neuropathy. Because of an increased risk of nephrotoxicity and ototoxicity, streptomycin should be avoided in patients with renal failure. If streptomycin is to be used, the dosage is 15 mg/kg, two or three times per week, to a maximum of 1 g per dose, and serum levels of the drug should be monitored.

Surgical Treatment

Surgical intervention is indicated in cases of advanced unilateral disease complicated by pain or hemorrhage and for bladder augmentation. Surgical excision of non-functioning kidneys or extensive lesions in partly functioning kidneys is controversial. Relief of ureteric obstruction by stenting or percutaneous nephrostomy may aid functional recovery, especially in patients with good renal cortical thickness, limited renal involvement and a GFR of more than 15 mL/min.[37]

REFERENCES

1. Teklu B, Ostrow JH. Urinary tuberculosis: A review of 44 cases treated since 1963. J Urol. 1976;115:507-9.
2. Weinberg AC, Boyd SD. Genitourinary tuberculosis. Urology. 1988;31:95-9.
3. Medical Reserch Council Tuberculosis and Chest Diseases Unit. BMJ. 1985;291:658-63.
4. Medlar EM. Cases of renal infection in pulmonary tuberculosis: Evidence of healed tuberculosis lesions. Am J Pathol. 1926;2:401-7.
5. Colabawalla BN. Diagnostic evaluation in renal tuberculosis. Indian J Surg. 1978;40:109-12.

6. Colabawalla BN. Reflections on urogenital tuberculosis. Indian J Urol. 1990;6:51-9.
7. Qunibi WY, Al-Sibai MB, Taher S, Harder EJ, de Vol E, Al Furayh O, et al. Mycobacterial infection after renal transplantation—A report of 14 cases and review of the literature. Q J Med. 1990;77:1039-60 .
8. Eastwood JB, Dilly SA, Grange JM. Tuberculosis, leprosy and other mycobacterial diseases. In: Infections of the Kidney and Urinary Tract. edited by Cattell WR. Oxford, Oxford University Press. 1996;pp.291-318 .
9. Lattimer JK: Renal tuberculosis. N Engl J Med. 1965;273:208-11.
10. Prasad R, Mukherjee PK, Agarwal SK, Verma KD. A study on renal tuberculosis among hospitalized patients of pulmonary tuberculosis. Ind J Surg. 1990;52:169-76.
11. Chugh KS. Pattern of renal amyloidosis in Indian patients. Postgrad Med J. 1981;57:31-5.
12. Mallinson WJW, Fuller RW, Levison DA, Baker LRI, Cattell WR. Diffuse interstitial renal tuberculosis—an unusual cause of renal failure. Q J Med. 1981;50:137-48.
13. Woeltje KF, Mathew A, Rothstein M, Seiler S, Fraser VJ. Tuberculosis infection and anergy in hemodialysis patients. Am J Kidney Dis. 1998;31:848-52.
14. Cheng IK, Chan PC, Chan MK. Tuberculous peritonitis complicating long-term peritoneal dialysis. Am J Kidney Dis. 1989;9:155-61.
15. Ong AC, Scoble JE, Baillod RA, Fernando ON, Sweny P, Moorhead JF. Tuberculous peritonitis complicating peritoneal dialysis: A case for early diagnostic laparotomy. Nephrol Dial Transplant. 1992;7:443-6.
16. Ekim M, Tumer N, Bakkaloglu S. Tuberculosis in children undergoing continuous ambulatory peritoneal dialysis. Pediatr Nephrol. 1999;13:577-9.
17. Singh N, Paterson DL. *Mycobacterium tuberculosis* infection in solid-organ transplant recipients. Impact and implications for management. Clin Infect Dis. 1998;27:1266-77.
18. Yildiz A, Sever MS, Turkmen A, Ecder T, Besisik F, Tabak L, et al. Tuberculosis after renal transplantation. Experience of one Turkish centre. Nephrol Dial Transplant. 1998;13:1872-5.
19. Lanjewar DN, Ansari MA, Shetty CR, Maheshwary MB, Jain P. Renal lesions associated with AIDS—An autopsy study. Indian J Pathol Microbiol. 1999;42:63-8.
20. Soriano-Rosas J, Avila-Casado MC, Carrera-Gonzalez E, Chavez-Mercado L, Cruz-Ortiz H, Rojo J. AIDS-associated nephropathy: 5-year retrospective morphologic analysis of 87 cases. Pathol Res Pract. 1998;194:567-70.
21. Prasad R, Mukherji PK, Agarwal SK, Verma KD. A study on renal tuberculosis in osteo-articular tuberculosis patients. J Bone and Joint Dis. 1987;3:1-6.
22. Cahill D, Dhanji A, Williams M, et al. Genitourinary tuberculosis in Middle England: look for it or miss it! BJU Int. 2001;87:273-4.
23. Cos LR, Cockett AT. Genitourinary tuberculosis revisited. Urology. 1982;20:111-7.
24. Fan ZM, Zeng QY, Huo JW, et al. Macronodular multi-organ tuberculoma. CT and MR appearances. J Gastroenterol. 1998;33:285-8.
25. Hamrick-Turner J, Abbitt PL, Ros PR. Tuberculosis of the lower genitourinary tract. Findings on sonography and MR. AJR Am J Roentgenol. 1992;158:919.
26. Serdar Arisan, et al. Polymerase chain reaction is a good diagnostic tool for *Mycobacterium tuberculosis* in urine samples. Journal of Cell and Molecular Biology. 2003;2:99-103.
27. Sechi LA, Pinna MP, Sanna A, Pirina P, Ginesu F, Saba F, et al. Detection of *Mycobacterium tuberculosis* by PCR analysis of urine and other clinical samples from AIDS and non-HIV-infected patients. Mol Cell Probes1. 1997;1:281-5.
28. Van Vollenhoven P, Heyns CF, de Beer PM, Whitaker P, van Helden PD, Victor T. Polymerase chain reaction in the diagnosis of urinary tract tuberculosis. Urol Res. 1996;24:107-11.
29. Aceti A, Zanetti S, Mura MS, Sechi LA, Turrini F, Saba F, et al. Identification of HIV patients with active pulmonary tuberculosis using urine based polymerase chain reaction assay. Thorax. 1999;54:145-6.

30. Lenk S, Schroeder J. Genitourinary tuberculosis. Curr Opin Urol. 2001;11:93-8.
31. Bisset RA, Khan AN. Differential diagnosis in abdominal ultrasound. 2nd ed. London. England. WB Saunders Co. 1992:326, 360:425–6.
32. Wasserman NF. Inflammatory disease of the ureter. Radiol Clin North Am. 1996;34:1131-56.
33. Wang JH, Sheu MH, Lee RC. Tuberculosis of the prostate. MR appearance. J Comput Assist Tomogr. 1997;21:639-40.
34. Muttarak M, Peh WC, Lojanapiwat B, Chaiwun B. Tuberculous epididymitis and epididymo-orchitis: Sonographic appearances. AJR Am J Roentgenol. 2001;176:1459-66.
35. Thukral A, Bhargava SK, Thukral KK. Diagnostic significance of excretory urography and ultrasonography in renal diseases. J Indian Med Assoc. 1997;95:579-81, 585.
36. Guidelines for the programmatic management of drug-resistant tuberculosis: emergency update 2008. Geneva, World Health Organization. 2008 (WHO/HTM/TB/2008.402).
37. Ramanathan R, Kumar A, Kapoor R, Bhandari M. Relief of urinary tract obstruction in tuberculosis to improve renal function. Analysis of predictive factors. Br J Urol. 1998;81: 199-205.

Chapter 47

Genitourinary Tuberculosis in Male

INTRODUCTION

Genitourinary tuberculosis is one of the most frequent non-pulmonary manifestations of tuberculosis. Genital involvement occurs in 50% of male patients with urogenital tuberculosis. This chapter aims to review epidemiology, pathogenesis, clinical features, diagnosis and management of male genital tuberculosis.

EPIDEMIOLOGY

The prostate and the epididymis are the most frequently affected genital sites in males for tuberculosis.[1] Testicles are less commonly infected followed by vas deferens, scrotal skin, seminal vesicles, urethra and penis. Epididymal TB most commonly develops in sexually active young men. Before the era of anti-TB therapy (ATT), the affected patients were in age group between 16–40 years but as the advancement in treatment has been achieved, now more than 70% of men with genital TB are older than 35, and 15–20% are above 65 years.[2,3]

PATHOGENESIS

The spread of tuberculosis to the epididymis is thought to occur hematogenously or by retrocanalicular descent of organisms from the hematogeneously infected prostate. As the incidence of epidydimal TB is more common than prostatic TB, the former mechanism seems to be more common. Distal spread through the genitourinary tract especially infection descending from the kidneys, may also occur. Pathologically, the characteristic finding of tubercular epididymitis is caseating granulomas, which may form the abscess cavity and contain yellow-green caseous materials. Initial involvement is confined to the tail of epididymis but either the disease regresses and heals, often with calcifications, or more commonly progressive involvement of entire organ. The disease is more frequently unilateral as it was once considered to be bilateral in the past.[4] The tubercular lesions are typically located in the peripheral part of the posterior and lateral lobes of the prostate in case of prostatic TB.

CLINICAL FEATURES

A painful urethral discharge, sometimes blood stained ejaculation in 20% cases, painful micturition and occasionally terminal hematuria. Per-rectal examination reveals that there is presence of well-defined nodules most often near upper/lower border of one or both lateral lobes. If cold abscess forms in the prostate then it is felt as soft swelling. Occasionally, cold abscess ruptures into urethra and rarely into perineum/rectum. Sometimes rectoprostatic fistula develops. However, symptoms may vary depending on the site of involvement.

Tuberculous Epididymo-orchitis

Tuberculosis may cause chronic epididymitis and epididymo-orchitis. Typical presentation is the gradual onset of swelling followed by pain. Complaints about voiding are generally absent unless associated involvement of kidney, bladder or prostate occur. Systemic symptoms are common. Tuberculous granulomas may develop within the testes and epididymis and rarely may be complicated by abscesses and discharging sinuses. Thickening of the scrotal wall and Tunica albuginea and moderate hydrocele may also be observed occasionally. Physical examination may reveal an enlarged, irregular, nodular and tender epididymis. Involvement is generally unilateral but if bilateral involvement occurs, association with male factor infertility may be observed.[14]

TB of Prostate and Seminal Vesicle

Tuberculosis of the seminal vesicles usually occurs as a result of hematogenous spread. Descending infection is unusual. The same pathologic processes occur as within the bladder (i.e. mucosal tuberculomas, ulceration and fibrosis). Calcification is present in only 10% of patients. Unlike seminal vesicle tuberculosis, tuberculosis of the prostate is usually secondary to descending infection from the kidney. However, the kidneys may occasionally appear normal, suggesting subclinical infection or a hematogenous prostatic infection. Patient may manifest with irritative voiding symptoms such as dysuria and frequency. Hematuria, hemospermia and male factor infertility may be other presenting symptoms. The tuberculous cavities or abscesses may discharge into the surrounding tissues forming sinuses or fistulae to the perineum or rectum, eventually resulting in a watering-can perineum. The scrotum and urethra may be involved, although rarely. Urethral involvement may be complicated by urethral strictures.

TB of Penis and Urethra

Penile tuberculosis is rare with less than 1% of patients having penile involvement.[5] Tuberculosis of the penis usually presents as ulcers, tubercular cavernositis or nodules. In most cases, the lesion appears as a superficial, solitary, painless ulcer on the glans penis. It can be clinically indistinguishable from malignant disease.[6] Rarely, lesions may persist as solid nodule or cavernositis with ulceration.[7,8] Papulonecrotic tuberculids may also present as an ulcer on the penis.[9] Penile involvement may occur secondary to coexisting urinary tract tuberculosis. The transmission occurs secondary to bacilluria in these patients. Infection of the penis may occur by direct contact at the time of intercourse with a partner having urogenital tuberculosis.[5]

Tuberculosis of male urethra is an uncommon condition and presents as urethral strictures, periurethral abscesses or fistula formation. Fistulas can occur in the perineum leading on to "water can" perineum.[10] Similar occurrence of fistulas in penis can aptly be designated as "water can" penis. Penile involvement occurred secondary to urethral tuberculosis. "Water can perineum" is also known to occur with gonorrhea. The strictures, fistulas and lymphoedema may lead to "saxophone" deformity of the penis. Such deformity is well-known with lymphogranuloma venereum but is unknown in tuberculosis.

INVESTIGATIONS

Urine Examination

Urinalysis may demonstrate microscopic hematuria or sterile pyuria raising the suspicion of disease but they do not definitively establish the diagnosis.

Bacteriological Examination

If genitourinary tuberculosis is suspected, 3–5 consecutive early morning urine samples should be cultured for *M. tuberculosis*. Prostatic TB diagnosis relies on culture and acid-fast bacilli (AFB) staining results of semen and 3–5 early morning urine specimens with reported sensitivity of only 52%.

Fine-needle Aspiration Cytology (FNAC)

FNAC has an important role in the differential diagnosis of epididymal nodules as it can rule out malignancy and other benign cytological diagnoses such as tubercular and pyogenic epididymo-orchitis.[11] By providing an accurate and rapid diagnosis, it prevents aggressive and potentially inappropriate surgical procedures.

Semen Analysis

Although not an essential test in routine use, but this investigation can be useful in the evaluation of male infertility associated with prostatic TB. It has been reported that of 53 patients with genital TB, 89% were having low semen volume and 53% were having azoospermia or oligospermia.[3] Significant leukocytospermia has been observed in patients with prostatic TB.

Polymerase Chain Reaction

Polymerase chain reaction (PCR) is becoming a useful diagnostic tool because of its rapid detection of organisms in urine and having high sensitivity and specificity of 95.59% and 98.12% respectively. It can be recommended for instant diagnosis and screening before further examination and cannot be the only one method in identification of urogenital TB.[12,13] It has a disadvantage that it fails to differentiate between active or latent TB infection.

Plain Radiograph

The findings in the prostate are tuberculous cavities or abscesses that may discharge into the surrounding tissues, forming sinuses or fistulae to the perineum or rectum and eventually resulting in a water-can perineum. These changes are demonstrated best on MRI. Plain radiographs may show dense calcification within the prostatic bed, which can also be demonstrated on ultrasound and CT scan. Urethrography or a micturating cystourethrogram typically demonstrates filling of variable dilated prostatic ducts associated with destruction of the prostatic parenchyma. Sloughing and irregular cavitation of the prostate eventually may result in a smooth-walled cavity that replaces the prostate. Prostatic calcification may be the aftermath of chronic prostatitis, prostatic carcinoma or diabetes mellitus. Calcification is depicted on plain abdominal radiographs in as many as 10% of patients with tuberculosis of the seminal vesicles. Calcification of the seminal vesicles is more common in patients with diabetes mellitus. Calcification of the epididymis and vas deferens may be visualized on plain radiographs of the male pelvis and must be differentiated from diabetes and schistosomiasis. Calcification of the epididymis and vas deferens may occur in patients with diabetes and schistosomiasis as well as in patients with tuberculosis.

Intravenous Urogram

This investigation should be obtained to determine the presence of concurrent renal tuberculosis. Of patients with prostatic TB, 72% have pathological evidence of renal tuberculosis during autopsy.

Ultrasonography

Tuberculosis is an unusual cause of chronic epididymitis and epididymo-orchitis. Scrotal ultrasonography can be helpful in assessing for complications of epididymal TB, such as fistula or abscess formation. In tuberculous epididymitis, the epididymis may appear heterogeneous and hypoechoic, associated with concomitant hypoechoic lesions in the testes and a discharging sinus. The most notable finding is an enlarged and heterogeneous epididymis, predominantly in the body and tail.[4] Other associated findings include thickened scrotal skin, hydrocele, intrascrotal extratesticular calcification, scrotal abscesses and sinus tract. Testicular involvement is shown as a diffusely hypoechoic testis or focal intratesticular areas. Thickening of the scrotal wall and tunica albuginea and moderate hydrocele may be observed occasionally. Follow-up scans may reveal intratesticular abscesses. The testes may become as hard as stone, which is associated with extratesticular calcification. Transrectal ultrasonography (TRUS) demonstrates hypoechoic areas with an irregular pattern in the peripheral zone of the prostate consistent with the findings of TB prostatitis. However, malignancy of prostate cannot be ruled out.[15] It allows demonstration and localization of the collection and can then guide transrectal aspiration and drainage of any fluid for culture and microscopic examination. TRUS guided biopsies can obtain tissues for definitive diagnosis of disease, monitoring of response to therapy and eradication of prostatic disease.

CT Scan

It shows hypoattenuating prostatic lesions, which probably represent foci of caseous necrosis and inflammation in case of TB prostatitis. Pyogenic prostatic abscesses have similar appearance, so its possibility cannot be excluded.

MRI

A prostatic abscess demonstrates peripheral enhancement on MRI differentiating from malignancy. In addition, it will display diffuse, radiating, streaky areas of low signal intensity in the prostate (Watermelon skin sign) on T2-weighted images.[16,17]

Cystourethrography

It is performed to confirm and delineate the extent of a vesicoperineal fistula associated with prostatic TB.

TREATMENT

Medical Treatment

Standard 6 months anti-TB drug treatment is the first line therapy in genital TB. They are based on an initial 2 months intensive phase of treatment in which, usually, four drugs—rifampicin, isoniazid, pyrazinamide and ethambutol (or streptomycin)—are given, and these destroy almost all tubercle bacilli. This is followed by a 4-month continuation phase in which only rifampicin and isoniazid are given, with the aim of eliminating the few remaining near-dormant, persisting bacilli. All patients should receive conventional antitubercular therapy for at least 6 months including initial 2 months of rifampicin, isoniazid, pyrazinamide and ethambutol given on daily basis or thrice weekly under DOTS (category I) under Revised National Tuberculosis Program (RNTCP). For success, all doses must be taken, and because failure to comply with therapy is the major cause for treatment failure, the World Health Organization (WHO) has stressed the importance of direct supervision of therapy. To render such observation easier for both patient and supervisor, the drugs may be given thrice weekly during the continuation phase. A 9-12 months course of therapy can be given in complicated cases.

Surgical Treatment

Surgical intervention is indicated in cases of abscesses, obstructive symptoms or failures of chemotherapy.[18] Although anti-TB chemotherapy must be the initial course of action in tuberculous epididymitis, epididymectomy is required when an intrascrotal abscess is identified not responding to chemotherapy and a firm swelling that has remained unchanged or slowly increased in size despite of conservative treatment. Orchidectomy is seldom required and ligation of the contralateral vas is not needed. Resection of prostate has been advised in patients having obstructive symptoms provided adequate ATT has been initiated prior to surgery. Surgical drainage of an abscess collection in prostate is required. TRUS guided needle drainage is an effective method.

REFERENCES

1. Gorse GJ, Belshe RB. Male genital tuberculosis:a review of the literature with instructive case reports.Rev Infect Dis. 1985;7(4):511-24.
2. Farer LS, Lowell AM, Meador MP. Extrapulmonary tuberculosis in the United States. Am J Epidemiol. 1979;109(2):205-17.
3. Pais V, Wagner A, Dahl D. Prostatitis, tuberculous. [online]. November 11, 2005. Available at URL:http://www.emedicine.com/med/topic 1921.htm.
4. Muttarak M, Peh WC, Lojanapiwat B, Chaiwun B. Tuberculous epididymitis and epididymo-orchitis: sonographic appearances. AJR Am J Roentgenol. 2001;176:1459-66.
5. Elkin M. Urogenital tuberculosis. In: Pollack HM (ed.). Clinical urography: an atlas and textbook of urological imaging. Philadelphia: WB Saunders. 1990;1030-52.
6. Gow JG. Genitourinary tuberculosis. In: Walsh PC, Ritik AB, Stamey TA (eds). Campbell's urology, Vol 1. 6th ed. Philadelphia: WB Saunders. 1992;951-81.
7. Venkataramaiah NR, van Raalte JA, Dutta SN. Tuberculous ulcer of penis. Postgrad Med J. 1982;58:59-60.
8. Ramesh V, Vasanthi R. Tuberculous cavernositis of the penis. Genitourin Med. 1989;65: 58-9.
9. Vijaikumar M, Thappa DM, Kaviarasan PK. Papulonecrotic tuberculid of the glans penis (correspondence). Sex Transm Infect. 2001;77:147.

10. Symes JM, Blandy JP. Tuberculosis of male urethra. Br J Urol. 1973;45:432-6.
11. Sah SP, Bhadani PP, Regmi R, et. al. Fine needle aspiration cytology of tubercular epididymitis and epididymitis and epididymoorchitis. Acta Cytol. 2006;50(3):243-9.
12. Lenk S, Schoereder J. Genitourinary tuberculosis. Curr Opin Urol. 2001;11(1):93-6.
13. Kamyashan IS, Stepanov PI, Ziablitsev SV, et. al. Role of Polymerase Chain Reaction in diagnosing tuberculosis of the bladder and male sex organs.Urologiia. 2003;3:36-9.
14. Lubbe J, Ruef C, Spirig W, et al: Infertility as the first symptom of male genitourinary tuberculosis. Urol Int. 1996;56:204-6.
15. Salmeron I, Ramirez-Escobar MA, Puertas F, et al. Granulomatous epididymoorchitis: sonographic features and clinical outcome in brucellosis, tuberculosis and idiopathic granulomatous epididymoorchitis. J Urol. 1998;159:1954-7.
16. Tajima H, Tajima N, Hiraoka Y, et al. Tuberculosis of the prostate: MR imaging. Radiat Med. 1995;13:171-3.
17. Wang JH, Sheu MH, Lee RC. Tuberculosis of the prostate: MR appearance. J Comput Assist Tomogr. 1997;21:639-40.
18. Carl P, Stark L. Indications for surgical management of genitourinary tuberculosis. World J Surg. 1997;21:505-10.

Chapter 48

Genitourinary Tuberculosis in Female

INTRODUCTION

Female genital tuberculosis, though known to have existed for centuries, was first described by Morgagni in 1744 during an autopsy on a 20-year-old girl known to have died of TB peritonitis.[1] It is almost always secondary to a focus elsewhere in the body. Large number of patients may remain asymptomatic and the finding of the disease may be incidental. This chapter aims to review epidemiology, pathogenesis, clinical features, diagnosis and management of female genital tuberculosis.

EPIDIMIOLOGY

Fallopian tubes are the first and most commonly affected genital organs, followed by endometrium, ovary and cervix.[2] There has been some change in trends in incidence of disease that has been observed in recent times, reasons responsible are improvement in economic standards in developed countries and global pandemic of the HIV infection. However, trend in developing countries are different. Incidence has been different in various parts of world ranging from 10.3% in India to being less than 1% in USA.[3,4] It has been observed that the worldwide incidence of genital TB in infertile women to be 5–10% whereas it has been estimated to range from 1–26.7% in several parts of India.[5,6] Sutherland described endometrial TB in 10 out of 1000 patients with abnormal uterine bleeding.[7] Schaefer reported that 80–90% of his patients were between 20 and 40 years of age.[8] However, further studies have shown a changing trend in the age at diagnosis. The mean age was 28.2 years in the initial decades as compared to 38.9 years observed in last decade in one of the studies. It has been reported from India that 68–69% of genital TB were between 20 and 30 years of age.

PATHOGENESIS

It is always secondary to primary tuberculosis infection elsewhere in the body. Although pulmonary tuberculosis is most commonly responsible but extrapulmonary organs can also be the source of infection.[9] The primary focus is found to be quiescent or healed by the time the genital lesion becomes evident. Many years may get evolved between the primary focus and appearance of genital TB. In 50% patients with genital TB, chest involvement is common. Hematogenous/lymphatic spread is the most common mode of transmission.

Fallopian Tube Tuberculosis

Fallopian tube is the most frequently involved part of genital tract seen in 90% of patients.[2,8] Ampullary portion is most commonly involved followed by isthmus and involvement of interstitial portion is rare. Bilateral involvement is more common. Various types of tubercular salpingitis have been recognized-tubercular endosalpingitis, tubercular exosalpingitis interstitial tubercular salpingitis.

TB of Ovaries

Ovarian involvement occurs in 15–25% cases.[2] It most often results from direct extension of the disease from the fallopian tubes. Clinically, these conditions present as tubo-ovarian mass or cyst.

Endometrial TB

Endometrial infiltration by tuberculosis is usually secondary to tubal involvement. It has been reported that endometrium is involved in 50–80% cases of genital TB.[10,11] A study was conducted in 156 hospitalized female patients of pulmonary tuberculosis and tuberculous endometritis was associated with 11.5% of patients.[12] The uterus may appear normal, but the endometrium may show giant cell microscopically. In more advanced cases, caseating material collects in the uterine cavity which may lead to pyometra. This is more commonly noted in postmenopausal women who have a stenosed cervix. Adhesions within the uterine cavity lead to formation of synechia. Rarely an abscess may also occur in myometrium.

TB of Cervix

TB of cervix may be seen in 5–15% cases of genital tuberculosis.[2] Cervix mostly gets involved by downward spread of the disease from the endometrium. Microscopic examination reveals granulomatous inflammation. Inflammatory atypia with frequent hyperplastic, mucosal changes may also be seen along with caseation.

TB of Vagina, Vulva and Bartholin Gland

TB of vulva and vagina has been observed in 1% of cases and is usually secondary to involvement of other parts of genital tract.[2] However, transmission of the disease by a male partner with involvement of epididymis or seminal vesicles has been reported.[13] Lesions may present as hypertrophic form and sometimes non-healing ulcers resembling malignancy for which histopathological examination is required for confirmation of diagnosis. There may be many different forms of skin lesions on the vulva including TB verrucosa cutis, lupus vulgaris, scrofuloderma and erythema indurata.

CLINICAL PRESENTATION OF FEMALE GENITAL TUBERCULOISIS

The most frequent presenting symptoms are primary and secondary infertility reported in 35–60% cases. Menorrhagia and secondary amenorrhea is reported in 40% and 10% patients respectively or even postmenopausal bleeding can occur. Lower abdominal or pelvic pain which is non-characteristic, chronic or dull aching in nature and occasionally it may be acute starting with tubercular peritonitis or by tubo-ovarian mass or pelvic inflammatory disease. Persistent and abnormal vaginal discharge seen in endocervical TB or TB of cervix and vagina. Amenorrhea was the most common menstrual complaint observed in 18 female patients having pulmonary tuberculosis with associated tuberculous endometritis.[12] Rarely patients may present with non-healing wounds/sinus/fistula, spontaneous vesico-vaginal fistulas and hour-glass bladder. No physical sign on abdominal or pelvic examination is characteristic of genital TB. Minimal induration in adnexal areas on both sides is most commonly noted finding during pelvic examination. Bilateral tubo-ovarian masses, especially in nullipara or unmarried girls in the absence of fever should raise a suspicion of genital TB.[2] Presence of ascites or doughy feel of abdomen with pyrexia and menstrual abnormalities should also raise the suspicion.

DIAGNOSIS

Genital TB is an elusive diagnosis and a high index of suspicion is the first step of the diagnostic process. A careful history with specific mention of previous exposure to or active TB is of prime importance. One has to rely on imaging and histopathology as genital TB is a paucibacillary disease. Endometrial biopsy for histopathological examination and mycobacterial culture remain the most commonly used procedures for the diagnosis of female genital TB. Laparoscopy, hysterosalpingography, ultrasonography of pelvic organs, CT scan and MRI are other investigations advised if the endometrial biopsy is inconclusive. However, diagnostic hysteroscopy and laparoscopy have emerged as the most useful investigations.

Endometrial Biopsy

Endometrial tissue obtained by biopsy, curette or dilatation of the cervix and curettage of endometrium is useful for the diagnosis of TB, performed best before the menstrual phase as lesions are located close to endometrium during this period.[2] Diagnosis of TB is established in 50–76% patients. Other findings such as dilatation of glands, destruction of epithelium and presence of inflammatory cells apart from granulomas and caseation necrosis on histopathology. A negative result does not rule out pelvic involvement suggesting involvement of adjacent organs.

Mycobacterial Isolation

Endometrial biopsy specimen, menstrual blood, cervical and vaginal secretions, tubal biopsy material or peritoneal fluid obtained during diagnostic laparoscopy have been subjected to mycobacterial smear and culture examination.

Plain Radiograph

Tuberculosis can affect any part of the female genital tract but more commonly involves the fallopian tubes.[14,15] Hydrosalpinx and pyosalpinx are usually large and may appear as soft tissue masses on plain abdominal radiographs. The pyosalpinx may be calcified. Tuberculous tubo-ovarian abscesses may calcify, are observed on either side of the pelvis and sometimes appear as well-defined homogeneous masses, occasionally with areas of increased density presumably due to the granuloma. Serpiginous or linear calcification can occur in the tubes.

Hysterosalpingography

Hysterosalpingographic (HSG) findings may suggest a diagnosis. HSG appearances vary as widely as the pathologic changes observed in this condition.[16] Tubal involvement is almost always bilateral but the degree of involvement varies between the two sides. HSG may demonstrate a flask-shaped dilatation of the fallopian tubes due to obstruction at the fimbria. Occasionally, the obstruction is at the uterine end of the tube; therefore, the tubes are not depicted. HSG may demonstrate sacculation with infiltration of contrast material resembling salpingitis isthmica nodosa. Infiltration around the tube, which creates a cloud-like appearance of the delicate sinus tracts, has also been described. A characteristic HSG feature suggestive of tuberculosis has been described; in which irregular contrast distribution occurs resembling a cotton-wool plug. Focal irregularity and areas of calcification may occur within the lumen of the fallopian tubes. Obstruction of the fallopian tubes is not pathognomonic for tuberculosis and may occur with other pathology. In end-stage disease, the tubes become rigid, lack peristalsis and resemble pipe-like conduits. Within the endometrial cavity, tuberculous endometritis findings include adhesions, which may vary from very thin to very thick synechiae. In end-stage disease, the uterine cavity may be obliterated completely. Within the pelvis calcified lymph nodes and ovaries may be observed. Blockage of the fallopian tubes is not pathognomonic for tuberculous salpingitis and may occur as a result of previous ectopic pregnancy, iatrogenic and developmental causes, pelvic inflammatory disease, and other forms of infective processes of the genital tract. In one series of 15 patients with genital tuberculosis and peritonitis, 12 patients had wet peritonitis and 3 had dry (adhesive) peritonitis. An adnexal mass was present in 93%, peritoneal thickening in 69%, omental thickening in 61%, and endometrial involvement in 83%. Associated ascites may be septated, particulated, and/or loculated.

Laparoscopy and Hysteroscopy

These procedures are essential in the diagnostic work-up of patients with infertility. Pelvic organs and peritoneal surfaces are directly visualized. It also helps in confirmation of tubal patency. Despite normal physical examination, several abnormalities can be detected in about 60% of the cases during laparoscopy.[17] The frequent use of these methods has led to diagnose large number of cases of genital TB among women with infertility and chronic pelvic pain.

Ultrasonography

Sonographic findings may suggest genitourinary tuberculosis in the appropriate clinical setting and findings may help eliminate the treatment choices using renal surgery or hysterectomy for benign disease. Demonstration of bilateral, predominantly solid, adnexal masses containing scattered small calcifications is highly indicative of TB involvement.[18] In patients with female genital tract tuberculosis, awareness of sonographic changes associated with the infection may improve diagnostic accuracy and avoid clinical mismanagement and surgical explorations in genital infections associated with wet-type (peritonitis) tuberculosis.[19]

Computed Tomography (CT)

CT-scan can reveal many findings suggestive of genital tuberculosis such as low density ascites, adenopathy, presence of multiple pelvic lesions, hepatic, adrenal and splenic lesions. All the features are suspected for TB especially encountered in young patients suffering from infertility, however possibility of malignancy cannot be ruled out.[18]

Magnetic Resonance Imaging (MRI)

MRI has been increasingly used for evaluation of pelvic and other abdominal masses and particularly useful in localizing soft tissue abnormalities in patients with the disease.[20]

Polymerase Chain Reaction (PCR)

The PCR is a useful supporting test for the diagnosis of female genital TB.[21] It is a rapid and sensitive molecular biologic method for detecting DNA of *Mycobacterium tuberculosis*. In a study reported from New Delhi,[22] endometrial aspirates as well as biopsies and fluid from pouch of douglas were investigated for mpt64 gene by PCR in 25 women with infertility and it was observed that 14 out of 25 patients were positive, correlated well with laparascopic findings. Multiple sampling from several sites increases the diagnostic yield.

TREATMENT

Standard anti-TB drug regimens are used to treat genital TB. It has been recommended that an initial 2 months intensive phase of treatment in which, usually, four drugs—rifampicin, isoniazid, pyrazinamide and ethambutol (or streptomycin)—are given followed by a 4-month continuation phase in which only rifampicin and isoniazid are given. Excellent cure rates have been reported with the standardized regimen. In India, patients with female genital TB receive DOTS category I under Revised National Tuberculosis Control Program (RNTCP).

Surgical intervention is required when there is persistence or increase of pelvic masses despite of adequate anti-TB treatment (ATT), recurrence of positive endometrial culture or histology, persistence of clinical symptoms such as pain or bleeding after conservative treatment and recurrence of pyometra due to TB in a postmenopausal patient.[2] Minimal disease is managed by conservative treatment including monthly examination. Dilatation and curettage is done after 6 months of ATT for histological and bacteriological examination. Advanced disease such as palpable tubo-ovarian masses are treated with total abdominal hysterectomy and bilateral salpingo-oophorectomy after 6 months of conservative therapy.[2] In vitro fertilization and embryo transfer (IVF-ET) can be an alternative option for successful pregnancies in young female patients with genital TB.[23] Tuboplasty can be performed after adequate medical treatment as infertility is the most common symptom. However, results are disappointing and very few successful pregnancies have been reported as most of pregnancies are likely to result in ectopic pregnancy or abortion.

REFERENCES

1. Anderson JR. Genital tuberculosis. In: Jones HW, Wentz AC, Burnett LS, (editors). Novak's text book of gynaecology. Eleventh edition. Baltimore: Williams and Wilkins. 1988;p.557-69.
2. Schaefer G. Female genital tuberculosis. In: Zuspan FP, Quillingan EJ, (editors). Current therapy in obstetrics and gynaecology. Fourth edition. Philadelphia: W.B.Saunders Company.1994;p.51-5.

3. Goldin AG, Baker WT. Tuberculosis of the female genital tract. J Ky Med Assoc. 1985;83: 75-6.
4. Krishna UR, Saathe AV, Mehta H, Wagle S, Purandare VN. Tubal factors in sterility. J Obstet Gynecol India. 1979;29:663-7.
5. Desmukh KK, Lopez ZA, Naidu TAK, Gaurkhede MD, Kashbhawala MV. Place of laparoscopy in pelvic tuberculosis in infertile women. Arch Gynecol. 1985;237(s):197.
6. Gupta S. Pelvic tuberculosis in women. J Obstet Gynecol India. 1956;7:181-98.
7. Sutherland AM. Functional uterine hemorrhage. A critical review of literature since 1938. Glasgow Med J. 1949;30:1-28.
8. Schaefer G. Female genital tuberculosis. Clin Obstet Gynecol. 1976;19:223-9.
9. Falk V, Ludviksson K, Agren G. Genital tuberculosis in women. Analysis of 187 newly diagnosed cases from 47 Swedish hospitals during the ten-year period, 1968-1977. Am J Obstet Gynecol. 1980;138:974-7.
10. Schaefer G. Tuberculosis of genital organs. Am J Obstet Gynecol. 1965;14:295-304.
11. Nogales-Ortiz F, Tarancon I, Nogales FF Jr. The pathology of female genital tuberculosis-a 31-year study of 1436 cases. Obstet Gynecol. 1979;53:422-8.
12. Mukerji PK, Misra VK, Nath J, Prasad R, Das K. A study of endometrial tuberculosis in hospitalized patients of pulmonary tuberculosis. Ind J Tub. 1991;38:197-9.
13. Lattimer JK, Colmore HP, Sanger G, Robertson DH, McLellan FC. Transmission of genital tuberculosis from husband to wife via the semen. Am Rev Tuberc. 1954;69:618-24.
14. Horne NW. Genitourinary tuberculosis. Br Med J. 1971; 2:587-8.
15. Johnson JD, Wolff HL, Nadig PW. Genitourinary tuberculosis in Texas. Tex Med. 1978;74: 90-7.
16. Korn AP, Ehrlich S. Images in infectious diseases in obstetrics and gynecology. Endometrial tuberculosis. Infect Dis Obstet Gynecol. 2000;8:118.
17. Ambiya VR, Sarogi RM, Rawal MY. Diagnostic laparoscopy. J Obstet Gynecol India. 1981;31: 623-5.
18. Walzer A, Koenigsberg M. Ultrasonographic demonstration of pelvic tuberculosis. J Ultrasound Med. 1983;2:139-40.
19. Thukral A, Bhargava SK, Thukral KK. Diagnostic significance of excretory urography and ultrasonography in renal diseases. J Indian Med Assoc. 1997;95:579-81.
20. Bankier AA, Fleischmann D, Wiesmayr MN, Hubsch P. Update:abdominal tuberculosis-unusual findings on CT. Clin Radiol. 1995;50:223-8.
21. Manjunath N, Shankar P, Rajan L, Bhargava A, Saluja S. Evaluation of a polymerase chain reaction for the diagnosis of tuberculosis. Tubercle. 1991;72:21-7.
22. Bhanu NV, Singh UB, Chakraborthy M, Suresh N, Arora J, Rana T. Improved diagnostic value of PCR in the diagnosis of female genital tuberculosis leading to infertility. J Med Microbiol. 2005;54:927-31.
23. Gurgan T, Urman B, Yarali H. Results of in vitro fertilization and embryo transfer in women with infertility due to genital tuberculosis. Fertil Steril. 1996;65:367-70.

Chapter 49

Non-tubercular Mycobacteria

INTRODUCTION

Mycobacterium other than human/bovine tubercle bacilli, occasionally causing human disease resembling tuberculosis, have been called atypical, anonymous, unknown, tuberculoid unclassified, non-tuberculous mycobacteria but best designated as mycobacteria other than tubercle bacilli (MOTT). They are also named environmental or opportunistic mycobacteria because their natural habitat appears to be soil and water. There is no definite evidence of their transmission directly from human being to human being and therefore they have been broadly grouped as "other mycobacteriosis". They are distinct from saprophytic mycobacteria e.g. *M. smegmatis, M. phlei.* Opportunistic mycobacteria are gaining more importance in developed countries where tuberculosis has been brought under control, some of them causing pulmonary disease but their morphology is different from *M. tuberculosis*. More increase in HIV infections led to marked increase in disease caused by atypical mycobacteria, mainly in Western country, but in developing countries like India where *M. tuberculosis* is more prevalent, opportunistic mycobacteria are gaining less importance. This current chapter deals with epidemiology, clinical features, diagnosis and management of non-tubercular mycobacteria.

EPIDIMIOLOGY

Most of the non-tubercular mycobacteria (NTM) are ubiquitous in environment, so that the true incidence is difficult to determine.

Notification system varies from country to country and none of them are accurate.[1] Two national surveys in last decades have helped to define the extent of non-tubercular mycobacteria in United States. The initial study based on states laboratory reports from 1979–1980 indicated that non-tubercular mycobacteria comprises one-third of the 32,000 mycobacteria isolates.[2] The most commonly recognized species were *Mycobacterium avium*-complex (61%), *Mycobacterium fortuitum*-complex (19%), and *Mycobacterium kansasii* (10%). Most of the reported isolates were from respiratory specimens. The second surveillance study between 1981–1983 revealed a similar distribution and showed higher rate of NTM among non-white, women and patients residing in urban areas. The prevalence of NTM disease in North America is 1.8/100, 000. In 1981, Communicable Disease Surveillance Center (CDSC) in England and Wales reported that 5% of all mycobacterial pulmonary disease is caused by NTM. In England and Wales, patients who do not have AIDS, *M. kansasii* and *M. malmoense* were producing pulmonary disease more commonly.[3]

In India, *Mycobacterium tuberculosis* is most common and proportion of NTM has varied from less than 1-28%,[4-11] and *M. avium* complex and *M. fortuitum* were isolated in different studies. *M. chelonae* and *M. fortuitum* were among the frequently isolated from clinical specimens in various hospitals from India. Author in one study reported atypical mycobacteria in 9.2% of 236 patients of active pulmonary tuberculosis in Lucknow, most common organism were *M. malmoense, M. gordonae, M. avium* intracelluare, *M. xenopi, M. fortuitum, M. gastri, M. terrae* and *M. flavescense.*[12] NTM needs culture with strict criteria and in developing country like India, it is not routinely performed, so there is usual tendency to ignore such isolates and in the absence of clear-cut guidelines, it is difficult to find out exact magnitude of atypical mycobacteria.

MODE OF INFECTIONS

Non-tubercular mycobacteria infections can be acquired by variety of mechanism including inhalation route, ingestion, direct inoculation after trauma and iatrogenically via syringe, needles, medical instrument such as bronchoscope, intravenous catheter and surgical skin lesions. Although animal to human transmission may occurs in some species, e.g. *M. simiae*. An increased risk of NTM infections seen in chronic obstructive pulmonary disese, healed tuberculosis, bronchiectasis, fungal disease, alveolar proteinosis, pneumoconiosis, rheumatoid disease, diabetes mellitus, heart disease, alcoholism, achalasia cardia and patients with partial gastrectomy, AIDS, malignancy and patients receiving corticosteroids and immunosuppresive drugs.[13,14]

CLASSIFICATIONS OF NTM

Based on Pigment Production and Rate of Growth

Environmental *Mycobacterium* have been classified into 4 groups by Runyon (1959)[15] based on pigment production and rate of growth.

Group-1: Photochromogen

These organisms produces a colony that produces no pigment in dark but when exposed to light for 1 hour in presence of air and reincubated for 24–48 hours, a yellow orange pigment appears. They are slow growing but growth is faster than *M. tuberculosis* for examination, *M. kansasii, M. marinum, M. simiae* and *M. asiaticum.*

Group-2: Scotochromogen

These organisms produce colonies and yellow-orange-red pigment in dark, e.g., *M. scrofulaceum, M. gordonae* and *M. szulgai.*

Group-3: Non-photochromogen

These organism produces colonies that produces no pigment in exposure to light colonies may resemble those of tubercle bacilli. For exmple, *M. avium, M. intracellulare* (Battey bacillus), *M. xenopi, M. ulcerans, M. malmoense, M. terrae, M. haemophilum, M. genavense.*

Group-4: Rapid grower

These organisms are capable of producing rapid growth, colonies appearing with in 7 days of incubation at 37 or 25°C. Some rapidly growing mycobacteria are considered "late pigmenter". For example, *M. chelonae, M. fortuitum, M. abscessus, M. smegmatis* and *M. flavescens* and *M. peregrium.*

Based on Location of Disease Production (Table 49.1)

- Pulmonary disease: *M. kansasii, M. avium complex, M. chelonae, M. fortuitum, M. xenopi, M. malmoense, M. szulgai, M. simiae*
- Lymph node: Lymph node involvement seen in infections in *M. avium*-complex, *M. scrofulaceum, M. malmoense*
- Skin and soft tissue disease: By most commonly seen in infections with *M. fortuitum, M. chelonae, M. marinum, M. ulcerans, M. abscessus*. All species of NTM can present as skin and soft tissue lesions
- Bone and joints disease: By most commonly seen in infections with *M. marinum*
- Crohn's disease: *Mycobacterium paratuberculosis*
- Disseminated in non HIV: *M. kansasii, M. avium*-complex, *M. chelonae, M. scrofulaceum, M. fortuitum, M. haemophilus*
- Disseminated in HIV: By most commonly *M. avium* complex

Table 49.1: Classification of non-tuberculosis mycobacteria according to disease in human

Sl. No.	Clinical Disease	Common Species	Growth Rate	Morphology	Rare Species
1.	Pulmonary	*M. avium* complex *M. kansasii* *M. chelonae* complex *M. xenopi*	Slow (> 7 days) Slow Rapid (< 7 days) Slow	Usually not pigmented Large and beaded AFB smear Not pigmented Pigmented	*M. malmoense* *M. szulgai* *M. simae*
2.	Lymph adenitis	*M. avium* complex *M. scrofulacum*	Slow Slow	Not pigmented Scotochromogen	*M. fortuitum* *M. chelonae*
3.	Skin lesions	*M. marinum* *M. fortuitum* *M. chelonae* *M. ulceranse*	Rapid Rapid Rapid Slow	Photochromogen requires low temperature for isolation Not pigmented Not pigmented Scotochromogen requires low temperature for isolation	*M. avium* complex *M. kansasii*
4.	Disseminated	*M. avium* complex *M. kansasii* *M. chelonae* *M. haemophilus*	Slow Slow Rapid Slow	Isolates from AIDS patients, usually pig-mented Photochromogen Not pigmented Not pigmented, requires hemin and low temperature	

DISTRIBUTION

Most NTM distributed freely in water and soil but some of them also isolated from house dust. *M. avium*[16,17] grows well in natural water while *M. kansasii*[18,19] has been found in tap water. Rapid grower species have been isolated from soil, natural water as well as tap water and water used for dialysis and surgical solution.

CLINICAL PRESENTATIONS

The most common clinical manifestation is chronic lung disease. Cough, expectoration, fever, weight loss, hemoptysis, malaise and breathlessness are most common complaints but 10–40% patients may be asymptomatic. Evaluation is often complicated by symptoms due to other pre-existing lung disease. However, lymphatic, skin/soft tissue, bone/joint involvement as well as disseminated disease are also important manifestations of infection. The propensity of a specific manifestation varies with the specific species and certain host factors. The most common form of NTM disease in children is cervical lymphadenitis. Involvement of lymph nodes is unilateral and non-tender with minimal systemic symptoms and can lead to sinus formation. Rapid growers can produce skin and soft tissue infection apart from lung involvement. Disseminated infections are most commonly associated with HIV infection and other forms of severe immunosuppression.

DIAGNOSIS

American Thoracic Society modifies laboratory functions that contribute to the diagnosis and treatment of disease caused by *Mycobacterium tuberculosis* and NTM divided into three major category of service offered. These are:

Level I: Collection and transport of specimen, prepration and examination of smears for acid-fast bacilli (AFB).

Level II: Procedure of level I plus, isolation and identification of *Mycobacterium tuberculosis.*

Level III: Procedure of level II, plus identification of NTM. Drug susceptibility should performed at level II, level III.

Culture Methods for NTM

The isolation of NTM presents the same problems as the isolation of *Mycobacterium tuberculosis.* As mycobacteria grows slowly, other bacteria have to be eliminated from the specimen by prior treatment with acid or alkali. Two common solid media are available: egg-potato-base (Lowenstein-Jensen medium) and agar based (Middle Brook 7H10 or 7H11). Specimen should be inoculated to both type of medium with additional use of broth medium being useful. This can be standard Middle Brook 7H9 or radio labeled 7H12 used for rapid isolation in BACTEC system. In slow growing NTM growth detectable in 2–4 weeks on solid media and 1 week in BACTEC system with the exception of *M. haemophilum* for that paper strip containing hemin (X-factor) used for identification.[20]

Table 49.2: Cultural characteristics of clinically important non-tubercular mycobacteria

Sl. No.	Species	Temperature Range			Pigment Production		Oxygen Preference	Tween Hydrolysis
		25	37	45	Light	Dark		
1.	*M. kansasii*	+	+	–	+	–	A	P
2.	*M. avium* complex	+	+	V	–	–	M	N
3.	*M. intracellulare*	+	+	V	–	–	M	N
4.	*M. scrofulaceum*	+	+	V	+	+	M	N
5.	*M. malmoense*	+	+	–	–	–	M	V
6.	*M. xenopi*	–	+	+	+	+	M	N

A, Aerobic; M, Microaerophilic; P, Positive; N, Negative; V, Variable

Identification on Nontubercular Mycobacteria

Several biochemical tests performed to identify species of NTM but principle test is niacin test that differentiate it from *Mycobacterium tuberculosis* as former is negative and latter is highly positive. Other biochemical tests such as Tween 80 degradation, arylsulphatase test, catalase test are positive for NTM (Table 49.2). These organisms display P-nitrobenzoate resistance and positive iron uptake in contrast to *M. tuberculosis*. Because of sluggish biochemical reaction several other tests have been reported that yields rapid identification of Atypical *Mycobacteruim* are—Thin layer chromatography, gas liquid chromatography and high pressure liquid chromatography (HPLC).[21] HPLC can also be used in the direct analysis of primary cultures of mycobacteria grown in BACTEC 7H12B medium (Becton Dickinson), MGIT as well as MB/BACT and the identification of MAC directly from samples with AFB smear-positive results. They can be classified at group, species and subspecies levels by analysis of lipids with such type of investigations. Strains can be identified with the help of serotyping and simple electrophoretic mobilities of proteins and isoenzymes. Two recent investigations that are currently in use to identify atypical *Mycobacterium*, more rapidly are specific DNA probe test and BACTEC Nap test (the average time for Nap test is 5 days). Former method can identify growth from solid and liquid media both. Acridium ester-labeled DNA probes specific for MAC, *M. kansasii*, and *M. gordonae* have been approved for the rapid identification of NTM. This technique is based on the release of target 16S rRNA from the organism. Testing can be performed using isolates from solid or liquid culture media and identification of these species can be achieved within 2 hours. Studies have shown 100% specificity with sensitivity between 85–100%. It has been suggested that there is no use of testing of sensitivity for rifampicin and isoniazid for rapid growers as they are usually resistant and other drugs must be taken into account.

The current PCR-RFLP method widely adopted for the identification of NTM is based on the coupling of the PCR of a 441-bp sequence of the gene encoding the 65-kD heat shock protein (HSP65) followed by restriction enzyme digestion. The size of the restriction fragments is generally species specific. DNA sequence analysis with16S rRNA can be of great help in recognition of various species.

Chest Radiography

There are some difference in the radiological feature of atypical *Mycobacteruim* and *M. tuberculosis*. These producing thin walled cavity with less surrounding parenchymal infiltrate, less bronchogenic and more contigous spread of disease and involving apical and anterior segment of upper lobes and involving pleura overlying the involved areas. Occasionally, they produce dense pneumonia or solitary pulmonary nodule without cavitations, basal pleural disease less common and pleural effusion are rarely observed.

Approximately 90% patients of *M. kansasii* disease and 75% patients of *M. avium* complex disease have cavitary infiltrates.[22]

High-Resolution Computed Tomographic (HRCT) Scan

HRCT scan is indicated if radiological findings are inconsistent with that of NTM infection such as no evidence of cavitation in radiograph. NTM pulmonary infections should be suspected when a patient presents with a compatible clinical picture and has multiple nodular or cavitary opacities with multifocal bronchiectasis.

Fine-needle Aspiration Cytology

Diagnosis is usually made by FNAC or excision biopsy of the involved lymph nodes. Only 50–80% of excised nodes will be culture positive.

Tissue Biopsies

Tissue biopsies that are cultured and examined histopathologically are the most sensitive way to diagnose infections due to rapid growers and *M. marinum*. It has been reported that visualization of organisms in the specimen from the involved site is seen in about 10% of cases and the yield of culture is not easy to be determined. Polymerase chain reaction can be useful in identification of NTM such as *M. ulcerans* apart from smear and culture of specimens as well as bronchial wash or bronchioalveolar lavage through bronchoscopy.

Diagnostic Criteria

Many atypical mycobacteria are colonizing the bronchial tree without causing any disease, so that their culture from sputum is having no pathological significance. Conventional criterion for diagnosis of disease depends of infiltrative lesions in radiology including chest radiograph as well as HRCT scan, isolation of *Mycobacterium* from sputum smear and culture and exclusion of other disorders, such as tuberculosis. As these organisms are commonly found in nature, contamination of culture or transient infection does occur. Thus, a single positive sputum culture is not sufficient to diagnose the disease. Culture of the organism from lung biopsy, bronchoalveolar lavage or pleural fluid or blood culture is of greater significance than an isolated sputum culture. The American Thoracic Society has recommended following criteria for diagnosing atypical *Mycobacterium* which fit best with *Mycobacterium avium* complex, *M. kansasii* and *M. abscessus*.[22]

1. Patients having cavitary infiltrate on the chest X-ray, NTM disease is considered to be present when:
    I. Two or more sputums (or sputum and bronchial washing) are AFB smear positive and/or result in moderate to heavy growth of NTM on culture.

II. Other reasonable causes for disease, e.g. fungal disease, malignancy, tuberculosis have been excluded.

Approximately 90% patients of *M. kansasii* disease and 75% patients of *M. avium* complex disease have cavitary infiltrates will be diagnosed by these criteria.[22]

2. In the presence of non-cavitary infiltrate not known to be due to another disease, NTM lung disease is considered to be present when:
   I. Two or more sputums (or sputum and bronchial washing) are AFB smear positive and/or result in moderate to heavy growth on culture.
   II. Failure of sputum cultures to convert negative with either bronchial hygiene or 2 weeks of specific mycobacterial drug therapy.
   III. Other reasonable causes for disease have been excluded.

   The second criterion is presumed to be to exclude colonization rather the disease state. *M. chelonae* lung disease is usually non-cavitary and would be diagnosed by these criteria.
3. In patients with low numbers of organism on sputum culture and/or concern about the presence of another disease to explain the radiographic abnormality, a lung biopsy is often required for diagnosis.
   I. If the TBLB, percutaneous or open lung biopsy is performed and biopsy tissue sample yields the organism and shows mycobacterial histopathology changes (i.e. granulomatous inflammation with or without AFB), this is sufficient to confirm diagnosis of NTM.
   II. If lung biopsy showing negative culture but demonstrates mycobacterial histopathology changes (in absence of a prior history of other granulomatous or mycobacterial disease), NTM lung disease is considered to be present when:
      — Two or more sputum (or sputum and bronchial washing) are culture positive for NTM, even if they are negative for AFB on smear and result in light growth on culture and other reasonable causes for granulomatous disease have been excluded.

FEATURES OF NTM

Mycobacterium avium Complex (MAC)

Overall MAC is most common NTM to cause human disease in immunocompetant patients and 50% of AIDS patients. MAC Includes commonly 2 organism first *M. avium* and *M. intracellure*. These are widely distributed in water (natural ponds, lakes, swamp, and bogs: public baths, and public drinking water system), soil and occasionally found in dust, plants, raw milk, and in cigarette also. Respiratory disease occurs primarily by aerosol inhalation. This organism also causes cervical lymphadenopathy. These organisms produce disease in animal also. Radiographic features are typically divided into primarily fibrocavitary and nodular bronchiectatic disease, former being more common in older men with overlying lung disease.

M. kansasii

It is most common organism after MAC in different parts of world and found uncommonly in Australia. This is widely distributed in water mainly tap water, in which able to survive for longer periods.[23-25] Respiratory disease occurs primarily by aerosol inhalation and occasionally causes lymphadenopathy. The disease is very similar to that caused by *M. tuberculosis*. Disease pattern in immunocompromized patients is disseminated. Radiographic appearance include upper lobe and thin walled cavitary opacities.

M. marinum

M. marinum is exclusively skin pathogens, occasionally there is extension into adjacent soft tissue or regional lymph nodes and causing chronic ulcers and granulomatous lesions in the skin. It has been regarded as a causative organism for swimming pool granuloma. Transmission of infections occurs by producing infection with contaminated fresh or salt water.[26] Most of reported cases are seen in the fishing industry.

M. xenopi

M. xenopi has been found in tap water[27,28] and shower heads and responsible to produce nosocomial infections due to contaminated water system. These organisms can grow at 45°C and isolated from hot and cold water. They are producing pulmonary disease frequently. Typically, patients present with underlying chronic obstructive pulmonary disease (COPD) and radiographic features similar to that of MAC infection.

M. chelonae

The *M. chelonae* complex which includes *M. chelonae, M. fortuitum* and *M. abscessus* and widely distributed in natural rivers, lakes, seas, human drinking and waste water and frequently responsible for nosocomial infections from several sources.[29] These organisms are producing commonly lung and skin manifestations.

M. scrofulaceum

M. scrofulaceum found in natural lakes and rivers also in raw milk or other dairy products and very rarely in drinking water.[25] This commonly causes cervical lymphadenitis in children's next to *M. avium* complex. Pulmonary infections seen less commonly and usually associated with underlying lung disease mainly COPD, pneumoconiosis and previous tuberculosis.

TREATMENT

The principles of treating NTM infections are different from that of *Mycobacterium tuberculosis*. The decision to treat is based on the potential risks and benefits for the individual patient. The clinician should know the limitation that in vitro susceptibility results for many NTM do not correlate with clinical response. There are various species of NTM for which different drugs and regimens are indicated. Duration of treatment is much longer than that of tuberculosis due to low bactericidal activity and high in vitro resistance. Surgical resection is more frequently indicated than medical management.

Most of the first line antituberculosis drugs with good in vitro activity against MTB has 10 to 100 times less activity against *Mycobacterium avium* complex, the diminished activity believed to result from the presence of lipophilic cell wall, which prevents drug penetration. The cornerstones of MAC therapy are primarily the macrolides such as clarithromycin and azithromycin, and ethambutol in combination with companion drugs, usually a rifamycin and injectable aminoglycoside possibly streptomycin or amikacin. Asymptomatic patients with stable radiological picture should be managed by observation only, if their sputum remains clear. However, the recommended initial regimen for patients with nodular/bronchiectatic lung disease is a three times weekly regimen including clarithromycin (1000 mg) or azithromycin (500 mg), ethambutol (25 mg/kg) and rifampin (600 mg). In cases having severe nodular/bronchiectatic lung disease or presence of fibrocavitation on radiography, daily regimen being prescribed. Injectable aminoglycosides can be used optionally depending on disease severity and treatment response. A more aggressive and less well-tolerated regimen including clarithromycin (1000 mg/day) or azithromycin (250–300 mg/day), ethambutol (15 mg/kg/day), a rifampin (450–600 mg/day) or rifabutin (150–300 mg/day) and injectable aminoglycoside for first 2 or 3 months of therapy is recommended for patients with severe and extensive disease or having previous treatment history. Surgery can be considered in such cases.

Macrolides should not be used as a single drug therapy in order to prevent emergence of drug resistant strains. In case of development of macrolide resistance, patient should be started on recommended therapy that comprises of four drug regimen of isoniazid (300 mg), rifampicin (600 mg) or rifabutin (300 mg), and ethambutol (25 mg/kg for first 2 months then 15 mg/kg) with streptomycin or amikacin preferably for initial 3–6 months and surgical resection (debulking) of disease.[47] The optimal regimen still requires further modification. The usual recommendation is that patients will be treated for 18–24 months and for atleast 12 months after sputum conversion. This four drug regimen has not been proved by comparative trials but shown sputum conversion up to 80%.[30,31] AFB smears and cultures of sputum should be done monthly during early part of therapy to assess response but these are not specific indicator of response. Occasionally, positive sputum culture after sputum conversion does not mean treatment failure or relapse as definite relapses while still receiving therapy or after discontinuation of therapy is common about 20% or higher with recommended four drug therapy.[30] Patients who fail to convert their sputum culture after 12 months of therapy should be reassessed. In these patients, drug therapy is more complex and higher incidence of toxicity. The alternative drugs are, cycloserine (250 mg twice a day), ethionamide (250 mg twice a day), rifabutin (600 mg daily), clofazimine (100–200 mg daily), ciprofloxacin (1000–1500 mg daily) or moxifloxicin (400 mg/day) but all of them are limited by little or no evidence of clinical efficacy and toxicity. Monitoring of the patients receiving above drugs is very essential. Patients whose disease is localized to one lobe of lung and who can tolerate resection surgery should be considered especially if there is poor response to drug therapy. Resected pulmonary nodules that prove to be due to MAC requires no further treatment in the absence of evidence of other MAC disease or immunosuppression.[32,33]

Disseminated MAC is a late opportunistic infection in immunosuppressed patients with AIDS. All patients should be treated with clarithromycin, 1000 mg/d or 500 mg twice daily or azithromycin as an alternative drug at a dose of 500 mg/day, ethambutol (15 mg/kg/day) and rifabutin (300 mg/day). Daily regimen is being preferred over intermittent therapy in such cases. Clarithromycin is more potent against *M. avium* and reducing bacillary count up to 99%[34]. Efficacy of drugs are limited for patients having macrolide resistant strains. Drugs that should be considered for inclusion are injectable aminoglycosides and a quinolone such as moxifloxicin. Clofazimine should not be used as it has been associated with excess mortality in patients having disseminated MAC.[48] Monitoring of treatment is highly recommended in patients with AIDS in order to prevent various complications related to adverse drug effects and pharmacokinetic interactions with antiretroviral therapy.

The recommended therapy for *M. kansasii* disease is the regimen of isoniazid 5 mg/kg/day (300 mg), rifampicin 10 mg/kg/day (600 mg), ethambutol (15 mg/kg) and pyridoxine (50 mg/day) given daily for 18 months. Intermittent therapy can be successful.[49] The regimen should be maintained for a further period of one year after achieving culture negative status. Pyrazinamide is not useful for *M. kansasii* as all isolates are resistant. Patients whose organism resistant to rifampicin as a results of previous therapy have shown response with high dose of isoniazid (900 mg), pyridoxine (50 mg), ethambutol (25 mg/kg) and sulfamethoxazole (3 g) for 18–24 months. The oral therapy has been combined with daily or five times per week streptomycin or amikacin for 2–3 months followed by intermittent streptomycin or amikacin for atleast 6 months. Results with this regimen showed 88% sputum conversion after 10 weeks. *M. kansasii* is second most common cause of disseminated lung disease.[35] The treatment regimen for disseminated disease should be the same as for pulmonary disease.

M. marinum causing skin diseases commonly. Treatment includes simple observation of minor lesions, surgical excision, antibiotics (clarithromycin, azithromycin as an alternative, doxycyclin or trimethoprim-sulfamethoxazole combinations) and antituberculosis drugs (rifampicin 600 mg and ethambutol 15 mg/kg daily), given for minimum 3 months durations.[38-41] Susceptibility testing is not routinely recommended and should be reserved for cases of treatment failure. Disease caused by *M. malmoense* is being treated by regimen containing isoniazid, rifampicin and ethambutol, with and without quinolones and macrolides for 18–24 months.[42,43] However, infection caused by this organism is difficult to treat and optimal chemotherapy needs to be considered. *M. xenopi* shows variable pattern of drug sensitivity in vitro often resistant to rifampicin, isoniazid, and ethambutol. Combination of clarithromycin, rifampicin and ethambutol is recommended and surgical resection is indicated in case of patients with sufficient lung function and who fails to respond to chemotherapy.[44-46] Efficacy can be improved by addition of quinolones particularly moxifloxicin and initial course of streptomycin. Therapy should be continued until the patient has maintained negative sputum cultures while on therapy for 12 months. *M. fortuitum, M. chelonae* and *M. abscessus* cause cutaneous diseases more commonly and are resistant to first line antituberculosis drugs (Table 49.3). All these organisms are susceptible to amikacin (100%), ciprofloxacin (100%), sulfonamides (100%), cefoxitin (90%), imipenem (100%), and doxycyclin (40%), erthromycin (30 to 80%), tobramycin (100%).[37] The only curative therapy is surgical resection of involved lung combined with multidrug chemotherapy. The optimal therapy seems to be questionable but a regimen can be prescribed including clarithromycin with a second agent being selected on the basis of in vitro susceptibilities. Success depends on the existence of negative sputum cultures throughout 12 months of treatment. For lymphadenitis in children recommended treatment is excisional surgery without chemotherapy.[36] The success rate with this procedure is about 95%. For children with recurrent disease, a second surgical procedure is usually performed. A multidrug therapy is recommended in patients with recurrence of disease two or more after surgical excisions.

Table 49.3: Sensitivity of NTM to individual antituberculosis drug in vitro

Sl. No.	Species	Streptomycin	INH	Rifampicin	Ethambutol	Ethionamide	Capreomycin	Cycloserine	Clarithromycin	Ciprofloxacin
1.	*M. kansasii*	B	R	S	S	S	B	S	S	V
2.	MAC	R	R	R	R	S	R	S	S	R
3.	*M. malmoense*	R	R	V	V	S	R	S	S	S
4.	*M. xenopi*	S	R	V	R	S	S	S	S	S

B, Borderline; R, Resistant; S, Sensitive; V, Variable

REFERENCES

1. Messiner G, Anz W. Sources of MAC infection resulting in human disease. Am rev respire dis. 1977;116:1057.
2. Good RC, Snider DE. Isolation of nontuberculous *Mycobacterium* in the United States, 1980. J infects Dis. 1982;146:829-33.
3. Woods GL, Washington JA II. *Mycobacterium* other than *Mycobacterium*: review of microbiologic and clinical aspects. Rev infect dis. 1987;9:275.
4. Thomas KL, Joseph S, Subbaih TV, Selkin JB. Identification of tubercle bacilli from Indian patients with pulmonary tuberculosis. Bull world Health organ. 1961;25:747-52.
5. Patel IU, D'Souza TJ, Sayed BA. A bacteriological study of *Mycobacterum tuberculosis* in Baroda. Indian J Med Sci. 1966;20;924-9.
6. Kulkarni KG, Frimodt-Moller J. Bacteriological study of mycobacteria isolated from cases of cervical lymphadenitis. Proceedings of the 24th TB and chest conference. Trivandrum, India, p391.
7. Parmasivan CN, Govindan D, Prabhkar R. Somasundaran R, Subbamal S, Tripathy SP. Species level identification of nontuberculous mycobacteria from south India BCG trial area during 1981. Tubercle. 1985;66:9-15.
8. Kaur H, Chitkara NL. A study of atypical acid fast bacilli (culture and biochemical characateristics). Indian J Tuberc. 1964;12:16-8.
9. Katoch K, Katoch VM, Dutta AK, Sharma VD, Ramu G. Chest infection due to *M. Fortuitum* in a case of lepromatous leprosy- a case report. Indian J Lepr. 1985;57:399-403.
10. Chakrabarti A, Sharma M, Dubey ML. Isolation rates of different mycobacterial species from chandigarh (north India.) Indian J Med Res. 1990;A91:111-4.
11. Singh S, Rattan A, Kumar S. Severe cutaneous *Mycobacterium chelonei* infection following a yellow jacket sting (letter). Tuber lung dis. 1992;73:305-6.
12. Babu KS, Mukerji PK, Prasad R, Aggarwal SK. Atypical mycobacteria in patients of pulmonary tuberculosis in Lucknow. Ind J Tub. 1997;44:56(Abstract).
13. Jonhson WG Jr, Nicholson DP. Pulmonary disease due to *M. k.*: an analysis of some factors affecting prognosis. Am rev respire dis. 1969;99:73.
14. Karsell PR. Achlasia, aspiration and atypical mycobacteria. Mayo clin proc. 1993;68:1025.
15. Runyan EH. Anonymous mycobacteria in pulmonary disease. Med Clin North Am. 1959; 43:273.
16. Paull A. An enviormental study of opportunistic mycobacteria. med lab technol. 1973;30:11.
17. Brooks RW, Parker BC, et al. Epidemiology of infection by NTM. V.Numbers in eastern united states soil and correlation with soil characteristics. Am rev respire dis. 1984;130:630.
18. Joyson DM.WATER: the natural habitat of *M. kansasii.* Tubercle. 1979;60:77.
19. Mc Swiggan DA, Collins CH, et al. The isolation of *M. kansasii* and *M. xenopi* from water system. Tubercle. 1974;55:291.
20. Vadney FS, Hawkins JE. Evaluation of a simple method for growing *Mycobacterum haemophilum.* J Clin Microbiol. 1985;22:884-5.
21. Butler WR, Ahearn DG, Kilburn JO. High performance liquid chromatography of myolic acids as a tool in the identification of *corynebacterium, Nocardia, Rhodococcus,* and *Mycobacterium species.* J clin Microbiol. 1986;23:182-5.
22. Ahn CH, McLarty JW, Ahn SS, Ahn SS, Hurst GA. Diagnostic Criteria for pulmonary disease caused by *Mycobacterium Kansasii* and *Mycobacterium intracellulare.* Am Rev Respir dis. 1982;12:5388-91.
23. Reich JM, Jhonson RE, et al. *Mycobacterium avium* complex pulmonary disease: incidence, presentation and response to therapy in a community setting. Am rev respire dis. 1991;143:1381.
24. Falkinham JO. Epidemiology of infection by non-tuberculosis mycobacteria. Clin microbial rev. 1996;9:177.

25. Eaton T, Falkinham JO, et al. Recovery of MAC from ciggarette. J.Clin Microbiol. 1995;33:2757.
26. Zeligman I. Mycobacterium granuloma: a disease acquired in the tributaries of Chesapeake Bay. Arch Dermatol. 1972;26:106.
27. Collins CH, Yates MD. Infection and colonization by *M. kansasii* and *M. xenopi*: aerosols as a possible source? J Infect. 1984;8:178.
28. Gross WM, Hawkins JE, Murphy DB. Origin and significance of *M. xenopi* in clinical specimens: I. Water as a source of contamination. Bull Int Union Tuberc. 1976;51:267.
29. Collins CH, Grange JM, Yates MD. A review *Mycobacterium* in water. J Appl Bacteriol. 1984;57:193.
30. Ahn CH, Ahn SS, Anderson RA, Murphy DT, Mammo A. A four drug regimen for initial treatment of cavitary disease caused by *Mycobacterium avium*-complex. Am Rev Respir Dis. 1984;134:438-41.
31. Seibert AF, Bass JB. Four drug therapy of pulmonary disease due to *Mycobacterium-avium complex* (abstract). Am Rev Respir Dis. 1989;139AJ.
32. Corpe RF. Surgical management of pulmonary disease due to *Mycobacterium avium intracellulare*. Rev Infect Dis. 1981;3:1064-7.
33. Moran JF, Alexander LG, Staub EW, Young WG, Sealy WC. Long-term results of pulmonary resection for atypical mycobacterial disease. Ann Thorac Surg. 1983;35:597-604.
34. Barradell LB, Plosker GL, et al. Clarithromycin. A review of its pharmacological properties and therapeutic use in *Mycobacterium avium- intracellulare complex* infection in patients with AIDS. Drugs. 1993;46:289.
35. Ahn CH, Wallace RJ Jr, Steele LC, Murphs DT. Sulfonamide containing regimens for discussed by rifampin-resistant *Mycobacterium sasii*. Am Rev Respir Dis. 1987;135:10-6.
36. Crawford JT, Bates JH. Analysis of Plasmids in *Mycobacterium avium-intracellulare* isolates from persons with acquired immunodeficiency syndrome. Am Rev Respir dis. 1986;134: 659-61.
37. Swenson JM, Wallace RJ Jr, Silcox VA, Thornsberry C. Antimicrobial susceptibility testing of 5 subgroups of *Mycobacterium fortuitum* and *Mycobacterium chelonae*. Antimicrob agent's chemo ther. 1985;28:807-11.
38. Kin R. Tetracycline therapy for atypical granuloma. Arch Dermatol. 1974;110:299.
39. Lorial PR. Minocycline hydrochloride treatment for atypical acid-fast infection. Arch Dermatol. 1976;112:517-9.
40. Black MM, Eykyn, S. The success ful treatment of tropical fish tank granuloma (*Mycobacterium marinum* infections). Arch intern Med. 1986;146:902-4.
41. Chow SP, Ip FK, Lau JHK, et al. *Mycobacterium marinum* infection of the hand and wrist. J Bone Joint surg (AM). 1987;69-A:1161-8.
42. Bollert FGE, Watt B, et al. Non-tuberculosis pulmonary infections in Scotland: a cluster in Lothion? Thorax. 1995;50:188.
43. France AJ, McLeod DT, Calder MA, Seaton A. *Mycobacterium malmoense* infections in Scotland: an increasing problem. Thorax. 1987:42:593.
44. Banks J, Hunter AM, Campbell IA, et al. Pulmonary infections with *M. xenopi*: review of treatment and response. Thorax. 1984;39:376.
45. Smith MJ, Citron KM. Clinical review of disease caused by *M. xenopi*. Thorax. 1984;39:376.
46. Costrini AM, Mahler DA, Gross WM, et al. Clinical and roentrographic features of nosocomial disease due to *M. xenopi*. Am rev respire dis. 1981;123:104.
47. Griffith DE, Brown-Elliott BA, et al. Clarithromycin-resistant *Mycobacterium avium* complex lung disease. Am J Respir Crit Care Med. 2006;174:928-34.
48. Chaisson RE, Keiser P, Pierce M, et al. Clarithromycin and ethambutol with or without clofazimine for the treatment of bacteremic MAC disease in patients with HIV infection. AIDS. 1997;11:311-7.
49. Griffith DE, Brown-Elliott BA, Wallace RJ Jr. Thrice-weekly clarithromycin-containing regimen for treatment of *Mycobacterium kansasii* lung disease: results of a preliminary study. Clin Infect Dis. 2003;37:1178-82.

Chapter 50

Infection Control in Tuberculosis

INTRODUCTION

Tuberculosis (TB) is endemic in India, and diagnosis is frequently delayed. Unsuspected TB cases contribute to TB transmission, because they are not being treated and may go unsuspected for days or weeks, and may visit multiple healthcare facilities or be admitted to wards. Unless TB is considered, available diagnostic tests may not be used, proper treatment might not be initiated, and proper TB infection control measures might not be in place. This chapter aims to describe various measures to infection control in tuberculosis.

MODE OF INFECTION IN TUBERCULOSIS

Tuberculosis is caused by *M. tuberculosis*. People who have TB disease in their lungs can release tiny particles containing *M. tuberculosis* into the air by coughing. These particles are called droplet nuclei which are invisible to the naked eye and are approximately 1-5 microns in size. Droplet nuclei can remain airborne in room air for many hours, until they are removed by natural or mechanical ventilation. To spread, there must be a source, a person with TB disease who produces *M. tuberculosis*, and an exposed person to inhale droplet nuclei containing the bacteria. Although TB is not usually spread by brief contact, anyone who shares air with a person with TB disease of the lungs in an infectious stage is at risk. A person who inhales one or more of the droplet nuclei can become infected with *M. tuberculosis*.

THE DIFFERENCE BETWEEN TB INFECTION AND TB DISEASE

TB Infection

TB infection is the state of having a small number of *M. tuberculosis* bacteria in the body which are unable to grow due to control by the immune system. The bacteria are inactive, but remain alive in the body and can become active later. This condition is also referred to as latent TB infection (LTBI). TB infection does not cause a person to feel sick, and there are no symptoms or signs detected on medical evaluation. A tuberculin skin test is the main method used to diagnose TB infection. A positive result usually means that TB infection is present, but persons with HIV-associated immunosuppression can have a false negative TB skin test even with TB infection. Also, persons who have received BCG vaccination may have a false positive skin test. Only one out of 10 people with TB infection and a normal immune system will develop TB disease in their lifetime. For persons with HIV infection and TB infection, one out of 10 each year will develop TB disease. Treatment for TB infection with the anti-TB drug such as isoniazid can reduce the risk of TB disease, though the protective benefit only lasts about 2 years.

TB Disease

Most of TB disease occurs in the lungs but it occurs in other sites such as bone, abdomen and brain in 15% of cases. In persons with HIV infection, up to half of TB cases have disease in other parts of the body. A person with TB disease of the lungs usually has a cough and sometimes coughs up blood. General symptoms of TB disease include fever, sweating at night, loss of appetite, weight loss, and fatigue. With standard treatment TB disease can be cured, even in persons with HIV infection. Untreated TB is often fatal, especially in persons infected with HIV. Any person with these symptoms should be evaluated by a healthcare provider as soon as possible. If TB is diagnosed or suspected, treatment will have to be prescribed.

When TB is Infectious?

TB can be infectious when it occurs in the lungs or larynx. In general, a person with TB disease of the lungs or larynx should be considered infectious until the person has completed at least 2 weeks of standard anti-TB therapy (ATT), preferably with direct observation with improvement of symptoms and has two consecutive negative sputum smears on 2 different days, with at least one morning specimen.

Problem of TB in HIV Care Settings

Persons with undiagnosed, untreated and potentially contagious TB are often seen in HIV care settings. TB is the most common opportunistic infection and a leading cause of death in persons living with HIV/AIDS (PLWHA).

In high TB burden settings, surveys have shown that up to 10% of persons with HIV infection may have previously undiagnosed TB at the time of HIV voluntary counseling and testing (VCT), including at centers providing prevention-of-mother-to-child HIV transmission (PMTCT) services.[1-3] Up to half of these may be infectious TB cases. Between 30% and 40% of PLWHA living in high burden TB settings will develop TB in their lifetime, in the absence of isoniazid preventive therapy or antiretroviral therapy.[4] The risk of developing TB disease doubles in the first year after becoming HIV-infected and gets progressively higher over time.[5] Persons without TB disease at the time of HIV diagnosis may still develop TB in later years, and will then be at risk of spreading *M. tuberculosis* in the community as well as to fellow patients, healthcare workers, and staff at their HIV care clinics and in community programs.

STANDARD PRECAUTIONS

Standard precautions is the term used for the group of infection control practices to reduce the risk of transmission of pathogens.[6] These are based on the principle that all blood, body fluids, secretions, excretions except sweat, non-intact skin, and mucous membranes may contain transmissible infectious agents. Standard precautions are applicable to all patients in all healthcare settings. Standard precautions combine the major features of universal precautions, body substance isolation, and airborne precautions. Implementation of these precautions requires risk assessment in all healthcare activities. Elements of standard precautions are—hand hygiene, selection of personal protective equipment based on assessment of risk, respiratory hygiene and cough etiquette, prevention of injury from needles and other sharp objects, cleaning of the patient care environment, linen and waste management and cleaning and disinfection of patient-care equipment.

HIERARCHY OF INFECTION CONTROL TO REDUCE RISK OF TRANSMISSION OF RESPIRATORY PATHOGENS

The selection of the combination of infection control methods will be based on assessment conducted by local epidemiological, climatic and socio-economic conditions.

Administrative Controls

Administrative controls are to identify persons with respiratory symptoms, separate them into appropriate environment, fast-track them through the healthcare facility to reduce exposure time to others, and diagnose/treat them with minimal delay. Hospitalization should be reduced or avoided to the greatest extent possible. At facility level, administrative controls play a major role in reducing the risk of TB transmission and are essential for the implementation of other controls (i.e. environmental controls and personal protective equipment). There are five components of administrative controls: 1. Infection control plan; 2. Administrative support for procedures in the plan, including quality assurance; 3. Training of staff; 4. Education of patients and increasing community awareness; and 5. Coordination and communication with the TB program.

Environmental Controls

The choice of environmental controls is largely determined by local factors and resources. Ventilation should be prioritized to reduce the number of infectious particles in the air. Effective ventilation may be achieved by natural ventilation where possible. In high-risk settings where optimal ventilation cannot be achieved through natural or mechanically-aided means, properly designed, placed and maintained ultraviolet germicidal irradiation (UVGR) devices should be considered as a complementary control.

Personal Protective Equipment

Personal protective equipment (e.g. particulate respirators certified as N95 or FFP2) should be available as required in high-risk situation, especially drug resistant tuberculosis, and during high-risk aerosol-generating procedures such as bronchoscopy or sputum induction.[6] Only N95 particulate respirator for healthcare worker, if properly fitted and used, provides some additional protection to the user against airborne infection. Masks for such workers may be useful for large respiratory droplets and protection of mucous membranes.

MANAGERIAL ACTIVITIES FOR NATIONAL, STATE, HOSPITAL ADMINISTRATION, AND LOCAL HEALTH OFFICIALS

Managerial activities should ensure political commitment and leadership at all levels (national, state district and facility level). The managerial activities are based on public health principles and represent the foundation of any public health program. Facility level managerial activities should be in line with and complement the national, state and district level managerial activities and should support and facilitate the implementation of the controls described later at facility level. Hospital administration plays a key role in creating the necessary conditions at the institutional level to prevent spread of health care associated pathogens. The physical separation of TB patients or people suspected of having TB requires rational design, construction or renovation of buildings. Controls aimed at reducing TB transmission in healthcare settings include triage, physical separation of TB patients or people suspected of having TB, cough etiquette and respiratory hygiene and minimize time spent in healthcare facilities. Facility Infection Control Committee should have a facility infection control/biomedical waste management plan in place.

The airborne infection control plan should be an integral part of this facility plan. The specific activities for healthcare facility administration: (a) Conduction of facility-risk assessment and development of a facility plan for airborne infection control. (b) Rethinking of using available spaces and consider renovation and/or construction to optimize implementation of controls. (c) Designating focal points for the facility-level activities, and support training of frontline healthcare workers. (d) Ensuring proper implementation of the administrative controls. (e) Framing of budget for maintenance of controls. (f) Supervision and monitoring of infection control activities, and (g) Addressing training and communication needs of health workers, patients and visitors. Broad areas of infection control suggested to be covered in facility infection control plan includes—facility procedures for standard precautions, facility biomedical waste management protocol, procedures for decompression of crowded areas, airborne infection control protocol, regular assessment of TB in all facility staff and infection control training of healthcare workers.

ADMINISTRATIVE CONTROL STRATEGIES FOR HEALTHCARE FACILITIES

Administrative control measures (policies and work practices) have the greatest impact on preventing TB transmission. They serve as the first line of defense for preventing the spread of TB in healthcare settings.

Administrative Controls for Outpatient Areas

The aim of administrative interventions in the outpatient area of any healthcare facility that manages patients with suspected tuberculosis is two-fold: (a) Reduce the total time period that such a patient stays in the healthcare facility, and (b) Reduce airborne transmission to other patients and healthcare workers in this limited time period. The implementation of the key administrative interventions (screening, education, segregation and fast tracking) would vary from facility to facility.

Screening

Screening for respiratory symptoms should occur as early as possible upon patient's arrival at the healthcare facility. Patients can be effectively screened at the registration counter itself by asking simple questions related to chronic respiratory symptoms, and those suspected to have tuberculosis can be given special cards or priority slips. This screening can be performed by physicians, nurses, paramedical staff and/or volunteers specially deputed for this purpose. If a separate screening counter is used, patients can be encouraged to first visit this counter if they have suggestive symptoms, by appropriate advertisements, posters or announcements in the registration area. Even if screening at registration is not possible, screening can occur when patients register at specific clinics or when in waiting areas.

Education on Cough Etiquette and Respiratory Hygiene

Another physical method that can prove useful for reducing airborne transmission is the provision of patient education on cough hygiene and sputum disposal. Where possible, disposable medical masks can be provided to patients by healthcare workers or volunteers. These workers should also explain to patients how and when to use masks. Cough etiquette should be reinforced by all staff members when poor cough etiquette is observed. Disposal of sputum at health settings need to be considered. Outpatient settings should include tissue papers and bins with disinfectants for easy accessibility to patients for disposal of sputum. Wall posters with instructions on cough etiquette and sputum disposal should be provided.

Patient Segregation

Segregation of patients with respiratory symptoms can be achieved by having a separate waiting area for chest symptomatics, within the overall outpatient area. This is particularly important in larger institutions with heavy OPD loads. If feasible, a separate doctor can be deputed to assess these patients in the segregated waiting areas, so that these patients do not mix with other patients waiting in the outpatient area. Another alternative is to implement a patient flow control mechanism at the entry point of the waiting area, so that chest symptomatics (who have been screened earlier and are carrying priority slips or other similar identification) are diverted to this special area rather than the common waiting area. The outpatient area, more so this segregated area, should be well-ventilated to reduce overall risk of airborne transmission.

Fast Tracking of Patients with Respiratory Symptoms

Those identified as patients with respiratory symptoms can be further fast-tracked in both their clinical and laboratory evaluation. One option could be to directly send these patients for sputum smear examination before they see a doctor. The other options are to allow these patients to jump the routine queue and be seen earlier than other patients, or to have totally segregated physician areas for these patients. The other important area where these patients can be given priority is while performing chest radiography. It is acknowledged that limited evidence is available to support the feasibility and effectiveness of these administrative interventions. In a setting of high patient load, it may prove difficult to screen and fast-track some patients at the expense of others, although with proper counseling and explanation, this may still be feasible. Patient misgivings, for instance in visiting the laboratory before the doctor, also need to be factored in. The site(s) of screening and the personnel involved need to be identified and/or created, and this may mean more administrative approvals. With all the ethnic, linguistic, social, economic and educational diversity existing in Indian patients, it is unlikely that a single measure will work well for all groups of patients. This field is an important area of operational research, and pilot projects need to be undertaken to identify what sets of administrative measures are likely to yield good results in a particular setting.

Administrative Interventions in the Inpatient Areas

Minimize Hospitalization of TB Patients

One of the most effective means to reduce the risk of transmission of airborne pathogens such as *M. tuberculosis* in hospital settings is to manage such patients in the outpatient setting whenever possible. Many patients can be managed entirely as outpatients, thereby avoiding hospitalization and the risk of exposing other patients and staff. If hospitalized, patients should be re-evaluated frequently for possible discharge with continuation of therapy as outpatients.

Establish Separate Rooms, Wards, or Areas Within Wards for Patients with Infectious Respiratory Diseases

When hospitalization is required, patients with infectious respiratory diseases should be physically separated from other patients, so that others are not exposed to the infectious droplet nuclei that they generate. Policies on patient separation inevitably generate concern about stigma, but with appropriate measures—such as training and public posting of separation rules—stigma can be minimized. Administrative procedures should ensure that separation happens promptly and automatically, similar to the automatic separation of men and women during inpatient admission. If sputum-smear microscopy or other relevant diagnostic tests are performed for patients with respiratory symptoms at the time of admission, then those who are most infectious can be quickly identified for separation from other patients. Suggested priorities for separation of patients are: (1) Separation of patients with confirmed or suspected diseases of public health concern, such as epidemic influenza, from all other patients. (2) Separation of sputum-smear positive TB patients from immune-compromised patients. (3) Separation of patients with known or suspected drug-resistant TB from immunecompromised patients. (4) Separation of patients with known or suspected TB from all other patients. The best choice for infectious or potentially-infectious patients is to house and manage them in airborne precaution rooms. Where such airborne precaution rooms are not feasible, other options for physical separation include: (1) Having a few small 'airborne precaution rooms for patients with infectious respiratory disease patients, (2) Having a separate ward designated for patients with infectious respiratory disease, (3) Keep a designated area with better ventilation available for the placement of potentially-infectious patients and where it is not possible to have a designated airborne precaution room, ward, or area of a ward, there can at least be an area designated as a "No immunocompromised patient area", where TB inpatients would be preferentially placed. This approach avoids specifically labeling patients as immunecompromised, HIV positive, or having infectious TB. If properly implemented, this approach would keep vulnerable immunocompromised patients safely away from areas where infectious TB patients might be housed.

Educate Inpatients on Cough Hygiene and Provide Adequate Sputum Disposal

Wards housing infectious patients should display sign boards in the ward demonstrating cough hygiene. All patients admitted in the ward/area should be issued surgical masks and counseled on their proper use, adequate measures for safe collection and disposal of sputum.

Establish Safe Radiology Procedures for Patients with Infectious Respiratory Disease, Including Smear-Positive TB Cases or TB Suspects

When caring for an infectious TB case/suspect, the radiology departments should attempt to schedule inpatient chest radiographs on infectious and suspect TB patients for nonbusy times, such as the end of the afternoon, provide coughing patients with a surgical mask to wear, or tissues or cloth to cover their mouths, provide priority service to potentially infectious TB patients to minimize the length of time spent in the department, restrict access to the radiology suite to patients and essential personnel only, and use the room with the best ventilation for taking images of potentially infectious TB patients.

ENVIRONMENTAL CONTROL MEASURES

Environmental control measures are the second-line of defense for preventing the spread of TB in healthcare settings. Environmental controls include ventilation (natural and mechanical), ultraviolet germicidal irradiation (UVGI), filtration and other methods of air cleaning. It is important to recognize that if administrative controls are inadequate, environmental controls may not eliminate all the risk. Some environmental control measures are simple and inexpensive while many others are technically complex and expensive. Environmental controls work on the same basic principle—dilution of infectious particles through real or 'effective' air exchange. In the case of ventilation, that dilution occurs through the introduction of fresh, uninfected air and the removal of infected air. In the case of UVGI or filtration, dilution is 'effective' through the creation and re-circulation of 'cleaned' air, in which infectious particles have been removed by irradiation or physical extraction. Certain circumstances may require directional control of airflow, so that air containing infectious particles is not introduced into clean air where staff or other patients are located.

Many environmental control measures are technologically complex and expensive, and therefore only practical for referral hospitals. Healthcare facilities should seek to achieve minimum standards for air exchange. High-risk settings should be prioritized for immediate assessment and implementation of improved ventilation.[7] In most settings, natural ventilation is the preferred method for ensuring adequate air exchange. In existing healthcare facilities, relying on natural ventilation, ensure effective ventilation at all times and in all climatic conditions through proper operation and maintenance, and by regular checks to ensure fixed, unrestricted openings. However, controlled natural ventilation can reduce the risk of spreading *M. tuberculosis*. Natural ventilation relies on open doors and windows to bring in air from the outside; "controlled ventilation" implies that checks are in place to make sure that doors and windows are maintained in an open position that enhances ventilation. Fans may also assist to distribute the air. When fresh air enters a room it dilutes the concentration of particles in room air, such as droplet nuclei containing *M. tuberculosis*. Designing waiting areas and examination rooms, so that they maximize natural ventilation can help reduce the spread of TB. In warm climates, this means open-air shelters with a roof to protect patients from sun and rain. Mechanical ventilation with or without climate control may be appropriate where natural ventilation cannot be implemented effectively or is inadequate in given local conditions (e.g. building structure, climate, regulations, culture, cost and outdoor air quality). If mechanical ventilation is used, the system should be well-designed, maintained and operated, to achieve adequate airflow rates and air exchange. In high-risk settings where it is not possible to achieve adequate air exchange using natural ventilation, a complementary option is to use upper room or shielded ultraviolet germicidal irradiation (UVGI) devices. Installation should seek to irradiate the maximal air volume with the highest intensity UV, while keeping staff and patient exposure to less than 6.0 mg/cm^2 over an 8-hour-period. Emphasis should be given on proper installation and maintenance. Optimal arrangement of patients and staff should be implemented in all outpatient departments, DOT centers, microscopy centers, and radiology. Directional control of air flow is recommended in specific high-risk settings where infectious patients with drug-resistant TB or other acute respiratory diseases of potential concern are likely to be managed, i.e. airborne precaution rooms, Multidrug-resistant TB (MDR-TB) wards and clinics, and bronchoscopy suites.

PROTECTION OF HEALTHCARE WORKERS AND STAFF

Increasing Awareness of TB in Healthcare Workers and Staff

Those at risk include not just healthcare providers, but any staff, including volunteers, who have contact patients with TB who have not yet been diagnosed and started on treatment. This could include porters and cleaners, as well as peer educators, adherence supporters, and volunteers working as counselors or in support groups. Persons living with HIV/AIDS in these roles are at particular risk of rapid progression to TB disease if they become infected or re-infected due to exposure to *M. tuberculosis* in the facility. They should be included in all training programs. Reminders that healthcare workers and other staff can develop TB, regardless of previous infection status or BCG vaccination, should occur with annual re-training on infection control. It is recommended that staff be investigated for TB free of charge if they have a cough for 2 weeks or more. The infection control plan should list designated staff members who should be contacted to initiate TB investigations, and reinforce that all services are confidential. Tuberculin skin testing can diagnose persons with TB infection who are most likely to develop TB disease, and who could potentially benefit from preventive treatment for TB infection. However, TB preventive therapy programs are not yet widely implemented in resource-limited settings.[8]

Increasing Access to Voluntary HIV Counseling and Testing

Encouraging and enabling healthcare workers and all staff to know their HIV status should be a priority of all healthcare services, and HIV care programs, in particular. The rate of HIV infection among healthcare workers and staff may be similar to that of the broader community.

MULTIDRUG RESISTANT TB

TB disease that is caused by organisms susceptible to the first-line anti-TB drugs can generally be treated effectively. TB disease caused by organisms resistant to at least the two most potent first-line drugs (isoniazid and rifampicin) is called MDR-TB. Treating MDR-TB takes longer and requires drugs that are more toxic, more expensive, often of limited availability in resource-limited settings, and generally less effective particularly in persons with HIV infection. Because of the risk of severe morbidity and mortality to HIV-infected persons from MDR-TB, persons with known MDR-TB should receive routine care in order to prevent spreading of infection to such persons. HIV care facilities can obtain estimates of the prevalence of MDR-TB in their community from the local TB program. Through joint coordination and communication, the TB and HIV programs can plan for how to care for these patients. In areas where MDR-TB is rare, special arrangements can be made to provide HIV care for an MDR-TB patient. In areas where MDR-TB is more prevalent, specialized clinics can be established.

DRUG REHABILITATION CENTERS AND CORELATIONS INSTITUTIONS

In many areas, the proportion of persons with HIV infection in drug rehabilitation centers and correctional institutions (e.g. jails and prisons) is much higher than in the general population. This is in part due to the high prevalence of HIV infection among injection drug users and sex workers, who in turn represent a large proportion of those in need of rehabilitation in some parts of the world. Additionally, TB is spread even more readily in these settings than in outpatient settings because of the longer duration of potential exposure, crowded environment, poor ventilation, and limited access to healthcare services. WHO has published guidelines for TB control in correctional institutions.[9] These guidelines emphasize effective administrative and environmental controls, including screening detainees upon entry into the facility, and on a regular basis during times of prolonged detention.

REFERENCES

1. World Health Organization. Report of a "Lessons Learnt" Workshop on the Six ProTest Pilot Projects I Malawi, South Africa and Zambia. Geneva, World Health Organization, 2004.
2. Nachega J, et al. Tuberculosis active case finding in a mother-to-child HIV transmission prevention programme in Soweto, South Africa. AIDS. 2003;17:1398-400.
3. Burgess A, et al. Integration of tuberculosis screening at an HIV voluntary counseling and testing center in Haiti. AIDS. 2001, 15:1875-9.
4. Corbett E, et al. The growing burden of tuberculosis: global trends and interactions with the HIV epidemic. Archives of Internal Medicine 2003;163:1009-21.
5. Sonnenberg P, et al. How soon after infection with HIV does the risk of tuberculosis start to increase? A retrospective cohort study in South African gold miners. J. Infec. Dis. 2005;191(2): 150-8.
6. Guidelines on Airborne Infection Control in Healthcare and Other Settings, In the context of tuberculosis and other airborne infections, Directorate General of Health Services, Ministry of Health and Family Welfare, Nirman Bhawan, New Delhi. April 2010 Accessed at www.tbcindia.org.
7. World Health Organization. WHO policy on TB infection control in health care facilities, congregate settings and households. WHO/HTM/TB/2009.419.
8. World Health Organization. Preventive therapy against tuberculosis in people living with HIV. Weekly Epidemiological Record 1999, 46:385-97.
9. Tuberculosis control in prisons: A Manual for Program Managers. Geneva, World Health Organization, 2000.

Index

Page numbers followed by *t* refer to table and *f* refer to figure.

J

K

L

M

N

O

P

T

V

W

X

Z